Heart Rate Variability

Edited by

Marek Malik PhD, MD, DSc, FACC, FESC

Professor, Department of Cardiological Sciences
St. George's Hospital Medical School

A. John Camm MD, BSc, FRCP, FACC, FESC, CSt

Chairman, Department of Cardiological Sciences
St. George's Hospital Medical School

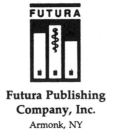

**Futura Publishing
Company, Inc.**
Armonk, NY

Library of Congress Cataloging-in-Publication Data

Heart Rate variability / edited by Marek Malik, A. John Camm.
p.   cm.
    Includes bibliographical references and index.
    ISBN 0-87993-607-X
      1. Pulse.   2. Heart beat.   3. Heart—Pathophysiology.   I. Malik,
      Marek. II.   Camm, A. John.
    [DNLM: 1. Heart Rate. WG 106 H436 1995]
    QP113.H43 1995
    612.1'71—dc20
    DNLM/DLC
    for Library of Congress

94-45665
CIP

Copyright 1995
Futura Publishing Company, Inc.

135 Bedford Road
Armonk, New York 10504-0418
LC #: 94-45665
ISBN: 0-87993-607-X

Printed in the United States of America.

This book is printed on acid-free paper.

Foreword

An appreciation of what is new and important depends upon an understanding of what has previously been discovered and learned. The earliest observations about disturbances in the heartbeat were made by feeling the pulse. The frequency and rhythms of the pulse have been of interest to physicians since the time of Hippocrates. In the early 1600s during the time of Sir William Harvey, Dr. Thomas Willis claimed that "cardiac contraction occurred as a response to a 'nervous liquor' produced in the cerebellum and brought to the heart via appropriate nerves." Over the course of nearly 400 years, an avalanche of clinical and physiologic studies established the foundation for our understanding of the heartbeat, from regular rhythms in health to complex arrhythmias in disease. Overlooked in this accumulating fund of knowledge was Dr. Willis' statement and the fact that the heart's supposedly regular rhythm was not precisely regular. The failure to appreciate this paradox was probably due to in vitro animal studies in which the heart and its cellular elements were dissociated from their intrinsic nerves, and to the use in patients of recording techniques that were relatively imprecise by today's standards.

The intervals between successive heart beats in quiescent, healthy individuals are not precisely of the same duration. Rather, there is a beat-to-beat variation that has an intrinsic oscillation reflecting a complex interplay between ionic membrane currents responsible for sinus node automaticity and the regulatory influences of the autonomic nervous system. In the absence of autonomic innervation to the heart, as occurs in patients with a transplanted heart, the heart rate is precisely regular with minimal, if any, variation in the intervals between successive beats. In the intact organism, the activity of the autonomic nervous system and possibly other factors modulate sinus node automaticity with a resultant microscopic oscillation in the heart beat that we call heart rate variability. Interest in and investigation of heart rate variability have increased exponentially in the past decade.

The fictitious British detective, Sherlock Holmes, would have been intrigued to deductively analyze the beat-to-beat variability in the heart rhythm for it provides clues about the activity of the autonomic nervous system on the heart, the functional status of the heart and the sinus node, arrhythmogenic mechanisms, the aging phenomenon, and the clinical course of patients with heart disease. By investigating heart rate variability with a magnifying lens in the time and frequency domains, the sympathetic, parasympathetic, and circadian oscillations are easily detected and, as Holmes would have said, "are elementary my dear Watson."

It is fitting and proper that two renowned cardiologists from St. George's Hospital Medical School in London have edited this comprehensive, timely, and up-to-date book on *Heart Rate Variability*. Drs. Malik and Camm have contributed significantly to our understanding of heart rate variability and have stimulated a large cadre of investigators—many of whom are contributors to this book—to enhance the scientific knowledge base and the clinical relevance of this new and exciting field.

ARTHUR J. MOSS, M.D.
Professor of Medicine
University of Rochester School of Medicine & Dentistry
Rochester, New York

Contributors

Philip B. Adamson, MD
Department of Internal Medicine, Cardiovascular Disease Section, The University of Oklahoma HSC, Oklahoma City

Solange Akselrod, PhD
Abramson Center for Medical Physics, School of Physics and Astronomy, Tel-Aviv University, Ramat-Aviv, Israel

Maria Alam
Autonomic Unit, National Hospital for Neurology and Neurosurgery/ Institute of Neurology, Queen Square, University of London, London, England

Dietrich Andresen, MD
Medizinische Klinik und Poliklinik, Abt. Kardiologie, Klinikum Benjamin Franklin, Freie Universität, Berlin

Guiseppe Baselli, MS
Department of Electronics for Automation, University of Brescia, Brescia, Italy

Stephen Behrens, MD
Medizinische Klinik und Poliklinik, Abt. Kardiologie, Klinikum Benjamin Franklin, Freie Universität, Berlin

Federico Bellavere, MD
Autonomic Physiopathology Unit, First Department of Medicine, Padua University Hospital, Padova, Italy

Luciano Bernardi, MD
Department of Internal Medicine, University of Pavia, Pavia, Italy

Anna M. Bianchi, MS
Laboratory of Biomedical Engineering, IRCCS H.S. Raffaele, Milano, Italy

Matthew S. Bosner, MD
The Jewish Hospital of St. Louis, Cardiology Division, St. Louis, Missouri

J. Brachmann, MD
Electrophysiological Laboratory, Department of Internal Medicine, Ruprecht-Karls-Universität, Heidelberg, Germany

Thomas Brüggemann, MSc
Medizinische Klinik und Poliklinik, Abt. Kardiologie, Klinikum Benjamin Franklin, Freie Universität, Berlin

A. John Camm, MD
Department of Cardiological Sciences, St. George's Hospital Medical School, London University, London, United Kingdom

Barbara Casadei, MD
John Radcliffe Hospital, University of Oxford, Oxford, England

Gian Carlo Casolo, PhD
Department of Cardiology, Ospedale San Giovanni di Dio, Florence, Italy

Didier Catuli, MD
Department de Cardiologie, Hopital Lariboisiere, Paris, France

Donatella Cerati, MD
Istituto di Clinica Medica Generale e Terapia Medica, Universita de Milano

Sergio Cerutti, MS
Department of Computer & System Sciences, University "La Sapienza," Roma, Italy

Philippe Coumel, MD
Department de Cardiologie, Hopital Lariboisiere, Paris, France

Kleber GC da Silva, MD
Department of Internal Medicine III, University of Heidelberg, Germany

Gaetano M. De Ferrari, MSc
Istituto di Clinica Medica, University of Milan, Milano, Italy

Marco Di Rienzo, MSc
LaRC, Centro di Bioingengeria, Fondazione Pro Juventute, Milano, Italy

Christoph Ehlers, MD
Medizinische Klinik und Poliklinik, Abt. Kardiologie, Klinikum Benjamin Franklin, Freie Universität, Berlin

Ernest L. Fallen, MD
Divisions of Cardiology and Neurology, Department of Medicine, McMaster University, Hamilton, Ontario, Canada

Lü Fei, MD
Department of Cardiological Sciences, St. George's Hospital Medical School, London, England

Giulia Ferrari, MS
Department of Electronics for Automation, University of Brescia, Brescia, Italy

Donald H. Glaeser, DSc
Sakowitz Computer Laboratory, Department of Surgery, Baylor College of Medicine, Houston, Texas

Antonella Groppelli,
Istituto Scientifico Ospedale S. Luca, Centro Auxologico Italiano, Milano, Italy

Roger Hainsworth, PhD
Research School of Medicine, University of Leeds, Leeds, UK

M. Hirsch, MD
Abramson Center for Medical Physics, School of Physics and Astronomy, Tel-Aviv University, Ramat-Aviv, Israel

Katerina Hnatkova, PhD
Department of Cardiological Sciences, St. George's Hospital Medical School, London, United Kingdom

Stephen S. Hull, Jr., PhD
Department of Physiology and Biophysics, The University of Oklahoma HSC, Oklahoma City

Markad V. Kamath, PhD
Department of Medicine, McMaster University, Hamilton, Ontario, Canada

J. Karin, BSc, MSc, PhD
Abramson Center for Medical Physics, School of Physics and Astronomy, Tel-Aviv University, Ramat-Aviv, Israel

Josef Kautzner, MD
Charles University General Hospital, Prague, Czech Republic

Harold L. Kennedy, MD
Department of Medicine, Rush Medical College, Rush-Presbyterian-St. Luke's Medical Center, Chicago, Illinois

Robert E. Kleiger, MD
The Jewish Hospital of St. Louis, Division of Cardiology, St. Louis, Missouri

Wolfgang Kübler, MD
Electrophysiological Laboratory, Department of Internal Medicine, Ruprecht-Karls-Universität, Heidelberg, Germany

Maria Teresa La Rovere, MD
Department of Cardiology, Centro Medico de Montescano, Foondazione Clinica del Lavoro, IRCCS, Montescano, Pavia, Italy

Federico Lombardi, MD
Associate Professor of Internal Medicine, University of Milan, Milan, Italy

Luca T. Mainardi, MS
Department of Biomedical Engineering, Polytechnic University, Milano, Italy

Pierre Maison-Blanche, MD
Departement de Cardiologie, Hopital Lariboisiere, Paris, France

Marek Malik, PhD
Department of Cardiological Sciences, St. George's Hospital Medical School, London, England

Alberto Malliani, MD
Professor of Medicine, Centro Ricerche Cardiovascolari, CNR, Medicina Interna II, Ospedale "L. Sacco," Università degli Studi, Milano, Italia

Giuseppe Mancia, MD
Centro Fisiologia Clinica e Ipertensione, Milano, Italy

Christopher J. Mathias
Professor of Neurovascular Medicine, Cardiovascular Medicine Unit, Department of Medicine, St. Mary's Hospital Medical School/Imperial College of Science, Technology & Medicine, London, England

Gregor E. Morfill, PhD
Director, Max-Planck-Institut für extraterrestrische Physik, Germany

Andrea Mortara, MD
Department of Cardiology, Centro Medico di Montescano, Fondazione Clinica del Lavoro, IRCCS, Montescano, Pavia, Italy

Olusola Odemuyiwa, MD
Wessex Cardiothoracic Centre, Southampton General Hospital, Southampton, United Kingdom

Zsolt Ori, MD
Department of Medicine, Meredia Huron Hospital, Cleveland, Ohio

Massimo Pagani, MD
Centro Ricerche Cardiovascolari, CNR, Medicina Interna II, Universita degli Studi, Opedale L. Sacco, Milano, Italy

Gianfranco Parati,
Istituto Scientifico Ospedale S. Luca, Centro Auxologico Italiano, Milano, Italy

Antonio Pedotti,
LaRC, Centro di Bioingengeria, Fondazione Pro Juventute, Milano, Italy

Gian Domenico Pinna, BME
Director of Department of Biomedical Engineering, Centro Medico de Montescano, Fondazione Clinica del Lavoro, IRCCCCS, Montescano, Pavia, Italy

Alberto Porta, MS
Graduate Student, Department of Electronics for Automation, University of Brescia, Brescia, Italy

Jeffrey N. Rottman, MD
The Jewish Hospital of St. Louis, Division of Cardiology, St. Louis, Missouri

Giulia Sandrone, MD
Assistant of Internal Medicine, Hospital "L. Sacco," Milan, Italy

J. Philip Saul, MD
Department of Cardiology, Children's Hospital, Harvard Medical School, Boston, Massachusettes

George Schmidt, MD
Director, Center for Nonlinear Dynamics, First Medical Clinic, Technical University of Munich, F.R.G.

Peter J. Schwartz, MD
Professor of Medicine, Istituto di Clinica Medica Generale e Terapia Medica, University of Milan, Milano, Italy

Mark Walter Franz Schweizer, MD
Medical University Hospital, Department of Cardiology, Angiology and Pulmonology, Heidelberg, Germany

Donald H. Singer, MD

Professor of Clinical Medicine, University of Illinois College of Medicine, Department of Medicine (Cardiology), Chicago, Illinois

Associate Attending Physician, Department of Medicine (Cardiology), Alexian Brothers Medical Center, Elk Grove Village, Illinois

Peter Sleight, MD

Cardiac Department, John Radcliffe Hospital, University of Oxford, Oxford, England

Phyllis K. Stein, PhD

The Jewish Hospital of St. Louis, Division of Cardiology, St. Louis, Missouri

Emilio Vanoli, MD

Assistant Professor, Dipartimento de Cardiologia, Universita de Pavia, Visiting Associate Professor, Department of Physiology & Biophysics, The University of Oklahoma, HSC, Oklahoma City

Tomas Vybiral, MD

Cardiology Section, Hugh Chatham Memorial Hospital, Bowman Gray School of Medicine, Wake Forest University, Elkin, North Carolina

Preface

The fact that the physiologic cardiac rhythm is not entirely regular has been widely appreciated for many years. However, until less than a decade ago, heart rhythm variations were virtually ignored in practical cardiology and it was generally believed that any irregularity of cardiac function is a pathological phenomenon. This was probably the result of clinical experience with atrial fibrillation and ventricular premature beats both of which indicate impaired intracardiac conduction and/or regulatory mechanisms and are negative prognostic factors in many cardiac diseases. Thus the observation that an absolutely regular sinus rhythm is also a negative prognostic factor came as a surprise to many clinical cardiologists.

Following successful clinical exploitation of fetal heart rate variations and the use of heart rate variability for the estimation of the degree of neuropathies, the first studies concerning variability of RR intervals in cardiac patients were published less than 20 years ago. Still, these 2 decades were sufficient for heart rate variability to become of wide interest. The number of published studies dealing with measurement, physiological interpretation, and clinical use of heart rate variability is increasing all the time and it seems that the state-of-the-art is just approaching the phase of deeper understanding when the recognition of different facts and facets of the problem starts to fit together. At such a phase of basic and clinical research, standards are usually being developed and books on the subject appear in order to both summarize the current knowledge and to teach and guide the scientific and professional community. The necessity of standards and widespread detailed understanding of heart rate variability is perhaps even more urgent than with other cardiological phenomena. Even before the clinical potential of heart rate variability was widely recognized, it became obvious that some of the precise analytical tools used to its assessment are too powerful to be used without proper and competent data preparation and without adequate understanding which only can make their precision valuable (G. H. Byford, 1979). Indeed, the significance and physiological meaning of the numerous indices and measures of heart rate variability and more complex than generally appreciated, thus there is a potential for incorrect conclusions and for excessive or unfounded extrapolations.

The need for standards of heart rate variability is not only widely appreciated by the specialists in the field but also recognized by the professional bodies of the cardiological and scientific community. The European Society of Cardiology jointly with the North American Society for Pacing and Electrophysiology have already initiated centralized standardization efforts to establish nomenclature, propose standard methods for measurement of heart rate variability, define its physiological and pathological correlates, critically review currently appropriate clinical applications, and identify ideas for future research. In order to achieve these goals, an international Task Force was established and the publication of the official document of the Task Force will shortly follow the publication of this book.

While the standards proposed by the Task Force should intensify the research in the field of heart rate variability and focus its clinical applications, the document produced by the Task Force cannot cover all the different facets of the field in a sufficient detail. Thus, in order to summarize the current state-of-the-art both in breadth and depth, we decided to assemble texts on individual aspects of heart rate variability and to produce this book.

The field of heart rate variability is broad. It includes aspects of mathematics, biomedical engineering, physiology, and clinical medicine. All these aspects are, of course, mutually interlinked. Nevertheless, in order to make the book structured according to the general foundations of heart rate variability, we distinguished three major components of the field which are reflected in the parts of this book. Thus, following a description of the background in the regulations of heart rate, the chapters of the book were sorted into three major groups: those dealing predominantly with the measurement of heart rate variability, with its physiological and pathophysiological interpretations, and with clinical applications. Although most the individual chapters can be read independently of others, the ordering of the chapters creates a continuous overview of the whole field. Thus, those readers who are interested in gaining a comprehensive knowledge on heart rate variability should read the book consecutively.

Finally, we would like to acknowledge the help and support which we received and which made this book possible. Our thanks go to all authors of individual chapters who accepted our invitation to contribute. The subject of heart rate variability is so extensive that a comprehensive review can only be achieved as a group effort; without the significant help of all contributors, the book would not have been written. Our thanks go also to the publisher. It was a pleasure to produce a book with a publisher as meticulous and caring as Futura.

February 1995,
Marek Malik and A. John Camm

Contents

Part III. Physiology of Heart Rate Variability

Part IV. Clinical Implications and Use of Heart Rate Variability

Part I

Background

Chapter 1

The Control and Physiological Importance of Heart Rate

Roger Hainsworth

Normal Heart Rate

Resting heart rate (HR) varies widely in different individuals. During various physiological stresses, particularly exercise, it can increase up to three-fold. Heart rate is dependent, among other things, on the level of physical fitness; highly trained endurance athletes, for example, have resting levels of HR which, in some people, might indicate the need for pacemaker implantation. The maximum level of HR achieved during physical exercise is dependent on the age of the subject, with 20-year olds typically able to achieve rates of 200 beats per minute (bpm) compared with maximum levels of 20 to 30 bpm less in older people.

Heart rate is normally determined by the rate of depolarization of the cardiac pacemaker. Pacemaker tissue is found in the sinuatrial node, the atrioventricular (AV) node, and the Purkinje tissue. However, because the rate of depolarization of the sinuatrial node is faster than that of other pacemaker tissue and the depolarizing impulse spreads via the heart's conducting mechanism to other pacemakers before they spontaneously depolarize, it is the sinuatrial node which normally determines the rate. If, for any reason, the normal pacemaker fails to generate an impulse, pacemaker tissue elsewhere usually takes over.

Autonomic Control of Heart Rate

The intrinsic HR, in absence of any neurohumoral influence, is about 100 to 120 bpm. In the intact, unblocked individual, the HR at any time represents the net effect of the parasympathetic (vagus) nerves which slow it and the sympathetic nerves which accelerate it. In resting conditions, both autonomic divisions are thought to be tonically active with the vagal effects dominant[1].

The motor neurons forming the vagus nerves originate in the dorsal motor nucleus and in the nucleus ambiguus. They run down the neck alongside the carotid arteries into the thorax. Sympathetic nerves origi-

From: Malik M., Camm AJ (eds.): *Heart Rate Variability*. Armonk, NY. Futura Publishing Company, Inc., © 1995.

nate in the intermediolateral column of the spinal cord in the upper thoracic region. White rami synapse in the sympathetic ganglia and the grey rami run with the preganglionic vagal fibers over the mediastinum, forming a plexus of cardiac nerves and parasympathetic ganglia, which supply the various parts of the heart, as well as many extracardiac structures. There is abundant evidence that both the vagal and sympathetic nerves carry not only efferent nerves including those to the heart, but also many afferent fibers which subserve various reflex functions[2].

Vagal Effects

The vagal nerves innervate the sinuatrial node, the AV conducting pathways, and the atrial muscle. The question of whether the vagi provide an efferent control of ventricular muscle remains controversial. It is possible that apparent depression of ventricular contraction by vagal stimulation reported in some studies may have been at least partly the result of decreased ventricular filling consequent on atrial depression. In some animals which are known to have a full efferent vagal innervation of the ventricles (duck and toad), vagal stimulation has been shown to have a large negative inotropic effect. In the dog, however, which like humans is thought to have little if any efferent ventricular innervation, vagal stimulation has only a trivial effect[3].

Stimulation of either vagus nerve slows the heart, although the right nerve is said to have a greater effect than the left[1]. This difference, however, has not been reported in all studies and may depend on the frequency of stimulation. In addition to its effect on the sinuatrial node, vagal activity also slows AV conduction. This effect seems to be greater in response to left rather than right vagal stimulation and high frequencies of left vagal activity are likely to result in complete AV conduction block[4].

The most obvious effect of vagal stimulation is to slow, or even stop, the heart. The latency of the response of the sinus node is very short, and the effect of a single vagal impulse depends on the phase of the cardiac cycle at which it is applied. After a single stimulus, the maximum response has been reported to occur within only 400 milliseconds[5]. Thus, vagal stimulation results in a peak response either in the first or the second beat after its onset. After cessation of vagal stimulation, HR rapidly returns to its previous level. The speed of recovery is a little slower than that of the onset, but HR is usually restored in less than 5 seconds.

Although there is no doubt that high levels of vagal activity slow the heart, there may be circumstances in which small increases in frequency may actually accelerate it[1]. This is because at vagal frequencies close to that of the heart, the cardiac pacemaker cells tend to become entrained by the vagal impulses and small increases in vagal frequency may cause the HR to increase. Whether this effect occurs in the intact animal is unknown and the physiological significance, if any, of this paradoxical vagal effect remains to be established.

The slowing of HR to vagal stimulation increases with the frequency of stimulation. Most of the change in HR is obtained at frequencies of up to 5 Hz, and the relationship between the change in HR and stimulus frequency can be fitted to a hyperbola[6]. The gross nonlinearity of this relationship suggests that HR may not be the appropriate variable to measure when quantifying efferent autonomic effects. If pulse-interval, which is a function of the reciprocal of HR, is plotted against stimulus frequency, the relationship then does become linear (Figure 1).[7,8]

One implication of the linearity of the relationship between pulse-interval and vagal stimulation frequency is that a given change in vagal activity causes quite different changes in HR when it starts from different initial levels. For example, a change in efferent vagal activity which causes a prolongation of pulse-interval by 333 milliseconds would result in a decrease in HR of 30 bpm when the rate is 90 bpm, but at 180

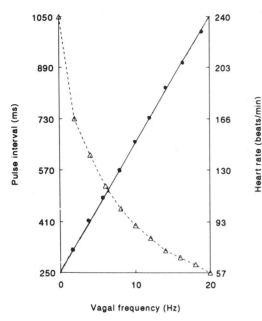

Figure 1. Chronotropic responses to graded efferent vagal stimulation. Responses expressed as HR (△...△) and as pulse-interval (•...•). Note the linear relationship of the pulse-interval plot in contrast to the hyperbolic relationship when HR is plotted. Results obtained from Parker et al.[7]

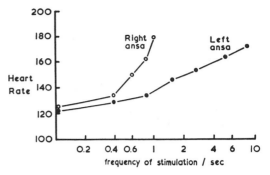

Figure 2. Responses of HR to graded stimulation of right and left ansae subclaviae (sympathetic nerves) in an anaesthetized dog. Note the much larger chronotropic responses to stimulation of the right compared with the left sympathetic nerves. Also note the approximate linearities of the relationships between the log stimulus frequency and the HR. From Furnival et al.[9]

bpm it would decrease the rate by as much as 90 bpm.

Sympathetic Effects

Sympathetic postganglionic fibers innervate the entire heart, including the sinuatrial node, the AV conducting pathways, and the atrial and ventricular myocardium. Increased activity in the sympathetic nerves results in increases in both HR and the force of contraction. In addition, the rate of conduction through the heart of the cardiac impulse is increased and the duration of contraction shortened.

An increase in sympathetic activity forms the principal method of increasing HR above the intrinsic level generated by the sinuatrial node (about 110 bpm) to the maximal levels achieved. These may be about 200 bpm in a young person. Following the onset of sympathetic stimulation, there is a latent period of up to 5 seconds followed by a progressive increase in HR which reaches a steady level in 20 to 30 seconds. Note the contrast with vagal responses which are almost instantaneous.

The relationship between frequency of sympathetic efferent activity and HR, like that for the response to vagal activity, is nonlinear. It can be approximately linearizd by use of pulse-interval instead of HR, or by plotting stimulus frequency on a semilogarithmic scale (Figure 2). Figure 2 also illustrates the consistent finding that there is a greater effect on HR from stimulation of the right sympathetic nerves than the left, particularly at low frequencies of stimulation. The left sympathetic nerves are more concerned with regulation of the cardiac inotropic state. The differential effect of the two sides on chronotropic and inotropic responses was examined by Furnival et al[9] who compared the effects on the maximum rate of change of left ventricular pressure (dP/dt max), at constant HR and mean aortic pressure, with the effects on the unpaced HR. Figure 3 shows a plot of the inotropic responses against the chronotopic responses for various frequencies of stimulation of the two sides. It emphasizes that right-sided sympathetic stimulation increases HR with little inotropic effect.

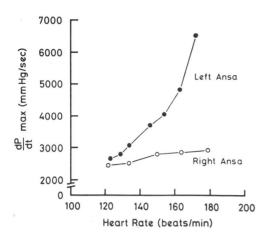

Figure 3. Comparison between the inotropic and chronotropic responses to stimulation of left and right sympathetic nerves at different frequencies. Each point relates the changes from control of dP / dt max (an inotropic index) and HR. These plots emphasize that stimulation of the right sympathetic nerves selectively increases HR whereas stimulation of the left nerves has much greater effect on inotropic state. From Furnival et al.[9]

Sympathetic-Vagal Interactions

In most circumstances, there is tonic activity in both divisions of the autonomic nervous system, and the net effect on HR represents the balance between the two antagonistic effects. Clearly, at rest the vagal influence is dominant, but with increasing levels of exercise, the vagal activity declines and that of the sympathetic increases. However, although the resulting HR is influenced by activity in both autonomic divisions, it cannot be computed by simple addition or subtraction of the separate effects. Levy and Zieske[10] emphasized that the effects of the vagus were more potent. They showed that the change in HR in response to vagal stimulation could be almost doubled when the initial rate had been accelerated by sympathetic stimulation. However, when their data are recalculated to express the responses in terms of pulse-interval, which is the variable actually to be controlled by the autonomic nerves, the apparent interaction between the two divisions is lost. It seems, therefore, that the effects of simultaneous sympathetic and vagal activ-ity are probably equal to the algebraic sum of their independent effects, but only as long as these effects are expressed as pulse-interval rather than HR.

Reflexes Influencing Heart Rate

Heart rate, at any instant in time, represents the resultant of many influences on the vagal and sympathetic centers (Table 1). Some reflexes may increase HR through a decrease in vagal tone, an increase in sympathetic activity, or both. Others exert the opposite effects. In the intact person or animal, several reflexes are likely to operate simultaneously and, for at least some of these, the interactions may be quite complex.

Baroreceptors

Arterial baroreceptors and their reflex effects have been studied very extensively both in animals and humans. Several recent books and reviews deal with arterial baroreflexes at length,[11-14] and only a brief summary will be given here. Baroreceptors are situated in the adventitia of some arteries, particularly the carotid sinuses and the aortic arch. Increases in blood pressure stretch these vessels and result in increases in discharge frequency in their afferent nerves. Following an increase in pressure, the discharge increases abruptly but then rapidly adapts to a rate which may be only moderately raised. Baroreceptors reset to change their operating range if a change in pressure is maintained. There is an early rapid resetting which occurs within minutes, and a chronic resetting which takes place over months[15].

Stimulation of baroreceptors results in increases in efferent cardiac vagal activity and decreases in sympathetic activity. Since the response of the sinuatrial node to vagal stimulation is very rapid, much of the latency of the HR response to a carotid sinus stimulus must be due to the time of the reflex transmission. The latency has been assessed in humans by recording the response of the electrocardiogram (ECG) to brief periods of

Table 1
Reflexes Influencing Heart Rate

Reflexes Causing Bradycardia	*Reflexes Causing Tachycardia*
Baroreceptors	Atrial receptors
Carotid chemoreceptors	Aortic chemoreceptors
Coronary chemoreflex (Bezold-Jarisch)	Muscle receptors
Lung hyperinflation	Lung inflation (moderate)

suction to the neck overlying the carotid sinuses, which increases carotid transmural pressure. Eckberg[16] showed that the response was dependent on the interval between the stimulus and the anticipated P wave. The maximum response was found to occur when the stimulus was applied 0.75 seconds before the anticipated P wave. The importance of this is that baroreceptors can modulate HR on a beat-to-beat basis. Baroreceptors may also regulate HR through modulation of sympathetic outflow but this has a much slower time-course.

The relationship between baroreceptor distending pressure and HR has the classical sigmoid shape. In dogs, aortic baroreceptor reflexes seem to operate over a higher range of pressures than carotid receptors.[17] This has prompted the suggestion that carotid receptors may protect against hypotension; aortic receptors, against hypertension. We have recently described another group of baroreceptors which are in the coronary arteries[18] however, these appear not to control HR.

The range of baroreceptor pressures which induce reflex cardiac responses is not necessarily the same as that causing vascular responses[17]. Clearly, the effects of baroreceptor inhibition must depend on the ongoing levels of autonomic activities. For example, if HR is already fast due to a low level of vagal activity and a high level of sympathetic activity, baroreceptor unloading would have a smaller effect than when HR was slow.

Aortic and carotid baroreceptors summate in their reflex effects. Because the relationship between total baroreceptor input and response is sigmoid, an increase in pres-

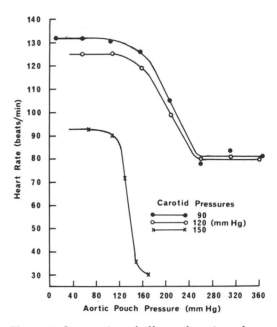

Figure 4. Summation of effects of aortic and carotid baroreceptors in control of HR. Increases in carotid sinus pressure lower the aortic threshold pressure for responses and increase the sensitivity of aortic baroreflex. These results can be explained by simple summation of two reflex inputs operating on a sigmoid relationship between total baroreceptor input and HR. From Hainsworth et al.[17]

sure in one region may cause this relationship to move to a steep part of the curve. This would result in an apparent increase in sensitivity to changes in input from the other baroreceptors (Figure 4).

In people, baroreceptor reflexes have been studied either by inducing changes in arterial blood pressure and recording changes in HR[19] or by applying negative or positive pressures to a neck chamber overlying the carotid sinuses[20]. The former technique changes the stimulus to all barorecep-

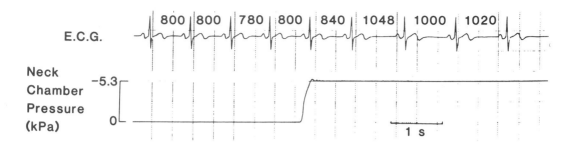

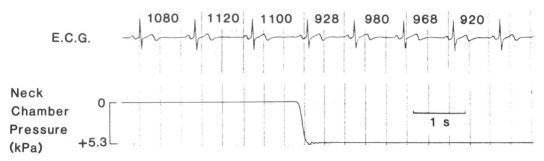

Figure 5. Responses to changes in carotid sinus transmural pressure in a healthy subject. Neck chamber pressure refers to the positive or negative pressures applied to a chamber made from thermoplastic, which seals to the anterior and lateral aspects of the neck and the lower border of the jaw. Numbers above ECG trace are of pulse-intervals. Note the very short latencies of the responses to increases and decreases in carotid transmural pressure (5.3 kPa = 40 mm Hg). Modified from Vukasovic et al.[20]

tors, whereas the latter affects only carotid baroreceptors with other receptors acting to 'buffer' the responses. However, because of the speed of the response of the heart, the neck chamber technique is suitable for investigating the carotid baroreceptor-HR reflex. The magnitude of the reflex is assessed by determining the maximum change in pulse-interval after application of the stimulus compared with the average interval before application of the stimulus (Figure 5).

Chemoreceptors

Peripheral arterial chemoreceptors are situated in the carotid and aortic bodies. Activity in their afferent nerves is increased by arterial hypoxia, hypercapnia or acidemia[21]. The most obvious effects of chemoreceptor stimulation are increases in the rate and depth of respiration. However, both sets of chemoreceptors also influence the

HR, but in different directions. Because HR is also influenced by respiratory efforts, the effects of chemoreceptor stimulation may be masked by the secondary effects of the respiratory response.

In animals, carotid chemoreceptors can conveniently be stimulated by intracarotid injections of sodium cyanide or nicotine[22]. Typically, this results in an increase in respiration with little effect on HR (Figure 6). The absence of a large consistent HR change is due to the respiratory response masking the cardiac response; if respiration is controlled, or particularly if it is stopped or the lung denervated, carotid chemoreceptor stimulation causes a large and consistent bradycardia (Figure 6).

Aortic body chemoreceptors also stimulate respiration, but in contrast to the carotid chemoreceptors, the primary effect on the heart is excitatory[23]. The reason why stimulation of aortic chemoreceptors

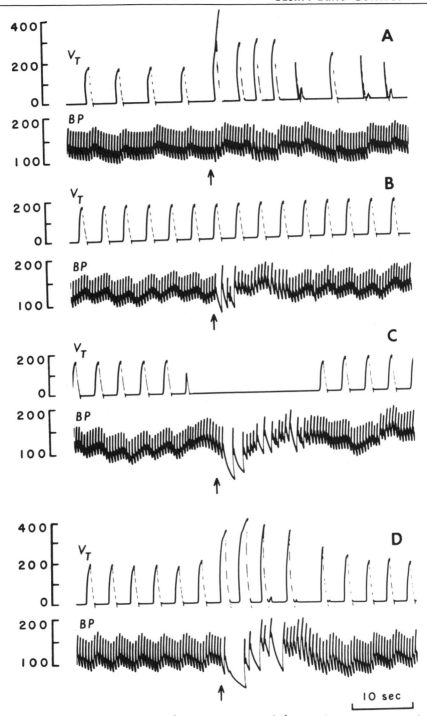

Figure 6. Interaction between carotid chemoreceptors and the respiratory response in control of HR in an anesthetized dog. Traces show tidal volume (mL) and blood pressure (mm Hg) responses to transient carotid body stimulation by injection into common carotid artery of 10 μg nicotine bitartrate during: A: spontaneous breathing; B: constant ventilation after neuromuscular blockade; C: interruption of ventilation; and D: after lung denervation. Results show masking by ventilatory response of bradycardia from chemoreceptor stimulation and enhancement of bradycardia by lung deflation or denervation. From Hainsworth et al.[22]

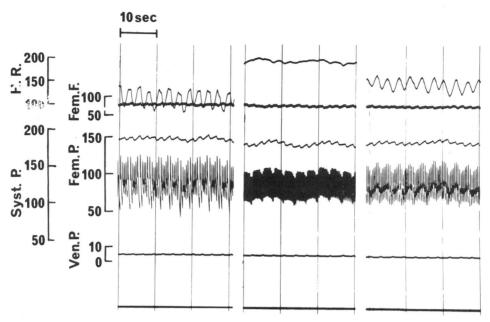

Figure 7. Responses in anesthetized dog to stimulation of left atrial receptors by inflation of balloons at pulmonary vein-atrial junctions. Traces of: beat-beat HR; femoral flow (mL/min); femoral arterial perfusion pressure; arterial blood pressure; femoral venous pressure (all mm Hg). In this preparation, a hind limb was perfused at constant blood flow, allowing its perfusion pressure to provide an index of femoral vascular resistance. During stimulation of atrial receptors, HR increased (by about 80 bpm) but there was no change in blood pressure or in femoral vascular resistance. From Carswell et al.[27]

should result in tachycardia when stimulation of the carotid receptors slows the heart is hard to explain.

Atrial Receptors

Atrial receptors are concentrated near the junctions of the superior and inferior venae cavae and the pulmonary veins with the atria[24]. They are stimulated mainly by stretching due to increases in atrial volume, but some are also excited by atrial contraction. Their discharge frequency is directly related to atrial pressure. The reflex response is to subserve the Bainbridge reflex, which is to increase HR in response to an increase in venous return[25]. The reflex effects can be studied experimentally by distending the pulmonary vein-atrial junctions with small balloons. This results in a reflex increase in HR mediated by an increase in activity in cardiac sympathetic nerves (Figure 7).[26-28] Largely because of the relatively slow time-course of sympathetic responses, the tachycardia to stimulation of atrial re-

ceptors requires up to 30 seconds to reach a stable level and the rate of offset tends to be even slower.

Atrial receptors are very slowly adapting, and reflex effects on the HR have been shown to be sustained for at least several hours.[29] Because distension of the atria is influenced, among other things, by the degree of circulatory filling, atrial receptors are often regarded as volume receptors. The reflex responses, an increase in HR, and an increase in urine flow have the effect of reducing the volume of the atria. It has been suggested that their reflex role is to ensure that ventricular size is maintained at an optimal level for ventricular function[30].

Coronary Chemoreflex (Bezold-Jarisch Reflex)

Well over a century ago, Von Bezold and Hirt observed that intravenous injections of Veratrum alkaloids elicited a powerful reflex depressor response[2]. The main reflexogenic area responsible for this effect

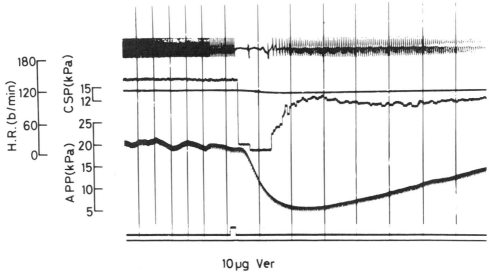

10 µg Ver

Figure 8. Responses to stimulation of coronary chemoreflex in an anesthetized dog. Traces of ECG, HR, carotid sinus pressure, and arterial perfusion pressure to vascularly isolated limb, which was perfused at constant blood flow. Injection into aortic root of 10µg veratridine promptly induced a profound reflex bradycardia as well as vasodilatation (decrease in arterial perfusion pressure)(1 kPa = 7.5 mm Hg). Modified from McGregor KH, Hainsworth R, Ford R. Hind-limb vascular responses in anaesthetized dogs to aortic root injections of veratridine. Quart J Exp Physiol 1986; 71: 577-587.

was subsequently localized to the heart and it was shown that minute injections of veratridine into the branches of the coronary arteries supplying the left ventricle caused the largest effects[31].

Injections of many stimulant chemicals into the coronary circulation result in bradycardia and hypotension (Figure 8). Chemicals causing this response include phenyl diguanide and capsaicin, as well as substances resulting from myocardial ischemia including bradykinin and prostaglandins[2]. Similar responses may also occur when radiopaque dyes are injected into the coronary arteries[32]. Both afferent and efferent pathways of this reflex involve the vagus nerves.

The coronary chemoreflex may be elicited in pathological states, particularly myocardial ischemia and infarction, and more particularly when this affects the inferolateral wall. There is no evidence, however, that this reflex has a normal physiological role. Some chemosensitive ventricular afferents are also stimulated by increasing ventricular pressure, but it is necessary to increase ventricular pressures to above the

physiological range,[18,33] or to cause ventricular dilatation and a large increase in ventricular end-diastolic pressure. Therefore, it seems that ventricular receptors are unlikely to be important in healthy individuals, although a role for them in myocardial ischemia and failure cannot be excluded.

Some chemosensitive nerves from the heart run in the sympathetic nerves and these are believed to cause excitatory responses including increases in HR[2]. They may contribute to the increases in HR and blood pressure that sometimes occur with myocardial ischemia and infarction, particularly when this involves the anterior wall of the heart. They also probably transmit cardiac pain.

Other Reflexes

Almost all parts of the body, when subjected to intense or noxious stimuli, may result in cardiovascular reflexes. However, several regions have been shown to be able to induce reflex cardiovascular effects in response to physiological stimuli. The lungs, including airways, pulmonary circulation and pulmonary artery, are richly innervated.[34] Lung inflation, with moderate pressures, stimulates airways stretch receptors which are attached to myelinated nerves. This results in a reflex increase in HR.[35,36] Pulmonary nonmyelinated nerves (C fibers) also innervate the bronchi and lung. They may be stimulated during hyperinflation of the lung and also during pulmonary congestion, embolism or following intravenous injections of stimulant chemicals including veratridine, capsaicin or bradykinin. The reflex response is to cause bradycardia, although its physiological significance is uncertain.

Stretch receptors also exist in the wall of the pulmonary artery and are excited by increases in pulmonary arterial pressure (AP). The reflex response is an increase in vascular resistance, but there seems to be no direct effect on the HR.[37]

The abdominal viscera are richly supplied with afferent nerves and the activity in these increases in response to venous congestion[38]. The resulting reflex is to increase sympathetic activity to the circulation, leading to hypertension and tachycardia. The question of the existence of mesenteric arterial baroreceptors has long been debated and, although it is possible to record from afferents which discharge with a cardiac pulsatility, these have not conclusively been shown to act as baroreceptors.

Influence of Complex Events on Heart Rate

Respiratory Influences

Sinus Arrhythmia

This refers to the cyclical variation in HR which is associated with respiration. Heart rate accelerates during inspiration and slows during expiration. The magnitude of the oscillation is variable, but usually it can be exaggerated by slow deep breathing.

The mechanism linking the variability of HR to respiration is complex and involves both central and reflex interactions. It is suggested that a 'gating' mechanism is involved in the central nervous pathways linking the respiratory control with the vagal motoneurons.[39] It is not necessary for breathing to actually occur, since it has been shown that sinus arrhythmia may persist in paralyzed, ventilated animals after stopping the ventilatory pump. Thus, the mechanism seems to be due partly to a central effect[40]. Reflexes arising from lung stretch receptors, probably those responsible for the Hering-Breuer reflex, are also likely to contribute because moderate degrees of lung inflation induce a reflex tachycardia[36]. Other reflexes are also likely either to contribute to or to modulate the respiratory HR variations. Cardiac filling varies with the oscillations of intrathoracic pressure, and this is likely to influence HR through various cardiovascular reflexes, in particular the atrial receptor-induced tachycardia and the baroreceptor-induced bradycardia.

The magnitude of the response of HR to baroreceptor stimulation varies throughout the respiratory cycle[41]. Figure 9 shows the responses of pulse-interval to brief periods

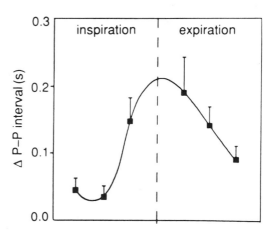

Figure 9. Responses to brief stimulations of carotid baroreceptors by applying neck suction at various phases of the respiratory cycle. Results are of means and SEM from six healthy subjects and show that baroreflex responses were greatest during early expiration and almost totally inhibited during the first part of inspiration. From Anrep et al.[40]

of baroreceptor stimulation in humans using a neck suction chamber. Responses are seen to be maximal during early expiration and almost totally inhibited during early inspiration.

Sinus arrhythmia is mainly, if not entirely, mediated through changes in efferent vagal activity. The magnitude of the sinus arrhythmia is claimed to provide an index of the level of efferent vagal activity to the heart.[42,43]

Valsalva

The Valsalva maneuver is another respiratory procedure which has a complex effect on the cardiovascular system. The various phases of this and the mechanisms thought to be involved have been described in detail by Sharpey-Shafer[44]. The subject takes a large inspiration followed by a maximal expiratory effort against an obstruction. This procedure generates an intrathoracic pressure of the order of 100 mm Hg. This is transmitted to the intrathoracic and intra-abdominal blood vessels and initially increases AP. Venous return from outside the thoraco-abdominal region is impaired so that cardiac output falls and blood pressure decreases. This decreases baroreceptor activity, resulting in reflex increases in HR and vascular resistance and a restoration of mean AP, although not pulse pressure. On release of the Valsalva, venous return from the region outside the thorax and abdomen is initially enhanced leading to a marked overshoot of blood pressure and a baro-reflex-mediated bradycardia.

The responses to the Valsalva maneuver provide a rough guide to the integrity of the autonomic neural pathways involved. For example, patients suffering from autonomic neuropathy show a sustained fall in pressure during the procedure with no compensatory tachycardia. Also, the overshoot at the end of the test and the accompanying bradycardia are reduced or absent.

Effects of Decreases in Venous Return

Return of blood to the heart is reduced when blood volume is decreased due to hemorrhage or other causes of hypovolemia. Venous return is also low if there is excessive pooling of blood in peripheral vessels during postural stress. Experimentally, postural decreases in venous return may be provoked by passive head-up tilting on a tilting table, or by subjecting the lower part of the body to subatmospheric pressures using a lower-body chamber. These stresses reduce cardiac filling pressures by not only altering the distribution of the intravascular volume towards the peripheral veins, but also substantially decreasing plasma volume due to increased capillary filtration.

There are three phases of responses of the cardiovascular system to decreases in venous return. Initially, blood pressure remains little changed, or may even be increased; this is associated with increases in vascular resistance and heart rate. Secondly, blood pressure may fall, despite further increases in vascular resistance and HR. Finally, there may be an abrupt fall in blood pressure and loss of consciousness. This severe hypotensive phase is accompanied by a decrease in vascular resistance and often also in HR, and is termed a vasovagal reaction.[45] These phases are illustrated in Figure 10, which shows the changes in arterial blood pressure and pulse-interval in a healthy subject who was first passively tilted head-up and then, while still head-up, lower body suction was applied.[46]

Moderate orthostatic stress (tilted phase in Figure 10) results in decreases in cardiac output and in cardiac filling pressure accompanied by tachycardia, but not hypotension. The mechanism responsible for this tachycardia and vasoconstriction is controversial. Many believe this to be a response to unloading of low pressure 'cardiopulmonary baroreceptors' because of the absence of any apparent decrease in the stimulus to arterial baroreceptors. However, there is no convincing evidence in sup-

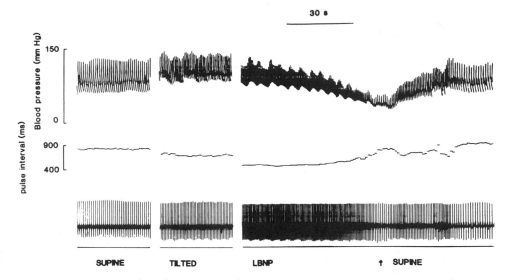

Figure 10. Responses in a healthy subject to head-up tilting alone and combined with application of a negative pressure of 20 mm Hg to the body below the iliac crests (LBNP). Tilting alone resulted in increases in both HR and blood pressure. Following the addition of LBNP blood pressure fell, followed by a decrease in the HR (a vasovagal reaction). From El-Bedawi et al.[46]

port of this and, in conscious primates, it has been shown that arterial baroreceptors are indeed essential for this response[47]. Furthermore, recent evidence has shown that there are changes in diameter of vessels containing baroreceptors even when no changes in pressure, including pulse pressure, are apparent[48,49].

The mechanism for inducing tachycardia and vasoconstriction during the early hypotensive phase (initial part of LBNP in Figure 10) is generally agreed to be mainly due to unloading of arterial baroreceptors because there is clearly a reduction in pulse pressure and, often, also in the mean level of pressure. The mechanism responsible for the acute hypotensive phase (vasovagal reaction) is not understood; earlier opinions that it was due to stimulation of cardiac ventricular receptors (a part of the Bezold-Jarisch reflex) are now largely discounted. This is because few ventricular receptors are excited this way[50], controlled animal experiments have not shown the existence of such a reflex[51] and similar reactions occur in patients who have had cardiac transplants and therefore have denervated ventricles[52]. The mechanism responsible remains a mystery.

However, it seems that the central nervous system is involved and opioids, probably of delta subtype, and serotonergic mechanisms may be mediators[53].

Exercise

The control of HR during exercise is a complex subject and no more than a brief summary can be given here. For more detail, the reader is referred to more comprehensive reviews[54-57].

Immediately at the onset of exercise, there is an increase in HR which, owing to its rapid onset, can only be of vagal origin. This immediate response is attributed to central command. Metaboreceptors within the muscle also become stimulated and these contribute to an afferent input which further increases HR. Many other mechanisms are also involved, including reflexes from lung inflation and possible inhibition of the baroreceptor reflex.

During exercise, the HR increases in direct relation to the work load up to the subject's maximum levels, which are related to age. A program of strenuous physical training increases the size of the heart and resting cardiac stroke volume, but resting HR is decreased and cardiac output is unchanged[58]. Inactivity has the opposite effect. The maximum HR is not greatly influenced by training, but because the resting level is lower, the relative increase is greater.

Physiological Importance of Heart Rate

The importance of HR lies in its contribution to cardiac output:

$$\text{Cardiac output} = \text{stroke volume} \times \text{HR}. \tag{1}$$

This equation is axiomatic and knowledge of any two of the variables readily permits calculation of the third. In terms of the physiological regulation of cardiac output, however, this equation can be misleading. This is because stroke volume and HR are not independent of each other and, in particular, changes in HR are liable to result in reciprocal changes in stroke volume.

There have been a number of studies with both animals and humans, which have examined the effect on cardiac output of inducing changes in HR by pacing, both at rest and during exercise[59-61]. The results of these studies are in general agreement that, at rest, changes in HR between about 80 and 150 bpm have little effect on the cardiac output because an increase in rate is almost exactly canceled by a corresponding reduction in stroke volume. Changes in rate between about 80 and 50 bpm do have a small influence on cardiac output, and below 50 bpm stroke volume tends to be fixed and changes in HR then result in proportional changes in flow.

The reason why changes in HR do not cause the expected change in cardiac output can be appreciated by reference to Figure 11. Changes in HR are effected mainly through changes in diastolic time, and so a reduction or acceleration in rate changes the time for venous filling and consequently has a minor influence on the output. At normal levels

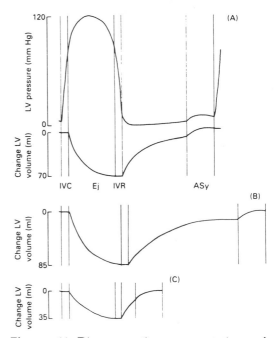

Figure 11. Diagrammatic representation of changes in left ventricular pressures and volumes during the cardiac cycle and the influence of HR. IVC: isovolumic contraction; Ej: ejection; IVR: isovolumic relaxation; ASy: atrial systole. In A, HR is 80 bpm (cycle length 0.75 s). Note that ventricular filling is greatest during early diastole and slows towards the end of diastole. Stroke volume is 70 mL and therefore cardiac output is 5.6 L/min. In B, HR has slowed to 60 bpm (cycle length 1.0 s). Diastole is prolonged and towards its end filling virtually ceases (diastasis). The decrease in rate and the increase in stroke almost cancel each other and cardiac ouput decreases only to 5.1 L/min. Further decreases in rate, however, because of the diastasis, would not result in compensatory increases in stroke volume and cardiac ouput would fall. In C, HR is 120 bpm (cycle length 0.5 s) and now atrial systole becomes important for the maintenance of ventricular filling. Stroke volume is reduced but cardiac output remains nearly unchanged from that depicted in A. From Hainsworth R. Syncope and Fainting. In: Bannister R, Mathias CJ (eds). Autonomic Failure, 3rd ed. Oxford, England: Oxford University Press, 1992; 761-781.

of venous filling pressure, diastolic volume is maximal at a rate of about 50 bpm, and so any further reduction in rate would indeed decrease the output. However, if venous filling pressure is low, for example during orthostasis or following loss of blood volume,

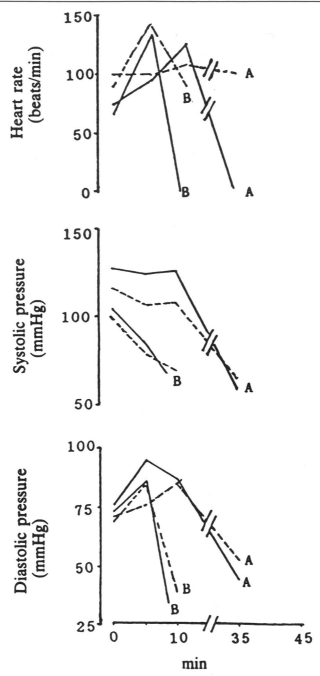

Figure 12. Effects of head-up tilting in two patients with orthostatic hypotension before and after implantation of sequential AV pacemakers. Before pacemaker implantation both patients lost consciousness accompanied by asystole and profound hypotension at about 10 min and 35 min after tilting. After pacemaker implantation syncope occurred in both patients at almost exactly the same time as previously and with almost exactly the same changes in blood pressure, but with the change in HR successfully prevented. From El-Bedawi KM, Wahbha MMAE, Hainsworth R. Cardiac pacing does not improve orthostatic tolerance in patients with vasovagal syncope. Clin Autonom Res 1994; 4:233-237.

it is likely that even lower HRs would fail materially to affect the output. One consequence of this is that prevention of bradycardia during tests of orthostatic tolerance have little or no influence on the time to syncope (Figure 12).

During severe physical exercise, the situation is quite different and the rapid HR is likely to contribute significantly to attaining high levels of cardiac output. Severe exercise is accompanied by a high level of efferent sympathetic nervous activity and this not only causes the tachycardia, it also increases the force of contraction, and importantly, reduces the duration of ventricular systole. The consequence of this is that diastolic time is reduced less than it would be by simple pacing. The high venous filling rate, the enhanced contribution to ventricular filling by atrial systole, and the partial preservation of ventricular diastolic time ensure that during exercise the ventricles are adequately filled despite tachycardia, and high levels of cardiac output are thereby achieved.

References

1. Levy MN, Martin PJ. Neural control of the heart. In: Berne RM (ed). Handbook of Physiology, Section 2, Volume 1. Bethesda, Md: American Physiological Society, 1979; 581-620.
2. Hainsworth R. Reflexes from the heart. Physiol Rev 1991; 71:617-658.
3. Furnival CM, Linden RJ, Snow HM. The inotropic effect on the heart of stimulating the vagus in the dog, duck and toad. J Physiol 1973; 230:155-170.
4. Hamlin RL, Smith CR. Effects of vagal stimulation on S-A and A-V nodes. Am J Physiol 1968; 215:560-568.
5. Levy MN, Martin PJ, Iano T, et al. Effects of single vagal stimuli on heart rate and atrioventricular conduction. Am J Physiol 1970; 218:1256-1262.
6. Rosenblueth A, Simeone FA. The interrelations of vagal and accelerator effects on the cardiac rate. Am J Physiol 1934; 110:42-55.
7. Parker P, Celler BG, Potter EK, et al. Vagal stimulation and cardiac slowing. J Auton Nerv Syst 1984; 11:226-231.
8. Mary DASG, Hainsworth R. Methods for the study of cardiovascular reflexes. In: Hainsworth R, Mark AL (eds). Cardiovascular Control in Health and Disease. London, England: Saunders, 1993; 1-34.
9. Furnival CM, Linden RJ, Snow HM. Chronotropic and inotropic effects on the dog heart of stimulating the efferent cardiac sympathetic nerves. J Physiol 1973; 230:137-153.
10. Levy MN, Zieske H. Autonomic control of cardiac pacemaker activity and atrioventricular transmission. J Appl Physiol 1969; 27:465-470.
11. Persson PB, Kirchheim HR. Baroreceptor Reflexes. Berlin, Germany: Springer-Verlag, 1991.
12. Zucker IH, Gilmore JP. Reflex Control of the Circulation. Boca Raton, Fla: CRC Press, 1991.
13. Hainsworth R, Mark AL. Cardiovascular Reflex Control in Health and Disease. London, England: Saunders, 1993.
14. Eckberg DL, Sleight P. Human Baroreflexes in Health and Disease. Oxford, England: Oxford University Press, 1992.
15. Chapleau MW, Abboud FM. Mechanisms of adaptation and resetting of the baroreceptor reflex. In: Hainsworth R, Mark AL (eds). Cardiovascular Reflex Control in Health and Disease. London, England: Saunders, 1993; 165-194.
16. Eckberg DL. Temporal response patterns of the human sinus node to brief carotid baroreceptor stimuli. J Physiol 1978; 258:769-782.
17. Hainsworth R, Ledsome JR, Carswell F. Reflex responses from aortic baroreceptors. Am J Physiol 1970; 218:423-429.
18. Drinkhill MJ, Moore J, Hainsworth R. Afferent discharges from coronary arterial and ventricular receptors in anaesthetized dogs. J Physiol 1993; 472:785-800.
19. Smyth HS, Sleight P, Pickering GW. Reflex regulation of arterial pressure during sleep in men. A quantative method of assessing baroreflex sensitivity. Circ Res 1969; 24:109-121.
20. Vukasovic JL, Al-Timman JKA, Hainsworth R. The effects of lower body negative pressure on baroreceptor responses in humans. Exp Physiol 1990; 75:455-469.
21. Sampson SR, Hainsworth R. Responses of aortic body chemoreceptors to physiological stimuli. Am J Physiol 1972; 222:953-958.
22. Hainsworth R, Jacobs L, Comroe JH Jr. Afferent lung denervation by brief inhalation of steam. J Appl Physiol 1973; 34:708-714.

23. Karim F, Hainsworth R, Sofola OA, et al. Responses of the heart to stimulation of aortic body chemoreceptors in dogs. Circ Res 1980; 46:77-83.

24. Nonidez JF. Identification of the receptor areas in the venae cavae and the pulmonary veins which initiate reflex cardiac acceleration (Bainbridge's reflex). Am J Anat 1937; 61:203-231.

25. Bainbridge FA. The influence of venous filling upon the rate of the heart. J Physiol 1915; 50:65-84.

26. Ledsome JR, Linden RJ. A reflex increase in heart rate from distension of the pulmonary vein—atrial junctions. J Physiol 1964; 170:456-473.

27. Carswell F, Hainsworth R, Ledsome JR. The effects of distension of the pulmonary vein—atrial junctions upon peripheral vascular resistance. J Physiol 1970; 207:1-14.

28. Hainsworth R. Atrial receptors. In: Zucker IH, Gilmore JP (eds). Reflex Control of the Circulation. Boca Raton, Fla: CRC Press, 1991; 273-289.

29. Ledsome JR. Renal responses to stimulation of left atrial receptors in anaesthetized dogs. In: Hainsworth R, McWilliam PN, Mary DASG (eds). Cardiogenic Reflexes. Oxford, England: Oxford University Press, 1987; 106-121.

30. Linden RJ, Kappagoda CT. Atrial Receptors. Cambridge, England: Cambridge University Press, 1982.

31. Dawes GS. Studies on veratrum alkaloids. VII. Receptor areas in the coronary arteries and elsewhere as revealed by the use of veratridine. J Pharmacol Exp Ther 1947; 89:325-342.

32. Perez-Gomez F, Garcia-Aguado A. Origin of ventricular reflexes caused by coronary arteriography. Br Heart J 1977; 39:967-973.

33. Drinkhill MJ, Moore J, Hainsworth R. Afferent discharges from coronary arterial and ventricular receptors in anaesthetized dogs. J Physiol 1993; 472:785-800.

34. Coleridge HM, Coleridge JCG. Afferent innervation of lungs, airway and pulmonary artery. In: Zucker IH, Gilmore JP (eds). Reflex Control of the Circulation. Boca Raton, Fla: CRC Press, 1991; 579-608.

35. Anrep GV, Pascual W, Rossler R. Respiratory variations of the heart rate. The reflex mechanism of the respiratory arrhythmia. Proc R Soc Lond 1936; 119:191-217.

36. Hainsworth R. Circulatory responses from lung inflation in anesthetized dogs. Am J Physiol 1974; 226:247-255.

37. Ledsome JR, Kan K. Reflex changes in hind limb and renal vascular resistance to disten-

sion of the isolated pulmonary arteries of the dog. Circ Res 1977; 40:64-72.

38. Longhust JC. Reflex effects from abdominal visceral afferents. In: Zucker IH, Gilmore JP (eds). Reflex Control of the Circulation. Boca Raton, Fla: CRC Press, 1991; 551-578.

39. Spyer KM, Jordan D. Electrophysiology of the nucleus ambiguus. In: Hainsworth R, McWilliam PN, Mary DASG (eds). Cardiogenic Reflexes. Oxford, England: Oxford University Press, 1987; 237-249.

40. Anrep GV, Pascual W, Rossler R. Respiratory variations of the heart rate. II. The central mechanism of the respiratory arrhythmia and the inter-relations between the central and the reflex mechanisms. Proc R Soc Lond 1936; 119:218-230.

41. Eckberg DL, Kifle YT, Roberts VL. Phase relationship between normal human respiration and baroreflex responsiveness. J Physiol 1980; 304:489-502.

42. Eckberg DL. Human sinus arrhythmia as an index of vagal cardiac outflow. J Appl Physiol 1983; 54:961-966.

43. Fouad FM, Tazazi RC, Ferrario CM, et al. Assessment of parasympathetic control of heart rate by a noninvasive method. Am J Physiol 1984; 246:H838-H842.

44. Sharpey-Shafer EP. Effects of respiratory acts on the circulation. In: Hamilton WF, Dow P (eds). Handbook of Physiology, Section 2, Volume 3. Washington, DC: American Physiological Society, 1964; 1875-1886.

45. Lewis T. Vasovagal syncope and the carotid sinus mechanism. Br Med J 1932; 1:873-876.

46. El-Bedawi KM, Hainsworth R. Combined head-up tilt and lower body suction: a test of othostatic tolerance. Clin Autonom Res 1994. In press.

47. Cornish KG, Gilmore JP, McCulloch T. Central blood volume and blood pressure in conscious primates. Am J Physiol 1988; 254:H693-H701.

48. Hartikainen J, Ahonen E, Nevalainen T, et al. Haemodynamic information encoded in the aortic baroreceptor discharge during haemorrhage. Acta Physiol Scand 1990; 140:181-189.

49. Lacolley PJ, Pannier BM, Cuche MA, et al. Carotid arterial haemodynamics after mild degrees of lower-body negative pressure in man. Clin Sci 1992; 83:535-540.

50. Oberg B, Thoren P. Increased activity in left ventricular receptors during haemorrhage or occlusion of the caval veins in the cat. A possible cause of vasovagal reaction. Acta Physiol Scand 1972; 85:164-173.

51. Al-Timman JKA, Hainsworth R. Reflex vascular responses to changes in left ventricular

pressures, heart rate and inotropic state in dogs. Exp Physiol 1992; 77:455-469.

52. Fitzpatrick AP, Bannder N, Cheng A, et al. Vasovagal reactions may occur after orthotropic heart transplantation. J Am Coll Cardiol 1993; 21:1132-1137.

53. Ludbrook J. Haemorrhage and shock. In: Hainsworth R, Mark AL (eds). Cardiovascular Reflex Control in Health and Disease. London, England: Saunders, 1993; 463-490.

54. Mitchell JH, Schmidt RF. Cardiovascular reflex control by afferent fibres from skeletal muscle receptors. In: Shepherd JT, Aboud FM (eds). Handbook of Physiology. The Cardiovascular System, Volume 3. Bethesda, Md: American Physiological Society, 1983; 623-658.

55. Astrand PO. Quantification of exercise capability and evaluation of physical capacity in man. Prog Cardiovasc Dis 1976; 19:51-67.

56. Vatner SF, Pagani M. Cardiovascular adjustments to exercise: hemodynamics and mechanisms. Prog Cardiovasc Dis 1976; 29:91-188.

57. Ray CA, Mark AL. Sympathetic adjustments to exercise: insights from microneurographic recordings. In: Hainsworth R, Mark AL (eds). Cardiovascular Reflex Control in Health and Disease. London, England: Saunders, 1993; 137-164.

58. Saltin B, Blomquist G, Mitchell JH, et al. Response to exercise after bedrest and after training. Circulation 1968; 37(supp 7):1-55.

59. Rushmer RF. Constancy of stroke volume in ventricular responses to exertion. Am J Physiol 1959; 196:745-750.

60. Miller DE, Gleason WL, Whalen RE, et al. Effect of ventricular rate in the cardiac output in the dog with chronic heart block. Circ Res 1962; 10:658-663.

61. Bevegard S, Jonsson B, Karlof I, et al. Effect of changes in ventricular rate on cardiac output and central pressures at rest and during exercise in patients with artificial pacemakers. Cardiovasc Res 1967; 1:21-33.

Chapter 2

Circadian Changes of the Cardiovascular System and the Autonomic Nervous System:
Observations in Autonomic Disorders

Christopher J. Mathias, Maria Alam

Introduction

Circadian rhythms affecting the circulation have been well documented, the most prominent being the fall in blood pressure and heart rate in normal man while asleep at night.[1,2] The mechanisms involved are likely to be multiple.[3,4] The endogenous oscillator within the central nervous system is probably the hypothalamus, while there are additionally a number of external factors, with varying degrees of influence. When blood pressure and heart rate are the measurement endpoints, a range of other factors need to be considered, including the autonomic nervous system, circulating and local hormones (which act either directly or indirectly to influence cardiovascular reactivity), and the target organs themselves. These multiple influences compound the difficulties in dissecting the mechanisms responsible for circadian changes affecting the cardiovascular

system, especially in disease states. There has been considerable progress in the detection, investigation and localization of the lesion in a variety of autonomic disorders which affect the cardiovascular system,[5] especially in diseases where the target organs themselves are not directly involved. Some of these subjects are clinical physiological models and have contributed to further knowledge of neural-cardiovascular interactions. This chapter will focus on such subjects. It will begin with a brief classification of autonomic disorders. This will be followed by a description of cardiovascular changes, as observed through 24-hour noninvasive ambulatory blood pressure and heart rate monitoring in subjects with well-defined lesions of the baroreceptor reflex arc. The role of various stimuli in daily life, which influence the circulation through autonomic or neurohormonal changes, will be discussed.

From: Malik M., Camm AJ (eds.): *Heart Rate Variability*. Armonk, NY. Futura Publishing Company, Inc., © 1995.

Classification of Autonomic Disorders

Autonomic dysfunction can be broadly divided into localized and generalized disorders. Examples of localized disorders are provided in Table 1. In cardiac transplantees, the external cardiac autonomic nerves are severed, but the intrinsic ganglia are preserved; this contrasts with cardiac involvement in Chagas' disease, where the cholinergic plexuses are targeted, probably by an autoimmune process. The generalized disorders (Table 2) can be divided into primary disorders, where the etiology is not known, and secondary disorders where the lesion has been clearly defined, or where there is a clear association with a disease such as diabetes mellitus. Drugs are a common cause of autonomic dysfunction, often as a side effect. Neurally mediated syncope, such as vasovagal syncope, probably belongs to the primary variety, but is tabled separately; in many subjects the precipitating factor may be known, but the precise mechanisms for the abnormal responses are often unclear.

Cardiovascular Circadian Rhythms in Different Autonomic Disorders

Ambulatory blood pressure and heart rate over a 24-hour period may be measured in a variety of ways. The previous techniques of using intra-arterial cannulation have now been largely superseded by noninvasive approaches; the majority of which provide intermittent recordings, although technological advances, as with the Portapres 2 (TNO Biomedical Instrumentation Research Unit, Amsterdam, The Netherlands), provide beat-by-beat finger arterial blood pressure and heart rate. The examples we provide have been based on intermittent recordings over a 24-hour period using the Spacelabs 90207 monitor (Redmond, Washington, USA). The machine was usually connected at 09.00 and programmed to take recordings at 30-minute intervals during the day and at 60-minute intervals at night, usually between 23.00 and 06.00 hours. In addition, these recordings were obtained after various stimuli, which included 5 minutes of lying, sitting and standing (usually at 10.00, 17.00 and 21.00 hours); before and after food ingestion; and before and after walking, while on the flat and after walking upstairs. This enabled recordings of circadian changes through the day and night, and also the influence of various other factors in daily life. In each of the subjects the autonomic disorder was defined on the basis of the history, clinical findings, and a series of autonomic investigations which included physiological, and where relevant, biochemical and pharmacological studies.[8]

Normal Subjects and Controls

Figure 1 provides the data obtained in a normal subject over a 24-hour period. At night, while in bed and when the subject was probably asleep, blood pressure usually fell. There was a clustering of measurements during the day at certain times, when multiple recordings were made to determine the effects of postural change, food and exercise. The recordings were noninvasive and used techniques which could be influenced by arm movement. Where ap-

---

Table 1

Examples of Localized Autonomic Disorders Affecting the Heart and/or Vasculature.

Cardiac transplantation
Chagas' disease (Trypanasomiasis cruzii)
Horner's syndrome*
Reflex sympathetic dystrophy*

---

*Denotes local vascular involvement in the face or hand. Adapted from Mathias.[6]

Table 2
Classification of Autonomic Disorders

Primary Autonomic Failure:
Chronic:
  Pure autonomic failure
  Shy-Drager syndrome
    —with Parkinsonian features
    —with cerebellar and pyramidal features
    —with multiple system atrophy (combination of above)
Acute or subacute dysautonomias
Secondary Autonomic Failure or Dysfunction:
Central:
  Brain tumors, especially of the third ventricle or posterior fossa
  Multiple sclerosis
  Syringobulbia
  Elderly
Spinal:
  Spinal transverse myelitis
  Transverse myelitis
  Syringomyelia
  Spinal tumors
Peripheral:
  Afferent:
    Guillain-Barré syndrome
    Tabes dorsalis
    Holmes-Adie syndrome
    Carotid sinus hypersensitivity
  Efferent:
    Diabetes mellitus
    Amyloidosis
    Surgery (such as splanchnicectomy)
    Dopamine β-hydroxylase deficiency
  Afferent/efferent:
    Familial dysautonomia (Riley-Day syndrome)
Miscellaneous:
  Autoimmune and collagen disorders
  Renal failure
  Neoplasia
  Human immunodeficiency virus infection
Drugs:
Neurally Mediated Syncope:
  Vasovagal syncope

From Mathias[7]

propriate, therefore, control subjects with similar additional problems but without autonomic dysfunction were studied. An example is provided in Figure 2 from a patient with Parkinson's disease, in whom the movement disorder (with rigidity and tremor) was similar to the neurological features observed in primary autonomic failure subjects with the Parkinsonian forms of the Shy-Drager syndrome. The subject in Figure 2 had no autonomic abnormalities and other than an increased variability in blood pressure, there was preservation of the circadian fall in blood pressure and heart rate at night, as occurs normally.

Baroreceptor Afferent Lesions

Subjects with a complete afferent lesion of the baroreceptor reflex arc are unusual. Figure 3 provides the data from one such

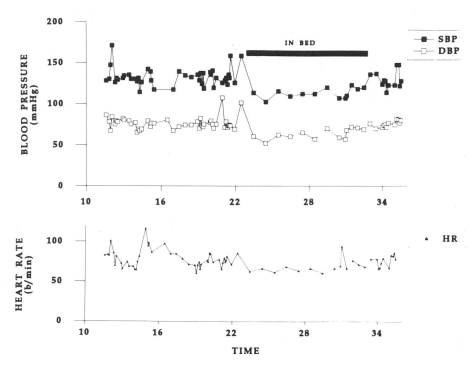

Figure 1. Blood pressure and heart rate profile in a normal subject over a 48-hour cycle period. 10 = 10.00hrs, 28 = 0400hrs the next morning.

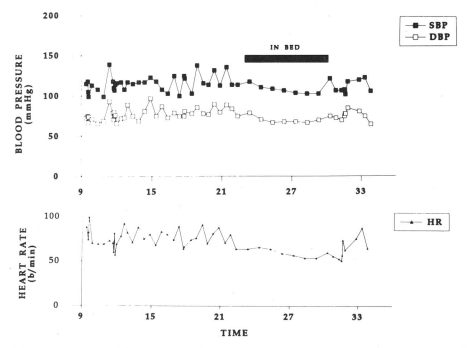

Figure 2. Blood pressure and heart rate profile in a subject with Parkinson's disease but without autonomic failure, over a 24-hour period.

patient, who, on detailed testing, had the equivalent of a chronic nucleus tractus solitarius lesion,[9] with virtually complete impairment of afferent inputs, but with preservation of the central and sympathetic efferent autonomic outflow. The patient had marked lability of blood pressure and heart rate, with postural hypotension. In addition, the patient also had severe hypertension, which was often associated with mental activation or physical exercise. The patient's heart rate rose when the blood pressure increased, presumably because of a centrally generated increase in sympathetic activity affecting the heart rate and blood vessels without appropriate buffering. When blood pressure fell, there was no rise in heart rate, in keeping with the baroreceptor afferent deficit. At night the patient's blood pressure and heart rate were lower, indicating that circadian rhythm remained. This was consistent with preservation of function of the central oscillator and efferent limbs of the baroreceptor reflex arc.

Cardiac Vagal Efferent Lesions

In certain disorders, such as diabetes mellitus, the autonomic neuropathy may initially involve the cardiac vagal outflow with the sympathetic efferent pathways affected later. The circadian responses in such subjects are of interest, since there may be preservation of certain changes such as the fall in blood pressure at night, as shown in Figure 4. In this subject, the autonomic tests indicated marked cardiac vagal failure with minimal change in heart rate when the blood pressure fell. This subject had minimal sympathetic involvement, with postural hypotension unmasked only when a hypotensive agent was used in an attempt to lower the subject's elevated supine blood pressure. As noted here, the circadian fall in blood pressure at night was maintained. On the occasions where the subject's blood pressure fell with postural change, there were few changes in heart rate. As the disease progresses, and when the sympathetic

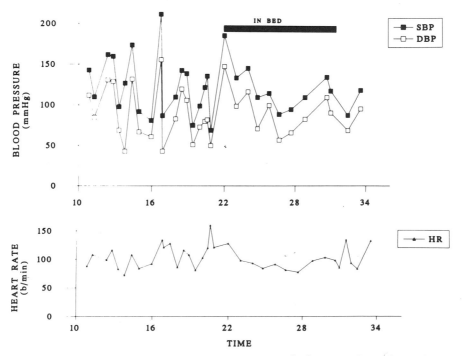

Figure 3. Blood pressure and heart rate profile in a subject with the equivalent of a nucleus tractus solitarius lesion.

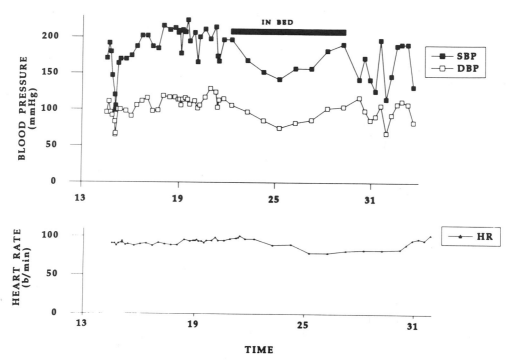

Figure 4. Blood pressure and heart rate profile in a subject with diabetes mellitus who had cardiac parasympathetic involvement but minimal sympathetic vasoconstrictor impairment.

efferent pathways are impaired, the responses in diabetic subjects may be similar[10,11] to those observed in chronic autonomic failure, as described below.

Sympathetic Efferent Lesions

In certain disorders, there is involvement of the sympathetic efferent pathways only, with sparing of the cardiac parasympathetic outflow. Dopamine β-hydroxylase deficiency is one such example, since the subjects have a selective inability to convert dopamine to noradrenaline, and thus, adrenaline.[12] They have sympathetic failure with postural hypotension and, characteristically, have elevated levels of plasma dopamine, with undetectable plasma noradrenaline and adrenaline. Electron microscopic studies indicate that the sympathetic nerve terminals are morphologically and otherwise biochemically intact.[13] Parasympathetic function to the heart, sweat glands, and urinary bladder is preserved. Figure 5

shows the changes in blood pressure in one such patient. There are frequent elevations in heart rate, mainly related to a fall in blood pressure, and there is no circadian fall in blood pressure at night.

Combined Sympathetic and Parasympathetic Efferent Lesions

In severe primary autonomic failure, both the sympathetic and parasympathetic nervous systems usually are involved. The lesion may be central, as in the Shy-Drager syndrome when there are associated neurological features with Parkinsonian and/or cerebellar signs, or peripheral as in pure autonomic failure where there are no additional neurological features. This can be confirmed by various tests[8,14] including the growth hormone response to the alpha 2 adrenoreceptor agonist, clonidine. This drug has predominantly central actions on alpha-adrenoreceptors in stimulating growth hormone release in normal subjects and in pure

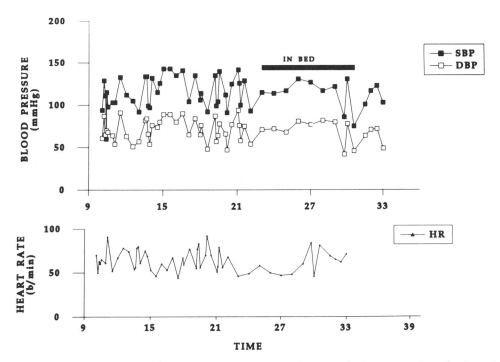

Figure 5. Blood pressure and heart rate profile in a subject with dopamine beta hydroxylase deficiency.

autonomic failure (with peripheral, but not central involvement). In the Shy-Drager syndrome with central involvement there is no rise in plasma growth hormone levels.[15]

Examples are provided of changes occurring in the Shy-Drager syndrome (Figure 6) and in pure autonomic failure (Figure 7). In both, there is hypotension during head-up postural challenge with minimal changes in heart rate. Hypertension occurs often while supine and particularly at night. The blood pressure is often lower in the morning, when postural hypotension and accompanying symptoms are at their worst, as seen in Figure 7. Reversal of the normal circadian rhythm in autonomic failure was observed during intra-arterial recordings by Mann et al.[16] They, however, were not aware at the time of a number of influences, as described below, which can influence blood pressure. Some of these, such as the vasodepressor effect of food ingestion, can be detected using noninvasive techniques.[17]

Factors in Daily Life Influencing the Circulation

There is increasing recognition that a number of factors in daily life affect the circulation. They may cause substantial regional effects, but modest systemic changes in normal subjects because of the homeostatic actions of the autonomic nervous system. The hormonal, autonomic, and cardiovascular effects of these stimuli are often unmasked in autonomic disorders; many of the stimuli enhance postural hyptotension, as listed in Table 3. A prime example is food ingestion, which causes minimal changes in blood pressure and a small rise in heart rate in normal subjects, but can result in severe postprandial hypotension in autonomic failure subjects.[18] The mechanisms of postprandial hypotension include the release of various hormones, both local and systemically, some of which have marked regional effects; these may contribute to postprandial angina. Other stimuli such as exercise,[19]

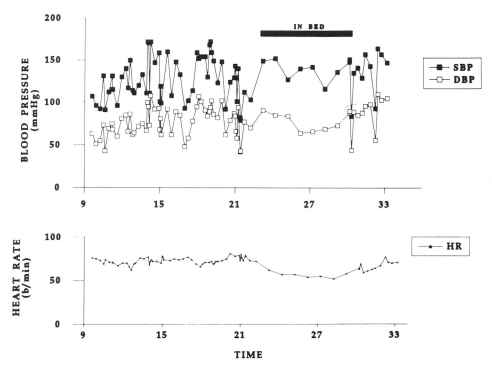

Figure 6. Blood pressure and heart rate profile in a subject with the Shy-Drager syndrome and central autonomic involvement causing both sympathetic and parasympathetic failure.

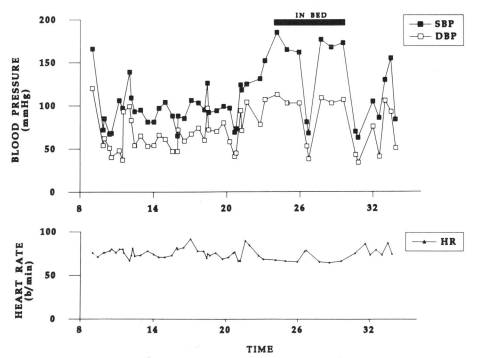

Figure 7. Blood pressure and heart rate profile in a subject with pure autonomic failure and peripheral involvement causing both sympathetic and parasympathetic failure. This subject has supine hypertension at night, while in bed. There is a marked fall in blood pressure after 26 hours (2 am), when he had to get up to micturate.

Table 3

Factors Influencing Postural Hypotension

Speed of positional change
Time of day—worse in morning
Prolonged recumbency
Warm environment (hot weather, central heating, hot bath)
Raising intrathoracic pressure—micturition, defecation or coughing
Food and alcohol ingestion
Physical exertion
Physical maneuvers and positions (bending forward, abdominal compression, leg crossing, squatting, activating calf muscle pump).*
Drugs with vasoactive properties (including dopaminergic agents)

*These maneuvers usually reduce the postural fall in blood pressure, unlike the others.

which raises blood pressure in normal subjects, can cause marked hypotension even while supine in autonomic failure.

Behavioral effects, including the presence of the doctor, are well recognized as influencing blood pressure.[4] Although this is not usually a problem in subjects with sympathetic failure, it relates to the majority of subjects with cardiovascular disease. This increases the complexity of analysis of blood pressure and heart rate, particularly over a 24-hour period. In the autonomic failure subjects, various forms of analysis have been performed, including the use of cumulative sums, which is one approach when there are marked variations in heart rate and blood pressure (Figure 8).[20]

Concluding Remarks

The study of the mechanisms responsible for circadian rhythms and their alteration in disease states is of importance for diagnosis, understanding the pathophysiological changes and in management. It is, however, a complex issue, because of the variety of both internal and external factors. The study of subjects with well-defined autonomic disorders has contributed to our understanding of such neural-cardiovascular interactions; with further work and newer investigative and analytical approaches, it is likely to help even further in understanding the basic principles behind a complex network of control.

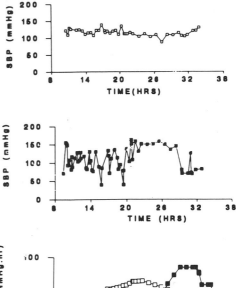

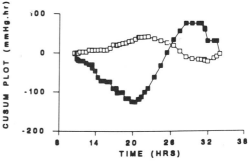

Figure 8. A: the 24-hour systolic blood pressure SBP profile of a normal subject; B: a patient with autonomic failure; C: the corresponding cumulative sums analysis (open squares: normal subject; filled square: autonomic failure). From Alam et al.[20]

Acknowledgments: We would like to acknowledge the support of the Wellcome Trust and Brain Research Trust, and the assistance of Mrs. Corinne Docherty.

References

1. Littler WA, Honour AJ, Carter RD, et al. Sleep and blood pressure. Br Med J 1975; 3:346-348.
2. Millar-Craig MW, Bishop CN, Raftery EB. Circadian variation of blood pressure. Lancet 1978; i:795-797.
3. Pickering TG. Strategies for the evaluation and treatment of hypertension and some implications of blood pressure variability. Circulation 1987; 76(suppl I):I-77-I-82.
4. Mancia G. Ambulatory blood pressure monitoring: research and clinical applications. J Hypertens 1190; 8(suppl 7):S-1-S-13.
5. Bannister R, Mathias CJ. Autonomic Failure: A Textbook of Clinical Disorders of the Autonomic System, 3rd ed. Oxford, England: Oxford Univerity Press.
6. Mathias CJ. Disorder of the autonomic nervous system. In: Bradley WG, Daroff RB, Fenchel GM, et al (eds). Neurology in Clinical Practice, Volume 2. Stoneham, Mass: Butterworths Publishers, 1991; 1661-1685.
7. Mathias CJ. Orthostatic hypotension—causes, mechanisms and influencing factors. Neurology. In press.
8. Mathias CJ, Bannister R. Investigation of autonomic disorders. In: Bannister R, Mathias CJ (eds). Autonomic Failure. A Textbook of Disorders of the Autonomic Nervous System, 3rd ed. Oxford, England: Oxford University Press, 1992; 255-290.
9. Mathias CJ, Anand P, Armstrong E, et al. A human equivalent of an experiment chronic nucleus tractus solitarious lesion. J Neurol 1990; 237(suppl 1):s54.
10. Hornung RS, Mahler RF, Raftery EB. Ambulatory blood pressure and heart rate in diabetic patients: an assessment of autonomic function. Diabetic Med 1989; 6:579-585.
11. Linger C, Favre L, Assal J.-Ph. Twenty-four hour blood pressure and heart rate profiles of diabetic patients with abnormal cardiovascular reflexes. Diabetic Med 1991; 8:420-427.
12. Mathias CJ, Bannister R. Dopamine-beta-hydroxylase deficiency and other genetically determined autonomic disorders. In: Bannister R, Mathias CJ (eds). Autonomic Failure. A Textbook of Disorders of the Autonomic Nervous System, 3rd ed. Oxford, England: Oxford University Press, 1992; 719-746.
13. Mathias CJ, Bannister R, Cortelli P, et al. Clinical autonomic and therapeutic observations in two siblings with postural hypotension and sympathetic failure due to an inability to synthesise noradrenaline from dopamine beta hydroxylase. Q J Med 1990; New Series 75; 278:617-633.
14. Polinsky RJ. Neuropharmacological investigation of autonomic failure. In: Bannister R, Mathias CJ (eds). Autonomic Failure. A Textbook of Disorders of the Autonomic Nervous System, 3rd ed. Oxford, England: Oxford University Press, 1992; 334-358.
15. Thomaides T, Chaudhuri KR, Maule S, et al. The growth hormone response to clonidine in central and peripheral primary autonomic failure. Lancet 1992; 263-266.
16. Mann S, Altman DG, Raftery EB, et al. Circadian variation of blood pressure in autonomic failure. Circulation 1983; 68:477-483.
17. Senard JM, Chamontin B, Rascol A, et al. Ambulatory blood pressure in patients with Parkinson's Disease with and without orthostatic hypotension. Clin Autonom Res 1992; 2:99-104.
18. Mathias CJ. Postprandial hypotension. Pathological mechanisms and clinical implication in different disorders. Hypertension 1991; 18:694-704.
19. Smith GDP, Bannister R, Mathias CJ. Post exercise dizziness as the sole presenting symptom in autonomic failure. Br Heart J 1993; 69:359-361.
20. Alam M, Pavitt DV, Mathias CJ. Cumulative sums analysis of 24 hour blood pressure profiles in patients with sympathetic denervation. J Hypertens 1993; 11(suppl 5):s286-287.

Part II

Measurement of Heart Rate Variability

Chapter 3

Time-Domain Measurements of Heart Rate Variability

Robert E. Kleiger, Phyllis K. Stein,
Matthew S. Bosner, Jeffrey N. Rottman

The heart is exquisitely designed to match cardiac output with the needs of the body. Thus, abrupt changes in heart rate (HR) are common and expected in response to physical or mental stress and exercise. In addition, even in the absence of external perturbations, the normal heart beat is not characterized by clockwork regularity.[1-3] Periodic changes in HR occur at a high frequency (HF) secondary to respiration (respiratory sinus arrhythmia) throughout the day and night. In addition, very slow circadian changes occur that are mediated by neural and hormonal influences[3,4] and various uncertain influences. Both the basic HR and its modulation are primarily determined by alterations in autonomic tone. Increased parasympathetic or vagal tone slows the HR, and increased sympathetic tone increases HR. It has been shown that normal aging results in a reduction of autonomic control of the heart.[5-10] Changes in HR (heart rate variability[HRV]) may be measured by a number of techniques, and since

changes in HR are autonomically mediated, these measurements reflect autonomic tone. In addition, it has been shown that information about the general health of the heart, including the propensity to malignant ventricular arrhythmias, and prognostic information about survival with various cardiac disease states may be gleaned from analysis of HRV.[11-21] Analysis of HRV using time-domain techniques will be elucidated in detail in this chapter.

Measurements Obtained from Short-Term Recordings

Variability in HR, reflecting autonomic tone, may be determined during brief periods of electrocardiographic monitoring. A number of techniques have been devised involving either manual analysis of electrocardiogram (ECG) strips or computerized analysis of digitized ECG signals.[8,12,13,16,22-26] These include the response of HR to spontaneous

From: Malik M., Camm AJ (eds.): *Heart Rate Variability.* Armonk, NY. Futura Publishing Company, Inc., © 1995.

and controlled ventilation at rates from 6 to 20 breaths per minute.[27-29] Other techniques involve assessing HR changes during tilt to an upright position,[10,30] standing to lying,[31,32] Valsalva maneuver,[33,34] in response to carotid sinus stimulation by suction cups,[35] in response to exercise,[36,37] and infusion of phenylephrine[38] or atropine.[6,39,40] Use of these techniques has demonstrated abnormalities in such diverse conditions as diabetic neuropathy,[26,28,41-50] alcoholism,[51-54] postmyocardial infarction,[25,55-59] and congestive heart failure [60-63] in humans and in animal models. The major advantage of such methods is the limited duration of electrocardiographic monitoring. Limitations include the necessity for interventions (sometimes invasive) and, in many instances, the requirement for patient cooperation, difficult to obtain in critically ill patients. Because of their limited duration, short-term recordings may fail to detect long-term trends or diurnal influences in HR that have clinical import.[17,50,64] Thus in groups of alcoholics[53] and in patients with diabetic neuropathy,[47] calculation of HR variables from 24-hour monitoring has been more sensitive in detecting abnormalities in autonomic function than short-term variables. Also the HR variables which have best predicted mortality following myocardial infarction have been those which can only be derived from longer term monitoring.[4]

Measurements Obtained from Long-Term Recordings

Long-term time-domain measurements are commonly performed utilizing 24-hour electrocardiographic recordings.[11,14,15,45,65] Holter tapes are scanned and QRS complexes identified. Artifact, ectopic beats, and normal beats are recognized and annotated. Individual cycle lengths between the QRS complexes are determined and variables describing the statistical distribution of the set of all cycle lengths (or instantaneous HRs), such as the mean and standard deviation, are calculated over the whole recording or segments of the recording.[42] Most common statistics are markedly perturbed by artifact and/or ectopic beats. For this reason most measurements of HRV attempt to exclude non-normal intervals from the analysis, ie, intervals between ectopic beats, between normal and ectopic beats, and intervals inaccurately measured because of artifact are excluded from analysis. Despite improvements in computer processing of tapes, human editing is required to detect mislabeled beats and artifacts. To reduce the degree of human overediting, a variety of approaches have been utilized to minimize erroneous calculations.[66] These include excluding from analysis intervals which are more than 20% different from preceding intervals,[15,67] and deriving bounds for the parameters of HRV which incorporate all cycles, including those with ectopic beats. The latter makes the assumption that such intervals represent an insubstantial minority of the total number of intervals, and will only marginally affect the final calculation. For most 'classic' parameters of HRV, this assumption appears to be valid only when ectopic beats are less than 10 per hour.[15] All such approaches are arbitrary to some extent, eg, the 20% rule will exclude some sinus intervals in which there are sudden large changes in sinus rate. On the other hand, calculations based on all RR intervals, while much simpler to implement, break down whenever there is an HF of ectopy as previously noted. A recent geometric approach that Malik and Camm and their group have taken is to construct a frequency plot or histogram of the measured intervals.[11,14,16,68,69] The modal frequency is determined, and using a variety of calculations, a measurement called 'baseline width,' dependent on the distribution of frequencies and excluding outliers, is calculated. Intervals outside the 'normal' ranges because of artifact (failure to detect a valid QRS or detection of artifact) or intervals including ectopics are thus potentially excluded from analysis without many 'normal-normal' intervals being excluded. Such a system may obviate or significantly reduce the need for human overediting. This approach is discussed in greater detail in Chapter 4 of this volume.

Alterations in tape speed could also potentially affect measurements of HRV. Such problems can be eliminated by using a Holter recorder that incorporates a timing signal and a scanner that recognizes and corrects for the timing signal. Most modern commercial systems have a timing track on Holter tapes.

Time-Domain Measures Based on Beat-to-Beat Intervals

Once a set of beat-to-beat intervals is obtained, a large number of variables can be measured. These are broadly divided into two classes. The first class is variables derived directly from the intervals themselves. In general, data are reported in terms of cycle lengths (in milliseconds), although heart period data can be calculated in terms of HR. Beat-to-beat interval-based variables include mean heart period (or HR) for the whole recording period, as well as standard deviation of the heart period or cycle length. If the standard deviation of heart period is reported for a 24-hour recording period, it is sometimes referred to as cycle length variability (CLV). Other terms are SDNN (standard deviation of normal-to-normal intervals) and SDRR (standard deviation of RR intervals). Standard deviations of mean cycle lengths over shorter segments of recording intervals are also commonly reported. One such variable is SDANN which is the standard deviation of the 5-minute mean cycle lengths over the entire recording. SDANN provides an index of the variability of the average of 5-minute intervals over 24 hours, but provides no information about short-term variability. Similarly, SDNNIDX, the mean of the standard deviation of 5-minute cycle intervals over the entire recording period is often measured. It provides no information about the variability due to cycle lengths over 5 minutes, but estimates the variability due to cycle lengths less than 5 minutes. Another interbeat interval-based measure is the difference in mean day versus night rates as heart periods.[56] Finally, because higher HRs are associated with decreased HRV, a coefficient of variance is sometimes calculated. This parameter is SDNN divided by the mean N-N interval. Its purpose is to detect changes in overall variability independent of changes in mean N-N interval. However, this variable is strongly correlated with SDNN and usually adds little additional information.

Time-Domain Measures Based on the Difference Between Adjacent Cycle Lengths

The second class of variables is based on the differences between adjacent cycles.[45,70] These measurements include rMSSD (the root mean square successive differences where each difference is squared, summed, the result averaged and then the square root obtained),[71-73] and the proportion or number of differences between adjacent cycles that exceed an arbitrary limit.[45,56] Variables which reflect the proportion of differences include pNN50 (the proportion of cycles where the difference is >50 milliseconds) and pNN6.25% (the proportion of cycles where the difference is >6.25% of the mean heart period). The number of instances where the difference between adjacent N-N intervals exceeds an arbitrary limit (eg, 50 milliseconds) is reported as 'counts.' Such measurements reflect, in essence, very short-term HRV measured over a much longer period of time. As such, these variables are virtually independent of diurnal or other long-term trends [71,73] and reflect, almost wholly, alterations in autonomic tone that are predominantly vagally mediated. It must be noted that SDNNIDX, the average of the 5-minute standard deviations, could be considered an 'intermediate' measure, reflecting both very short-term and somewhat longer term (up to 5-minute) variability.

Table 1 lists some of the time-domain measures which have been reported. The

Table 1
Definitions for Time Domain Measures of Heart Period Variability

Variable	Domain	Units	Definition
Night/day difference	time	msec	Difference between the average of all the normal RR intervals at night and the average of all the normal RR intervals during the day
CLV	time	msec	Standard deviation of all normal RR intervals in the entire 24-hr ECG recording (Also referred to as SDRR or SDNN)
SDANN	time	msec	Standard deviation of the mean of normal RR intervals for each 5 min period of the 24 hr ECG recording
SDNNIDX	time	msec	Mean of the standard deviations of all normal RR intervals for all 5 min segments of a 24-hr ECG recording
pNN50	time	%	Percent of difference between adjacent normal RR intervals that are greater than 50 msec. computed over the entire 24-hr ECG recording
r-MSSD	time	msec	Root mean square successive difference, the square root of the mean of the sum of the squares of differences between adjacent normal RR intervals over the entire 24-hr ECG recording
SDSD	time	msec	The standard deviation of successive differences between adjoining normal cycles
Counts	time	beats	The number of time that the difference between adjacent normal RR intervals is greater than 50 msec, computer over the entire 24 hr recording

list is not all-inclusive since many other time-domain measures have been used. In addition, there is still little uniformity in naming many of these variables.

Correlations Among the Time-Domain Variables

The previously cited time-domain variables are all positively correlated with each other, but the strength of correlation varies greatly. Table 2 shows the correlations obtained for some of these variables in 14 recordings obtained from normal subjects receiving placebo medication. As might be expected, SDNN and SDANN (not shown) are highly correlated. The variables calculated from the differences between adjacent cycles such as rMSSD, PNN50, and counts have correlations well above 0.9 and may be considered surrogates for each other[55,72]; these variables strongly reflect vagal tone.

Bigger et al[55] showed that pNN50 and rMSSD in patients with low CLV <50 milliseconds and high CLV >100 milliseconds following myocardial infarction had correlations greater than 0.9. In subsequent studies in normal subjects, the strong positive correlation of rMSSD and pNN50 was confirmed.[72] The more broadly based time-domain measures such as CLV, or baseline width, have weaker correlations with the 'short-term' time-domain variables since they are primarily influenced by diurnal and secular trends and short-term sympathetic influences, and less by vagal tone. In general, the weakest correlations are found between night/day difference and the other variables.

As a result of the strong correlation between time-domain variables, alterations in basal state by either disease, pharmacological, or physiological interventions, will usually alter time-domain variables in the same

Table 2
Correlations for 14 Placebo Records

	r-MSSD	pNN50	SDNN	NDDiff	RR	RR.N	RR.D	SDNNIDX
pNN50	0.96							
24-Hour standard deviation of NN intervals (msec) (CLV)	0.78	0.71						
Night/day difference	0.52	0.36	0.78					
Average NN interval for 24-hours (msec)	0.84	0.89	0.80	0.40				
Average nighttime NN interval (msec)	0.87	0.84	0.92	0.72	0.92			
Average daytime NN interval (msec)	0.76	0.88	0.66	0.19	0.97	0.82		
Mean of standard deviation of 5-min. NN intervals over 24 hours (SDNN Index)	0.97	0.94	0.85	0.53	0.89	0.91	0.85	
Total power	0.94	0.92	0.87	0.57	0.86	0.90	0.85	1.0
Low frequency power	0.91	0.81	0.85	0.71	0.72	0.86	0.63	0.92
High frequency power	0.98	0.92	0.68	0.45	0.74	0.77	0.71	0.90

Table 3
Correlations for 14 Placebo Records (continued)

	Total Power	Low Frequency Power
Low frequency power	0.93	
High frequency power	0.88	0.89

CLV = cycle length variability, NDDDiff = Night/day differences, NN = normal cycle interval, pNN50 = percent of difference between adjacent normal cycle intervals >50 ms computed over the entire 24-hour electrocardiogram recording, r-MSSD = root mean square successive difference
*From Kleiger RE, Bigger JT, Bosner MS, et al: Stability over time of variables measuring heart rate variability in normal subjects. Am J Cardiol 68:626, 1991; with permission.

direction. However, it is possible to alter some without affecting all. For example, in a population of normals, atenolol markedly increased rMSSD and pNN50 without any significant effect on CLV.[74] This occurred because CLV is dependent not only on vagally mediated short-term effects on HR (predominantly sinus arrhythmia) but also on the differences between night and day time HRs, and between maximal and minimal HR. While both night/day and maximum/minimum HR differences are markedly reduced by β-blockers, this change is balanced by the increase in short-term variability produced by β-blocker.

Relationship Between Frequency-Domain and Time-Domain Measures

Theoretically heart period *variance*, a time-domain measure equal to (SDNN),[2] and *total power*, a frequency-domain measure, are mathematically identical. However, 'total power' has often been used as a synonym for combined HF and low-frequency (LF) power, reflecting only a portion of the total spectrum. Also, earlier investigations by Bigger, Kleiger et al estimated total power over 24 hours by calculating the total power of successive 5-minute periods.[55,72] This method does not account for variance associated with cycle lengths between 5 minutes and 24 hours. The variance associated with cycle lengths over 5 minutes includes diurnal cycles which are a major determinant of 24-hour variability. Thus, the mathematical relationship between $(SDNN)^2$ and total power may not always hold in published data. This may produce seemingly paradoxical results. For example, in the previously cited study of the effect of atenolol on HRV in normals,[74] atenolol was shown to markedly increase 'total power' but not affect SDNN. Total power, in this case, was determined from 5-minute segments, and since the variance at cycle lengths less than 5 minutes increased with atenolol, 'total power' appeared to increase. However, as previously mentioned, diurnal variation (measured at cycle lengths greater than 5 minutes) was significantly reduced. With the exception of circumstances like that observed with atenolol, total power estimated from 5-minute segments and SDNN should be closely correlated.

In practice, few studies have examined the relationship between time- and frequency-domain variables measuring HRV.[19,55] Kleiger et al[72] showed that pNN50 and rMSSD had very strong (>0.85) positive correlations with HF power, a measurement of variance in the range of frequencies associated with breathing (0.15 to 0.40 Hz or 9 to 24 cycles per minute). Since the majority of short-term variance in HR is mediated by respiratory sinus arrhythmia, this close relationship is not surprising. Another frequency-domain variable, very low-frequency (VLF) power represents variance in the 0.04 to 0.0033 Hz range (25 seconds to 5 minutes). SDNNIDX correlates strongly with VLF power. This is because of the 18% of total power found in cycle lengths under 5 minutes; on average, VLF power accounts for 12%, LF power (0.04 to 0.15 Hz) accounts for 4%, and HF power for 2%.[75] Thus, the majority of 5-minute variance (measured by SDNNIDX) is accounted for by VLF power. This has been found to be the case in both postinfarct and normal subjects. Moreover, since SDNNIDX is the average of the 5-mi-

nute SDNNs, and total power calculated over 5-minute intervals is the average of total powers (ie, variance) for all of the 5-minute segments, SDNNIDX and 5-minute total power should be perfectly correlated. Indeed, Kleiger et al[72] found a correlation of 1.0 between these variables in 14 normals. The authors concluded that certain time-domain variables may serve as surrogates for the more difficult to measure frequency-domain variables, particularly r-MSSD and pNN50 for HF power (see Table 2). Moreover, it is clear that SDNN is a surrogate for total power and that SDNNIDX is a surrogate for VLF power.

Stability of Time-Domain Measurements

There have been few studies in which repeat measures of HRV have been performed over time. Studies of spectral measures, as well as baroreceptor sensitivity, have been performed in patients and in experimental animal models which document a decrease in HRV at the time of myocardial infarction with subsequent recovery following infarction.[57] A number of studies have addressed the influence of drugs on measures of HRV, but there is a paucity of data on the reproducibility of HRV measures on repeated measurements. This is analogous to the problem of interpreting changes in ectopic frequency or the number of ischemic episodes on recording which show marked change variation from recordings to recording.[76,77] A study from Washington University and Columbia College of Physicians and Surgeons examined 14 normal patients with repeat monitoring, one recording at baseline, and one on placebo medication.[72] The intervals between recordings ranged from 3 to 65 days. Various time-domain measures were determined including CLV, rMSSD, pNN50, SDNNIDX, mean RR interval, and mean difference between night and day RR interval. The authors calculated the mean and standard deviations for these measures and the intraclass correlation coefficient, a measure of individual variability. They showed that the group means and standard deviations for the variables were virtually identical for the baseline and placebo recordings. Moreover, for some of the time-domain variables such as pNN50 and rMSSD, the intraclass correlations exceeded 0.9, demonstrating not only group stability but individual stability in measurement. They concluded that the stability of these variables over time, the lack of placebo effect, and the limited individual variability in their measurement made them suitable variables for the study of interventions on autonomic tone. This study was replicated in 17 stable patients with Class II and III congestive heart failure (CHF).[78] HRV was measured at baseline and 2 weeks later. Time-domain indices of HRV were stable (no significant mean differences, r>0.86) for mean heart period, SDNN, SDANN and SDNNIDX. However, because distributions of values for pNN50 and rMSSD were skewed towards low values, these data were log transformed. Transformation resulted in correlation coefficients of 0.85 for ln pNN50 and 0.67 for ln rMSSD. Thus, these variables are also suitable for studying patients with CHF, although in the case of time-domain indices of vagal tone, care must be taken to account for low values.

Drugs and Heart Rate Variability

A variety of cardioactive drugs have been investigated for effects on HRV. These include antihypertensive agents,[23,35,79-82] cardiac glycosides,[23,62,83] antiarrhythmics,[84,85] anticholinergics such as atropine[86] and scopolamine,[87,88,125] calcium channel blockers,[74] and β-blockers.[74,89] It is clear from these studies that many cardioactive agents of diverse classes have profound effects on autonomic tone, and that the direction and magnitude of these effects can be estimated by time-domain measures of HRV. The clinical significance of these findings is, as of yet, not fully known but warrants further study. The

effects of drugs on HRV are discussed at length in Chapter 22 of this volume.

Indices of Heart Rate Variability and Sudden Death and Malignant Ventricular Arrhythmias

As mentioned at the beginning of this chapter, decreased HRV is a powerful risk stratifier for overall mortality,[15,45] induced and spontaneous ventricular tachycardia, and sudden death following myocardial infarction.[3,19,84,90-92,124,127] Decreased HRV has also been found in the same ambulatory ECGs as ventricular fibrillation in recordings from patients demonstrating this rhythm.[18] HRV is significantly decreased in patients with inducible ventricular tachycardia compared to age-matched controls with frequent ectopic ventricular beats. These findings are compatible with a number of experimental studies showing that decreased parasympathetic and increased sympathetic tone decreased ventricular fibrillation threshold and increased spontaneous ventricular tachycardia in ischemic animal models and in humans.[93-99] Alterations in autonomic tone in these animal models could be measured by various techniques including measurements of baroreceptor sensitivity,[74,100,101] or by HRV measures using time-domain parameters such as standard deviations of cycle intervals. This topic will be covered at length in Chapters 32 and 33 of this volume.

Predictive Value of Time-Domain Variables in Heart Disease

The data from post-MI studies clearly demonstrate that decreased indices of HRV such as CLV[15] baseline width,[45] or baroreceptor sensitivity are associated with increased mortality and increased arrhythmic death following infarction. This topic will be covered in great detail in Chapters 25 to 29 and 31 of this volume. Although most studies of HRV in cardiac disease concern patients who are postinfarction, a number of other conditions have been studied including coronary artery disease,[102] hypertension,[103-106] congestive heart failure,[60,61] cardiomyopathy, posttransplant patients[107] and others.[108,109] Details of these studies are reported in other parts of this volume.

Heart Rate Variability in Noncardiac Diseases

Measurement of time-domain indices of HRV has been used to assess autonomic function in patients with many noncardiac conditions including: neurological disorders such as stroke, multiple sclerosis[110,111,128] and myotonia, in diabetes, alcoholism,[51,52] at-risk neonates,[129] cancer,[112,113] glaucoma,[114] and others.[115-118] Most studies have relied on short-term assessment techniques, eg, baroreceptor sensitivity, measuring respiratory sinus arrhythmia by controlled ventilation, and responses to tilt. Several studies have utilized long-term ambulatory electrocardiographic monitoring to assess autonomic tone. Ewing et al,[42] investigating patients with diabetes, showed that a decrease in the number of successive cycle differences greater than 50 milliseconds was a more sensitive indicator of autonomic dysfunction than conventional tests for autonomic dysfunction. Likewise, Malpas et al[47] showed that rMSSD was more sensitive than traditional tests in detecting abnormalities in these patients. Malpas et al[53] also reported similar findings in chronic alcoholics. Further information about HRV in noncardiac diseases will be found in Chapter 37. Interestingly, as discussed in Chapter 38 of this book, a large body of evidence demonstrates that prognosis for fetal and neonate survival can be predicted by HRV with an adverse effect seen with low variability.[24,119-123] Many of the conditions noted above are characterized by a high incidence of sudden death. It seems probable, based on experimental data, that the decreased parasympathetic and increased sympathetic tone implicit in a decrease in HRV predisposes to malignant ventricular arrhythmias.

Summary

Measurement of time-domain variables is a simple and practical tool to assess autonomic function. Their utility has been demonstrated in a diverse number of both cardiac and noncardiac pathological states as well as in normal subjects. Time-domain variables can be used to assess the autonomic effects of drugs and other interventions including exercise and psychological and physical stress. It has been shown to be useful in assessing risk following myocardial infarction and in other disease states. Time-domain indices of HRV are and will remain an active field of research.

Acknowledgments: The authors gratefully acknowledge Marge Leaders for expert secretarial assistance, and Jill Griffin for editorial assistance.

References

1. Appel ML, Berger RD, Saul JP, et al. Beat to beat variability in cardiovascular variables: noise or music? J Am Coll Cardiol 1989; 14:1139-1148.
2. Denton TA, Diamond GA, Helfant RH, et al. Fascinating rhythm: a primer on chaos theory and its application to cardiology. Am Heart J 1990; 120:1419-1440.
3. Molgaard H, Sorensen KE, Bjerregaard P. Circadian variation and influence of risk factors on heart rate variability in healthy subjects. Am J Cardiol 1991; 68:777-784.
4. Bigger JT, Fleiss J, Steinman RC, et al. Frequency domain measures of heart period variability and mortality after myocardial infarction. Circulation 1992; 85:164-71.
5. Chipps DR, Kraegen EW, Zelenka GS, et al. Cardiac beat to beat variation: age related changes in the normal population andabnormalities in diabetics. Aust N Z J Med 1981; 11:614-629.
6. Gautschy B, Weidmann P, Gnädinger MP. Autonomic function tests as late; red to age and gender in normal man. Klin Wochenschrift 1986; 64:499-505.

7. Gribbin B, Pickering TG, Sleight P, et al. The effect of age and high blood pressure on baroreflex sensitivity in man. Circ Res 1971; 29:424.

8. O'Brien IA, O'Hare P, Corrall RJM. Heart rate variability in healthy subjects: effect of age and the derivation of normal ranges for tests of autonomic function. Br Heart J 1986; 55:348-354.

9. Pfeifer MA, Weinberg CR, Cook D, et al. Differential changes of autonomic nervous system function with age in man. Am J Med 1983; 75:249-258.

10. Waddington JL, MacCulloch MJ, Sambrooks JE. Resting heart rate variability in man declines with age. Experientia 1979; 35:1197-1198.

11. Cripps TR, Malik M, Farrell TS, et al. Prognostic value of reduced heart rate variability after myocardial infarction: clinical evaluation of a new analysis method. Br Heart J 1991; 65:14-19.

12. Eckberg DW. Parasympathetic cardiovascular control in human disease: a critical review of methods and results. Am J Physiol 1980; 239:H581-H593.

13. Ewing DJ. Heart rate variability: an important new risk factor in patients following myocardial infarction. Clin Cardiol 1991; 14:683-685.

14. Farrell TG, Bashir Y, Cripps T, et al. Risk stratification for arrhythmic events in postinfarction patients based on heart rate variability, ambulatory electrocardiographic variables and the signal-averaged electrocardiogram. J Am Coll Cardiol 1991; 18:687-697.

15. Kleiger RE, Miller JP, Bigger JT, et al. Decreased heart rate variability and its association with increased mortality after acute myocardial infarction. Am J Cardiol 1987; 59:256-262.

16. Malik M, Camm J. Heart rate variability. Clin Cardiol 1990; 13:570-576.

17. Malik M, Farrell T, Camm AJ. Circadian rhythm of heart rate variability after acute myocardial infarction and its influence on the prognostic value of heart rate variability. Am J Cardiol 1990; 66:1049-1054.

18. Martin GJ, Magid NM, Myers G, et al. Heart rate variability and sudden death secondary to coronary artery disease during ambulatory electrocardiographic monitoring. Am J Cardiol 1987; 60:86-89.

19. Myers GA, Martin GJ, Magid NM, et al. Power spectral analysis of heart rate variability in sudden cardiac death: comparison to other methods. IEEE Trans Biomed Eng 1986; 33:1149-1156.

20. Odemuyiwa O, Malik M, Farrell T, et al. Comparison of the predictive characteristics of heart rate variability index and left ventricular ejection fraction for all-cause mortality, arrhythmic events and sudden death after acute myocardial infarction. Am J Cardiol 1991; 68:434-439.

21. Pipilis A, Flather M, Ormerod O, et al. Heart rate variability in acute myocardial infarction and its association with infarct site and clinical course. Am J Cardiol 1991; 67:1137-1139.

22. Gunderson HJC, Neubauer B. A long term diabetic autonomic nervous abnormality. Reduced variations in resting heart rate measured by a simple and sensitive method. Diabetologia 1977; 13:137-140.

23. Katona PG, Jih F. Respiratory sinus arrhythmia: noninvasive measure of parasympathetic cardiac control. J Appl Physiol 1975; 39:801-805.

24. Parer WJ, Parer JT, Holbrook RH, et al. Validity of mathematical methods of quantifying fetal heart rate variability. Am J Obstet Gynecol 1985; 153:402-409.

25. Persson A, Solders G. R-R variations, a test of autonomic dysfunction. Acta Neurol Scand 1983; 67:285-293.

26. Pfeifer MA, Cook D, Brodsky J, et al. Quantitative evaluation of cardiac parasympathetic activity in normal and diabetic man. Diabetes 1982; 31:39-345.

27. Eckberg DL. Human sinus arrhythmia as an index of vagal cardiac outflow. J Appl Physiol 1983; 54(4):961-966.

28. Ewing DJ, Borsey DQ, Bellavere F, et al. Cardiac autonomic neuropathy in diabetes: comparison of measures of R-R interval variation. Diabetologia 1981; 21:18-24.

29. Grossman P, Van Beek J, Wientjes C. A comparison of three quantification methods for estimation of respiratory sinus arrhythmia. Psychophysiology 1990; 27:702-714.

30. Levine TB, Francis GS, Goldsmith SR, et al. The neurohumoral and hemodynamic response to orthostatic tilt in patients with congestive heart failure. Circulation 1983; 67:1070-1075.

31. Bellavere F, Cardone C, Ferri M, et al. Standing to lying heart rate variation. A new simple test in the diagnosis of diabetic autonomic neuropathy. Diabet Med 1987; 4(1):41-43.

32. Ewing DJ, Hume L, Campbell IW, et al. Autonomic mechanisms in the initial heart rate response to standing. J Appl Physiol 1980; 49:809-814.

33. Bennett T, Farquhar IK, Hosking DJ, et al. Assessment of methods for estimating autonomic nervous control of the heart in pa-

tients with diabetes mellitus. Diabetes 1978; 27:1167-1174.

34. Levin AB. A simple test of cardiac function based upon heart rate changes induced by the Valsalva manoeuvre. Am J Cardiol 1966; 18:90-99.

35. Ebert TJ. Captopril potentiates chronotropic baroreceptor responses to carotid stimuli in humans. Hypertension 1985; 7:602-606.

36. Billman GE, Dujardin JP. Dynamic changes in cardiac vagal tone as measured by time-series analysis. Am J Physiol 1990; 258:H896-H902.

37. Jennett S, Lamb JF, Travis P. Sudden large and periodic changes in heart rate in healthy young men after short periods of exercise. BMJ 1982; 285:1154-1156.

38. Bigger JT, LaRovere MT, Steinman RC, et al. Comparison of baroreflex sensitivity and heart period variability after myocardial infarction. J Am Coll Cardiol 1989; 14:1511-1518.

39. Fouad FM, Tarazi RC, Ferrario CM, et al. Assessment of parasympathetic control of heart rate by a noninvasive method. Am J Physiol 1984; 246:H838-842.

40. Hayano J, Sakakibara Y, Yamada A, et al. Accuracy of assessment of cardiac vagal tone by heart rate variability in normal subjects. Am J Cardiol 1991; 67:199-204.

41. Ewing DJ. Practical bedside investigation of diabetic autonomic failure. In: Bannister R (ed). Autonomic Failure. Oxford, England: Oxford University Press, 1983; 371.

42. Ewing DJ, Borsey DQ, Travis P, et al. Abnormalities of ambulatory 24-hour heart rate in diabetes mellitus. Diabetes 1983; 32:101-105.

43. Ewing DJ, Campbell IW, Clarke BF. The natural history of diabetic autonomic neuropathy. Q J Med 1980; 49:95-108.

44. Ewing DJ, Martyn CN, Young RJ, et al. The value of cardiovascular autonomic function tests: ten years experience in diabetes. Diabetes Care 1985; 8:491-498.

45. Ewing DJ, Neilson JMM, Travis P. New method for assessing cardiac parasympathetic activity using 24 hour electrocardiograms. Br Heart J 1984; 52:396-402.

46. Kitney RI, Byrne S, Edmonds ME, et al: Heart rate variability in the assessment of autonomic diabetic neuropathy. Automedica 1982; 4:155.

47. Malpas SC, Maling TJB. Heart-rate variability and cardiac autonomic function in diabetes. Diabetes 1990; 39:1177-1181.

48. Masaoka S, Lev-Ran A, Hill LR, et al. Heart rate variability in diabetes: relationship to age and duration of the disease. Diabetes Care 1985; 8:64-68.

49. Murray A, Ewing DJ, Campbell IW, et al. RR interval variations in young male diabetics. Br Heart J 1975; 37:882.

50. Rothschild AH, Weinberg CR, Halter JB, et al. Sensitivity of RR variation and Valsalva ratio in assessment of cardiovascular diabetic autonomic neuropathy. Diabetes Care 1987; 10:735-741.

51. Duncan G, Lambie DG, Johnson RH, et al. Evidence of vagal neuropathy in chronic alcoholics. Lancet 1980; 2:1053-1057.

52. Johnson RH, Robinson BJ. Mortality in alcoholics with autonomic neuropathy. J Neurol Neurosurg Psychiatry 1988; 51:476-481.

53. Malpas SC, Whiteside EA, Maling TJB. Heart rate variability and cardiac autonomic function in men with chronic alcohol dependence. Br Heart J 1991; 65:84-88.

54. Zuanetti G, Latini R, Nielson JMM, et al. Heart rate variability in patients with ventricular arrhythmias: effect of antiarrhythmic drugs. J Am Coll Cardiol 1991; 17:604-612.

55. Bigger JT, Albrecht P, Steinman RC, et al. Comparison of time- and frequency-domain based measures of cardiac parasympathetic activity in Holter recordings after myocardial infarction. Am J Cardiol 1989; 64:536-538.

56. Bigger JT, Kleiger RE, Fleiss JL, et al. Components of heart rate variability measured during healing of acute myocardial infarction. Am J Cardiol 1988; 61:208-215.

57. Lombardi F, Sandrone G, Pernproner S, et al. Heart rate variability as an index of sympathovagal interaction in patients after myocardial infarction. Am J Cardiol 1987; 60:1239-1245.

58. Rothschild M, Rothschild A, Pfeifer M. Temporary decrease in cardiac parasympathetic tone after acute myocardial infarction. Am J Cardiol 1988; 62:637-639.

59. Ryan C, Hollenberg M, Harvey D, et al. Impaired parasympathetic responses in patients after myocardial infarction. Am J Cardiol 1976; 37:1013-1018.

60. Casolo G, Balli E, Taddei T, et al. Decreased spontaneous heart rate variability in congestive heart failure. Am J Cardiol 1989; 64:1162-1167.

61. Eckberg DL, Drabinsky M, Braunwald E. Defective cardiac parasympathetic control in patients with heart disease. N Engl J Med 1971; 285:877-883.

62. Ferguson DW, Berg WJ, Sanders JS, et al. Sympatho-inhibitory responses to digitalis glycosides in heart failure patients. Circulation 1989; 80:65-77.

63. Lombardi F, Gnocchi-Ruscone T, Montano N, et al. Restraining effect of captopril on

cardiovascular sympathetic efferent neural activity. J Hypertens 1989; 7(suppl):S55-56.

64. Malik M, Farrell TG, Camm AJ. Evaluation of receiver operator characteristics. Optimal time of day for the assessment of heart rate variability after acute myocardial infarction. Int J Biomed Comput 1991; 27:175-192.

65. Saul JP, Albrecht P, Berger RD, et al. Analysis of long term heart rate variability: methods, 1/f scaling and implications. Comput Cardiol 1988; 419-422.

66. Bernston GG, Quigley KS, Jang JF, et al. An approach to artifact identification: application to heart period data. Psychophysiology 1990; 27:586-598.

67. Kleiger RE, Miller JP, Krone RJ, et al. The independence of cycle length variability and exercise testing on predicting mortality of patients surviving acute myocardial infarction. Am J Cardiol 1990; 65:408-411.

68. Malik M, Cripps T, Farrell T, et al. Prognostic value of heart rate variability after myocardial infarction: a comparison of different data-processing methods. Med Biol Eng Comput 1989; 27:603-611.

69. Malik M, Farrell T, Cripps TR, et al. Heart rate variability in relation to prognosis after myocardial infarction: selection of optimal processing techniques. Eur Heart J 1989; 10:1060-1074.

70. McEwen TA, Sima AAF. Autonomic neuropathy in BB rat. Assessment by improved method for measuring heart-rate variability. Diabetes 1987; 36:251-255.

71. Heslegrave RJ, Ogilvie JC, Furedy JJ. Measuring baseline-treatment differences in heart rate variability: variance versus successive difference mean square and beats per minute versus interbeat intervals. Psychophysiology 1979; 16:151-157.

72. Kleiger RE, Bigger JT, Bosner MS, et al: Stability over time of variables measuring heart rate variability in normal subjects. Am J Cardiol 1991; 68:626-630.

73. Von Neumann J, Kent RH, Bellinson HR, et al. The mean square successive difference. Ann Math Stat 1941; 12:153-162.

74. Cook JR, Bigger JT, Kleiger RE, et al. Effect of atenolol and diltiazem on heart rate variability in normal persons. J Am Coll Cardiol 1991; 17:480-484.

75. Bigger JT, Fleiss LJ, Steinman RC, et al. Correlations among time and frequency domain measures of heart period variability two weeks after acute myocardial infarction. Am J Cardiol 1992; 69:891-898.

76. Deanfield JE. Holter monitoring in assessment of angina pectoris. Am J Cardiol 1987; 59:18C-22C.

77. Morganroth J, Michelson EL, Horowitz LN, et al. Limitations of routine long-term electrocardiographic monitoring to assess ventricular ectopic frequency. Circulation 1978; 58:408-414.

78. Stein PK, Rich MW, Rottman JN, et al. Stability of heart rate variability in stable patients with congestive heart failure. PACE 1994; April. Abstract.

79. jayi AA, Campbell BC, Howie CA, et al. Acute and chronic effects of the converting enzyme inhibitors enalapril and lisinopril on reflex control of heart rate in normotensive man. J Hypertens 1983; 53:47.

80. Campbell BC, Sturani A, Reid JL. Evidence of parasympathetic activity of the angiotensin converting enzyme inhibitor, captopril in normotensive man. Clin Sci 1985; 68:49-56.

81. Giudicelli JF, Berdeaux A, Edouard A, et al. The effect of enalapril on baroreceptor mediated reflex function in normotensive subjects. Br J Clin Pharmacol 1985; 20:211-218.

82. Raman GV, Waller DG, Warren DJ. The effect of captopril on autonomic reflexes in human hypertension. J Hypertens 1985; 2(suppl):S111-115.

83. Quest JA, Gillis RA. Effect of digitalis on carotid sinus baroreceptor activity. Circ Res 1974; 35:247. Abstract.

84. Singer DH, Martin GL, Magid N, et al. Low heart rate variability and sudden cardiac death. J Electrocardiol 1988; 21:S46-55.

85. Stein PK, Conger BM, Kleiger RE. The effect of pindolol and labetalol on heart rate variability in normal subjects. JACC 1993; 21:286A. Abstract.

86. Siemens P, Hiller HH, Frowein RA. Heart rate variability and the reaction of heart rate to atropine in brain death patients. Neurosurg Rev 1989; 12:282-284.

87. Dibner-Dunlap ME, Eckberg DL, Magin NM. Transcutaneous scopolamine: a potential defense against sudden cardiac death. J Clin Invest 1984; 32:473A. Abstract.

88. Vybiral T, Bryg RJ, Maddens ME, et al. Effects of transdermal scopolamine on heart rate variability in normal subjects. Am J Cardiol 1990; 65:604-608.

89. Stein PK, Bosner MS, Kuru T, et al. The effect of moricizine on heart rate variability in normal subjects. J Ambulatory Monitoring 1992; 5(suppl):17. Abstract.

90. Magid NM, Martin GJ, Kehoe RF, et al. Diminished heart rate variability in sudden cardiac death. Circulation 1985; 72:III-241. Abstract.

91. Schwartz PJ, Stone HL. The analysis and modulation of autonomic reflexes in the

prediction and prevention of sudden death. In: Zipes DP, Jalife J (eds). Cardiac Electrophysiology and Arrhythmias. Orlando, Fla: Grune & Stratton, 1985; 167.

92. Schwartz PJ, Stone HL. The role of the autonomic nervous system in sudden coronary death. Ann NY Acad Sci 1982; 382:162-180.

93. Billman GE, Hoskins RS. Time-series analysis of heart rate variability during submaximal exercise. Evidence for reduced cardiac vagal tone in animals susceptible to ventricular fibrillation. Circulation 1986; 80:146-157.

94. Corr PB, Yamada KA, Witkowski FX. Mechanisms controlling cardiac autonomic function and their relation to arrhythmogenesis. In: Fozzard HA, Haber E, Jenning RB, et al (eds). The Heart and Cardiovascular System. New York, NY: Raven Press, 1986; 1343.

95. Hull SS Jr, Evans AR, Vanoli E, et al. Heart rate variability before and after myocardial infarction in conscious dogs at high and low risk of sudden death. J Am Coll Cardiol 1990; 16:978-985.

96. Lown B. Sudden cardiac death: the major challenge confronting contemporary cardiology. Am J Cardiol 1979; 43:313-328.

97. Myers RW, Pearlman AS, Hyman RM, et al. Beneficial effects of vagal stimulation and bradycardia during experimental acute myocardial ischemia. Circulation 1974; 49:943. Abstract.

98. Schwartz PJ, Brown AM, Malliani A, et al. Neural Mechanisms in Cardiac Arrhythmias. New York, NY: Raven Press, 1978; 75.

99. Sharma AD, Corr PB. Adrenergic factors in arrhythmogenesis in the ischemic and reperfused myocardium. Eur Heart J 4(suppl D):D79-90.

100. Higgins CB, Vatner SF, Eckberg DL, et al. Alterations in the baroreceptor reflex in conscious dogs with heart failure. J Clin Invest 1972; 251:715-724.

101. Schwartz PJ, Vanoli E, Stramba-Badiale M, et al. Autonomic mechanisms and sudden death. New insights from analysis of baroreceptor reflexes in conscious dogs with and without a myocardial infarction. Circulation 1988; 78:969-979.

102. Tibblin G, Eriksson CG, Bjuro T, et al. Heart rate and heart rate variability a risk factor for the development of ischaemic heart disease (IHD) in the 'men born in 1913 study'—a ten year follow-up. IRCS Medical Science: Cardiovascular System. Soc Occupational Med 1975; 3:95.

103. Conway J, Boon N, Davies C, et al. Neural and humoral mechanisms involved in blood pressure variability. J Hypertens 1984; 2:203-208.

104. Furlan R, Guzzetti S, Crivellaro W, et al. Continuous 24-hour assessment of the neural regulation of systemic arterial pressure and RR variabilities in ambulant subjects. Circulation 1990; 81:537-547.

105. Mancia G, Parati G, Pomidossi G, et al. Arterial baroreflexes and blood pressure and heart rate variables in humans. Hypertension 1986; 8:147-153.

106. Pagani M, Furlan R, Dell'Orto S, et al. Simultaneous analysis of beat by beat systemic arterial pressure and heart rate variabilities in ambulatory patients. J Hypertens 1985; 3:S83-85.

107. Bernardi L, Keller F, Sanders M, et al. Respiratory sinus arrhythmia in the denervated human heart. J Appl Physiol 1989; 67:1447-1455.

108. Guzetti S, Iosa D, Pecis M, et al. Effects of sympathetic activation on heart rate variability in Chagas' patients. J Auton Nerv Syst 1990; 30(suppl):S79-81.

109. Guzzetti S, Iosa D, Pecis M, et al. Impaired heart rate variability in patients with chronic Chagas' disease. Am Heart J 1991; 121:1727-1734.

110. Neubauer B, Gundersen JG. Analysis of heart rate variations in patients with multiple sclerosis. A simple measure of autonomic nervous disturbances using an ordinary ECG. J Neurol Neurosurg Psychiatry 1978; 41:417-419.

111. Pentland B, Ewing DJ. Cardiovascular reflexes in multiple sclerosis. Eur Neurol 1987; 26:46-50.

112. Bruera E, Chadwick S, Fox R, et al. Study of cardiovascular autonomic insufficiency in advanced cancer patients. Cancer Treat Rep 1986; 70:1383-1387.

113. Gould GA, Ashworth M, Lewis FTR. Are cardiovascular reflexes more commonly impaired in patients with bronchial carcinoma? Thorax 1986; 41:372-375.

114. Clark CV, Mapstone R. Autonomic neuropathy in ocular hypertension. Lancet 1985; 2:185-187.

115. Forsström J, Forsström J, Heinonen E, et al. Effects of haemodialysis on heart rate variability in chronic renal failure. Scand J Clin Lab Invest 1986; 46:665-670.

116. Marin Neto JA, Marciel BC, Gallo L, et al. Effect of parasympathetic impairment of the haemodynamic response to handgrip in Chagas' heart disease. Br Heart J 1986; 55:204-210.

117. Niklasson U, Olofsson BO, Bjerle P. Autonomic neuropathy in familial amyloidotic polyneuropathy. A clinical study based on

heart rate variability. Acta Neurol Scand 1989; 79:182-187.

118. Sachs C, Conrad S, Kaijser L. Autonomic function in amyotrophic lateral sclerosis: a study of cardiovascular responses. Acta Neurol Scand 1985; 71:373-387.

119. Gaziano EP, Freeman DW. Analysis of heart rate patterns preceding fetal death. Obstet Gynecol 1977; 50:578-582.

120. Mazza NM, Epstein MAF, Haddad CG, et al. Relation of beat-to-beat variability to heart rate in normal sleeping infants. Pediatr Res 1980; 14:232-235.

121. Modanlou HD, Freeman RK, Braly P. A simple method of fetal and neonatal heart rate beat-to-beat variability quantification. Am J Obstet Gynecol 1977; 127:861-868.

122. Schechtman VL, Harper RM, Kluge KA, et al. Heart rate variation in normal infants and victims of the sudden infant death syndrome. Early Hum Dev 1989; 19:167-181.

123. Valimaki IA, Nieminen T, Antila KJ, et al. Heart rate variability and SIDS. Examination of heart rate patterns using an expert system generator. Ann NY Acad Sci 1988; 533:228-237.

124. Billman GE, Schwartz PJ, Stone HL. Baroreceptor reflex control of heart rate: a predictor of sudden cardiac death. Circulation 1982; 66:874-880.

125. Eckberg DL, Cavanaugh MS, Mark AL, et al. A simplified neck suction device for activation of carotid baroreceptors. J Lab Clin Med 1975; 85:167-173.

126. Kaufman ES, Bosner MS, Stein PK, et al. The effect of enalapril and digoxin in heart period variability in normal subjects. Am J Cardiol 1993; 72:95-99.

127. Kolman BS, Verrier RL, Lown B. The effects of vagus nerve stimulation upon the vulnerability of the canine ventricle: role of sympathetic-parasympathetic interactions. Am J Cardiol 1976; 37:1041-1045.

128. Vybiral T, Bryg RJ, Maddens ME, et al. Effect of passive tilt on sympathetic and parasympathetic components of heart rate variability in normal subjects. Am J Cardiol 1989; 63:1117-1120.

129. Weise F, Krell D, Brinkhoff N. Acute alcohol ingestion reduces heart rate variability. Drug Alcohol Depend 1986; 17:89-91.

Chapter 4

Geometrical Methods for Heart Rate Variability Assessment

Marek Malik

The conventional time-domain methods for heart rate variability (HRV) measurement utilize different statistical formulae and provide a scale of measures which express the most important facets of HRV. The major limitation of these statistical methods is their dependency on the quality of data of RR interval series which are analyzed by the statistical formulae. This dependency was fully appreciated when the conventional statistical methods were applied to RR data obtained by an automatic analysis of long-term electrocardiograms (ECGs). Although a high quality of long-term, eg, 24-hour ECGs is in principle achievable, it requires not only careful maintenance of the recording equipment and appropriate subject-specific positioning of the electrodes, but also a high degree of cooperation from the patient who is the subject of the recording in respect to the electrode contact, lead stability, etc. This makes high-quality, long-term ECGs difficult to sustain in clinical settings. It is well known that the quality of long-term ECGs recorded during clinical studies is poorer

than that of recordings in physiological laboratory investigations, especially of those involving well-motivated, healthy volunteers.

In principle, there are two practical methods for assessing HRV from imperfect long-term records. Firstly, the RR interval sequence obtained from such records can be 'filtered' using different physiologically based requirements of the data. For instance, it has been proposed that the durations of neighboring RR intervals of sinus rhythm should never differ by more than 20%.[1] In addition, the maximum and minimum duration of a valid RR interval may be postulated and a simple preprocessing of the sequence of all RR intervals can remove all intervals which are dubious and likely to be wrong. Only the subset of RR intervals which satisfy the logical 'filter' are then used in the statistical formulae of the time-domain methods. Unfortunately, this logical filtering is not always successful and in some cases may make the sequence RR intervals even less valid.[2] This leads to a second possibility for processing imperfect records which is based on

From: Malik M., Camm AJ (eds.): *Heart Rate Variability*. Armonk, NY. Futura Publishing Company, Inc., © 1995.

the idea of using completely different methods that are substantially less affected by the quality of the data. In searching for such techniques, the so-called geometrical methods were invented.

Principles of Geometrical Methods

As the name suggests, the geometrical methods use the sequence of RR intervals to construct a certain geometrical form and extract the assessment of HRV from this form. The geometrical forms used in different methods vary. In most cases, the methods are based on the sample density histogram of RR interval durations, the sample density histogram of differences between successive RR intervals, and on the so-called Lorenz plots or Poincarè maps which plot the duration of each RR interval against the duration of the immediately preceding RR interval.

The way in which the HRV measure is extracted from the geometrical form also varies from method to method. In general, three approaches are used:

1. some measurements of the geometrical form are taken, eg, the baseline width or the height of a sample density histogram, and the HRV measure is derived from these numbers;
2. the geometrical pattern is approximated by a mathematically defined shape and the HRV measured are derived from the parameters of this shape; and
3. the general pattern of the geometrical form is classified into one of several predefined categories and the HRV measure or characteristic is derived from the selected category.

Methods Based on the RR Interval Histogram

The most studied geometrical methods include the sample density histogram of RR interval durations. The incorrect RR inter-

vals are usually either substantially shorter or substantially longer than the population of correct RR intervals. The short incorrect intervals are frequently obtained when the computerized analysis of a long-term ECG recognizes a tall T wave or recording noise as a QRS complex; the long incorrect intervals are most frequently acquired when the analysis fails to identify one or several QRS complexes and measures an RR interval, which is in reality composed of two or even more interbeat intervals. Such incorrect measurements of RR interval fall outside the major peak of the distribution histogram and can frequently be clearly identified (Figure 1A-B). This is an important feature of the distribution histogram, which is also often utilized in commercial systems for the analysis of long-term ECGs.

The geometrical methods processing the histogram reduce the effect of the incorrect RR intervals by concentrating on the major (eg, the highest) peak of the sample density curve. The simplest method is the so-called *HRV triangular index*, which is based on the idea that if the major peak of the histogram were a triangle, its baseline width would be equal to its area divided by its height.[3] The height H of the histogram can easily be obtained as the number of RR intervals with modal duration, while the area A of the histogram equals the number of all RR intervals used to construct it. Thus, the HRV triangular index approximates the baseline width of the histogram by a simple fraction A/H. The numerical value of the HRV triangular index depends on the sampling applied to construct the histogram, that is, on the discrete scale used to measure the RR intervals. Most experience with the method has been obtained with sampling of 128 Hz, ie, when measuring the RR intervals on a scale with steps of approximately 8 milliseconds (precisely 7.8125 milliseconds).[4] However, slight departures from this sampling frequency do not affect the results of the method greatly.

The so-called *triangular interpolation* of RR interval histogram (the TIRR method or the TINN method when processing the his-

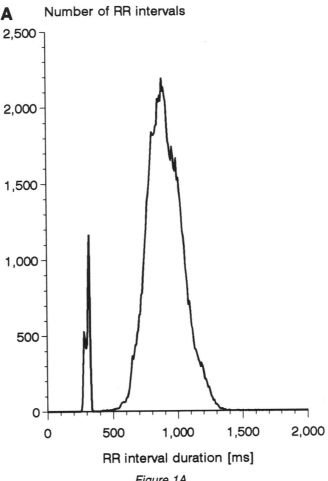

A Number of RR intervals

RR interval duration [ms]

Figure 1A

tograms of normal-to-normal RR intervals) is a modification of the HRV triangular index method which is less dependent on (but not completely independent of) the sampling frequency. Using the method of minimum square difference interpolation, the highest peak of the sample density histogram is approximated by a triangle, and the HRV is expressed as the length of the base of this triangle (Figure 2).[5]

Both of these methods are particularly suited when the RR interval histogram contains only one dominant peak. This is frequent in recordings obtained from subjects exposed to a stable environment without physical and mental excesses. Such an environment is often present during in-hospital recordings which makes these geometrical methods easily applicable to many clinical studies. On the contrary, 24-hour recordings of normally active, healthy individuals frequently register two distinct populations of RR intervals corresponding to active day and resting night periods. In such situations, the geometrical algorithms concentrate on the most dominant peak of the histogram and lead to underestimation of global HRV. The HRV triangular index method underestimates all bimodal histograms, the TIRR method is more stable in this respect and only leads to significant underestimation of the global HRV if the two major peaks of the histogram are substantially separated (Figure 3A-B).

In addition to these 'triangular' methods, other approaches have also been suggested, eg, the assessment of the sharpness of the dominant peak of the histogram.

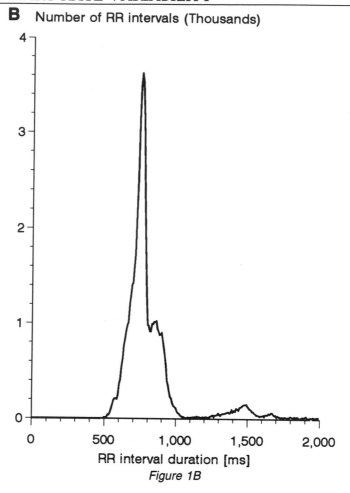

B Number of RR intervals (Thousands)

RR interval duration [ms]

Figure 1B

Figure 1A-B. Examples of RR interval histograms obtained from 24-hour Holter recordings when automatic analysis of the recordings was not working satisfactorily. **Panel A** shows a histogram in which the analysis recognized repeatedly tall T waves as supraventricular QRS complexes. **Panel B** shows a histogram obtained when the analysis failed to identify several thousands of QRS complexes. Note in this panel that the secondary peak of the histogram appears at RR interval durations which equals approximately to double RR intervals of the main peak of the histogram. In reality, these measured RR intervals were composed of two cardiac cycles in which the middle QRS was not recognized.

However, little is known about the practical value of these proposals.

Methods Based on the Histogram of Successive Differences

Approaches similar to those used to process the histograms of RR interval durations can be applied to the histograms of differences between successive intervals. However, the differential histograms are much narrower than the interval histograms and

their approximation by triangles is not as appropriate as in the case of interval histograms. Thus, those geometrical methods which are proposed for the processing of differential histograms concentrate on the sharpness of the peak of the differential histogram.

A very simple method for such an assessment proposes to measure the width of the histogram at two selected heights, eg, at the level of 1000 and 10 000 pairs of intervals, (Figure 4) and to express HRV as the

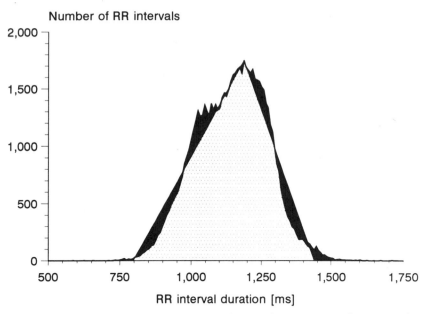

Figure 2. The Triangular Interpolation method interpolates the RR interval histogram by a triangle which has its base on the horizontal axis of the histogram and the peak on the maximum point of the histogram. The computation of the method identifies such a triangle for which the square of the difference between the histogram and the triangle is the minimum among all possible triangles. The length of the base of such a triangle is taken as the measure of HRV.

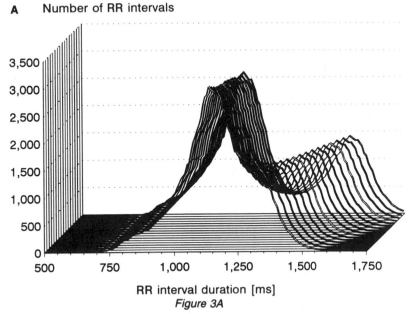

Figure 3A

difference between or the proportion of these widths.[6] Understandably, the width of the histogram at a selected height depends not only on the sampling frequency with which the RR intervals are measured, but also on the absolute duration of the rec-

ording. However, the experience with the method shows that analyzing recordings of standardized length, eg, nominal 24-hour ECGs, and when using the usual sampling frequency of 128 Hz (which is currently the most common precision of commercial

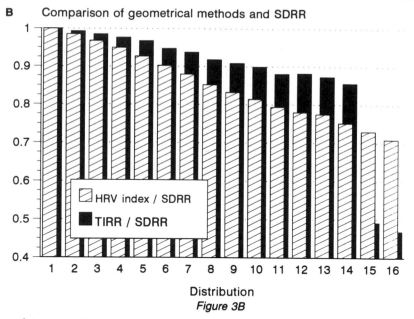

B Comparison of geometrical methods and SDRR

Distribution

Figure 3B

Figure 3A-B. This figure illustrates a technical investigation of the performance of the HRV triangular index and the triangular interpolation methods in cases of strongly bimodal distributions of RR interval duration. **Panel A** shows 16 histograms obtained artificially by mixing two populations of RR intervals. The two geometrical methods and the statistical method computing the standard deviation of all RR intervals were applied to these histograms. The comparison of the geometrical methods with the statistical method is shown in **Panel B** which shows a proportion between the geometrical and statistical method (normalized by taking the proportion for the first histogram equal to 1). In this panel, the histograms are numbered from the least bimodal (#1) to the most bimodal (#16). Note that for histograms #15 and #16, the triangular interpolation measures of HRV were related exclusively to the dominant peak of the histogram.

Holter systems), the methods provides practically applicable assessment of HRV.

Interpolation of differential histograms by a mathematically defined curve was also proposed. For this purpose, the histogram composed of absolute values of inter-interval differences is used. The method expects that in such a histogram, the variability of the genuine sinus rhythm will create a smooth sharply falling curve, while errors in the assessment of the RR intervals and premature atrial or ventricular beats (as well as their compensatory pauses) will lead to additional secondary peaks of the tail of the histogram. The dominant curve of the histogram can be extracted by a negative exponential interpolation of the histogram which is equivalent to a linear interpolation of the histogram if drawn on a semilogarithmic scale. The degree of HRV is then characterized by the slope of such an interpolation

(Figure 5).[7] This method seems to be appealing especially for fully automatic assessment of HRV. However, its performance has not been investigated in sufficiently large sets of ECGs.

Lorenz Plots

Simple visual judgment of HRV in a long-term ECG is perhaps best facilitated by the Lorenz plot, which is a map of dots in Cartesian coordinates. Each pair of successive RR intervals is plotted as a dot with coordinates (duration R_iR_{i+1}, duration $R_{i+1}R_{i+2}$).

The incorrectly measured RR intervals or the coupling intervals and the compensatory pauses of atrial and ventricular premature beats lead to clear outliers in the map of the plot which are easily visible (Figure 6A-B). Thus, compared to the histograms

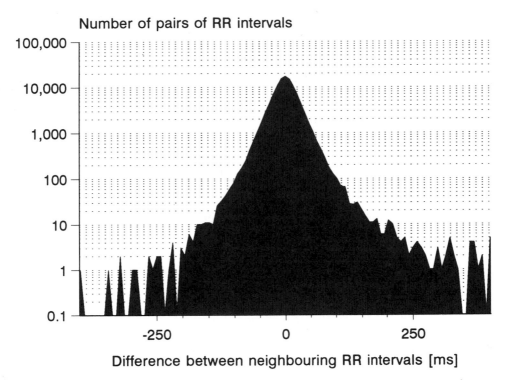

Number of pairs of RR intervals

Difference between neighbouring RR intervals [ms]

Figure 4. The width of a histogram of absolute differences between successive RR intervals measured at two specified levels of histogram height. The histogram is plotted at a semilogarithmic scale which enhances the outliers caused by errors in the analysis of long-term ECG.

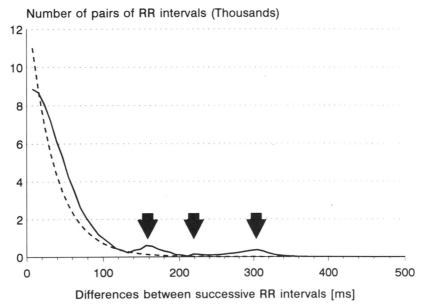

Number of pairs of RR intervals (Thousands)

Differences between successive RR intervals [ms]

Figure 5. The figure shows a histogram of absolute differences between successive RR intervals of a 24-hour recording (full line). The arrows indicate secondary peaks of the histogram which were caused by errors in RR interval recognition. Such secondary peaks would strongly affect statistical computation of HRV but do not affect the mathematically defined interpolation of the histogram (dashed line).

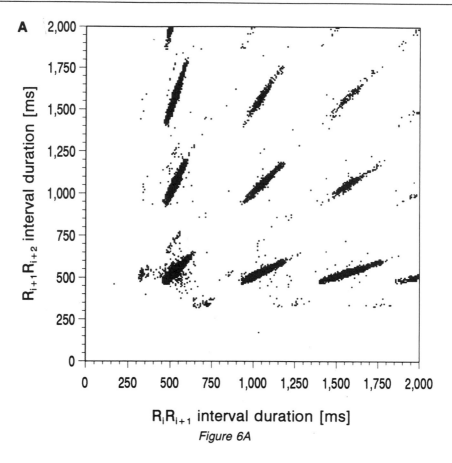

A

Figure 6A

R$_i$R$_{i+1}$ interval duration [ms]

of RR durations, the Lorenz plots are even more appropriate to judge the quality which the RR intervals were identified in a long-term ECG. Similarly, various rhythm disturbances such as paroxysmal atrial fibrillation can easily be identified on a Lorenz plot.

Preserved physiological HRV leads to a wide spreading Lorenz plot, while records with markedly reduced HRV produces a compact pattern of the plot (Figure 7A-F). Based on such a visual judgment, some studies have led to proposals for classification of patterns of Lorenz plots and distinguished, for instance, 'comet' and 'torpedo' shapes (note the shapes shown in Figure 7).[8] While such approaches are valid for initial visual judgment, they lack a precise definition of each category, and as different plots create a continuous spectrum between the 'comet' and 'torpedo' shapes, are subject to a significant operator bias. Thus, these simple classifications of the shape of the plots

are not very well suited for systematic studies of large clinical populations and therefore, the practical experience with them is limited. More complex and mathematically precise classifications of Lorenz plots have also been proposed, usually based on computing several time-domain HRV indices of the plot and classifying the shape of the plot according to these indices. This, unfortunately, means that the Lorenz plot is used only as an additional graphics expression of the results of the time-domain methods and does not have any superiority over these methods used on their own.

Recent investigations have also disputed a direct link between HRV of a long-term recording and the two-dimensional pattern of the corresponding Lorenz plot.[9] It has been suggested that 'height' of the plot, ie, the number of pairs of RR intervals corresponding to the same dot of the plot, should be considered. Indeed, it is possible

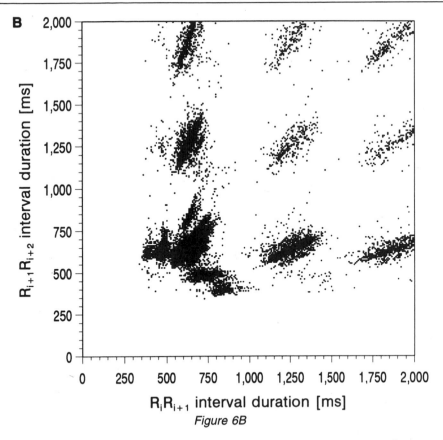

B

Figure 6B

Figure 6A-B. Examples of Lorenz plots obtained from improperly recognized 24-hour Holter recordings. **Panel A** shows a plot in which a substantial number of measured RR intervals corresponds to couplets, triplets, etc. of real RR intervals. Different combinations of such incorrect intervals produce patterns which appear at multiples of the dominant length of RR intervals which is approximately 500 ms in this case. **Panel B** shows a Lorenz plot in which the same error is combined with incorrect recognition of ventricular premature beats. Note that the left bottom part of the plot is not symmetric. This was caused by combinations of premature beats and their compensatory pauses.

to find recordings with markedly different HRV which lead to a very similar pattern of the plot (Figure 8A-D). The more complex analyses of the plots which have been proposed following these observations are both typical geometrical methods (eg, interpolation of the plots with the height used as the third dimension by mathematically defined shapes) and methods which are a mixture of geometrical and nonlinear approaches.

Advantages, Limitations and Use of Geometrical Methods

From what has been said earlier, the advantages of the geometrical methods are obvious. They are capable of providing a reasonable assessment of HRV even when the quality of data does not permit the use of conventional time-domain and spectral methods. This does not mean that the geometrical methods can replace the other methods entirely. Their results are only approximate and they are not as precise as the more exact statistical and spectral analyses.

The approximate nature of the results of geometrical methods is, of course, their limitation. Another important limitation of the methods lies in the fact that in general, a substantial number of RR intervals is needed to construct a representative geo-

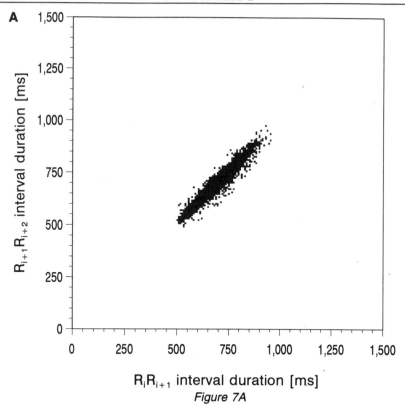

Figure 7A

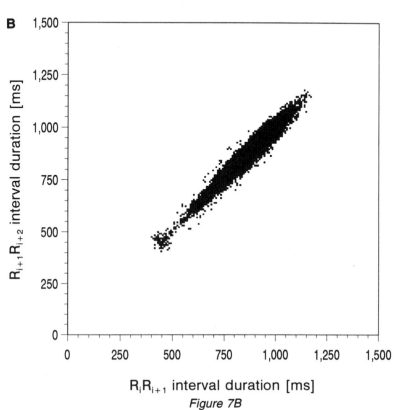

Figure 7B

C

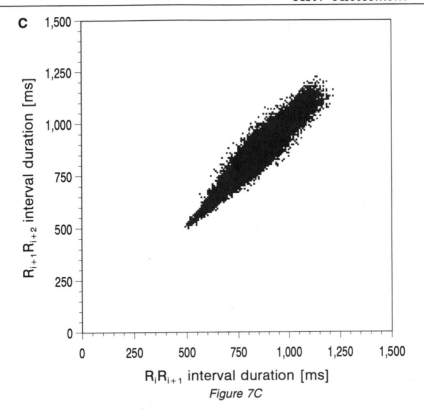

Figure 7C

D

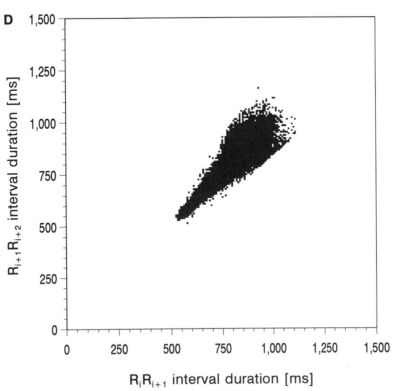

Figure 7D

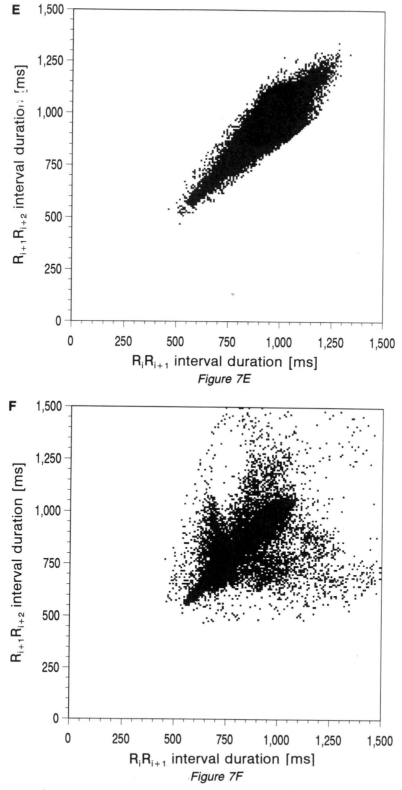

Figure 7E

Figure 7F

Figure 7A-F. This figure shows a scale of Lorenz plot patterns ordered from minimum **(Panel A)** to maximum **(Panel F)** HRV.

A

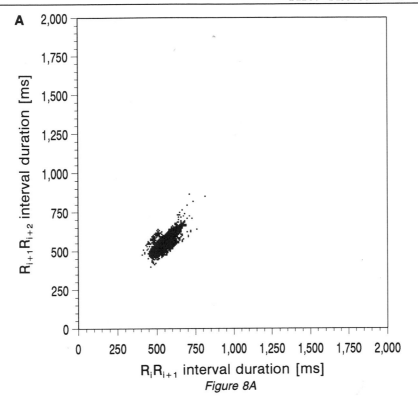

Figure 8A

B

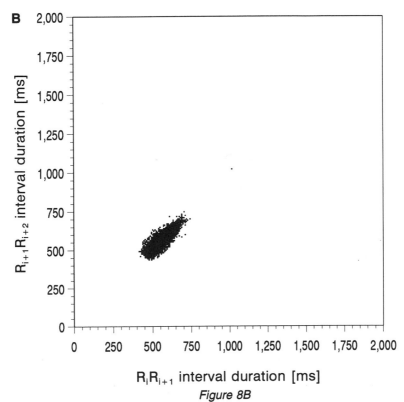

Figure 8B

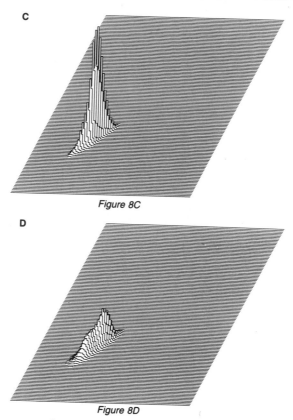

Figure 8C

Figure 8D

Figure 8A-D. Panels A and B show conventional Lorenz plots of long-term ECGs of two different patients. **Panels C and D** show the three-dimensional representations of these plots in which the number of pairs of RR intervals corresponding to each dot of the plot is used at the third coordinate of the plot. **Panels C and D** show that despite the substantial similarity of the patterns of two-dimensional plots shown in A and B, HRV was different in both cases. When HRV triangular index method was applied to both recordings, the results 8.13 and 12.34 were obtained for cases (A-C) and (B-D), respectively.

metrical pattern. Experience shows that at least 20-minute recordings are needed to create a valid histogram of RR interval durations and an even longer record is needed to obtain a satisfactory shape of the Lorenz plot. Naturally, the longer the recording, the better the definition of the derived geometrical pattern. Thus, it is optimum to apply geometrical methods to 24-hour or even longer recordings.

The need to record a sufficient number of cardiac cycles excludes the geometrical methods from being used in physiological studies which investigate short-term recordings made under specific conditions. However, the accuracy and quality of recordings obtained during such studies is usually high and careful manual editing of

short records can easily be performed. In principle, this removes the need to use geometrical methods in physiological studies and makes the statistical and spectral methods more appropriate.

Thus, the application of geometrical methods should be restricted to clinical investigations and to cases in which obtaining an error-free sequence of RR intervals is impractical. Those geometrical methods which analyze the histogram of RR durations provide assessment of overall HRV, and for error-free sequences of RR intervals without clear bimodal distribution, provide results comparable with the standard deviations of all RR intervals. The methods of processing the histogram of difference between successive RR intervals assess short-term HRV comparable to the rMSSD and pNN50 statistical methods. It has been proposed that some measurements taken from Lorenz plots are able to approximate both overall and short-term HRV (eg, the length and the width of the pattern of the plot, respectively) but no systematic investigation involving a sufficient number of recordings has provided confirmation. At present, sufficient experience exists only with the methods analyzing histograms of RR interval durations. Clinical studies which employed these methods demonstrated that the practical value of their assessment of global HRV is not inferior to that of the statistical and spectral methods.

References

1. Kleiger RE, Miller JP, Bigger JT, et al. Decreased heart rate variability and its association with increased mortality after acute myocardial infarction. Am J Cardiol 1987; 59:256-262.
2. Malik M, Cripps T, Farrell T, et al. Prognostic value of heart rate variability after myocardial infarction—a comparison of different data processing methods. Med Biol Eng Comput 1989; 27:603-611.
3. Malik M, Farrell T, Cripps T, et al. Heart rate variability in relation to prognosis after myocardial infarction—selection of optimal processing techniques. Eur Heart J 1989; 10:1060-1074.
4. Cripps TR, Malik M, Farrell TG, et al. Prognostic value of reduced heart rate variability after myocardial infarction: clinical evaluation of a new analysis method. Br Heart J 1991; 65:14-19.
5. Farrell TG, Bashir Y, Cripps T, et al. A simple method of risk stratification for arrhythmic events in post-infarction patients based on heart rate variability and signal averaged ECG. J Am Coll Cardiol 1991; 18:687-697.
6. Bjökander I, Held C, Forslund L, et al. Heart rate variability in patients with stable angina pectoris. Eur Heart J 1992; 13(suppl):379. Abstract.
7. Scherer P, Ohler JP, Hirche H, et al. Definition of a new beat-to-beat parameter of heart rate variability. PACE 1993; 16:939. Abstract.
8. Woo MA, Stevenson WG, Moser DK, et al. Complex heart rate variability and serum norepinephrine levels in patients with advanced heart failure. J Am Coll Cardiol 1994; 23:565-569.
9. Hnatkova K, Staunton A, Camm AJ, et al. Numerical processing of Lorenz plots of RR intervals is superior to conventional time-domain measures of heart rate variability for risk stratification after acute myocardial infarction. PACE 1994; 17:767. Abstract.

Chapter 5

Spectral Analysis of the Heart Rate Variability Signal

Sergio Cerutti, Anna M. Bianchi, Luca T. Mainardi

Introduction

The control mechanisms of the heart rate (HR), as well as of the arterial blood pressure (BP) and other cardiovascular variables, are reflected in rhythmic oscillations on a beat-to-beat basis of different parameters: the RR interval durations on electrocardiographic (ECG) signal; the systolic and diastolic values of arterial pressure; blood flow values, etc. Even in stationary control conditions these parameters, in normal subjects, are characterized by a variability in the order of 10% of their mean value. The variability is due to the synergistic action of the two branches of the autonomic nervous system, the sympathetic and the parasympathetic, which act in balance through neural, mechanical, humoral, and other different physiological mechanisms, in order to maintain cardiovascular parameters in their optimal ranges, and to react optimally to modified external or internal conditions, in order to set the controlled process to a new working point.[1-3]

Measures of the beat-to-beat changes in HR, BP values, etc., in both stationary conditions and in response to external standardized stimuli, may constitute an objective and noninvasive quantification of the state of the autonomic nervous system in both physiological and pathological conditions.

For these reasons, in the last years, interest has grown in the study of such changes, mainly in the HR,[4,5] with the aim of achieving new indices and criteria able to lead to a better diagnosis of various, important pathologies with which an alteration of the autonomic nervous system may be associated (hypertension, cardiac ischemia, myocardial infarction, diabetic neuropathy and other autonomic dysfunctions) and, hence, to a more specific therapy.

In addition, a quantitative study of these changes, as a consequence of external standardized stimuli, or after drug administration, is fundamental in physiological studies, for a better comprehension of the complex mechanisms underlying these oscillations.[6,7]

From: Malik M., Camm AJ (eds.): *Heart Rate Variability*. Armonk, NY. Futura Publishing Company, Inc., © 1995.

The first step in the analysis is the correct choice of the fiducial point on the ECG signal, that can well represent the trigger point on a beat-to-beat basis. This point should theoretically be the onset of the P wave, which corresponds with the start of activation of the cells of the sinoatrial node. However, it is acceptable to use the RR time interval as a measure of the heart period, as the R peak is more easily identifiable on the ECG tracing and the PR interval is relatively constant in the absence of conduction disorders.

Thus, the heart rate variability (HRV) signal is obtained, in the simplest way, as the sequence of the RR durations expressed as a function of the beat number: the time is measured in cardiac beats, instead of seconds (such a series is generally called an *RR interval tachogram* or, more concisely, *tachogram*). In order to operate in the more common time scale, some authors, express the HRV signals as a function of time, by interpolating and resampling the RR sequence. A complete review and comparison of the different techniques for achieving HRV signals is provided by DeBoer and colleagues.[8] Classical approaches of quantification of the variability phenomena are in the time domain: histograms, scattergrams of the series, analysis of the mean value and variance, difference or ratio between the longest and the shortest RR values after a stimulus and others, have been successfully applied in different clinical and research areas.[4,6]

For a deeper insight into the dynamics underlying the beat-to-beat RR variations and for understanding how the overall variance is distributed in different frequency contributions, more advanced techniques have to be applied, based on second order statistics, through the calculation of the autocorrelation function (ACF) and mainly its Fourier transform, the Power Spectral Density (PSD).

Spectral Analysis of the Heart Rate Variability Signal

From the earliest studies by Penaz et al,[9] Sayers,[10] and Akselrod et al,[11] it was clear that the HRV signal contains well-defined rhythms, which have been successfully shown to contain physiological information. Figure 1a shows the RR tachogram series relative to a normal subject in control conditions (relaxed on a bed): the PSD of the series (Figure 1c) shows three main contributions to the total power which are well identifiable in three different frequency ranges.

Long period rhythms are contained in the very low-frequency (VLF) range, between DC and 0.03 Hz. They account for the long-term regulation mechanisms probably related to thermoregulation, to the renin-angiotensin system and to other humoral factors.[12] These rhythms cannot be satisfactorily resolved and quantified by the traditional spectral analysis that is performed on records of few minutes; different techniques and specific methodologies have to be applied for a correct understanding and quantification of these complex and not yet clarified mechanisms.

In the low-frequency (LF) range, between 0.03 and 0.15 Hz, there is a rhythm, generally centered around 0.1 Hz. Its physiological interpretation is still controversial. Both sympathetic and parasympathetic contributions can be involved in this activity. However, an increase in its power has always been observed as a consequence of sympathetic activation (rest-tilt maneuver, mental stress, hemorrhage, coronary occlusion, etc.). Thus, an increase in the LF power is accepted by many authors as a marker of sympathetic activation.[5,13]

At the respiratory frequency, generally in a wide range between 0.18 and 0.4 Hz, it is possible to identify a high-frequency (HF) component in the PSD of the HRV signal. Such a rhythm, synchronous with the respiration rate, is due to the intrathoracic pressure changes and mechanical variations caused by the breathing activity. It is mediated by the vagus nerve on the heart; such activity is therefore generally accepted as a marker of parasympathetic activation.[14,15] With this background, it is obvious that the power related to these various components

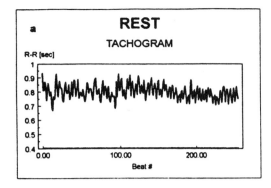

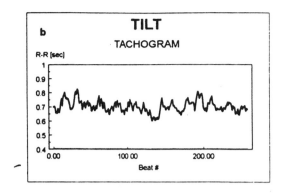

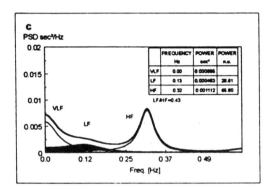

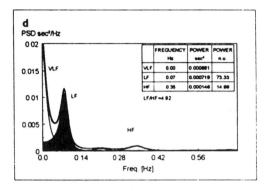

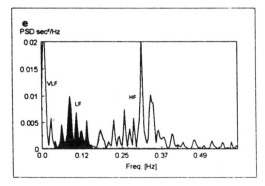

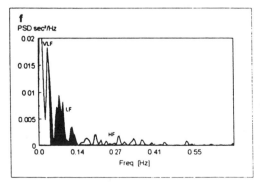

Figure 1. a: Tachogram of a normal subject in resting condition; b: after a tilting maneuver. The related PSDs, calculated through an AR model are shown in 'c' and 'd'; the spectral parameters are reported in the tables. 'e' and 'f' show the PSDs of 'a' and 'b,' respectively, evaluated through an FFT algorithm. The LF is shaded in dark grey, while the HF is in light grey.

may be used to quantify the sympatho-vagal balance in controlling HR.

LF and HF powers may be expressed in absolute values (*seconds²*), or in normalized units (*nu*, ie, as percentage value over the total power after the subtraction of the VLF power). Figure 1c illustrates the overall PSD with the three components mentioned above. For each component, the central frequency and power in absolute as in nu are calculated. Figure 1b shows the same patient after tilt stimulation: the relevant PSD (shown in Figure 1d) demonstrates an increasing of the LF component and a decrease of the HF component when changing from rest to tilt; the LF/HF ratio increases from 0.43 to 4.92, accordingly. Since an antagonist relation exists between the LF and HF powers, ie, similar to that characterizing the sympatho-vagal balance, it is possible to quantify such a balance by the LF/HF ratio between the power of the LF and HF components, respectively.

In the following section different algorithms, commonly employed for the frequency analysis of the HRV will be presented. Advantages and disadvantages of the methods will be elaborated in order to stress the importance of understanding the methods in order to achieve a reliable calculation of the spectral parameters and to correctly comprehend and interpret the results.

Algorithms for Calculating the Spectral Parameters

Spectral analysis of the HRV signal is traditionally performed on stationary records of at least 200 to 500 consecutive heartbeats (256 or 512 when the PSD is calculated through the Fast Fourier Transform[FFT] algorithm), corresponding to a time window of a few minutes. This choice was initially imposed by the need to obtain a good compromise between a sufficient frequency resolution (that may be achieved with long data records, at least with traditional methods) and the stationarity condition of the signal which is required for a reliable spectral esti-

mation. This cannot be maintained for a long time, especially on biological signals.

The classical frequency analysis is based upon the Fourier Transform which can be easily evaluated through the FFT algorithm.[16] The expression of the PSD as a function of the frequency, $P(f)$, can be directly obtained from the time series y(k), where 'k' is the discrete time index, by using the periodogram expression:

$$P(f) = \frac{1}{N\Delta t}\left|\Delta t\sum_{k=0}^{N-1}y(k)e^{-j2\pi fk\Delta t}\right|^2 = \frac{1}{N\Delta t}|Y(f)|^2,$$

where Δt is the sampling period, N is the number of samples, and Y(f) is the discrete time Fourier transform of y(k). PSD is also obtainable in two steps from the FFT of the ACF of the signal.

FFT based methods are widely diffused for their easy applicability, computational speed and direct interpretation of the results. However, ACF and Fourier Transform are theoretically defined on infinite data sequences, thus, errors are introduced by the need to operate on finite data records in order to obtain estimates of the true functions. In addition, the finite data set makes it necessary to make assumptions, sometimes not realistic, about the data outside the recording window: commonly, they are considered to be zero. This implicit rectangular windowing of the data results in a spectral leakage in the PSD. Different windows, that smoothly connect the side samples to zero, are most often used in order to solve this problem, but they may introduce a reduction in the frequency resolution. In fact, the frequency resolution is strictly related to the record data length ($\Delta f=1/T$ where T is the recording period in seconds) and this is reduced by the windowing operation. Furthermore, the estimates of the signal PSD are not statistically consistent and need various techniques for improving their statistical performances. This is obtained, for example, by smoothing the rapid fluctuations of the spectrum. Various methods are mentioned in the literature:

1. averaging over adjacent spectral frequencies;
2. dividing the data sequence in nonoverlapping segments and then averaging the pseudo-ensemble of the obtained PSD; and
3. averaging as in point #2, but using windowing techniques and overlapping data segments.

Of course, all these procedures cause a further reduction in frequency resolution.[16]

The above methods are known as *nonparametric* approaches for the PSD calculation, in opposition to the *parametric* ones. Parametric approaches assume the time series under analysis to be the output of a given mathematical model and no drastic assumptions are made on the data outside the recording window. The PSD is calculated as a function of the model parameters according to appropriate expressions. A critical point in this approach is the choice of an adequate model to represent the data sequence. The model is completely independent from the physiological, anatomical and physical characteristics of the biological system, but simply provides the input-output relationships of the process in the so-called black-box approach.

Among the numerous possibilities of modeling, linear models, characterized by a rational transfer function, are able to describe a wide number of different processes. In the most general case, they are represented by the following linear equation that relates the input driving signal $w(k)$ and the output of an AutoRegressive Moving Average (ARMA) process:

$$y(k)=-\sum_{i=1}^{p}a_iy(k-1)+\sum_{j=1}^{q}b_jw(k-j)+w(k)$$

where $w(k)$ is the input white noise with null mean value and variance λ^2, p and q are the orders of AR and MA parts, respectively, and a_i, b_j are the proper coefficients.

The ARMA model may be reformulated as an AR or an MA if the coefficients b_j or a_i are respectively set to zero.

Since the estimation of the AR parameters results in linear equations, AR models are usually employed in place of ARMA or MA, also on the basis of the Wold decomposition theorem [17] that establishes that any stationary ARMA or MA process of finite variance can be represented as a unique AR model of appropriate order, even infinite; likewise any ARMA or AR process can be represented by an MA model of sufficiently high order.

The AR PSD is then obtained from the following expression:

$$P(f)=\frac{\lambda^2\Delta t}{\left|1+\sum_{i=1}^{p}a_iz^{-i}\right|^2_{z=\exp(j2\pi fi\Delta t)}}.$$

Parametric methods are methodologically and computationally more complex than the nonparametric ones, as they require an a priori choice of the structure and of the order of the model of the signal generation mechanism. Different criteria have been proposed for the choice of the optimal order, which may help in the determination of the value of p (order of the model) (AIC and FPE due to Akaike, RIS due to Rissanen and PAR due to Parzen) are generally employed. The value of $\bar{p}$ by which the figure of merit is minimal is chosen as an optimal value of the model order. They generally take into generally take into account the complexity and the numerosity of the model (given by the order and by the number of samples) and the fitting to the data (measured through the variance of the prediction error).[18,19] Some tests are required a posteriori to verify the whiteness of the prediction error, such as the Anderson test (autocorrelation test),[20] in order to test the reliability of the estimation. Different criteria have been proposed for the choice of the optimal order, which may help in the determination of the value of $\bar{p}$ (order of the model) (AIC and FPE due to Akaike, RIS due to Rissanen and PAR due to Parzen) are generally employed. The value of $\bar{p}$ by which the figure of merit is minimal is chosen as an optimal value of the model order. A correct identification of the model implies that p be higher than the value of p by which the Anderson test is satisfied. In the same way, too low (or too high) values of P may yield scarcely informative spectra (or cause too many spurious peaks in the spectra).

When the methods of spectral estimation are employed for the spectral analysis of the HRV signal, some other considerations must be taken into account. As it was pointed out in the above section, physiological and clinical information is achieved from the spectral analysis of the HRV signal through a postprocessing of the PSD, and the calculation of spectral parameters able to quantify the sympatho-vagal balance, in particular the LF and HF powers and frequencies, and the LF/HF ratio.

In this regard, the AR modeling has the advantage of allowing a spectral decomposition for a direct and automatic calculation of the power and frequency of the spectral components. In the z-transform domain the ACF, $R(k)$ and the PSD of the signal are related by the following expression:

$$R(k)=\frac{1}{2\pi j}\int\limits_{|z|=1}P(z)z^{k-1}dz$$

If the integral is calculated by means of the residual method, the ACF is decomposed into a sum of dumped sinusoids, each one related to a pair of complex conjugate poles, and of dumped exponential functions, related to the real poles. The Fourier Transform of each one of these terms gives the expression of each spectral component that fits the component related to the relevant pole or pole pair. The argument of the pole gives the central frequency of the component, while the i-th spectral component power is the residual γ_i in case of real poles and $2\text{Re}(\gamma_i)$ in case of conjugate pole pairs. γ_i is computed from the following expression[21,22]:

$$\gamma_i=z^{-1}(z-z_i)P(z)\big|_{z=z_i}.$$

Figure 1c shows the PSD of the interval tachogram displayed in Figure 1a. The LF component is filled in dark grey, while the HF is in light grey and their central frequency and power are reported in the table.

When using the FFT, the same spectral parameters are evaluated by integrating the PSD in predefined frequency bands, as shown in Figure 1e (the same convention as in Figure 1c is maintained for LF and HF). The integration procedure may introduce some errors linked to the choice of the integration band; a large integration band makes much power, not related to the relevant oscillation, to be evaluated, while narrow bands may disregard much power of interest, and may miss the relevant component when the frequency is shifted with respect to the previously chosen range.

In Figure 1f the LF power, calculated by integration of the PSD between 0.03 and 0.15 Hz, comprises some power external to the relevant rhythm, especially towards the lower frequencies, where the VLF power partially masks the LF one.

After the tilting maneuver the respiration power component markedly decreased. While the AR spectral estimation is able to well identify the HF power through the spectral decomposition, (Figure 1d), the predefined frequency range in the FFT makes the HF power to be misrecognized (Figure 1f).

Each method (parametric or nonparametric) has advantages and disadvantages and the user should be well aware of them.

Time Variant Spectral Identification

Traditional spectral analysis requires that the signal is stationary in order to provide reliable results. But even wide-sense stationarity is not a strictly physiological condition and may be achieved only by paying particular attention during the experimental protocol and the signal recording phase. On the other hand, in particular experiments, or during particular pathological events, the interest may be in the evolution of the sympatho-vagal balance, not only in its static determination. In fact, a large number of phenomena take place in a short time, too short for reaching a good frequency resolution by means of traditional batch spectral estimation. For those reasons, many research groups are actually proposing methods and algorithms able to detect transient phenomena, and able to describe a signal both in terms of frequency and time.

Nonparametric approaches are generally based on the Wigner-Ville distribution.[23] Different similar distributions have been successively introduced with the aim of eliminating some disadvantages, like the cross-terms due to the nonlinearity of the transformation (a summary of these techniques is reported in Cohen[24]).

Actually, a great interest is given to the Wavelet Transform which, among the broad field of possible applications, allows an attractive time-frequency representation of the signal: it is possible to obtain HF or time resolution in the same plot for better evidencing the different characteristics of the signal at the same time.[25]

In the parametric field it is possible to track the spectral modification of a signal by means of AR models in recursive form.[26] In correspondence of each new sample in the signal (an RR interval in case of the HRV signal), a new set of model parameters $a(k)$ is obtained from the preceding ones and from the prediction error:

$$a(k)=a(k-1)+K(k)[y(k)-\hat{y}(k)]$$

where $\hat{y}(k)$ is estimated by the model through the coefficients evaluated at time k-1 and $K(k)$ is the gain of the algorithm. $K(k)$ may assume different formulations on the basis of different algorithms (RLS, directional, Fortesque) [27] and contains a forgetting factor w that exponentially weighs the *past* of the signal, in such a way that the more recent terms mostly contribute in the innovation, while the oldest ones are pro-

gressively forgotten. The value of the forgetting factor determines how fast the adaptation must be and how sensitive the algorithm must be to the signal changes.[26]

Figure 2a shows a tachogram of an ischemic episode detected on a high-fidelity Holter recording in correspondence with an ST segment depression on the ECG. The horizontal line under the tachogram denotes the time interval (expressed in number of RRs) during which the ST episode is present. The corresponding sequence of spectra is in Figure 2b in contour plot representation (time is on the horizontal axis in term of beat number, and frequency on the vertical one), while the Compressed Spectral Array (CSA) form is in Figure 2c: the frequency is reported on the horizontal axis, the PSD on the vertical, while the time is represented from the top downward. On the side, in correspondence of each spectrum, the spectral parameters are plotted (LF and HF power together with the LF/HF ratio). A horizontal arrow (B) indicates the beginning of the ST depression. In the few minutes before the onset of the ischemic episode (about two minutes in this case), it is possible to note an increase in the LF power and a decrease in the HF power, with a consequent increase in the LF/HF ratio, that denotes a sympathetic activation before the onset of the attack (at least as traditionally detected on ECG tracing).

Besides the previously mentioned advantages of the parametric approaches with respect to the nonparametric, the recursive implementation allows continuous monitoring of the spectral parameters, and hence the sympatho-vagal balance, while nonparametric techniques require the time series under analysis to be known over the entire temporal window and can only be applied off-line.

In parametric models, as the quantification of the sympatho-vagal balance is obtained through the evaluation of the spectral parameters which are directly obtained from the poles of the AR transfer function, a more effective on-line monitoring of the sympatho-vagal balance is obtained by the

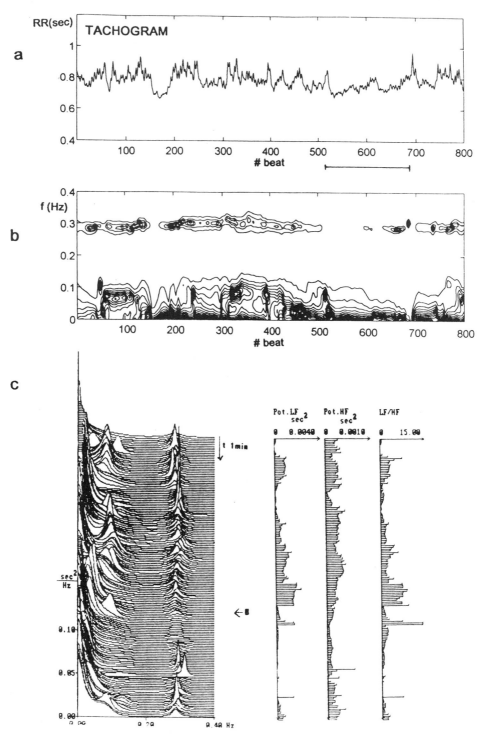

Figure 2. a: Tachogram during an ischemic attack; b: the contour plot of the spectra calculated on a beat-to-beat basis (see text). The horizontal line in 'a' marks the time of ST depression on the ECG signal. The same spectra are plotted in CSA form in 'c' (from top downward) where the arrow B denotes the onset of the attack. LF, HF and LF/HF parameters are shown side-by-side on a beat-to-beat basis.

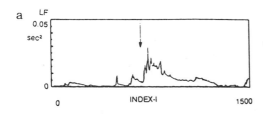

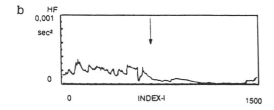

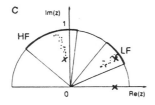

Figure 3. a: LF; b: HF beat-to-beat values of power during a tilt maneuver; c: beat-to-beat position of the poles in the complex z-plane. After the tilt the LF and HF frequency ranges are marked.

direct updating of the poles z_i of the model. This is achieved by means of the following expression:

$$\Delta z_i = \sum_{k=1}^{p} \frac{\partial z_i}{\partial a_k} \Delta a_k$$

that directly evaluates the innovation of the position of the poles z_i, in the z-transform plane, once the set of the coefficients a_i is updated, without zeroing the corresponding equation at each step.[28] Such a procedure may be carried out even on-line. As an example, in Figure 3c, the beat-to-beat position of the poles of the AR model is shown relative to 1500 consecutive RRs. Figures 3a and b show LF and HF beat-to-beat powers (in seconds[2]), respectively, in correspondence with a tilt maneuver whose beginning

is indicated by the arrow. After the tilt, it is possible to look at the trend of pole position inside the unitary circle. Only the poles relative to LF and HF regions along the unitary circle are indicated. The trajectories of the pole positions are clearly evidenced. The increasing of LF power is accompanied by a movement of the pole towards the unitary circle, while the decreasing of HF is characterized by the movement of the pole towards the center of the circle. It is then possible to evaluate whether their central frequencies go out from the defined regions.

Long-Term Analysis

As already mentioned, in order to maintain the hypothesis of stationarity of the signal, the traditional spectral analysis is generally performed on temporal windows of few minutes (generally containing 200 to 500 consecutive heart cycles), but analysis over longer periods have also been performed (ie, up to 24-hour recordings). A first method consists in dividing the whole record (about 100 000 RR values in 24 hours) in consecutive or overlapping windows of 200 to 500 beats, and in calculating the PSD on each of them by means of the traditional batch techniques. The spectra are then plotted in a CSA form, together with the spectral parameters, in order to evidence their trend during the day. Still, the resolution of the spectra depends obviously on the number of points considered in each spectrum. In this way, it is possible to follow the changes of spectral parameters along the 24-hour period and to quantify day-night differences, circadian variations and so on.[29]

An interesting spectral measurement may be obtained over long-term records of HRV signal (typically from 20 000 RRs, up to the ones over the entire 24-hour period). Since evidence[30] has been obtained that long-term HRV signal has a spectrum which follows $\frac{1}{f^\alpha}$ law (in log-log scale), where $\alpha =$

1. $\frac{1}{f}$ processes are self-similar and present a

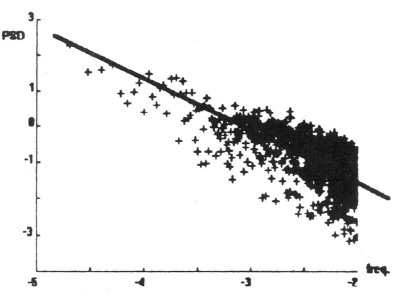

Figure 4. FFT plot of 24-hour tachogram on a log-log scale. The regression line is superimposed. From Calcagnini, et al[31].

fractal (fractionary) dimension. Chaotic behavior may be associated to this kind of process. Such a behavior may be assessed through the measurements typical of nonlinear dynamics which are not intended to be dealt with in this chapter. Disclosure of α from 1 (with $\alpha > 1$) is typical of some pathologies, ie, hypertension.[31] Figure 4 reports the $\frac{1}{f^{\alpha}}$ spectrum of a normal subject. The difference of α from normal to hypertensive is significant (p <0.02) over the considered cases (20 young hypertensive patients and 20 healthy subjects).

Conclusion

The HRV signal contains much information regarding the control mechanism elicited by the autonomic nervous system. The frequency-domain analysis of such a signal is widely employed both in physiological and clinical studies. In this paper we have described the algorithms more commonly used for obtaining PSD from the HRV signal and the techniques which are able to extract suitable spectral parameters for quantifying the phenomenon under study. The basic characteristics of the two approaches (nonparametric and parametric) which are generally employed are described below. The latter (parametric) has advantages with respect to the former:

1. it has a more statistical consistency even on short segments of data, ie, under certain assumptions, a spectrum estimated through autoregressive modeling is a maximum entropy spectrum (MES);
2. the spectrum is more easily interpretable with an 'implicit' filtering of what is considered random noise;
3. an easy and more reliable calculation of the spectral parameters (postprocessing of the spectrum), through the spectral decomposition procedure, which is directly interpretable from a physiological point of view;
4. there is no need to window the data, in order to decrease the spectral leakage;
5. the frequency resolution does not depend upon the quantity of data; and

6. a recursive implementation can be realized, that performs on-line monitoring of the sympatho-vagal balance through direct updating of the spectral parameters of physiological interest.

On the other hand the parametric approach:

1. is more complex from a methodological and computational point of view; and
2. requires an a priori definition of the model (AR, MA, ARMA or others) to be fitted, and its complexity (ie, the number of parameters). Some figures of merit introduced in literature and already mentioned may be of help in determining their value. Still, this procedure may be difficult in some particular cases.

In conclusion, it is essential to analyze the HRV signal correctly, especially in the frequency domain, when parameters can be obtained which are directly correlated to the patho-physiology of the system. On the other hand, such an analysis should be made in the context of the appropriate knowledge of the relevant spectral techniques.

References

1. Cannon B. The Wisdom of the Body. New York, NY: WW Norton, 1932.
2. Mayakawa K, Koepchen HP, Polosa C. Mechanisms of Blood Pressure. Berlin, Germany: Springer Verlag, 1984.
3. Chess GF, Tam RMK, Calaresu FR. Influence of cardiac neural inputs on rhythmic variations of heart period of the cat. Am J Physiol 19; 128:775-789.
4. Kleiger RE, Miller JP, Bigger JT, et al. Decreased heart rate variability and its association with increased mortality after acute myocardial infarction. Am J Cardiol 1987; 59:256-262.
5. Kamath MV, Fallen EL. Power spectral analysis of HRV: a noninvasive signature of cardiac autonomic functions. Crit Rev Biomed Eng 1993; 21(3):245-311.
6. Ewing DJ, Martin CN, Young RJ, et al. The value of cardiovascular autonomic function tests: ten years experience in diabetes. Diabetes Care 1985; 8:491-498.
7. La Rovere MT, Specchia G, Mortara A, et al. Baroreflex sensitivity, clinical correlates and cardiovascular mortality among patients with a first myocardial infarction. A prospective study. Circulation 1988; 78:816-824.
8. DeBoer RW, Karemaker JM, Strackee J. Beat-to-beat variability of heart rate interval and blood pressure. Automedica 1983; 4:217-222.
9. Penaz J, Roukenz J, Van der Waal HJ. Spectral analysis of some spontaneous rhythms in the circulation, Biokybernetik. Bd.I, In: Drischel H, Tiedt N (eds). Leipzig, Germany: Karl Marx University, 1968; 233.
10. Sayers B Mc A. Analysis of heart rate variability. Ergonomics 1973; 16:85-97.
11. Akselrod S, D Gordon S, Ubel FA, et al. Power spectrum analysis of heart rate fluctuations: a quantitative probe of beat-to-beat cardiovascular control. Science 1981; 213:213-220.
12. Kitney RI, Rompelman O. Analysis of the human blood pressure and thermal control systems. In: Perkins J (ed). Biomedical Computing. Pitman Medical, 1977; 49-50.
13. Malliani A, Pagani M, Lombardi F, et al. Cardiovascular neural regulation explored in the frequency domain. Circulation: Research Advanced Series 1991; 84:482-492.
14. Pagani M, Lombardi F, Guzzetti S, et al. Power spectral analysis of a beat-to-beat heart rate and blood pressure variability as a possible marker of sympatho-vagal interaction in man and conscious dog. Circ Res 1986; 159:178-193.
15. Hirsch JA, Bishop B. Respiratory sinus arrhythmia in humans: how breathing pattern modulates heart rate. Am J Physiol 1981; 241:11620-11629.
16. Marple SL. Digital Spectral Analysis with Applications. Englewood Cliffs, NJ: Prentice Hall, 1987.
17. Kay SM, Marple SL. Spectrum analysis: a modern perspective. Proc IEEE 1981; 69:1380-1418.
18. Akaike H. Statistical predictor identification. Ann Inst Statist Math 1970; 22:203-217.
19. Akaike H. A new look at the statistical model identification. IEEE Trans Autom Contr 1974; AC-19:716-723.
20. Box GEP, Jenkins GM. Time Series Analysis: Forecasting and Control. San Francisco, Ca: Holden-Day, 1976.

21. Zetterberg LH. Estimation parameters for a linear difference equation with application to EEG analysis. Math Biosci 1969; 5:227-275.

22. Baselli G, Cerutti S, Civardi S, et al. Heart rate variability signal processing: a quantitative approach as an aid to diagnosis in cardiovascular pathologies. Int J Biomed Comput 1987; 20:51-70.

23. Novak P, Novak V. Time-frequency mapping of the heart rate, blood pressure and respiratory signal. Med Biol Eng Comput 1993; 31:103-110.

24. Cohen L. Time-frequency distribution—a review. Proc IEEE 1989; 177, 7:941-981.

25. Rioul O, Vetterli M. Wavelets and signal processing. IEEE SP Mag 1991; 26:14-38.

26. Bianchi AM, Mainardi LT, Petrucci E, et al. Time-variant power spectrum analysis for the detection of transient episodes in HRV signal. IEEE Trans Biomed Eng 1993; 40:136-144.

27. Bianchi AM, Cerutti S, Mainardi LT, et al. Time-variant spectral estimation of heart rate variability signal. Comp in Cardiol Conf; September 23-26, 1991; Venice, Italy.

28. Mainardi LT, Baselli G, Bianchi AM, et al. Time-variant estimation of the spectral parameters of the heart rate variability. Proc. 14th Annual Intern. Conf. of the IEEE Engin. Med. and Biol. Soc.; 1992; Paris, France.

29. Cerutti S, Bianchi AM, Baselli G, et al. Compressed spectral arrays for the analysis of 24-h heart rate variability signal: enhancement of parameters and data reduction. Comp Biomed Res 1989; 22:424-441.

30. Kobayashy M, Musha T. 1/f fluctuations of heartbeat period. IEEE Trans Biomed Eng 1982; 29:456-464.

31. Calcagnini G Jr, Lino S, Starno S, et al. 1/f spectrum of 24 hour heart rate variability signal in normal and hypertensive subjects. Comp in Cardiol Conf; September 5–8, 1993; London, England.

Chapter 6

Correction of the Heart Rate Variability Signal for Ectopics and Missing Beats

Markad V. Kamath, Ernest L. Fallen

Introduction

The sinoatrial (SA) node is the source of repetitive electrical impulses which generate the electrocardiogram (ECG) waveforms. In addition to the primary pacemaker in the sinus node, latent pacemakers exist throughout the heart, particularly in the atrioventricular (AV) node and the His-Purkinje system.[1] These latent pacemakers may interpose additional electrical impulses which appear as ectopic beats. Therefore, disturbances due to either abnormal impulse formation or impaired conduction gives rise to extra electrical wavelets or nonsinus beats, disrupting normal sinus-conducted RR interval variability. Since modulatory signals from the brain to the heart are embedded as variations in the beat-to-beat intervals of sinus rhythm, a locally generated aberrant beat will appear to temporarily disrupt neurocardiac modulation. The ectopic beat, often premature, produces a short beat-to-beat interval followed by a compensatory delay and hence, a longer than normal interval. Therefore, a sharp transient appears in the heart rate variability (HRV) signal. Ectopic beats can appear in ECGs recorded from both normal subjects and heart disease patients and, therefore, represent a major source of error when analyzing HRV data in both the time and frequency domain.

The issue of ectopics becomes relevant usually after QRS detection has been performed on the analog ECG signal and before the RR interval (or heart rate) time series undergoes HRV computation. Computation of either short- or long-term HRV indices is adversely affected by the presence of even a small number of ectopic beats. Figure 1 provides an example of the effects of a single ectopic beat on the power spectrum of HRV.[2]

Another source of error while computing the HRV signal occurs during detection and identification of the RR interval. If the software or the hardware which processes the raw ECG waveform misses a QRS complex or detects an extra RR interval, then a sharp transient appears in the HRV data. If

From: Malik M., Camm AJ (eds.): *Heart Rate Variability*. Armonk, NY. Futura Publishing Company, Inc., © 1995.

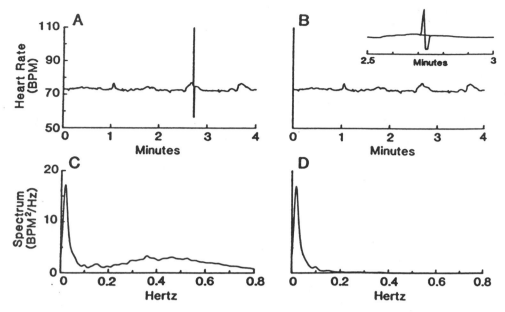

Figure 1. A single premature beat causes an abrupt increase followed by a decrease in heart rate. A: Frequency content of the impulse-like 'artifact' is broad; C: is eliminated; D: by removing the spike in time series; B: with a nonlinear computer filtering algorithm (inset). From Saul, et al. Am J Cardiol 1988; 61:1292-1299. Reprinted with Permission.

these errors are contained within a small number of beats, then it is possible to correct for these missing or additional beats and obtain a smooth HRV signal consistent with sinus conducted RR intervals, or more correctly, NN intervals.

This chapter addresses the issues that arise from the presence of ectopic and missing beats in the ECG signal and suggests techniques which should help correct sudden variations in the HRV signal due to ectopic or missing beats. We begin by examining the origin and prevalence of ectopic beats. The next section discusses how ectopic beats are identified and tagged. The significance of correcting ectopic beats is then explained. Algorithms for correcting ectopic and missing beats are described in the next section, and the final section discusses the limitations and recommendations for handling ectopic and missing beats.

Origin and Prevalence of Ectopic Beats

Ectopic beats can arise due to anomalies in the genesis of the pacemaking im-

pulse or because of impaired propagation of electrical impulses through the heart.[1] Abnormal impulse generation can give rise to atrial fibrillation, sinus tachycardia, sinus bradycardia, AV junctional premature beats, ventricular premature beats, ventricular tachycardia, and ventricular fibrillation. Conduction disturbances can result in rhythm disruption by introducing pauses due to a variety of blocks, ie, AV block, SA block, sinus arrest, etc. It is generally accepted that heightened adrenergic autonomic tone and psychological stressors may play a role in the generation and perpetuation of cardiac arrhythmias.[3,4] Ventricular ectopic beats (in runs or in isolation) can result in a momentary reduction in stroke volume, diminished systemic arterial blood pressure and reflex sympathetic stimulation.[5] Welch et al[6] reported a study where they recorded efferent sympathetic activity from the peroneal nerve using microneurographic techniques. It was observed that sporadic premature beats with coupling intervals less than 80% of sinus cycle length were consistently followed by a burst of sympathetic activity, which was significantly higher in amplitude and duration than were bursts of such activity during sinus rhythm. The magnitude of this burst activity increased as the coupling interval of the premature beat decreased. However, it is generally believed that an isolated ectopic beat does not cause any phase change in the HRV signal or its power spectrum.[2,7]

Cardiac dysrhythmias occur at one time or another in 90% to 95% of patients with acute myocardial infarction[1] and 70% to 95% of patients with congestive heart failure due to cardiomyopathy.[8] A recent study reports that approximately one third of healthy men have one or more ventricular premature beats during a 1-hour recording and 12% had frequent or complex ventricular arrhythmias.[9] Therefore, one encounters ectopic beats frequently among patients undergoing tests for HRV. There is therefore, a need to develop tools to correct the HRV data which contains ectopic beats.

Identification of Ectopic, Missing or Spurious Beats

An aberrant QRS complex in an ECG tracing gives rise to a nonsinus-conducted RR interval. This is due to the fact that while the true sinus rate ought to be measured by the PP interval, the RR intervals are detected with a greater degree of confidence in practice. In general, most QRS detection algorithms ignore the presence or absence of P waves while computing the RR interval and therefore, an ectopic beat can give rise to a spurious nonsinus, short RR interval which is followed by a long compensatory pause. This appears as a sharp transient spike in the HRV time series.

Apart from ectopic beats, two other types of errors can arise with any QRS detector, whether it is implemented through hardware or a function subroutine. If a QRS complex is detected prematurely when in fact a sinus conducted R wave has not occurred, this error is labeled as a Type A error.[10] A Type A error occurs when the threshold for identifying the R wave is set too low. In ef-

fect, this would subdivide an RR interval into additional inter-event intervals due to sensing of the T and/or P waves. Alternatively, a threshold detector set too high may fail to detect the occurrence of an R wave, an error which is labeled a Type B error. This type of error would merge two consecutive RR intervals and would result in an exceptionally wide inter-event interval.

Visual inspection of both ECG and HRV data is strongly recommended while processing the HRV signal. In acute studies lasting a few minutes, the ECG should be viewed continuously during the recording period. Many data acquisition software packages have tagging and annotation facilities to mark ectopics. During QRS detection the ectopics are clearly identified and the corresponding data segment may be either discarded or corrected. For 24-hour studies, where the ECG data is recorded on a Holter tape and analyzed off-line, the technologist performing the analysis has to assure strict quality control. Most Holter analysis software packages perform automatic ECG recognition and classification of all beats and annotate a class against each individual beat (Figure 2). The technologist scans different morphologies of beats and ascertains their accuracy, a procedure which can be time consuming. Often, an individual tape may require up to 45 minutes for thorough analysis, annotation and editing. Thus, an analysis of Holter tapes for deriving the HRV indices is labor intensive and prone to errors. Therefore, a well-trained Holter technologist plays a critical role by identifying and delineating aberrant beats. Once the ectopic, missing or spurious beats are identified and tagged, segments containing these are either corrected or rejected. Thereafter, it is up to the automated HRV analysis software to incorporate the corrected RR intervals in the computational algorithms.

Significance of Identifying and Correcting Aberrant Beats in the Heart Rate Variability Signal

Whether one is dealing with time-domain or frequency-domain analysis, ectopic

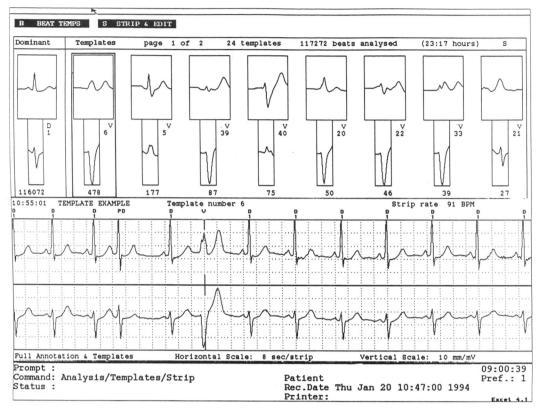

Figure 2. Typical annotated output of a Holter ECG analysis program. Top half of the figure displays two channels of the various templates and the number of beats in each template. Dominant beat morphology has 116,072 beats over a 23:17 hour period. Lower half displays sample annotation which includes two premature beats. The interbeat intervals can be downloaded onto a floppy for off-line signal processing. D: dominant; V: ventricular; PD: premature depolarization.

or missing beats introduce significant errors into the HRV statistics. During time-domain analysis of HRV, data is passed through various filters which incorporate only normal sinus beats. Additional logical conditions are imposed on the data to eliminate beats which appear before and after an ectopic beat.[11] For power spectral analysis, it has been suggested that one may correct the HRV signal for ectopic beats in one of the following two ways:

1. If the HRV time series contains occasional ectopic or anomalous beats, one can interpolate around the extra beat(s) and then perform the subsequent power spectral analysis; and
2. If there are frequent ectopics, it is better to eliminate the segments of

the HRV signal that contain the ectopics.

The first procedure assumes that the beat-to-beat control exerted by the autonomic nervous system did not play a significant role in the generation of ectopics and hence ignores such effects. The second procedure simply reduces the number of useful data segments for estimation of HRV indices. Meyers et al[5] estimated the number of useful 4-minute segments that can be derived from an hour's Holter ECG record for computing power spectra by employing Welch's overlapped method. They note that even a small number of ectopic beats can significantly decrease the amount of ectopy-free data available. For a patient with a 0.2% incidence of ectopy (about 7 ectopic beats/

hour), with a 50% overlap of HRV data, only 30% of the data is useful. In patients whose ECG contains ectopic beats, an aggregation or cluster of ectopy may actually increase the number of useable segments, as opposed to when extra beats appear at random intervals. Molgaard [12] states that both the standard deviation of the 24-hour heart rate and root mean square of SD (r-MSSD) are very sensitive to missed beats, especially in patients with reduced HRV.

Algorithms for Correcting Ectopic, Missing and Spurious Beats

In the case of ectopic beats, one can substitute an ectopic beat by computing the average of neighboring normal RR intervals without causing undue bias in the data. In this section we present algorithms which correct the HRV signal for ectopics or extra beats generated by errors in detection. Of these algorithms, the first two are appropriate for correcting the HRV signal containing ectopics, before computing a power spectrum of HRV.[13] Type A and Type B errors can be corrected by algorithm described by Cheung[10]. We present an algorithm developed in our laboratory, which is based on Cheung's algorithm, for correcting both ectopic beats and beats generated due to Type A and Type B errors.[14]

Algorithm 1[13]

Let R(k) be the autocorrelation function (ACF) of the given time series, for lags 1..k. for the HRV signal x(n), where n is the sample number 0...N. In the absence of ectopic beats, R(k) is estimated to be:

$$R(k) = 1/(N-k) \sum_{n=0}^{N-k-1} x(n)*x(n+k) \quad (1)$$

If there are ectopics, then estimate R(k) from only those beats which are normally conducted:

$$R(k) = 1/N_k \sum_{n} x(n)*x(n+k) \quad (2)$$

where N_k is defined as the number of terms

for which x(n)*x(n+k) is computed without ectopics. If there are no ectopics equation 2 reduces to equation 1. Once the ACF is computed using equation 2, the estimation of power spectrum proceeds through a computation of the fast Fourier transform of the windowed ACF.

Algorithm 2[13]

Use linear spline interpolation to compute the value of the heart rate at any instant where an ectopic beat appears. If x(n) is the HRV signal for which an ectopic beat exists at instant, n, then estimate:

$$x(n) = x(n0) \quad (3)$$
$$+ (x(n1)-x(n0))*(n-n0)/(n1-n0)$$

where x(n0) is the value of the signal at instant immediately prior to n and x(n1) is the value of HR at an instant subsequent to n. Computation of the autocorrelation and power spectrum then proceeds as before.

Albrecht and Cohen[13] state that algorithm 2 performs better than algorithm 1 because it introduces less high-frequency noise into the computation process. Confidence intervals for power spectral components estimated by both methods are given.[13] The mathematical basis for these algorithms are detailed in reports by Parzen[15] and Scheinok.[16]

Algorithm 3

An implicit assumption that underlies the correction of ectopic or erroneously detected beats is that the RR interval during sinus rhythm does not oscillate significantly from the mean value.[10] Secondly, variability of inter-event intervals containing errors is greater than the variability of the corresponding RR intervals. Based on these assumptions, Cheung[10] describes an algorithm suitable for correcting HRV signal for beats generated by false triggering (Type A or Type B error). Recovery of the actual RR interval is then attempted before comparison of further inter-event intervals is to proceed.

The basis of this algorithm is to compare each inter-event interval to the preceding one. If the difference in width exceeds certain percentages, an error is detected. Figure 3 presents a flow chart of the algorithm. The recovery procedure consists of iteratively summing into or subdividing the inter-event interval in question and comparing the outcome to the preceding inter-event interval until an acceptable reconstruction is achieved. Thus, assuming that the inter-event interval used as the standard for the first comparison is not in error, the algorithm processes each consecutive inter-event interval to correct detected errors, and then uses the processed inter-event interval as the standard for the next comparison (Figure 4). It is recommended by Cheung that the corrections using his algorithm be applied for any HRV signal where the maximum expected increase over a single RR interval and the maximum expected decrease over a single RR interval are less than 32.5% and 24.5%, respectively of the previous interval.

Algorithm 4[14]

In our laboratory we have developed an algorithm that works with RR intervals downloaded from a Holter analysis computer system. The algorithm combines the error detection part of algorithm 3 with the interpolation part of algorithm 2. The annotation file provided by the Holter is examined to see if the interval is an irregular interval. Secondly, the value of the RR interval is verified to be within 30% of at least four previous intervals which have passed this test. If the RR interval does not meet this criterion, it is considered an error. Once an error is detected, the program will find the first correct beat

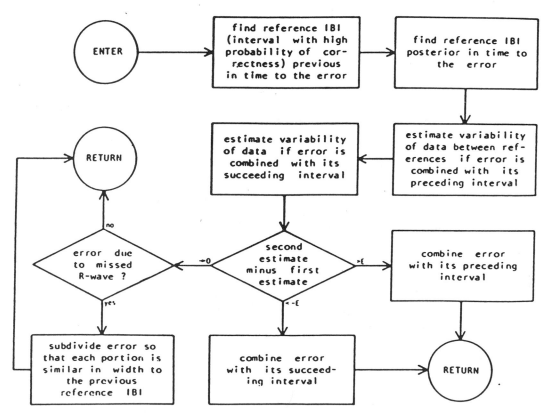

Figure 3. Algorithm to recover missing beats. The symbol E denotes the minimum expected difference between the two variability estimates if a false trigger error has occurred. From Cheung[10].

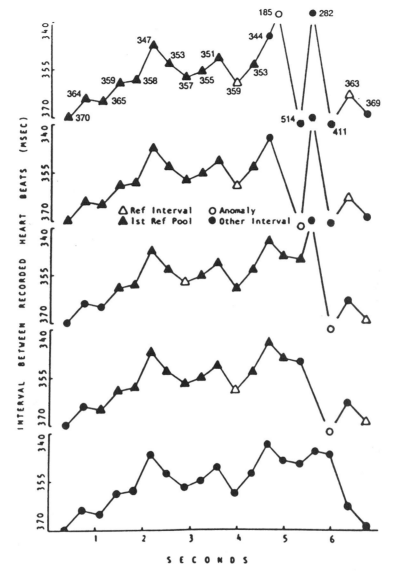

Figure 4. Example of the error processing algorithm. The top band shows the original data from a pediatric subject containing four errors in four consecutive beats, with actual intervals noted next to each data point. Each remaining band shows the outcome of one iteration through the algorithm. From Cheung[10].

before and after the beat(s) in question, using the RR interval and morphology information. If there are more than one irregular intervals in succession, a check is made of the number of erroneous beats and their total duration. If this duration represents more than the sum of four recent correct beats, then we tag that interval as an error that cannot be corrected and terminate the time series at the last correct beat. If the interval is less than four beats, the time duration between the two correct beats is now replaced with a combination of either the sum of two adjacent beats, or divided into two beats (algorithm 3) or interpolated with a linear spline (algorithm 2) . A flow chart for this procedure is shown in Figure 5. Figures 6A and B show the results of applying ectopic

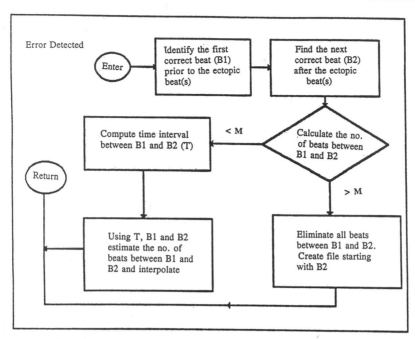

Figure 5. An algorithm to recover ectopic and missing beats. M: maximum number of errors that can be encountered in a row. We set M = 4 empirically.

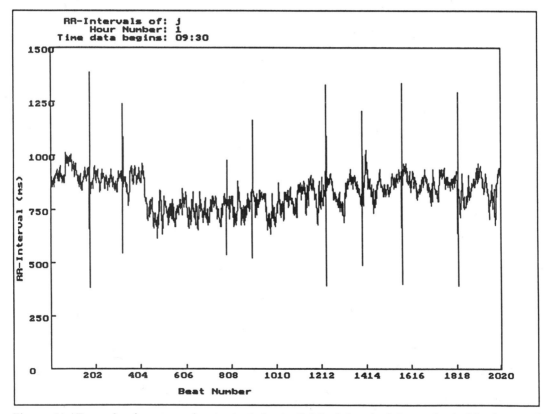

Figure 6A. Example of recovery from ectopic beats. Original data had 8 ectopics in 30 minutes of HRV signal.

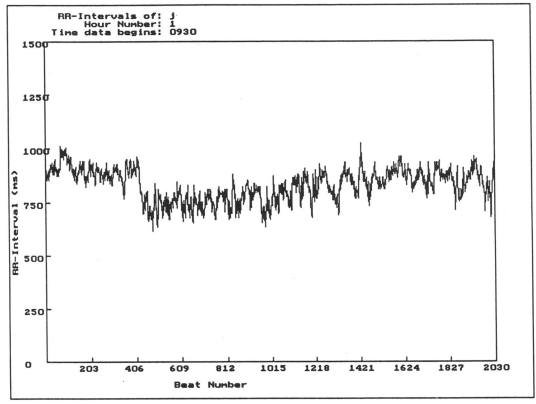

Figure 6B. Example of recovery from ectopic beats. The HRV data after correction using algorithm given in Figure 5.

correction algorithm to an HRV time series from a patient.

Recommendations and Limitations

If ectopic beats occur frequently (say every few seconds) in the ECG signal, then one is not able to evaluate a patient's neurocardiac control through HRV techniques. If the data is nonstationary and there are a number of ectopics in the ECG, one is advised to reject the signal segment altogether. It is interesting to note that there are no specific recommendations in the literature as to the maximum number of ectopics one can interpolate or accept.[17-19] Most investigations in the HRV field generally reject signal segments containing ectopics.[20] Huikuri et al[21] reject all ectopic complexes and all 5-minute complexes with <30 sinus beats. However, no interpolation techniques were employed. Bigger et al[22] reject segments if they contain >3 seconds (consecutively) of noise or more than two consecutive atrial or ventricular premature complexes. Kleiger et al[23] accept only those sinus intervals which do not exceed 20% of the previous beat.

While laboratory conditions may be closely controlled, artifacts are present in almost all Holter ECGs. There are two basic considerations for handling artifacts in the Holter ECG record. The first of these arises out of the need for obtaining stationary data and the second relates to the issue of identifying the artifacts and correcting them. In any acute laboratory study, if steady state conditions are maintained for the prescribed duration, artifacts are unlikely to occur, except perhaps during exercise. In uncooperative subjects, infants, or during longer term ECG recordings lasting several hours, it is virtually impossible to achieve steady state conditions and therefore, artifacts present a serious problem. Identification of artifacts can be carried out by visual editing of the raw ECG data or after QRS detection. An algorithm which automatically identifies and corrects the HRV signal for artifacts may be employed.[24] However, this correction must be viewed from the perspective of preserving the physiological and statistical stationarity of the data under question, ie, if the HRV data is nonstationary, it is unlikely to be suitable for power spectral analysis.

With more than a decade of experience in handling HRV data in our laboratory,[19] we suggest there be no more than two or three ectopic beats in a short-term study (less than 5 minutes), with no more than two beats occurring in succession. In longer data sets lasting several minutes to hours, investigators are urged to verify that there are no runs of ectopic beats, or periodic interposition of nonsinus beats. In our laboratory, we arbitrarily limit our analysis to those data sets which have less than 20 ectopic beats/hour. In a period containing more than 3000 beats, this represents less than 0.7% of the total number of beats. If there are more frequent ectopics, as occurs not infrequently in patients with severe coronary disease, it is suggested that the longest ectopic-free data segments be examined first followed by interpolation of those segments which contain less than five ectopics for every 15 minutes. Whatever the algorithm used for correcting HRV data containing abnormal intervals, it should be stressed that the investigator ensure that:

1. characteristics of the underlying physiological process is reflected in the computation;
2. data is not distorted by preprocessing; and
3. it is preferable to use data segments that are free of ectopics.

Acknowledgments: The authors wish to thank Dr. A.R.M. Upton, Professor of Medicine at McMaster, for his generous support and advice. We acknowledge the support of the DeGroote Foundation and the Heart and Stroke Foundation of Ontario.

References

1. Chung EK. Principles of Cardiac Arrhythmias, 4th ed. Baltimore, Md: Williams and Wilkins, 1989; 3-4.
2. Saul JP, Arai Y, Berger RD, et al. Assessment of autonomic regulation in chronic congestive heart failure by heart rate spectral analysis. Am J Cardiol 1988; 61:1292-1299.
3. Coumel P. Rate dependence and adrenergic dependence of arrhythmias. Am J Cardiol 1989; 64:41J-45J.
4. Lown B, DeSilva R. Roles of psychologic stress and autonomic nervous system changes in provocation of ventricular premature complexes. Am J Cardiol 1979; 41:979-985.
5. Myers G, Workman M, Birkett C, et al. Problems in measuring heart rate variability of patients with congestive heart failure. J Electrocardiol 1992; 25(suppl):214-219.
6. Welch WJ, Smith ML, Rea RF, et al. Enhancement of sympathetic nerve activity by single premature ventricular beats in humans. J Am Coll Cardiol 1989; 13:69-75.
7. Birkett CL, Kienzle MG, Myers GA. Mechanisms underlying alterations in power spectra of heart rate variability associated with ectopy. Proceedings of Annual Conference on Computers in Cardiology. Washington, DC: IEEE Computer Society Press, 1992; 19:391-394.
8. Podrid PJ, Fogel RI, Fuchs TT. Ventricular arrhythmia in congestive heart failure. Am J Cardiol 1992; 69:82G-96G.
9. Bikkina M, Larson MG, Levy D. Prognostic implications of asymptomatic ventricular arrhythmias: The Farmingham Heart Study. Ann Intern Med 1992; 117:990-996.
10. Cheung MN. Detection of recovery from errors in cardiac interbeat intervals. Psychophysiology 1981; 18:341-346.
11. Malik M, Cripps T, Farrell T, et al. Prognostic value of heart rate variability after myocardial infarction. Med Biol Eng Comput 1989; 27:603-611.
12. Molgaard H. Evaluation of the Reynolds Pathfinder II system for 24h heart rate vari-

ability analysis. Eur Heart J 1991; 12:1153-1162.

13. Albrecht P, Cohen RJ. Estimation of heart rate power spectrum bands from real-world data: dealing with ectopic beats with noisy data. Comp in Cardiol., Washington, DC, 1988; 15:311-314.

14. Ramnauth L, Sarvanandan S. Twenty-four Hour Heart Rate Variability Analysis Software. Hamilton, Canada: McMaster University, Department of Computer Science and Systems, 1993. BSc Thesis.

15. Parzen E. On spectral analysis with missing observations and amplitude modulation. Sankhya A 1963; 25:383-392.

16. Scheinok PA. Spectral analysis with randomly missed observations: the binomial case. Ann Math Stat 1965; 36:971-977.

17. Kleiger RE, Stein PK, Bosner MS, et al. Time domain measures of HRV. Cardiol Clin 1992; 10:487-498.

18. Ori Z, Monir G, Weiss J, et al. Heart rate variability—frequency domain analysis. Cardiol Clin 1992; 10:499-533.

19. Kamath MV, Fallen EL. Power spectral analysis of heart rate variability: a noninvasive signature of cardiac autonomic function. Crit Rev Biomed Eng 1993; 21:245-311.

20. Myers GA, Martin GJ, Magid NM, et al. Power spectral analysis of heart rate variability in sudden cardiac death. IEEE Trans Biomed Eng 1986; BME-33:1149-1156.

21. Huikuri HV, Kessler KM, Terracall EL, et al. Reproducibility and circadian rhythm of heart rate variability in healthy subjects. Am J Cardiol 1990; 65:391-393.

22. Bigger TJ, La Rovere MT, Steinman RC, et al. Comparison of baroreflex sensitivity and heart period variability after myocardial infarction. J Am Coll Cardiol 1989; 13:1511-1518.

23. Kleiger RE, Miller JP, Bigger JT, et al. Decrease heart rate variability and its association with increased mortality after acute myocardial infarction. Am J Cardiol 1987; 59:256-262.

24. Berntson GG, Quigley KS, Jang JF, et al. An approach to artifact identification: application to heart period data. Psychophysiology 1990; 27:586-598.

Chapter 7

Nonlinear Methods for Heart Rate Variability Assessment

Georg Schmidt, Gregor E. Morfill

Rhythmicity, a major feature of the electrocardiogram (ECG) signal, is a characteristic of biological systems and deviations from rhythmicity are often associated with information transfer. RR intervals describe the cardiac rhythm and are a very interesting data subset, although they constitute only a small fraction of the entire ECG signal. They contain a great deal of information about intracardiac and extracardiac processes. This information includes the active function control by the autonomic nervous system. Figure 1 shows the RR intervals plotted over 24 hours for two patients suffering from coronary artery disease. The plots illustrate the complexity as well as the transient character of the structures found in such a data set. One can clearly see the fuzzy dark bands of the sinus rhythm as well as structured and apparently structureless arrhythmias. Obviously, the tachograms contain a great deal of information on cardiac function.

In recent years, analysis of heart rate variability (HRV) has become a standard tool for the prediction of cardiac mortality with the general 'rule of thumb' that a reduced variability is a signature for disease and enhanced risk.[1-13] However, the clinical value of the methods employed (eg, the calculation of averages, standard deviations and variances of RR interval subsets, analysis of the frequency content) is limited: false positive results cut the positive predictive value down to 30%. A possible reason for this disappointing value might be found in the data analysis technique—the standard methods truncate the available information considerably, as is exemplified in Figure 2.

Within the last years, significant progress has been achieved in the theory and analysis of 'complex systems.' The methods of nonlinear dynamics are gaining a great deal of momentum, sparked by the advances made on a fundamental information theoretical level in the study of chaotic systems, and by the great interest in physics,

From: Malik M., Camm AJ (eds.): *Heart Rate Variability*. Armonk, NY. Futura Publishing Company, Inc., © 1995.

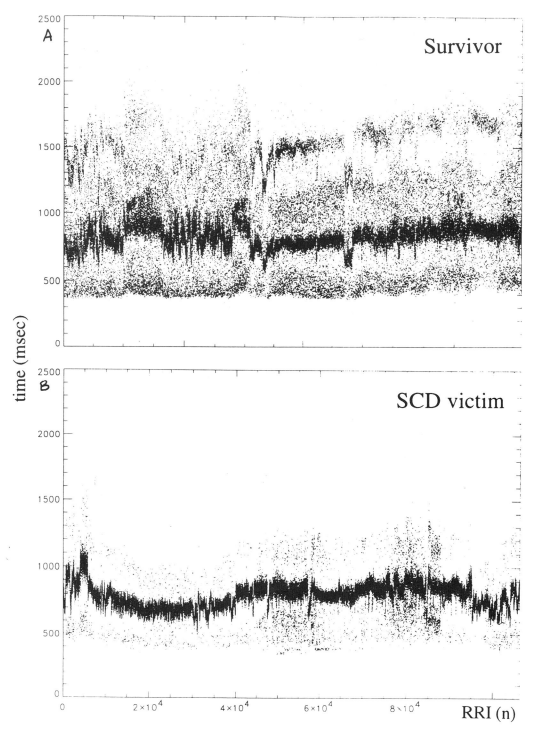

Figure 1. Tachograms of two patients suffering from coronary artery disease associated with frequent ventricular arrhythmias: The first patient (A) has survived now for more than 8 years, the second patient (B) died suddenly a few months after the ECG was recorded.

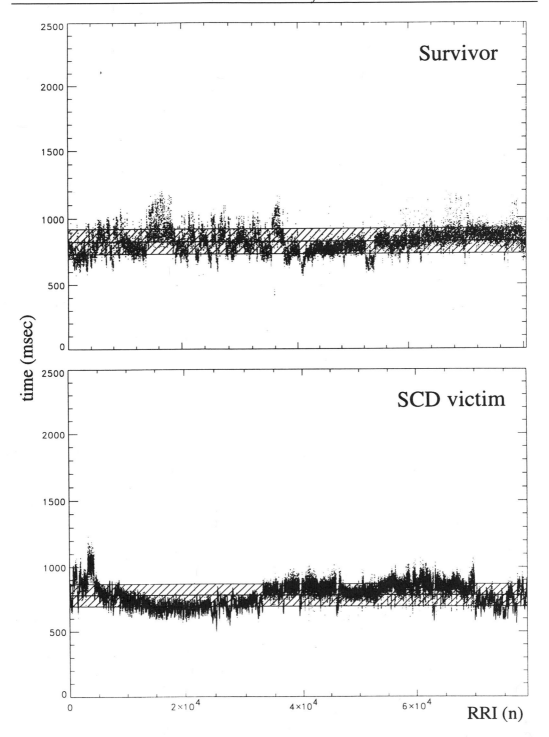

Figure 2. Truncation of the tachogram information of Figure 1 by filtering out all ventricular ectopies and calculating HRV as standard deviation around the 24-hour mean (9).

chemistry, engineering, information science etc. to characterize complex systems quantitatively.

Phase Space Representation

Nonliving Systems

Many-body systems, such as gases, may be regarded as being among the most complex physical (ie, nonliving) systems. Very successful methods have been developed for their description, starting from the basic kinetic theory, statistical mechanics and thermodynamics. The great achievement has been to link the dynamics of all the individual particles to the macroscopic state variables (ie, pressure, temperature), although the individual particles can only be described by their position and their velocity and consequently, do not possess a 'pressure' or a 'temperature.'

One major concept is to represent the system *at a given moment in time* as a single point in a so-called 'phase space.' This point defines the 'state' of the system at that moment. To be able to do this, a phase space has to be constructed, which includes six dimensions (or coordinates) for each particle of the system (three space or position coordinates and three velocity coordinates). For a system of N particles (for gases N is of the order of 10^{19}) this requires a phase space with 6N dimensions. Since the particles continuously move and collide, the 'state' of the system continuously changes, ie, its position in phase space moves in time along a characteristic trajectory. If this evolution is followed for a sufficiently long period of time, a representative distribution of states (points along the trajectory) has been sampled (this is the ergodic hypothesis). Observing for a very much longer period improves the statistics but does not conjure up any new dynamics. The system can then be characterized by this distribution of 'states' in phase space.

The distribution of points (states) in phase space is described by a 'distribution function' $f_{6N}(\underline{x})$, where $\underline{x}$ is a 6N-dimensional 'position' vector. Appropriate statistical analyses can be performed (eg, ensemble averages) to obtain macroscopic quantities that are measurable. This makes the microscopic theory subject to observational tests and thus opens the way to improve the basic kinetic theory (eg, mixtures of gases, molecules). In this iterative way, the theory has been developed to a high level of sophistication, including relativistic and quantum effects.

Biological Systems

For the analysis of complex biological systems we propose a similar approach however, there have to be some conceptual adaptations which have important consequences for the subsequent analysis[14,15]:

1. In contrast to nonliving systems, biological systems not only passively react to external influences but also employ active control mechanisms. These include various *sensors*, an *information transmission system*, a central *data processing unit* and peripheral *effectors* (Figure 3).
   Thus, the complexity of a biological system is not only caused by the number of interacting independent components, but also by a number of feed-back and feed-forward mechanisms in order to optimize the survival chances. Within the system, information is both created and destroyed (see below). The transfer of the analysis methods from nonliving to living systems must therefore be done with great care. Any interpretation requires close collaboration between the disciplines involved (eg, mathematics, physics, medicine).
2. In the case of the cardiovascular system, there are no obvious dynamical variables which correspond to those that define the phase space in physical systems. Recourse is taken to using an 'artificial phase space,' a procedure which is commonly used in complex physical systems where

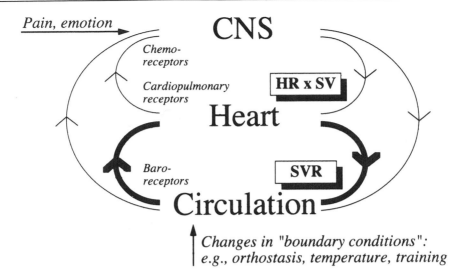

Figure 3. Simplified schematic diagram of relevant 'control circuits' in the cardiovascular system. The central parameter is the cardiac output, the product of stroke volume (SV) and heart rate (HR). The thin curved arrows describe the information transfer through the autonomous nervous system. In case of a dysfunction of one of the system's components, compensatory changes in the other components will try to keep the entire system within its normal 'operating limits.' These compensatory mechanisms affect all components on different reaction time scales.

only one measurement quantity is available as a time series. In our case, points or 'states' of the system in such an artificial phase space are constructed from RR interval trains of length 'n' which are represented on 'n' orthogonal axes in an n-dimensional artificial phase space (Figure 4). The usefulness of artificial phase space is discussed in Takens.[16]

3. 'States' of biological systems include all the usual functions and operations of the system under consideration—its response to external stimuli, work loads, temperature, training, psychological effects, sleep etc. This means using long-term (eg, 24-hour) ECGs in order to ensure a 'representative' sampling.

4. It is important to make sure that the phase space dimension 'n' is sufficiently large to embed the underlying dynamics of the system without 'distorting' projections. If the phase space dimension is not sufficiently high, the structure of the points representing the 'states' of the system

is seen in a projection, ie, only part of the information is available. If the projection angle happens to be chosen badly, there could be overlaps, for instance, leading to interpretative problems (see Figure 5).

The appropriate phase space dimension can be determined by evaluating the structural complexity measure α (see below for the definition) for increasing phase space dimensions (longer RR interval trains). The $N(\alpha)$ histogram eventually registers no change (within statistical limits) above a certain value, 'n.' This then is the required artificial phase space dimension, which has to be used for the data analysis.

5. The artificial phase space dimension for dynamical biological systems is generally low compared to the 6N of many-body systems. In a sense, the required phase space dimension, 'n,' which embeds the biological system, is an expression of its complexity. For most ECGs we have found

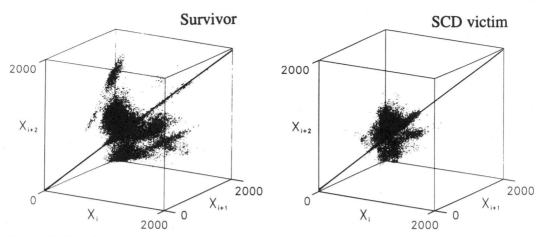

Figure 4. The phase space diagrams of the RR interval data shown in Figure 1. Each point in this diagrams signifies three successive RR intervals plotted along the x_i, x_{i+1}, and x_{i+2} axes of the phase space cube respectively. The distribution of points corresponds to the distribution of 'states' of the cardiovascular system. The central club-shaped structure along the diagonal signifies the sinus rhythm, slow heart rates at the top, fast rates at the bottom. Arrhythmias produce additional structures.

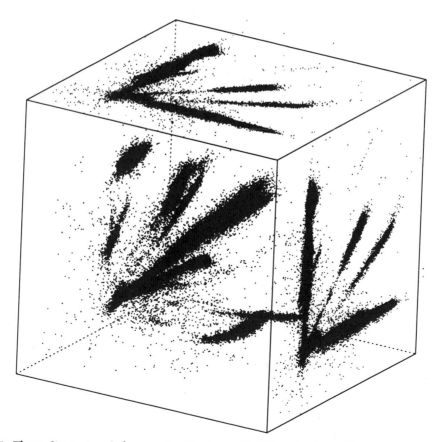

Figure 5. Three-dimensional phase space diagram with 2-D projections. The projections appear less complex than the 3-D structure. This is due to overlapping features.

that n = 3 is sufficient for a clean analysis.

6. The complexity is governed by practical limitations. For a given measurement accuracy, small influences can be overlooked and the system might appear less complex than it really is. This possibility emphasizes the need for high accuracy in biological data sensors. In the same vein, if a change in the phase space dimension is observed from one measurement cycle to the next, one should be aware that this could have different origins. For instance, a decrease in dimensionality may reflect a real evolution change, but may equally well or even more likely not be associated with a real decrease in the complexity of the system. In the latter case, it could be caused by a *transient domination of a single component* over others, whose fluctuations may have dwindled below the measurement accuracy. This again emphasises the need for long data sets.

Complexity Measures—General Comments

Any quantity derived from measured data of a given system, which characterizes that system, may be termed a 'measure' of that system (eg, average properties, standard deviation, variance). When this measure incorporates aspects of the complex dynamics of the system, we may describe it somewhat more accurately as a 'complexity measure.' These complexity measures may be 'differential' or 'integral'—a well-known example of a differential complexity measure is the Fourier spectrum—a corresponding integral measure could be the bandwidth or the integrated power.

For the analysis and characterization of complex systems, differential complexity measures are almost invariably required, in particular those that allow the correlations to be quantified on all scales of interest. Attempts to characterize complex systems with, eg, two-point correlation analyses or by specifying their correlation dimension, Ljapunov exponent or Kolmogorov entropy (to name a few possibilities), are unlikely to be wholly successful, because these measures emphasize the dominant mode or structure in the data set. The finer details, which may well carry the significant information, could be overlooked.

On the other hand, using, eg, Fourier analysis or power spectra does give information on the whole spectrum of the modes present however, this is obtained at the expense of losing the correlation. These techniques are very useful for picking out important rhythms (eg, diurnal, respiration) but not for identifying complex patterns. For this more general problem, we have to employ new approaches.

Structures in the Phase Space Distribution

When we look at a picture or a landscape, for instance, we observe 'structures.' These structures have certain forms, eg, they may be clumpy, have straight lines, curvy lines, diffuse cloudy shapes etc.—a complex picture will generally have a combination of such 'structures.' It has been demonstrated that for many natural systems (eg, certain leaves, flowers, trees), their fractal geometry can be used to characterize their structure quantitatively and efficiently.[17]

In our case we want to characterize a cloud of points (states) in an n-dimensional phase space. It seems expedient to do this utilizing this concept. Of course, we have to be aware that the phase space distribution may (and generally will) contain many structures and features—this means we have to use an approach which emphasizes the multifractal nature for a structural measure of complexity.

There is one aspect to be kept in mind, however, the *scale*. A diffuse structure on a fine scale may look point-like on a coarse scale—it clearly matters at what resolution a 'picture' is viewed. The optimum choice for this resolution is difficult to assess generally. There are practical limitations in trying to make too fine a resolution—these are statistical uncertainties in defining an adequate structure parameter. There are other limitations in making the resolution too coarse—one may overlook the important smaller scale aspects. Some compromise has to be found which avoids both pitfalls—this is usually the major problem in quantitative structure analysis, and clear 'prescriptions' or 'rules' do not exist. One way is to try different resolution scales and to compare the computed structural complexity measures. When the measures are 'stable' to variations in resolution and still reflect the complex structure adequately (this can be checked by reconstruction, for instance), the characterization may be regarded as 'good' and becomes acceptable.

For our purposes, structural complexity measures have to be able to characterize a whole range of different forms and shapes in n-dimensional phase space quantitatively and the resolution (or scale) has to be chosen in a way commensurate with the complexity of the problem under study. The most successful technique known to us so far for doing this is the 'scaling index method' (SIM), which was developed by the MPE and patented by the Max Planck Society.

Dynamics of Information Flow in Phase Space

Regarding the dynamical evolution of the system, we could for instance, characterize the trajectory in phase space in some suitable way. This turns out to be almost impossible (with as many as 100 000 data points) and in any case may be too detailed to be of practical interest (or too long-term, whichever the case may be). An approach which has been used in statistical quantum mechanics, and which has been very useful for predicting quantum states and spectroscopic signatures, has been the concept of 'transition probabilities.' Borrowing from this concept, we coarse-grain the phase space

into subvolumes (cells denoted by the letter $i = 1$ to i_{max}) and calculate the occupation probability, P_i, as well as the transition probability from each subvolume to each other one, $P_i \rightarrow j$, as well as the probability of being accessed by a given subvolume, $P_i \leftarrow j$. From these probabilities we can calculate the 'net information change,' Δ_i, of a given cell 'i.' This information may be a 'gain' (if it is positive) or a loss (if it is negative).

For biological systems, this choice of dynamical variable or complexity measure appears particularly well suited. We mentioned earlier that biological systems not only process information but that they must be able to create and destroy it as well. The act of *creating* information may be associated with some positive reaction (eg, to a special demand or as a consequence of a pathological behavior). There may be instances when a great deal of information is produced (usually associated with special or extreme circumstances) and there will be (far more) instances when the system is preceding well within its normal operating limits and very little information change (positive or negative) is necessary to keep it going. The act of *destroying* information can be associated with the return path of the system into its normal operating mode—akin to, eg, electrical shutdown when idling or going into standby mode. For the cardiovascular system, such situations occur, eg, during recovery from physical or mental activity or pathological states. Being able to quantitatively characterize these aspects of biological system behavior allows us to investigate both normal and abnormal appearing signatures in detail—by first identifying them and then examining all aspects closely in the original ECG.

Naturally, the same procedure can be followed with the structural complexity measures or, even better, by employing a combination of the two. This would appear to be the most powerful and theoretically well-founded (from complex system theory) technique for characterizing complex data sets quantitatively, identifying special

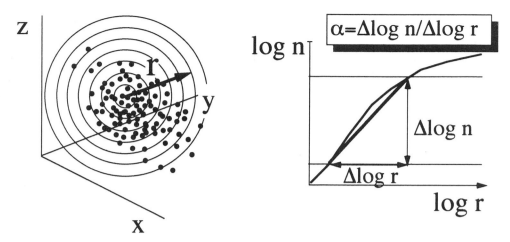

Figure 6. Computation of α: In the left panel the computation $N_i(r)$ is shown, the right panel depicts the fitting of the scaling index α. For a complete description see text.

features and investigating them in the fullest available detail.

Let us add a note of caution, however. The research field of 'complexity characterization' of dynamical systems is young and new discoveries abound. The complexity measures that can be used are to some extent still a matter of choice and personal preference—no theory exists yet, which can give a clear guideline. See, however, Wackerbauer et al, for an attempt at ordering.[18]

Definition of Complexity Measures

Scaling Index α

The *scaling index* α makes use of the local fractal structure of the state distribution in phase space. It is calculated by counting the number of states 'N,' which occur within an n-dimensional sphere of radius 'r' around a point 'i,' located at ξ_i in phase space. By varying 'r,' we obtain the function $N_i(r)$, which can be represented (in a particular 'scaling' region) as a power law $\sim r^{\alpha}i$. The quantity α_i is the scaling index characterizing the structure in which the point 'i' is embedded (Figure 6). It is a property of that point. The distribution function is $f_n(\alpha_i, \xi_i)$ and by performing the appropriate

sums (or integrals) we can determine the $N(\alpha)$ histogram (Figure 7), which describes the structural complexity of the entire cardiac rhythm.

These $N(\alpha)$ histograms can be used to characterize RR intervals in a far more general and physiologically far more meaningful way than has been possible previously. Figure 7 shows the $N(\alpha)$ histograms of the patients whose tachograms are given in Figure 1. The first peak (at lower α's) represents the complexity of the sinus rhythm; the other(s), the complexity of the ectopies. In a clinical study on 59 patients suffering from CAD and frequent ventricular arrhythmias, patients with impaired left ventricular function and large complexity differences, $\Delta\alpha$, between sinus peak and that due to ectopies had an extremely increased risk for sudden death.[19,20]

Net Information Flow Δ

The *net information flow* Δ is derived as follows: the phase space is 'coarse grained' into cells of a given size (eg, 40 milliseconds) located at a mean position ξ_i. The choice of the cell size is again limited by statistical probabilities and resolution requirements, as in the case of structural complexity determination. Then the probabilities, P_i, of a given state being in any given subcell, 'i,'

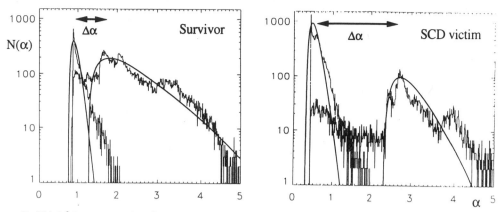

Figure 7. N(α) histograms for the same patients shown in Figure 1.

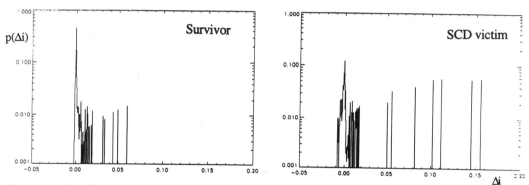

Figure 8. N(Δ) histograms for the same patients shown in Figure 1.

and the transfer probabilities, P_{ij}, of consecutive states occupying subcell 'i' and 'j,' respectively, are calculated. The net information flow for cell 'i' is then calculated from

$$\Delta_i = \sum P_{ij} \log P_i / P_j$$

As mentioned earlier, Δ_i can be positive or negative depending on the different transfer probabilities—representing information gain or loss respectively. Thus, the distribution function is $f_n(\Delta_i, \xi_i)$ and by performing the appropriate sums we can determine the N(Δ) histogram.

When an arrhythmia appears, information is created (positive Δ), when this arrhythmia terminates, this information will be destroyed (negative Δ). The net information flow during one such 'arrhythmia cy-

cle' is generally found to be small. In patients prone to sudden death, the amount of information created by arrhythmias and destroyed by their termination was significantly higher than in survivors. Figure 8 shows the N(Δ) histograms for the patients already described in Figures 1 and 7.

Concluding Remarks

The methods of nonlinear dynamics open up new and principally different ways to analyze HRV and cardiac arrhythmias. We can now separately quantify the complexity of sinus rhythm and that of ectopies. According to our observations, CAD patients with variably coupled arrhythmias

---

Note that the term 'complexity of arrhythmias' in this context is different to the concept of the Lown classification. We employ the structural and dynamical complexity measures described above for our definition.

and an invariable sinus rhythm, have an extreme sudden death risk, if the function of the left ventricle is impaired.

The pathophysiological mechanisms responsible for the observed arrhythmia complexity variations is up to now speculative. We do believe, however, that the complexity of arrhythmias is linked to their underlying electrophysiological mechanism. According to this view, low complexity arrhythmias possess a sound electrophysiological substrate (probably a reentry within a stable myocardial scar), whereas high complexity arrhythmias indicate an unstable substrate (eg, transient ischemia, early and late after-depolarizations). These are preliminary conclusions, which have to be followed up with detailed analyses, using the diagnostic tools which are being developed right now. In any case, it is not unlikely that the analysis of HRV with methods of nonlinear dynamics might open the way for a new classification of ventricular arrhythmias, which takes into consideration both the quantity of PCs and their complex interplay.

Acknowledgments: This chapter was written by us as representatives of the members of the *Zentrum für nichtlineare Dynamik in der Kardiologie.* These are Petra Barthel, Peter Brandl, Anna Goeldel, Horst Herb, Robert Ivancic, Heinz Kreuzberg (1. Medizinische Klinik der Technischen Universität München) and Wolfram Bunk, Valentin Demmel, Herbert Scheingraber, Renate Wackerbauer, Gerda Wiedenmann (Max-Planck-Institut für extraterrestrische Physik).

References

1. Algra A, Tijssen JG, Roelandt JR, et al. Heart rate variability from 24-hour electrocardiography and the 2-year risk for sudden death. Circulation 1993; 88(1):180-185.
2. Bigger JT Jr, Kleiger RE, Fleiss JL, et al. Components of heart rate variability measured during healing of acute myocardial infarction. Am J Cardiol 1988; 61(4):208-215.
3. Cripps TR, Malik M, Farrell TG, et al. Prognostic value of reduced heart rate variability after myocardial infarction: clinical evaluation of a new analysis method. Br Heart J 1991; 65(1):14-19.
4. Dougherty CM, Burr RL. Comparison of heart rate variability in survivors and non-survivors of sudden cardiac arrest. Am J Cardiol 1992; 70(4):441-448.
5. Ewing DJ. Heart rate variability: an important new risk factor in patients following myocardial infarction. Clin Cardiol 1991; 14(8):683-685.
6. Farrell TG, Bashir Y, Cripps T, et al. Risk stratification for arrhythmic events in post infarction patients based on heart rate variability, ambulatory electrocardiographic variables and the signal-averaged electrocardiogram. J Am Coll Cardiol 1991; 18(3):687-697.
7. Gomes JA, Winters SL, Ip J, et al. Identification of patients with high risk of arrhythmic mortality. Role of ambulatory monitoring, signal-averaged ECG, and heart rate variability. Cardiol Clin 1993; 11(1):55-63.
8. Huikuri HV, Kessler KM, Terracall E, et al. Reproducibility and circadian rhythm of heart rate variability in healthy subjects. Am J Cardiol 1990; 65(5):391-393.
9. Kleiger RE, Miller JP, Bigger JT Jr, et al. Decreased heart rate variability and its association with increased mortality after acute myocardial infarction. Am J Cardiol 1987; 59(4):256-262.
10. Malik M, Camm AJ. Significance of long term components of heart rate variability for the further prognosis after acute myocardial infarction. Cardiovasc Res 1990; 24(10):793-803.
11. Malik M, Cripps T, Farrell T, et al. Prognostic value of heart rate variability after myocardial infarction. A comparison of different data-processing methods. Med Biol Eng Comput 1989; 27:603-611.
12. Pipilis A, Flather M, Ormerod O, et al. Heart rate variability in acute myocardial infarction and its association with infarct site and clinical course. Am J Cardiol 1991; 67(13):1137-1139.
13. van Hoogenhuyze D, Martin GJ, Weiss JS, et al. Heart rate variability. An update. J Electrocardiol 1989; 22(1):204-208.
14. Schmidt G, Morfill G. Complexity diagnostics in cardiology: fundamental considerations. PACE 1994; 17:1174-1177.
15. Schmidt G, Morfill G. Complexity diagnostics in cardiology: methods. PACE 1994; 17:2336–2341.

16. Takens F. Detecting strange attractors in turbulence. Lecture Notes in Mathematics 898, 366, 1980.
17. Mandelbrot BB. The Fractal Geometry of Nature. New York, NY: WH Freeman and Co., 1982.
18. Wackerbauer R, Witt A, Atmanspacher H, et al. A comparative class of complex measures. Chaos, Solitons und Fractals 1994; 4:133-173.
19. Morfill G, Schmidt G. Komplexitätsanalyse in der Kardiologie: Fahndung nach Frühzeichen des Plötzlichen Herztodes. Physikalische Blätter 1994; 50:156-160.
20. Morfill G, et al. Der Plötzliche Herztod, Neue Erkenntnisse durch die Anwendung komplexer Diagnoseverfahren. Bioscope. 1994; 2:11–19.

Chapter 8

Effect of Electrocardiogram Recognition Artifact on Time-Domain Measurement of Heart Rate Variability

Marek Malik

Several studies by different research groups have clearly demonstrated the importance of heart rate variability (HRV) in both physiological investigations and clinical studies.[1-5] While the measurement of HRV in physiological and laboratory investigations is most frequently based on short-term recordings made under specific controlled circumstances, the clinical use of HRV, eg, its application among predictors of arrhythmic complications during the convalescent phase of myocardial infarction,[5-7] requires its estimation in long-term electrocardiograms (ECG). Although the values of HRV assessed from short-term ECGs carry clinically useful information,[8,9] the values of HRV derived from a complete 24-hour ECG recording appear to be more clinically useful than those obtained from short recordings.[9]

The measurement of HRV in long-term ECGs conforms to a standard procedure. Following an analogue-digital conversion of the ECG record, the recognition phase identifies all QRS patterns of ventricular activation, classifies them according to their morphology, and establishes their physiological interpretation (ie, classifies the complexes as belonging to normal sinus nodal rhythm, as supraventricular or ventricular ectopics, etc.). The result of the recognition phase is a digital record of the classification of each QRS complex and of the duration of each RR interval.

The sequence of QRS classifications and of the RR intervals may be used in many ways in order to measure HRV. Reported studies have used various time-domain and spectral-domain methods for expressing the value of HRV in numerical terms. The spectral-domain methods are known to be sensitive to artifact in automatic recognition of long-term ECGs. The use of spectral-domain methods is also more appropriate with short-term recordings in which the prerequisites of the spectral analysis, eg, the sta-

From: Malik M., Camm AJ (eds.): *Heart Rate Variability.* Armonk, NY. Futura Publishing Company, Inc., © 1995.

tionarity of the signal, can be more easily maintained. No study has so far demonstrated a clear advantage of spectral HRV measurement for its clinical use. Thus, clinical studies predominantly utilize time-domain methods. Some of the time-domain methods are believed to be less sensitive to artifact in automatic recognition of long-term ECGs and others have only been used together with visual checking and manual editing of the automatic recognition.

The visual verification and manual correction of the automatic recognition of a long-term ECG can be extremely time-consuming for 24-hour recordings. A perceived need for such a manual intervention discourages, to a certain degree, the assessment of HRV in routine clinical practice and confines the investigation of HRV to an academic setting. There is, therefore, a practical demand for fully automatic methods of HRV measurement which are robust and which provide clinically useful results for recordings of typical quality.

This chapter describes a study which evaluated the effects of the misrecognition artifact of the automatic ECG analysis on six methods for time-domain HRV measurement which have previously been shown to provide clinically relevant data.

Patients and Methods

Patients and Recordings

The study examined long-term ECGs recorded in 548 survivors of the acute phase of myocardial infarction. In each patient, a 24-hour ECG was recorded prior to discharge at a median of 7 days after infarction, the diagnosis of which was based on previously published criteria.[10] Patients with atrial fibrillation and permanent pacemaker implant were excluded, but as the study examined only the technical performance of different methods of HRV measurement, no other diagnostic selection criteria were applied to the patient population. However, 26 patients in whom the ECG record was

imperfect to the extent that its automatic recognition failed completely (details in following section), were not included into the studied population. Thus, the studied ECG records represented a typical mixture of good, average, and moderately poor quality long-term recordings obtained in a population of postinfarction patients. Similarly, the number of ectopic beats and other rhythm disturbances recorded in the studied ECGs should have been typical of such patients.

Analysis of Long-Term Electrocardiograms

The recordings were made on tape based Reynolds Tracker 2-channel recorders (leads II and modified CMS). An analysis of each record was obtained in two different ways. A visually checked recognition with a thorough manual correction was made using the Laser XP 8000 system of Marquette Electronics Inc, USA by a qualified operator. One computer file of QRS classification and RR intervals was produced before the visual and manual correction, and another file after completing the visual and manual correction.

As the Marquette system export the durations of RR intervals as a one byte value with the maximum value of 2 seconds in 8 bits, the intervals between adjacent QRS complexes were measured in arbitrary units corresponding to steps of 1/128 seconds (approximately 8 milliseconds).

Exclusion Criteria

The technical criteria, on the grounds of which the 26 ECG records mentioned in the previous section were excluded, required that the fully automatic recognition contained enough intervals between QRS complexes of normal supraventricular morphology belonging to the physiological sinus rhythm (the so-called 'normal-to-normal' RR intervals, or the NN intervals). Very small numbers of normal-to-normal RR intervals were unacceptable, since they did not permit the construction of a representative histogram of NN interval durations which was used in some of the HRV measurement methods. Thus, 26 ECG recordings were excluded because their automatic recognition contained fewer than 1000 NN intervals. The limit of 1000 NN intervals was selected arbitrarily. Most of these recordings were those in which one of the automatic recognition algorithms was unable to distinguish between QRS complexes of supraventricular and ventricular origin and diagnosed an 'unclassified' QRS morphology throughout the complete recording.

Measurement of Heart Rate Variability

The sequences of durations of the intervals between adjacent QRS complexes were analyzed using six different algorithms for time-domain measurement of HRV. All methods analyzed only the NN intervals. The following methods were used:

1. standard deviation of the durations of normal-to-normal RR intervals (SDNN);
2. standard deviation of 5-minute averages of normal-to-normal RR intervals (SDANN);
3. root mean square difference between immediately successive normal-to-normal RR intervals (rMSSD);
4. percentage of Normal to Normal Prolongation >50 milliseconds (pNN50), that is the relative number of normal-to-normal RR intervals which were shorter by more than 50 milliseconds than the immediately following NN interval;
5. Heart Rate Variability Triangular Index (HRV index), that is the total number of normal-to-normal RR intervals divided by the largest number of equally long NN intervals, ie, the number of NN intervals with modal duration;
6. Triangular Interpolation of the Normal to Normal Histogram (TINN),

that is the baseline width of a triangular peak function which is the minimum square difference interpolation of the frequency distribution histogram of the normal-to-normal RR intervals.

Statistics and Data Manipulation

The analysis of the ECG records and the subsequent measurement of HRV by the various methods provided 12 values for each patient (6 methods applied to 2 records of NN interval sequences). The study investigated to what extent the recognition artifact imposed by the automated ECG recognition influenced the HRV values provided by each of the 6 methods. In order to perform this investigation, the results based on the automated recognitions were compared with those based on the manually verified recognition which was taken as a 'gold standard' analysis of the long-term ECGs.

Correlation Coefficients

The correlation between the values provided by the calculation of HRV from nonedited and edited ECG recognitions were computed for all six HRV formulae. As the distribution of the HRV values in the study population was not Normal (especially for the pNN50 method), the Spearman rank correlation coefficient was used. In order to investigate whether the misrecognition artifact influences more lower or higher values of HRV, the correlations between the values of nonedited and edited recognitions were also computed separately for the inter-50 percentile and inter-25 percentile range of the values of the edited results. In other words, for each method of the HRV analysis, the total population was divided into four parts according to the values of the edited results and the correlation coefficients were computed separately for the half of the population with lowest and highest HRV values, respectively, and similarly for each quarter of the population.

Relative Bias and Errors

Correlation coefficients are of course merely a measure of association between ranks of values from both measurements. That is, they express to what extent the small and large values obtained without editing correspond to the small and large values obtained with ECG editing, which is what is needed when using the depressed values of HRV as a risk predictor. Theoretically, a more appropriate approach is to compute the bias and relative errors.[11]

Thus, for each method, the relative errors of the nonedited measurements of HRV were also calculated. That is, for each patient and for each method, the value $(HRV_{be} - HRV_{ae})/HRV_{ae}$ was computed where the values HRV_{be} and HRV_{ae} represent the HRV measurement before and after editing of the long-term ECG, respectively.

Reproducibility of Patient Stratifcation

The correlation coefficients and the relative errors represent only indirectly the influence of the artifact on the clinical meaning of the HRV values, if the measurement is intended merely to distinguish between patients with normal and depressed HRV. Such a distinction is the most common practical goal in clinical studies which utilize HRV as a predictor of complications.

In order to evaluate the influence of the artifact in a more direct way, the stratification of patients with high- and low-edited values of HRV was compared with the stratification of patients with low- and high-nonedited values of HRV. The same procedure was applied to all six methods: for a given number 'n' ranging from 5% to 50% of the total population, two groups $M_{(n)}$ and $M^{(n)}$ of 'n' patients were selected with the lowest and highest edited HRV values, respectively, and two other groups $m_{(n)}$ and $m^{(n)}$ of 'n' patients were selected with the lowest and highest nonedited HRV values, respectively. The size of the overlap between the groups $M_{(n)}$ and $m_{(n)}$ and between the groups $M^{(n)}$ and $m^{(n)}$ was then expressed as the percentage of 'n' (the higher this percentage, the higher the agreement between the automatic and manually verified measurement). The results obtained were plotted in the form of graphs showing the dependency of the agreement between the measurements on 'n.'

Results

Correlation Coefficients

Scatter diagrams of pairs of values obtained when applying individual methods for HRV assessment to the sets of edited and unedited RR interval sequences are presented in Figure 1A-F. The corresponding rank correlation coefficients are shown in Figure 2A-B.

Note in Figure 1 that the SDNN method and, to some extent, the SDANN method provided systematically higher values for the nonedited than for the edited Holter recognitions. This was caused by the operational mode of the Marquette system. If the voltage of the QRS complex is too low, it is omitted by the automatic phase and the resulting 'normal-to-normal' interval consists of two or even more genuine NN intervals. When correcting this recognition artifact, which is by far the most frequent, the standard deviation of durations of corrected NN intervals is smaller than that of uncorrected intervals. This problem is, however, more general and applies equally to other Holter systems.[12]

Both the scatter diagrams and the correlation coefficients show that the methods HRV index and TINN, which were originally designed to be independent of low-level misrecognition artifact, performed slightly better than the other three methods. The scatter diagrams and correlation coefficients in subsets of the patient population also show that correlations of the two geometrical methods are better than those of the other methods in regions of low HRV values. This was confirmed when evaluat-

A   Before editing [ms]

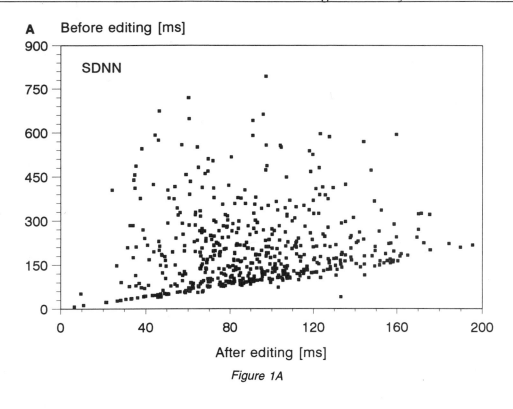

After editing [ms]

Figure 1A

B   Before editing [ms]

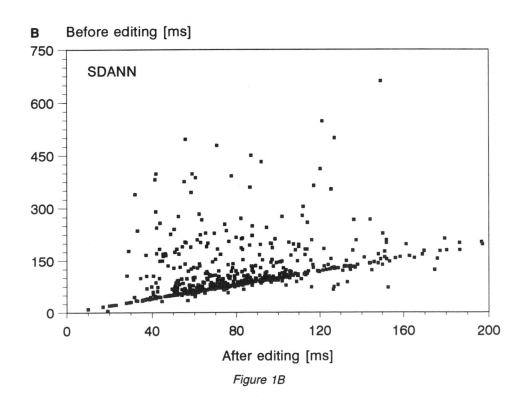

After editing [ms]

Figure 1B

C Before editing [ms]

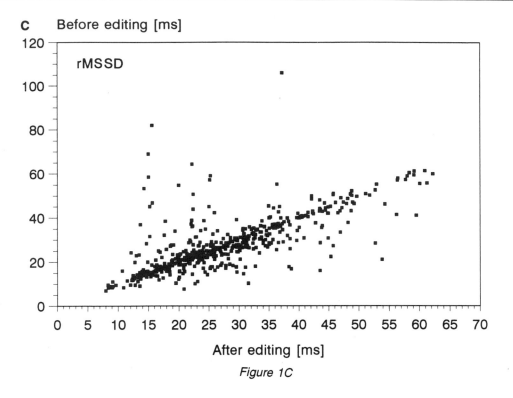

Figure 1C

D Before editing [%]

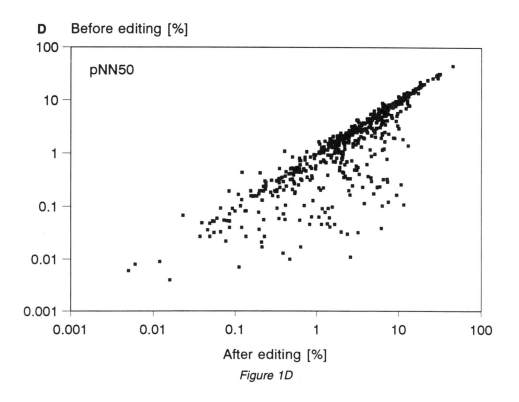

Figure 1D

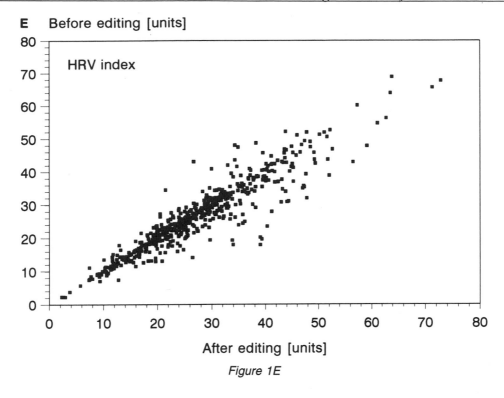

Figure 1E

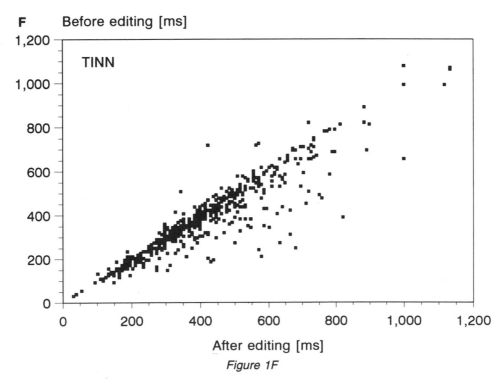

Figure 1F

Figure 1A-F. Scatter diagrams of pairs of values obtained when applying individual methods to edited and nonedited sequences of NN intervals.

A Spearman correlation coefficients

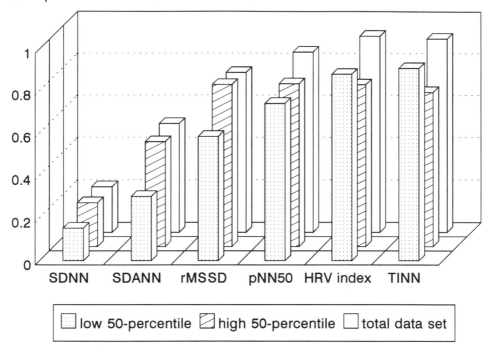

Figure 2A

B Spearman correlation coefficients

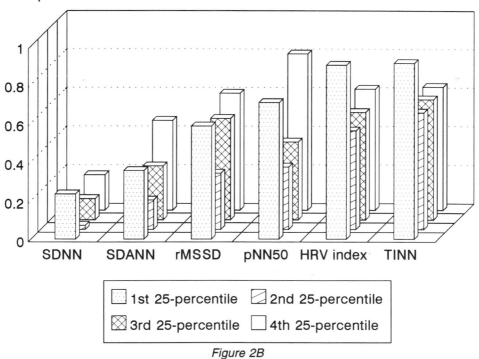

Figure 2B

Figure 2A-B. Spearman correlation coefficients between results of HRV methods applied to edited and nonedited sequences of NN intervals. The correlation coefficients are shown for the total population as well as for different inter-percentiles.

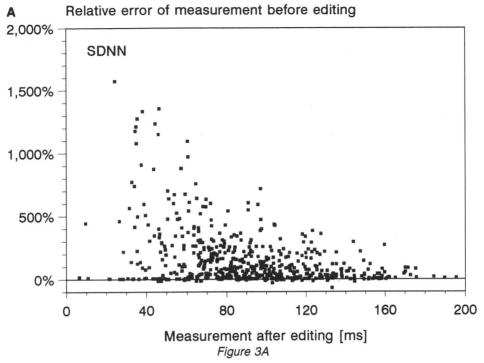

A   Relative error of measurement before editing

Figure 3A

ing the relative errors and the reproduction of patient stratification.

Relative Errors

Scatter diagrams of relative errors of nonedited HRV values are shown in Figure 3A-F. Since the scatter diagrams do not permit an easy judgment of the bias introduced by using the nonedited data, the averages of the relative errors and their standard deviations computed in moving 5-percentiles of the complete population are shown in Figure 4A-F (see the figure legend for technical details).

In this figure, we can easily observe the large bias introduced by the nonedited data into the results of the SDNN and SDANN methods, especially at the low values of HRV. For groups of patients with the lowest values of the true (ie, edited data based) HRV, the bias of the SDNN methods reaches up to 500%. This is probably caused by the fact that survivors of myocardial infarction who have a very low value of overall HRV have also a higher frequency of ventricular

ectopy which influences the quality of automatic ECG recognition.

Note also that while the bias introduced into the results of the rMSSD method fluctuates around zero, being higher with lower values of true HRV (probably for the same reason as just mentioned with the SDNN method), we observe a systematically negative bias of the pNN50 method. This has probably been caused by changes in the proportions of NN interval prolongations and the total number of NN intervals recognized automatically and after manual editing of the data.

Reproducibility of Patient Stratification

Figure 5A-F presents graphs showing the agreement between measurements based on edited and nonedited data in identifying patients with low and high values of HRV. Note that the methods HRV index and TINN performed better than the other methods (especially in a clinically important region of 20% to 40% of low HRV values) and that the rMSSD and pNN50 methods addressing the short-term variations were,

B Relative error of measurement before editing

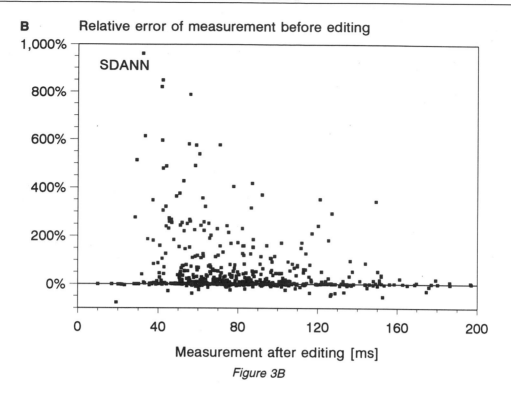

Figure 3B

C Relative error of measurement before editing

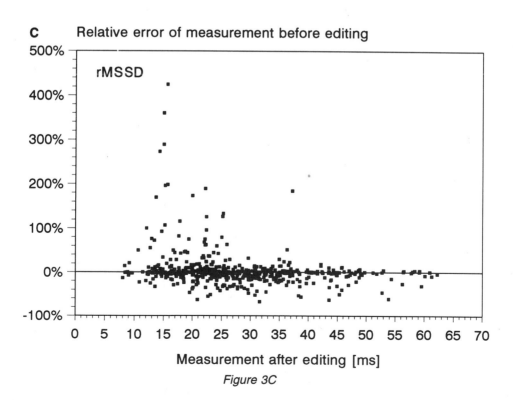

Figure 3C

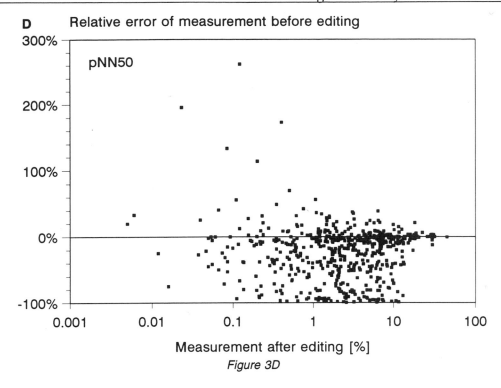

Figure 3D

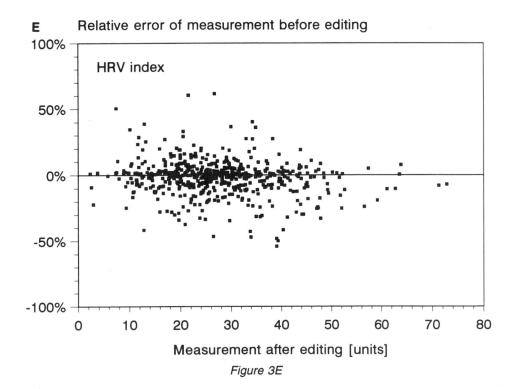

Figure 3E

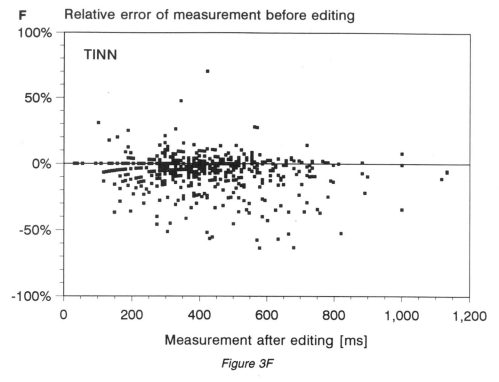

Figure 3F

Figure 3A-F. Scatter diagrams of relative errors of HRV measurements based on nonedited NN interval data plotted against the 'true' values of HRV (ie, values obtained from edited NN sequences).

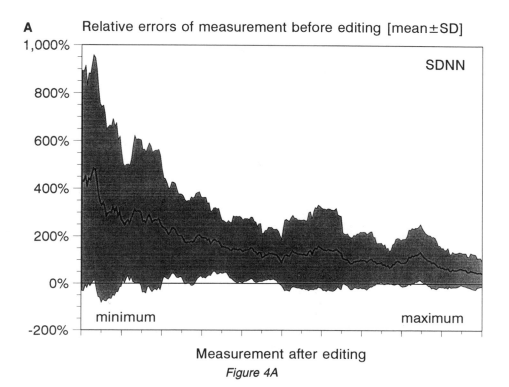

Figure 4A

B Relative errors of measurement before editing [mean±SD]

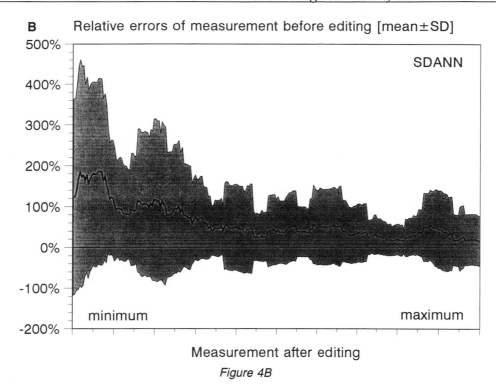

Figure 4B

C Relative errors of measurement before editing [mean±SD]

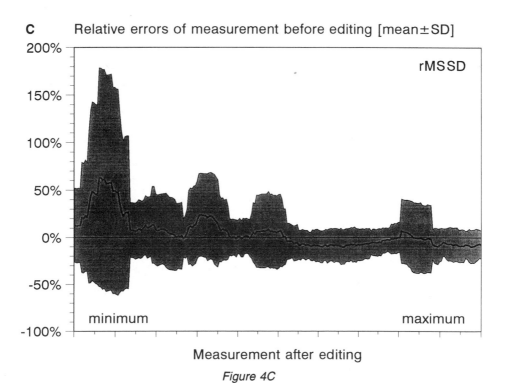

Figure 4C

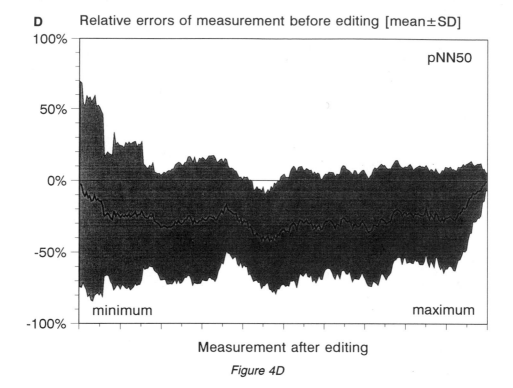

D Relative errors of measurement before editing [mean±SD]

Figure 4D

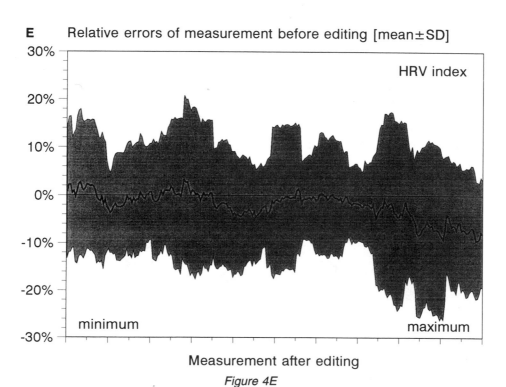

E Relative errors of measurement before editing [mean±SD]

Figure 4E

F   Relative errors of measurement before editing [mean±SD]

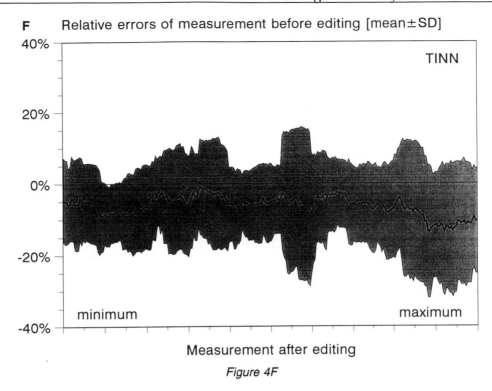

Figure 4F

Figure 4A-F. For each method of HRV measurement, a moving window of 5% of the total population was used to scan through the sequence of edited HRV data sorted from the minimum to the maximum value. For each window, the mean and standard deviation of the relative error of HRV measurements based on nonedited NN interval data were computed. The graphs show the results of these computations for each position of the window.

A   Agreement between measurements before and after editing

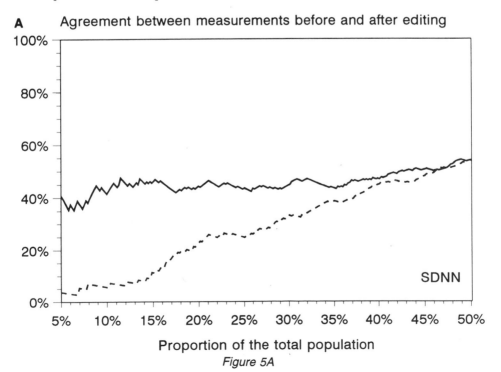

Figure 5A

B Agreement between measurements before and after editing

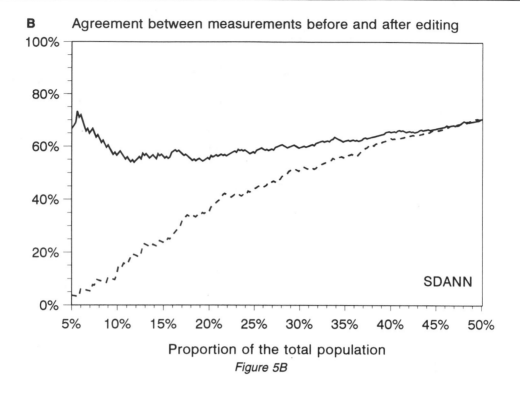

Proportion of the total population

Figure 5B

C Agreement between measurements before and after editing

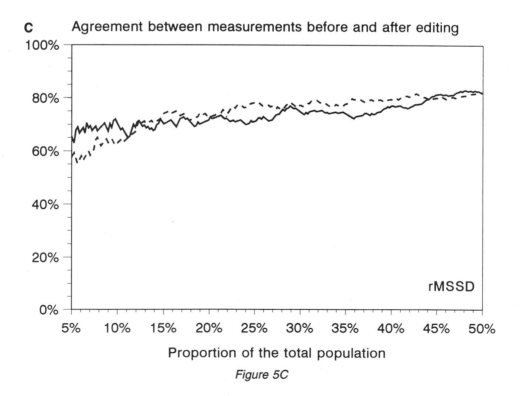

Proportion of the total population

Figure 5C

D   Agreement between measurements before and after editing

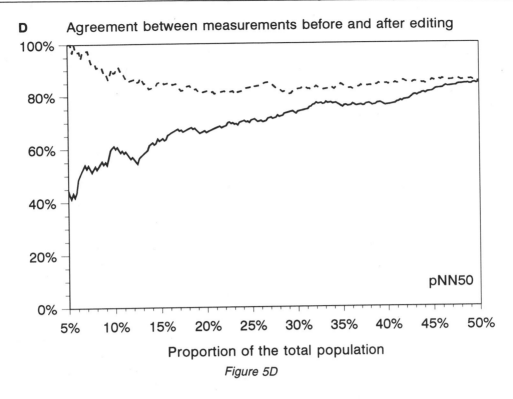

Figure 5D

E   Agreement between measurements before and after editing

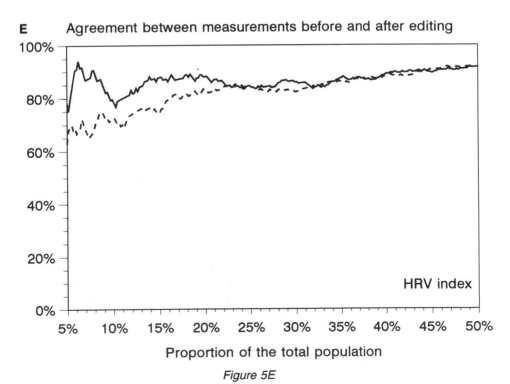

Figure 5E

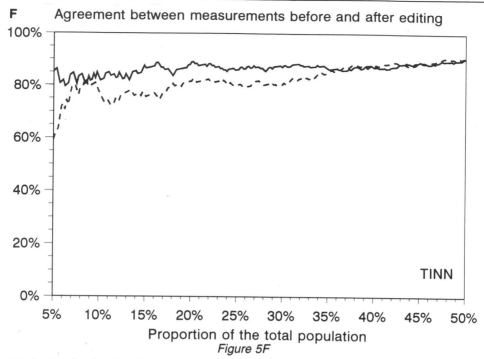

Figure 5A-F. Graphs showing the agreement between patient stratification based on automatic and manually verified assessments of HRV (see the text for details). The full lines correspond to the agreement of stratification of patients with lowest values of HRV; the dashed lines, to the agreement of stratification of patients with highest values of HRV.

in this respect, clearly superior to the SDNN and SDANN methods which reflect the overall HRV.

Discussion

The study examined only the 'technical' performance of the individual methods for HRV measurement. Important information could be obtained from the assessment of the performance of these methods in predicting clinical events, ie, from a similarly designed study examining the influence of the misrecognition artifact on the clinical predictive characteristics of sets of HRV values provided by different methods. However, this would entail a sufficient number of endpoints, such as sudden cardiac death or sustained ventricular tachycardia among patients for whom the methods disagreed.

The influence of the recognition errors on other methods for HRV measurement should also be considered. The spectral methods have not been addressed here on purpose, but it is possible that some of the numerous special methods for time-domain HRV measurement,[13] which have never been evaluated in a larger population of postinfarction patients, might be robust against recognition artifact as well as providing clinically relevant prognostic information.

The overall findings of the study are in a good agreement with previously published clinical studies.[6,7] Clinically useful exploitation of the more conventional methods for HRV measurement, such as the SDNN, required manual validation of the computerized analysis of long-term ECGs, while more robust methods provided clinically useful results even when operating on fully automated ECG recognitions.

There are several possible explanations for the comparatively large influence of noise on the methods based on the calculation of standard deviation of normal-to-normal intervals. The most probable explanation lies in the fact that the formula for calculating the standard deviation is more robust against error values near to the mean of the true values than against errors far from the mean. Hence, this formula is susceptible to the most usual misrecognition mistakes in automatic Holter analysis.

The most frequent errors in computerized analysis of long-term ECGs are related to mistriggering of the QRS pattern detection and recognition algorithms. Some of the sinus rhythm QRS complexes which have a low voltage of the R peak may not be recognized by the analysis, while sharp T waves, as well as closely coupled ventricular premature beats, can be detected and classified as QRS complexes of supraventricular morphology. In such cases, the error data produced by the recognition phase contain values which are both much shorter and much longer than the mean value of the sinus rhythm RR intervals. Some authors employed logical filters in order to remove the extreme values from the sequence of NN interval duration[6] but other studies showed that clinical applicability of the results cannot rely on such filtering techniques. In some cases, a repeated recognition error occurs and logical filters, eg, those excluding all RR intervals which differ by more than, say, 20% from the previous RR or the latest accepted NN interval, may distort the sequence of NN intervals to such an extent that the 'filtered' HRV measurement is even less correct than the 'unfiltered' one.[14,15]

The way in which the automatic recognition phase operates may also play an important role. If the QRS complexes of borderline morphology and/or coupling are left unclassified, as is the case with the automated part of the Marquette system, the automatic recognition results in fewer and more regular normal-to-normal RR intervals than the manually corrected recognitions and, therefore, leads to a lower value of the SDNN measure. This also accounts for the errors in the SDANN formula when the unedited NN data left in a 5-minute segment of the ECG are not representative for this segment.

On the contrary, the precision of the measurement of individual RR intervals is unlikely to influence the results of the study. The sampling of the record at 128 Hz is very common among different manufacturers of Holter tape equipment and substantially higher frequencies cannot be reconstructed from the Holter tape for simple technical reasons.[16]

In summary, the study showed that careful selection of the processing method may overcome the practical necessity of manual verification of the automatic recognition of long-term ECG records. Among the investigated formulae for HRV calculation, the HRV index and TINN methods were influenced less by computer error in automatic recognitions of the long-term ECGs than were the other measurements, especially the SDNN and SDANN methods.

References

1. Akselrod S, Gordon D, Ubel FA, et al. Power spectrum analysis of heart rate fluctuations: a quantitative probe of beat-to-beat cardiovascular control. Science 1981; 213:220-223.
2. Pagani M, Lombardi F, Guzzetti S, et al. Power spectral analysis of heart rate and arterial pressure variabilities as a marker of sympatho-vagal interaction in man and conscious dog. Circ Res 1986; 59:178-193.
3. Bigger JT, Kleiger RE, Fleiss JL, et al. Components of heart rate variability measured during healing of acute myocardial infarction. Am J Cardiol 1988; 61:208-215.
4. Ewing JE, Neilson JMM, Travis P. New method for assessing cardiac parasympathetic activity using 24-hour electrocardiograms. Br Heart J 1984; 52:396-402.
5. Cripps TR, Malik M, Farrell TG, et al. Prognostic value of reduced heart rate variability after myocardial infarction: clinical evaluation of a new analysis method. Br Heart J 1991; 65:14-19.
6. Kleiger RE, Miller JP, Bigger JT, et al. Decreased heart rate variability and its association with increased mortality after acute myocardial infarction. Am J Cardiol 1987; 59:256-262.

7. Farrell TG, Bashir Y, Cripps T, et al. Risk stratification for arrhythmic events in post-infarction patients based on heart rate variability, ambulatory electrocardiographic variables and the signal-averaged electrocardiogram. J Am Coll Cardiol 1991; 18:687-697.

8. Bigger JT, Fleiss JL, Rolnitzky LM, et al. The ability of several short-term measures of RR variability to predict mortality after myocardial infarction. Circulation 1993; 88:927-934.

9. Malik M, Camm AJ. Significance of long term components of heart rate variability for the further prognosis after acute myocardial infarction. Cardiovasc Res 1990; 24:793-803.

10. Odemuyiwa O, Malik M, Farrell T, et al. A comparison of the predictive characteristics of heart rate variability index and left ventricular ejection fraction for all-cause mortality, arrhythmic events and sudden death after acute myocardial infarction. Am J Cardiol 1991; 68:434-439.

11. Bland JM, Altman DG. Statistical methods for assessing agreement between two methods of clinical measurement. Lancet 1986; 1(8476):307-310.

12. Malik M, Xia R, Odemuyiwa 0, et al. Influence of the recognition artefact in the automatic analysis of long term electrocardiograms on time-domain measurement of heart rate variability. Med Biol Eng Comput 1993; 31:539-544.

13. Parer WJ, Parer JT, Holbrook RH, et al. Validity of mathematical methods of quantitating fetal heart rate variability. Am J Obstet Gynecol 1985; 153:403-409.

14. Malik M, Farrell T, Cripps T, et al. Heart rate variability in relation to prognosis after myocardial infarction—selection of optimal processing techniques. Eur Heart J 1989; 10:1060-1074.

15. Malik M, Cripps T, Farrell T, et al. Prognostic value of heart rate variability after myocardial infarction—a comparison of different data processing methods. Med Biol Eng Comput 1989; 27:603-611.

16. Brüggemann Th, Andresen D, Schröder R. Technical problems in detecting ST segment changes with ambulatory ECG monitoring systems. Eur Heart J 1989; 10(suppl):98. Abstract.

Chapter 9

Correspondence of Different Methods for Heart Rate Variability Measurement

Josef Kautzner, Katerina Hnatkova

It is well recognized that heart rate (HR) is governed by two factors: the intrinsic rate of discharge of automatic pacemaker cells in the sinus node; and, probably the more predominant of the two, the influence of the autonomic nervous system and its modulation. It has been shown that the heart responds rapidly to parasympathetic stimulation, while more gradually to sympathetic stimuli. This ability of the vagus nerves to regulate HR beat-by-beat can be explained by the speed at which the neural stimulus is transformed to cardiac response and, simultaneously, by the speed of acetylcholine removal after cessation of vagal activity.[1]

As mentioned in other technical chapters of this book, cyclical changes in HR over time or heart rate variability (HRV) may be measured by multiple techniques, some of which provide specific physiological or pathophysiological information. This chapter reviews the current knowledge on how different methods of HRV measurement correspond each to the other, both in terms of the numerical values provided and in terms of regulatory mechanisms addressed.

Recording Strategy

Not only the technique for HRV measurement, but also the length of recording significantly influences the results of quantitative HRV assessment. For instance, time-domain analysis performed on short electrocardiographic recordings lasting only minutes generally reflect modulation of vagal activity. However, for long-term, eg, 24-hour recordings, the situation appears to be more complex, and clinical studies have shown that the predictive value of reduced heart variability is not a simple reflection of depressed vagal antiarrhythmic defense.[2] The employment of spectral techniques have demonstrated that both high-frequency (HF) and low-frequency (LF) components account for less than 10% of the total power spectrum. The remaining part is represented by ultra low and very low-

From: Malik M., Camm AJ (eds.): *Heart Rate Variability*. Armonk, NY. Futura Publishing Company, Inc., © 1995.

frequency (VLF) components, the physiological mechanism of which has yet to be identified. Hypotheses about the background for these VLF components include thermoregulation, changes in the activity of the renin-angiotensin system, as well as environmental changes.[3,4] Some investigators have also suggested that power <0.04 Hz is practically only noise, possibly associated with characteristics of the Holter recorders used for ECG recordings.[5,6] In this respect, very limited experience exists about the influence of recording procedures[7] and some researchers suggested that physical activity is a major determinant of the VLF component of HRV, demonstrating the dependence of the VLF power on the amount and natural variations of physical activity.[8]

Short-Term Recordings

Studies examining short-term HRV can either use simple time-domain estimates such as a ratio or a difference between maximum and minimum RR interval, or statistical time-domain measures like the standard deviation of RR intervals.[9-11] Although these techniques have been successfully used for assessment of autonomic tone both in experimental models and in clinical studies, their value as a measure of changes in sympathovagal balance is limited. These components of cardiac neural control can be separated by evaluation of harmonics of HRV, using frequency-domain analysis.[12,13] Moreover, short-term recordings are preferable for application of spectral analysis because acquisition of biological signals during a brief period of time can better comply with the theoretical prerequisites of spectral analysis, especially in the respect of data stationarity.[12,13]

Long-Term Recordings

In addition to short-term recordings, very valuable and clinically relevant information was also obtained when HRV was assessed from long-term, ie, nominal 24-hour ECG recordings.[14-17]

There are several time-domain methods addressing different components of HRV:

1. overall HRV can be easily assessed using the standard deviation of the NN intervals (SDNN) or triangular HRV index;
2. long-term oscillatory components, ie, cycles longer than 5 minutes, can be estimated by the standard deviation of the average NN intervals calculated over 5-minute periods; and
3. short-term components of HRV can be expressed in terms of NN50 counts, which reflect the number of pairs of adjacent NN intervals differing by more than 50 milliseconds, pNN50, which reflects the percentage of NN50 counts with respect to the total number of NN intervals, and rMSSD or root mean square of differences between adjacent NN intervals.[17,18]

Of these time-domain methods, both NN50 counts and pNN50 parameters are dichotomized variables; this fact influences their statistical properties.

In parallel, power spectral analysis of HRV has been successfully used to predict the risk of mortality after myocardial infarction.[19,20] However, the information provided by spectral methods applied to long-term recordings is not more useful than that obtained from simpler time-domain methods which are easier to implement and which are less dependent on strict requirements regarding data quality and character.

Correlations Among Time-Domain Measures

The relationship between various commonly used statistical measures of HRV was comprehensively studied by Kleiger et al[21] in a group of 14 normal subjects. It has been shown that the variables calculated from the differences between adjacent cycles such as rMSSD and pNN50 are highly correlated (r = 0.96) and thus, may be considered as surrogates for each other. These parameters are widely accepted as estimates of short-term components of HRV, strongly reflecting modulations of vagal tone. On the other hand, approximates of overall HRV such as SDNN have been demonstrated to relate less significantly with previous ones. This may be explained by dependence of overall HRV measures on multiple influences such as circadian patterns, differences between day and night, physical and mental activity, etc. In a subsequent study, Bigger et al[18] evaluated correlations among time-domain statistical measures and frequency-domain parameters 2 weeks after myocardial infarction (Table 1). For time-domain indices, they confirmed previous observation in normal individuals, specifically strong correlation between rMSSD and pNN50 parameters (r = 0.93) and also between overall measures of HRV such as SDNN and SDANN (r = 0.98). As a part of our study in survivors of acute myocardial infarction,[22] we showed good correlation between statistical measures of overall HRV and both geometrical indices (Figure 1).

Correlation coefficients in the range of >0.85 demonstrate that geometrical HRV indices may serve as an alternative for less easily obtainable statistical parameters (Table 2).

Comparison Between Time-Domain and Frequency-Domain Parameters

Based on mathematical theory, HR variance (which is equal to the squared standard deviation of the NN intervals) and total spectral power are identical. Therefore, it is not surprising that comparisons between frequency- and time-domain measures have shown that for every band of the 24-hour HR power spectrum there is at least one time-domain correlate (Table 1).[18] Specifically, parameters shown previously to reflect mainly parasympathetic activity (ie, pNN50 and rMSSD) correlated well with HF power. SDNN index had very strong correlation with VLF, LF and HF measures, suggesting that it is influenced by both vagal and sympathetic tone. SDNN and SDANN indices correlated significantly with total power and ultra LF component (Table 3). These strong correlations suggest that the two variables can be used interchangeably in clinical studies.

Table 1
Correlations Between Time and Frequency-Domain Measures of HRV in Patients after Myocardial Infarction

Time Domain	Frequency Domain				
	TP	ULF	VLF	LF	HF
SDNN	0.96	0.95	0.78	0.72	0.67
SDANN	0.94	0.96	0.68	0.61	0.57
SDNN index	0.79	0.71	0.90	0.89	0.82
pNN50	0.56	0.50	0.59	0.64	0.89
rMSSD	0.58	0.52	0.60	0.65	0.92

Abbreviations: SDNN: standard deviation of all NN intervals over a 24-hour period; SDANN: standard deviation of the average NN intervals for all 5-minute segments of a 24-hour recording; SDNN index: mean of the standard deviations of all NN intervals for all 5-minute segments of a 24-hour recording; pNN50: proportion of adjacent NN intervals >50ms different over the entire 24-hour recording; rMSSD: root mean square of differences between adjacent NN intervals in a 24-hour recording; TP: total power of the heart power spectrum (0 to 0.40 Hz); ULF: ultra low frequency power (0 to 0.0033 Hz); VLF: very low frequency power (0.0033 to 0.04 Hz); LF: low frequency power (0.04 to 0.15 Hz); HF: high frequency power (0.15 to 0.40 Hz). Adapted from Bigger et al.[18]

A SDANN [msec]

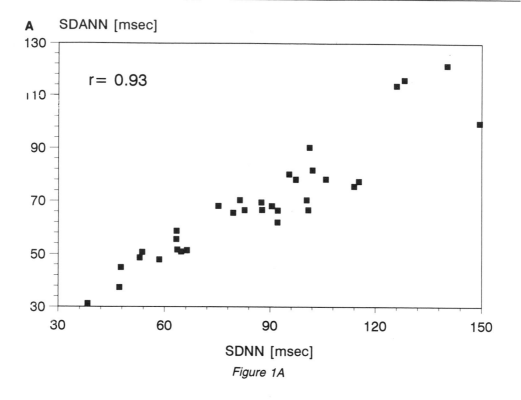

Figure 1A

B SDNN index [msec]

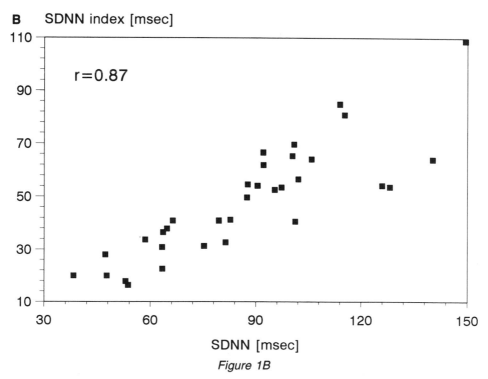

Figure 1B

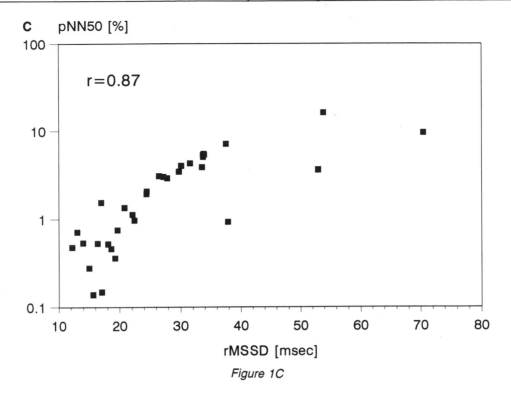

Figure 1C

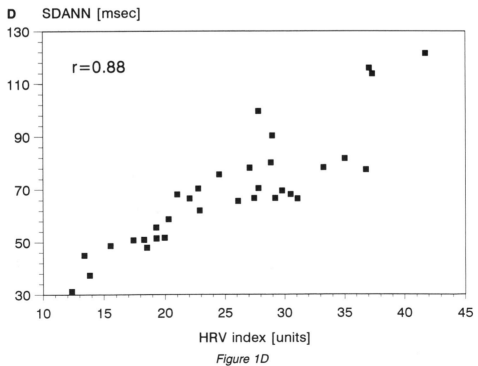

Figure 1D

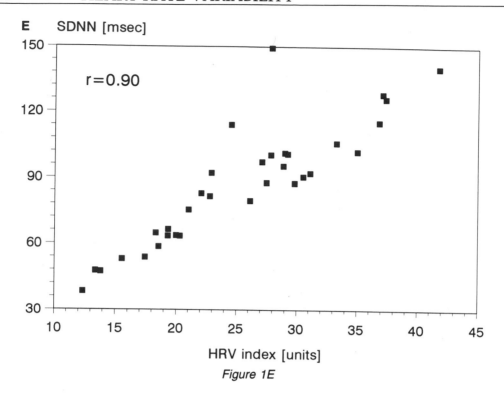

Figure 1E

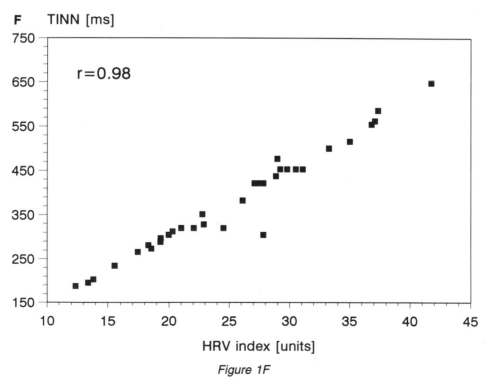

Figure 1F

Figure 1A-F. Relationship between individual time-domain HRV parameters assessed in 33 survivors of the acute phase of myocardial infarction. The 'r' values correspond to Spearman correlations coefficients. The abbreviations are same as in Table 2.

Table 2
Spearman Correlation Coefficients among Time-Domain HRV Indices
in 33 Survivors of Acute Myocardial Infarction

Parameter	SDNN	SDANN	SDNN index	pNN50	rMSSD	HRV index
SDNN	—					
SDANN	0.93	—				
SDNN index	0.87	0.68	—			
pNN50	0.57	0.38	0.70	—		
rMSSD	0.71	0.54	0.83	0.87	—	
HRV index	0.90	0.88	0.76	0.45	0.56	—
TINN	0.84	0.85	0.67	0.40	0.49	0.98

Abbreviations: HRV index: the integral of the density distribution divided by the height of the distribution; TINN: the baseline width of the distribution measured by its minimum square difference triangular interpolation; other abbreviations same as in Table 1.

Table 3
Components of Heart Rate Variability

Spectral Component	Frequency Band (Hz)	Optimal Length of Recording	Time-Domain Correlate[18,21,23]
HF	0.15-0.40	1-5 minutes	rMSSD, pNN50
LF	0.04-0.15	2-5 minutes	SDNN index
VLF	0.0033-0.04	12-24 hours	SDNN index
ULF	<0.0033	12-24 hours	SDNN, SDANN, HRV index
TP	0-0.40	24 hours	SDNN, HRV index

Abbreviations same as in Tables 1 and 2.

Conclusion

It is indisputable that for stationary short-term recordings the spectral analysis of HRV provides specific information about sympatho-vagal balance. This is a major advantage over time-domain techniques.

On the other hand, physiological interpretation of individual spectral components derived from long-term (24-hour) rec-
ordings is difficult and to a large extent, unknown. Therefore, the time-domain analysis based on statistical or geometrical methods gives more reliable results. From a pathophysiological point of view, more comprehensive studies of VLF and ultra LF components of HR spectrum are desirable. Furthermore, the influence of recording procedures and the performance of different recording media on HRV measurement needs detailed investigation.

References

1. Levy MN, Yang T, Wallick DW. Assessment of beat-by-beat control of heart rate by the autonomic nervous system: molecular biology techniques are necessary, but not sufficient. J Cardiovasc Electrophysiol 1993; 4:183-193.

2. Malik M, Camm AJ. Heart rate variability: from facts to fancies. J Am Coll Cardiol 1993; 22:566-568.

3. Sayers BA. Analysis of heart rate variability. Ergonomics 1973; 1:17-32.

4. Akselrod S, Grodon D, Ubel FA, et al. Power spectrum analysis of heart rate fluctuation: a quantitative probe of beat-to-beat cardiovascular control. Science 1981; 213:220-223.

5. Pagani M, Lombardi F, Guzzetti S, et al. Power spectral analysis of heart rate and arterial pressure variabilities as a marker of

sympatho-vagal interaction in man and conscious dog. Circ Res 1986; 59:178-193.

6. Furlan R, Guzzetti S, Crivellaro W, et al. Continuous 24-hour assessment of the neural regulation of systemic arterial pressure and RR variabilities in ambulant patients. Circulation 1990; 81:537-547.

7. Pinna GD, Maestri R, Di Cesare A, et al. The accuracy of power-spectrum analysis of heart-rate variability from annotated RR lists generated by Holter systems. Physiol Meas 1994; 15:163-179.

8. Bernardi L, Valle F, Coco M, et al. Physical activity is a major determinant of heart rate variability, its 'very low' frequency component and 1/f (chaotic) distribution. Eur Heart J 1994; 15:242.

9. Wheeler T, Watkins PJ. Cardiac denervation in diabetes. Br Med J 1973; 4:584-586.

10. Eckberg DW. Parasympathetic cardiovascular control in human disease: a critical review of methods and results. Am J Physiol 1980; 239:H581-H593.

11. Ewing DJ, Martin CN, Young RJ, et al. The value of cardiovascular autonomic function tests: ten years experience in diabetes. Diabetic Care 1985; 8:491-498.

12. Malliani A, Lombardi F, Pagani M. Power spectrum analysis of heart rate variability: a tool to explore neural regulatory mechanisms. Br Heart J 1994; 71:1-2.

13. Malliani A, Pagani M, Lombardi F, et al. Cardiovascular neural regulation explored in the frequency domain. Circulation 1991; 84:482-492.

14. Kleiger RE, Miller JP, Bigger JT Jr, et al. Decreased heart rate variability and its association with increased mortality after acute myocardial infarction. Am J Cardiol 1987; 59:256-262.

15. Martin GJ, Magid NM, Myers G, et al. Heart rate variability and sudden death secondary to coronary artery disease during ambulatory electrocardiographic monitoring. Am J Cardiol 1987; 60:86-89.

16. Malik M, Camm AJ. Significance of long term components of heart rate variability for the further prognosis after acute myocardial infarction. Cardiovasc Res 1990; 24:793-803.

17. Cripps TR, Malik M, Farrell TG, et al. Prognostic value of reduced heart rate variability after myocardial infarction: clinical evaluation of a new analysis method. Br Heart J 1991; 65:14-19.

18. Bigger JT Jr, Fleiss JL, Steinman RC, et al. Correlations among time and frequency domain measures of heart period variability two weeks after acute myocardial infarction. Am J Cardiol 1992; 69:891-898.

19. Lombardi F, Sandrone G, Pernpruner S, et al. Heart rate variability as an index of sympathovagal interaction after acute myocardial infarction. Am J Cardiol 1987; 60:1239-1245.

20. Bigger JT Jr, Fleiss JL, Steinman RC, et al. Frequency domain measures of heart period variability and mortality after myocardial infarction. Circulation 1992; 85:164-171.

21. Kleiger RE, Bigger JT Jr, Bosner MS, et al. Stability over time of variables measuring heart rate variability in normal subjects. Am J Cardiol 1991; 68:626-630.

22. Kautzner J, Hnatkova K, Staunton A, et al. Day to day reproducibility of time domain measures of heart rate variability in survivors of the acute phase of myocardial infarction. In press.

23. Stein PK, Rottman JN, Kleiger RE. Time domain measures of heart rate variability as surrogates for frequency domain measures in stable congestive heart failure patients and normals. Circulation 1994; 90(part2):I-331.

Chapter 10

Heart Rate Variability Instruments from Commercial Manufacturers

Harold L. Kennedy

Introduction

Since the clinical value of changes in response to physiological alterations in heart beats was first realized with the absence of normal beat-to-beat variability of fetal heart rate (HR) (indicative of abnormal pregnancy conditions)[1], attention has focused on the clinical value of following such physiological perturbations. After the pioneer work of Akselrod et al,[2,3] early investigative studies of HR changes were directed at patients with cardiovascular disease.[4] Subsequently, clinical studies and the evolution of technology have grown to assess heart rate variability (HRV) in two distinct ways: by calculation of indices based on statistical operations (time-domain analysis) of the RR intervals, or by spectral (frequency-domain) analysis of a series of RR intervals.[3,5] These methods require accurate timing of electrocardiographic R waves, and can be performed on short electrocardiograms (ECGs) (from 0.5 to 5 minutes) or on 24-hour ambulatory ECG recordings.

As with the evolution of ambulatory ECG recordings for arrhythmia analysis, the emergence of computer technology has facilitated automatic detection of the normal RR beat intervals, calculation of their precise measurement in milliseconds, and examination of these data by both time- and frequency-domain measurements. Similar to other developments in ambulatory electrocardiography, after the emergence of clinical investigations which characterized HRV as a method of diagnosis and prognosis in some patient populations, commercial manufacturers of ambulatory ECG instrumentation focused their attention on this new ambulatory ECG parameter. As with all new innovations in the commercial marketplace, this development has been nonguided and left to free-market forces. However, because HRV has generated a rather high level of clinical and scientific interest and can be obtained at a relatively modest cost, there has occurred a rapid introduction of HRV instruments by commercial manufacturers with limited information or guidance con-

From: Malik M., Camm AJ (eds.): *Heart Rate Variability*. Armonk, NY. Futura Publishing Company, Inc., © 1995.

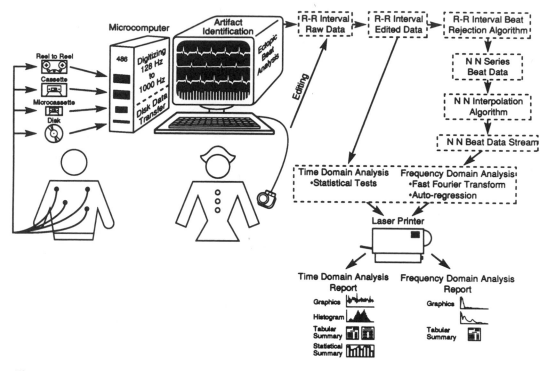

Figure 10.1.

cerning the validity of the measurements they report. This chapter focuses on those technical components which are common to all HRV instruments of commercial manufacturers, presents available descriptions of such instrumentation as obtained from manufacturers, and discusses what standards or guidelines should perhaps be developed and adopted to result in accurate and reproducible data from such instrumentation in the future.

Components of Heart Rate Variability Instrumentation

Components of HRV instrumentation common to all instruments is a playback component which examines the 24-hour ambulatory ECG recording tape (cassette, microcassette or reel-to-reel) and digitizes the analog electrocardiographic signal for digital data examination by the ambulatory ECG instrument (Figure 1). More recent technology, digitizes the analog electrocardiographic signal directly to disk storage, and the data is simply transferred to the

computer storage (Figure 1). Digitizing rates have varied from 128 to 1000 Hz and most commonly, in order to facilitate other ambulatory ECG functions, are performed at 128 or 256 Hz. Once the ambulatory ECG instrument receives such data, it must employ its software algorithms to recognize artifactual noise, identify ectopic beats (ventricular and supraventricular), correctly annotate normal cardiac R wave beats (RR intervals), selectively edit normal RR beat files to obtain selected NN beat data, and then perform selected NN data analysis by both time- and frequency-domain analysis. Selected NN data is commonly identified by excluding the preceding and succeeding RR interval contiguous to noise or ectopic beats. The instantaneous heart period function during those periods of excluded data is estimated by linear interpolation. Most manufacturers examine RR beat data in 5 minute increments of epoch of time. Some manufacturers require that at least 80% of the RR interval data in a 5 minute epoch constitute selected RR interval or NN intervals, otherwise that epoch is excluded from the total analysis. This process of ambulatory ECG instrument identification of artifact, ectopic beats, and rejection of selected RR intervals, of course, is instrument specific, and will be subject to the techniques and accuracy of a variety of manufacturers. Thus, in early publications of HRV clinical studies, some investigators called attention to a second stage of custom editing being performed to find and correct errors not detected by commercial instruments that could adversely affect heart variability measurements.[6-8] Whether or not such methods are currently needed for any or all commercially manufactured HRV instruments is unknown. Once the RR interval data is submitted to the ambulatory ECG instrument and completes the process of interpolation, selected beat rejection and perhaps secondary editing, the resulting RR or NN beat-to-beat series of time measurements then are processed to time-domain statistical testing or frequency-domain spectral analysis (Fast Fourier Transform or autoregressive) (Figure 1). Other factors which may influence these final analysis data include the sampling rate, length of time of epochs, or filters used in spectral analysis. For example, commercial instruments that sample at 128 Hz can localize a specific QRS with an 8 millisecond accuracy. Thus, higher sampling rates (eg, 256 Hz) would require more computer memory and processing time (perhaps), but would be more accurate. Manufacturers may also vary as to what epoch (measurement of time) they use to examine a series of NN intervals to determine either their time-domain or frequency-domain measurements. Whereas some may examine data as a matter of epoch time (eg, 2 or 5 minutes), others may examine a specific number of beats (eg, 512 beats). Theoretical problems are encountered in computing the frequency spectrum of HRV data, and every method must be a balance or compromise between achieving scientific rigor and practical measurements. Accurate noise rejection criteria are the fundamental basis which allows consistent processing to avoid long periods of arbitrary computer interpolation. Thus, a threshold requiring greater than 80% of the RR intervals in a 5 minute epoch to be acceptable NN interval data has been touted as optimal to achieve a balance between the competing objectives of minimizing both interpolation and data segment rejection.[9] This 80% criteria is the most stringent criteria that is thought to yield both consistent results and a large fraction of accepted data.[9] Making such computations on 5 minute epochs requires only 1/250th of the total memory that would be required for examining a stream of NN intervals over an entire 24-hour period. Thus, recommendations have been made in the literature to use 5 minute epoch data for application to commercial ambulatory ECG Holter instruments.[9]

Calculation of the frequency analysis by Fast Fourier Transform or autoregressive methods also may bring about various alterations.[10] Variations of the Fast Fourier Transform and autoregressive methods employ filters (eg, boxcar, Hanning window, etc.) that modulate or de-emphasize specific characteristics of the data to provide more specific measurement of a given frequency.

Manufacturers of ambulatory ECG instruments which purport to have some form of HRV measurements are shown in Table 1. In reality, HRV is a software program incorporated into a Holter instrument system or another electrocardiographic product (Table 1). Apparently in the United States, FDA approval and the release of such products was halted in HRV in 1993. In all likelihood this resulted from the investigational nature of HRV data [11] and the nonexistence of validation methods to attest to the accuracy and validity of the methodologies employed by the manufacturers. It is extremely unusual for a commercial manufacturer to document the validity of their measurements as was done in the Reynolds Pathfinders System. [12] However, some manufacturers have published their own quality assurance methodology in the form of technical service manuals.[10,13]

Table 1
Commercial Instrumentation for Heart Rate Variability

Manufacturer	Instrumentation	Digitizing Rate	Time Domain	Parameters	Frequency Domain	Epoch Options
ACS	Response pending					
ANSAR	ECG instrument	160	Yes	HR, R-R measured	FFT	32 sec
ART	ECG instrument	User defined	Yes	Total R-R, Mean R-R, Accepted R-R, SDANN, SD of accepted R-R, rMSSD, pNN50, CVr, coeff. of variation	FFT, AR	User defined (2 min minimum)
	SAECG	125	Yes	SD, Mean R-R, nInt, SDANN, rMSSD, pNN50	FFT	2 min, 5 min
Biomedical Systems	Ambulatory ECG	128, 400	Yes	SDNN, SDNN5, pNN50, rMSSD, SDANN index, HRVI index, Mean R-R, Modal R-R, Modal Freq.	FFT, AR	2 min, 5 min, 1 hr, 24 hr
Biosensor	Ambulatory ECG	250	Yes	NN (mean), SDNN	FFT	User defined (1 min minimum)
Burdick	Ambulatory ECG	200, 400, 1000	Yes	NN (mean), NN (total), NNN (total), CLV5, SDNN, rMSSD, pNN50	FFT, AR	User defined (2 min minimum)
Del Mar Avionics	Ambulatory ECG	128, 256, 1000	Yes	SD, Min R-R, Max R-R, SDNN, SDANN, rMSSD, pNN50, Avg HR of qualified beats, Epoch Min-Avg, Epoch Max-Avg	FFT	User defined (2 min minimum)
	ECG instrument	1000	Yes	SD, Mean HR, Variance	FFT	5 min
DMI	Ambulatory ECG	200, 400, 1000	Yes	NN (mean), NN (total), NNN (total), CLV5, SDNN, rMSSD, pNN50	FFT, AR	User defined (2 min minimum)
DMS	Ambulatory ECG	128	Yes	NN, SDNN, SDNN index, SDANN, SDANN index, mean R-R, rMSSD, pNN50, Qualified beats, Count of valid epochs	FFT	5 min, 1 hr, 24 hr
Hewlett Packard*	Ambulatory ECG	User defined	Yes	Total R-R, Mean R-R, Accepted R-R, SDANN, SD of accepted R-R, rMSSD, pNN50, CVr coeff. of variation	FFT, AR	User defined (2 min minimum)

Mortara	Ambulatory ECG	128	Yes	SDNN, pNN50, rMSSD	FFT	5 min
Oxford	Response pending					
Marquette Electronics	Ambulatory ECG	128	Yes	NN, SDNN, SDANN, SD, rMSSD, pNN50	FFT	User defined (2 min minimum)
Reynolds Medical	Ambulatory ECG	128, 256, 500, 1000	Yes	Mean R-R, SD, SDNN, rMSSD, sNN50, sNN50 increases, sNN50 decreases, St. George's (Triangular) index	FFT	User defined (2 min minimum)
Rozinn Electronics	Ambulatory ECG	180	Yes	SD, pNN50, rMSSD	FFT	User defined (2 min minimum)
	SAECG*	1000	Yes	SD, pNN50, rMSSD	FFT	5 min, 1 hr
SpaceLabs	Ambulatory ECG	128	Yes	SD, rMSSD, pNN50, SDANN, SDNN, Count of valid epochs	FFT	User defined (2 min minimum)
Zymed	Response pending					

FFT = Fast Fourier Transform; AR = Autoregression; * = utilizes Corazonics software

Guidelines and the Standards Needed

Commercial manufacturers of HRV currently are in need of a defined standard of performance relevant to the following characteristics:

1. issues that involve acceptable ECG recording noise (eg, baseline wander, electrical artifact, etc);
2. identification of ectopic beats;
3. determination of stationarity and measurement artifact;
4. sampling rate;
5. cost-effective time epochs to be examined;
6. recommended filter procedures to be used in spectral frequency identification and analysis;
7. optimal short-time and long-term segments of data for time- and frequency-domain analysis; and
8. guidelines applicable to the autoregressive model (permitting estimation) relative to the Fast Fourier Transform (relies on observation).

A recent American College of Cardiology position statement [11] has called for prospective multi-center studies to determine the sensitivity, specificity, and predicted accuracy of HRV in various clinical states, and they recognized that normal values and determination of optimal time- and frequency-domain measurements must also be defined. Interestingly, in addition to the need for study of normal populations stratified for age and gender, the guidelines recognized the need to determine both Fast Fourier analysis and the autoregressive methods to attempt to examine the issues.

References

1. Hon EH, Lee ST. Electronic evaluation of the fetal heart rate patterns preceding fetal death: further observations. Am J Obstet Gynecol 1965; 87:814-826.
2. Akselrod S, Gordon D, Ubel FA, et al. Power spectrum analysis of heart rate fluctuations: a quantitative probe of beat-to-beat cardiovascular control. Science 1981; 213:220-223.
3. Akselrod S, Gordon D, Madwed JB, et al. Hemodynamic regulation: an investigation by spectral analysis. Am J Physiol 1985; 249:4867-4875.
4. Wolf MM, Varigos GA, Hunt D, et al. Sinus arrhythmia in acute myocardial infarction. Med J Aust 1978; 2:52-53.
5. Parer WJ, Parer JT, Holbrook RH, et al. Validity of mathematical methods of quantitating heart rate variability. Am J Obstet Gynecol 1985; 153:402-409.
6. Bigger JT, Fleiss JL, Steinmann RC, et al. Correlations among time and frequency domain measures of heart rate variability two weeks after acute myocardial infarction. Am J Cardiol 1992; 69:891-898.
7. Birman KP, Rolnitzky LM, Bigger JT. A shape oriented system for automated Holter ECG analysis. Comp Cardiol 1978; 5:217-220.
8. Xia R, Odemyyiwa O, Gill J, et al. Influence of recognition errors of computerized analysis of 24-hour electrocardiograms on the measurement of spectral components of heart rate variability. Int J Biomed Comput 1993; 32:223-235.
9. Rottman JN, Steinman RC, Albrecht P, et al. Efficient estimation of the heart period power spectrum suitable for physiologic or pharmacologic studies. Am J Cardiol 1990; 66:1522-1524.
10. Marquette Electronics. Heart Rate Variability Physician's Guide. 2nd ed. Software version 002A. 1992.
11. ACC Position Statement. Heart rate variability for risk stratification of life-threatening arrhythmias. J Am Coll Cardiol 1993; 948-950.
12. Molgaad H. Evaluation of the Reynolds Pathfinder II system for 24 hour heart rate variability analysis. Eur Heart J 1991; 12:1153-62.
13. Mortara Instrument, Inc. Heart rate variability issues and implementation. 1991.

Part III

Physiology of Heart Rate Variability

Chapter 11

Models for the Analysis of Cardiovascular Variability Signals

Giuseppe Baselli, Alberto Porta, Giulia Ferrari

Introduction

Short-term cardiovascular variability has been addressed by means of signal processing methods, starting with spectral analysis.[1] This gave the opportunity to quantify rhythmic components of beat-to-beat variabilities, which had been studied since the earliest recordings of arterial pressure (AP) and the electrocardiogram (ECG).[2] In this field, emphasis is given to the relationships between the variability spectrum and the activity of the autonomic nervous system.[3,4] This presentation will refer to two main classes of oscillations detected in the band of short-term variability (ie, from 0.03 Hz, up to a half of heart rate ~0.5 Hz):

1. a high frequency (HF) rhythm at respiratory frequency (~0.25 Hz); and
2. lower frequency (LF) spontaneous oscillations around 0.1 Hz.[4]

When several recordings of variability and related signals are available, signal processing methods such as cross-spectral analysis[5-7] and multivariate[8-11] parametric methods are used to analyze phase relationships and causal interactions. At the same time, these analyses address questions about the genesis of variability rhythms and about their physiological meaning; namely, questions relevant to the relationships between respiratory sinus arrhythmia and the respiratory (second order) AP waves, and also to the interactions between central and vasomotor mechanisms in the generation mechanisms of LF (third order or Mayer, in AP) waves.[2]

Signal processing methods are (more or less explicitly) based on models which imply hypotheses necessary to focus the specific characteristics to be measured and to simplify the processing algorithms. Compared to simulation models, which try to provide an exhaustive description, data analysis models have the characteristics to define the least a priori hypotheses in order

From: Malik M., Camm AJ (eds.): *Heart Rate Variability*. Armonk, NY. Futura Publishing Company, Inc., © 1995.

to fix the basic structure of the problem and then leave to the identification procedure the task of extracting quantitative parameters. Nonetheless, it is important to have a clear (even pictorial) representation of the model assumed in order to understand the potentials and limits of the method applied. In the authors' opinion, data models are particularly useful for the analysis of cardiovascular variability, as the complexity of the interactions among the physiological systems involved [12] has prevented the elaboration of univocal theories concerning the underlying mechanisms.[2] So, it can be useful to provide data processing tools able to quantify different mechanisms which can change according to the experimental condition or subject. In other words, these models are used as 'filters' for extracting specific features from data.

This chapter will try to present, in a simple way, the most usual structures relevant to the processing of RR interval variability, AP variability and respiration data, and also to trace the links among different models and algorithms, starting from single-channel models and autospectral analysis up to multivariate (multichannel) models. It will concentrate on linear methods (either parametric or not). Therefore, the features considered are those relevant to the autocorrelation and cross-correlation properties (second order characteristics) of the signals, while the information contained in higher order moments is neglected. These methods permit the representation of second order characteristics in terms of spectral content, frequency responses, and causal relationships, which can be given more easily a physical interpretation.

In order to keep notation as simple and uniform as possible, in the following it will be referred only to the beat-to-beat variability series of RR interval duration, $\{t(i)\}$, and of systolic arterial pressure (SAP), $\{s(i)\}$, and to the beat-by-beat sampled respiration signal, $\{r(i)\}$. This criterion will be kept even if some of the referenced models were proposed for different heart rate variability, AP variability, or respiration signals. The con-

cepts presented are quite general, as they are based on cross-correlations and causal interactions among signals; hence, they can be easily converted for the application to continuous time or sampled signals.

For the sake of simplicity, only the discrete time domain of beat count, 'i,' and the frequency domain, 'f,' of Hz equivalents (obtained from cycles/beat units) will be mentioned, omitting the complex z-transform domain which links both. In addition, similar blocks in different models will be indicated by the same symbol; even if the exact meaning of the block depends on the context in which it appears; eg, $H_{ts}(f)$ will always indicate the transfer function from s to t. Generally, the blocks represent rational transfer functions (ratio of polynomials); when they are constrained to simple polynomials (all-zero blocks), in order to evidence the parametric structure and to relate poles with closed-loops, this will be indicated in the text.

Spectral Analysis

As an introduction, spectral analysis and single-channel identification will be briefly illustrated, in order to show that even elementary methods do imply a priori assumptions and, therefore, a model which underlies the data analysis.

The Fourier analysis, provided by a Fast Fourier Transform (FFT), describes a signal as the sum of several sinusoids at fixed and equally spaced frequencies; ie, the output of several sinusoidal oscillators, the amplitudes and phases of which are described by the FFT. In order to translate it into the spectral estimate provided by a smoothed periodogram, further assumptions are required. First, stationarity permits consideration of the phases provided by the FFT as random features and use of the squared amplitudes to compute a periodogram. Next, adjacent frequencies are considered as related to the same phenomenon, so that smoothing permits the spectral shape to be rendered more readable; this assumption also permits division of the spectral power according to bands relevant to the frequency ranges of higher activity where peaks are detected. In this way, the variability data are interpreted as the linear superposition of several oscillating sources occupying different frequency bands. This is the most common application of the spectral analysis of beat-to-beat variability signals, when nonlinear interferences between different oscillating mechanisms can be neglected.[13]

Autoregressive identification is based on a linear prediction model for which the actual sample of the signal, eg, t(i), is derived by a linear combination of 'p' samples of its own past plus a random (white) error $w_t(i)$: $t(i) = a_1t(i-1) + a_2t(i-2) +....a_pt(i-p) + w_t(i)$; the linear parameters ($a_1, a_2...., a_p$) are estimated by means of a linear regression. This concept is sketched in Figure 1a, where the linear combination of 'p' past samples is performed by the block H_{tt}, which (through the mathematics of z-transforms) has also the meaning of a transfer function and of a frequency response (filter) in the frequency domain f: $H_{tt}(f)$. This filter has no poles and a finite impulse response; but the self-loop of the autoregression creates an all-pole filter $M_t(f) = 1/\{1-H_{tt}(f)\}$, which describes the spectral peaks and components of the signal.

The autoregressive spectral estimate is obtained by multiplying the squared modulus of the all-pole filter by the variance of w_t: $S_{tt}(f) = |M_t(f)|^2 \cdot \lambda_t^2$. This spectrum is smooth as the positions of a limited number of peaks are determined by pairs of conjugate poles and it can be accordingly divided into components, as shown in Figure 1c, through the residual method.[14] Therefore the autoregressive model implies the assumption of a few superimposed oscillating mechanisms, the power and frequency of which are experimentally determined through the autoregressive analysis, without any a priori definition of frequency bands. The behavior of these oscillators is not sinusoidal, but is more or less modulated as shown by the bandwidth of the relevant components, which present a peak

at their central frequency with a smooth descent over a wide frequency range. In other words, the autoregressive filter $M_t(f)$ describes resonances, which are excited by the random input w_t, and fluctuate around their central frequency.

Autospectral analysis neglects all phase information, which is either lost after the periodogram computation in the nonparametric analysis, or confined in the white noise in parametric models. Passing to multivariate analysis, phase differences between different signals gain importance: the evaluation of their value and persistency at each frequency is the base for cross-spectral analysis in the frequency domain and for multivariate parametric identification in the time domain, as will be discussed in the next sections.

Analysis of Baroreceptive Mechanisms

Models are more explicitly useful when relationships among different variability signals are explored. In this field, the most common application is in the analysis of RR interval changes corresponding to AP changes (usually SAP changes) in order to assess the activity of baroreceptive mechanisms.

Classically, this activity is evaluated by inducing a change in SAP with a pharmacological stimulus and observing the reflex RR changes; eg, the vasoconstriction induced by a phenylephrine bolus causes a progressive SAP increase lasting several (10 to 20) heartbeats and a reflex bradycardia.[15] In this experimental condition, it is clear that the RR change is caused by the induced SAP change. In other words, an open-loop model can be considered, as in Figure 2a. The block from SAP to RR is usually considered as a linear gain with eventually a delay of few (1 to 2) beats; other superimposed effects (mainly respiratory arrhythmia) are considered in order to be eliminated. This perspective is implicit in the linear regression algorithm most often applied to evaluate the

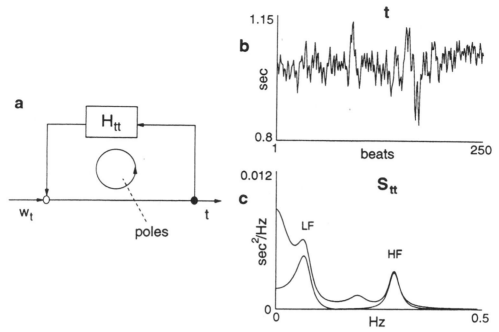

Figure 1. Single-channel autoregressive analysis of RR interval variability. a: autoregressive model; b: beat-to-beat series of RR interval variability, 't,' of a resting human; c: relevant autoregressive spectrum, $S_{tt}(f)$, and spectral decomposition.

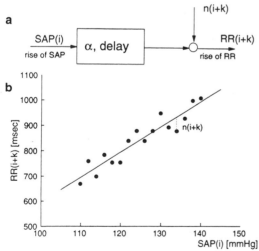

Figure 2. Measurement of cardiac baroreflex inducing an AP rise. a: implied model; b: estimate of gain α.

reflex gain as α slope in milliseconds/mm Hg of RR changes versus SAP changes, as shown in Figure 2b. A delay of 'k' beats can be estimated and compensated for simply searching the value of k (k = 0,1,2...) which optimizes the linear regression coefficient in the regression of RR(i+k) versus SAP(i). Superimposed effects n(i+k) are confined in the regression residual or error according to the model RR(i+k) = SAP(i) + n(i+k) (i = onset of pressure change, ..., end of pressure change). Well-recognized nonlinear effects (such as threshold and saturation in the response, different response to positive or negative pressure changes, and interference of respiration phase) are disregarded in this approximation.

The utility to generalize the above approach to the analysis of spontaneous variability is evident: the measurement is less invasive; continuous monitoring can be obtained; and the normal behavior of cardiovascular control in the absence of external perturbations is observed. Unfortunately, the simple scheme of Figure 2a is less reliable in this condition. In fact, the investigated control mechanisms are based on closed-loop feedback actions, rendering it difficult to disentangle a reflex response from the effectiveness of the changes induced by the reflex itself. In other words,

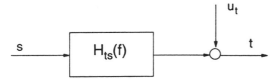

Figure 3. Open-loop model of cardiac baroreflex.

after a phenylephrine bolus, the SAP rise is governed almost entirely by the external stimulus and feedbacks can be disregarded; on the contrary, during normal control activity RR and SAP variability do continuously follow each other. Furthermore, in the absence of a simple transient, such as the ramp-like pressure rise induce by phenylephrine, the dynamics of the reflex may not be disregarded, and the simple regression of RR on a single SAP value has to be substituted with a multiple regression of $t(i)$ over several preceding SAP variability values: $s(i), s(i-1), ..., s(i-p)$.

Nonetheless, simplified approaches were proposed in order to evaluate the baroreflex based on an open-loop scheme. In a time-domain approach, sequences with a contemporaneous rise or reduction of both SAP and RR are searched and used to assess the baroreflex, assuming that this mechanism dominates RR variability during these short (3 to 4 beats) time intervals.[16] In a frequency-domain approach, Robbe et al[17] proposed estimating the SAP to RR transfer function as the ratio between the cross-spectrum and the input spectrum: $H_{ts}(f)=C_{ts}(f)/S_{ss}(f)$. This formula implies a model as in Figure 3, very similar to that of Figure 2a, except that the dynamics of the baroreflex is described by the transfer function $H_{ts}(f)$, so that different frequency bands can be distinguished. Robbe et al proposed using the amplitude of $H_{ts}(f)$ to assess the baroreflex gain only at frequencies in which variability is driven by pressure in order to fulfill the hypothesis implied by the model of Figure 3; namely, LF was hypothesized to be a valid stimulus to the baroreflex.

A closed-loop approach recognizes that, while pressure variability reflexly affects RR variability, RR changes do contrib-ute to pressure changes as in the scheme of Figure 4a first formalized by Askelrod et al.[18] When a closed-loop identification procedure is applied, no a priori hypothesis about variability being driven by SAP rather than by RR is necessary.[9] It is only required that the input u_s is effective at all the considered frequencies (ie, persistently exciting),[19] so that $H_{ts}(f)$ can be disentangled from the closed-loop. This is particularly useful as the nature of the HF respiratory arrhythmia and of the LF spontaneous waves change according to different experimental models and conditions.[10] As shown in Figure 4b, once $H_{ts}(f)$ has been evaluated, it can be extracted from the loop and excited by a ramp which mimics the pressure rise given by a phenylephrine bolus; so a single gain parameter, α_{cl}, is obtained by means of a regression of the simulated 't' rise versus the ramp of 's,' as in Figure 4c.

Askelrod et al proposed a simplified closed-loop analysis of $H_{ts}f)$, which holds when variability is almost entirely driven by AP so that u_t can be neglected as in Figure 5. Under this condition, the amplitude of baroreceptive response can be computed simply as the square root of the ratio of the RR spectrum over the SAP spectrum:

$$|H_{ts}(f)| = \{S_{tt}(f)/S_{ss}(f)\}^{1/2}.$$

This model was found[18] to be valid in conscious dogs at LF. On the contrary, it was found[18] that at HF in conscious dogs, variability is almost entirely driven by RR; accordingly it was stressed that in the latter and in similar conditions, the spectral ratio described above would yield $|1/H_{st}(f)|$, which is obviously not a measure of baroreceptive response, but rather relies on mechanical effects. Pagani et al[20] proposed a similar algorithm based on the same model but using a ratio of autoregressive spectral components either at LF or at HF: $\alpha_{LF}=\{P_{tt}(LF)/P_{ss}(LF)\}^{1/2}$ and $\alpha_{HF}=\{P_{tt}(HF)/P_{ss}(HF)\}^{1/2}$ respectively. This modification renders the results more robust as main components rather than single frequencies are considered, and can also immediately follow a spectral decomposition of RR and

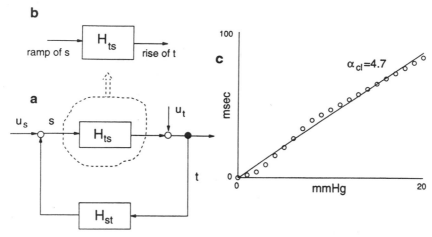

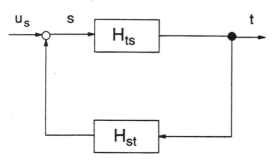

Figure 4. a: closed-loop model of RR interval and SAP variability interaction; b: after closed-loop identification block $H_{ts}(f)$ is considered separately to simulate a response to a pressure rise; c: estimate of the gain parameter from the simulation (same subject of Figure 1).

Figure 5. Simplified closed-loop model for the estimate of cardiac baroreflex through a spectral ratio.

SAP beat-to-beat series. Both α_{LF} and α_{HF} were found[20] to follow baroreceptive activity in man suggesting that in these subjects both LF and HF variability is mainly driven by AP.

It can be interesting to compare the results of the open-loop approach by Robbe et al,[17] $|H_{ts}(f)|_{OL}$ with that of the simplified closed-loop approach by Askelrod et al,[18] $|H_{ts}(f)|_{SCL}$:

$$|H_{ts}(f)|_{OL} = |C_{ts}(f)| / S_{ss}(f) = K(f) \cdot \{S_{tt}(f)/ S_{ss}(f)\}^{1/2} = K(f) \cdot |H_{ts}(f)|_{SCL}$$
$$\text{where } K(f) = |C_{ts}(f)| / \{S_{tt}(f) \cdot S_{ss}(f)\}^{1/2}$$

is the cross-spectral coherence (ie, the degree, from 0 to 1, of linear correlation at each frequency). Usually, values of squared-coherence higher than 0.5 are required to validate an interaction between RR and SAP variabilities[5] and are most often found in the major bands [6]; so, $0.7 < K(f) < 1$; ie, in the worst case $|H_{ts}(f)|_{OL}$ can be 70% smaller than $|H_{ts}(f)|_{SCL}$. In conclusion, both methods can be applied only when variability is driven mainly by AP and depend on the choice of a specific band or spectral component; they lead to similar numerical values. The open-loop approach disregards the mechanical effects of RR on SAP (ie, $H_{st}(f)$) while the simplified closed-loop approach disregards variability inputs on RR (u_t). The necessity to adopt either simplification can be avoided by closed-loop identification.

Effects of Respiration

Respiration is one of the main sources of cardiovascular variability and is unique in that it can be measured directly. As shown in the model of Figure 6, respiration can often be considered to be an exogenous input to short term variability (ie, LF and HF bands); since, the small beat-to-beat changes in cardiovascular function are not likely to affect respiration.[21] On the contrary, long-term variability is likely to be driven by mechanisms that also modulate breathing. The assumption that respiration is exogenous is not valid, also when a common

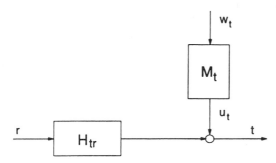

Figure 6. Model with respiration considered as exogenous signal affecting a variability signal, eg, 't.'

central drive modulates both breathing and cardiovascular control, such as during periodic breathing and synchronous slow Mayer waves.

The model of Figure 6 can be useful in assessing the mechanisms which contribute to respiratory sinus arrhythmia, through transfer function $H_{tr}(f)$, and also to analyze that part of spectral content of 't' depending on 'r.' Both nonparametric and parametric methods can be applied. Via nonparametric methods, after the computation of the spectrum of respiration $S_{rr}(f)$ and of RR, $S_{tt}(f)$, and the cross-spectrum between RR and respiration, $C_{tr}(f)$, the transfer function is readily obtained: $H_{tr}(f) = C_{tr}(f)/S_{rr}(f)$. Hence, the partial-spectrum of 't' depending on 'r' is: $S_{t/r}(f) = |H_{tr}(f)|^2 \cdot S_{rr}(f)$. Substituting the formula of $H_{tr}(f)$ and considering that the squared coherence between 't' and 'r' is $K_{tr}(f)^2 = |C_{tr}(f)|^2/\{S_{tr}(f) \cdot S_{tt}(f)\}$ results: $S_{t/r}(f) = K_{tr}(f)^2 \cdot S_{tt}(f)$. The partial-spectrum not depending on 'r' is obtained by difference: $S_{t/wt} = S_{tt}(f) - S_{t/r}(f) = \{1 - K_{tr}(f)^2\}S_{tt}(f)$. Therefore, the two partial-spectra can be referred to as coherent and noncoherent parts of $S_{tt}(f)$ with respect to respiration.[22]

Parametric methods require choosing a suitable model structure and order. They provide directly the parameters of $H_{tr}(f)$ and $M_t(f)$ and also the variance, λ_t^2, of the white prediction error w_t. $S_{rr}(f)$ requires a separate estimate. Afterwards, $S_{tt}(f)$ is readily obtained as sum of the partial-spectra:

$$S_{tt}(f) = S_{t/r}(f) + S_{t/wt}(f) = |H_{tr}(f)|^2 \cdot S_{rr}(f) + |M_t(f)|^2 \cdot \lambda_t^2.$$

The most simple parametric structure is the autoregressive with exogenous input (ARX) one shown in Figure 7a, in which the sample of $t(i)$ is linearly predicted from 'p' past values of 't' and 'p' past values of 'r' plus a random error $w_t(i)$:

$$t(i) = a_1 t(i-1) + a_2 t(i-2) + ... + a_p t(i-p)$$
$$+ b_1 r(i-1) + b_2 r(i-2) + ... + b_p r(i-p) + w_t(i).$$

So the parameters of $H_{tt}(f)$ ($a_1, a_2, ..., a_p$) and those of R_t ($b_1, b_2, ..., b_p$) can be easily obtained by means of a multiple regression. Next, $H_{tr}(f) = R_t(f)/\{1 - H_{tt}(f)\}$ and $M_t(f) = 1/\{1 - H_{tt}(f)\}$ are obtained. The spectral content of 'r' is identified by an autoregressive model. Other structures such as dynamic adjustment (illustrated in the next session) and ARMAX do require more complex identification algorithms. Figure 7b displays a spectral decomposition of $S_{tt}(f)$ into $S_{t/wt}(f)$ and $S_{t/r}(f)$, performed after ARX identification. Note that $S_{t/wt}$ contains mainly a peak at LF and almost no HF activity; $S_{t/r}(f)$ contains the HF peak at respiratory frequency, but also LF activity related to some resonating mechanism which enhances any input at LF, even if this input (respiration in this case) has very low power in this band. So the partial-spectrum coherent with 'r' does enhance the HF activity but also contains components related to cardiovascular control. These components can be separated according to the poles of the ARX model in Figure 7a distinguished from the poles of the autoregressive model of respiration with a procedure analogous to that illustrated in detail in the next section.

In the case of normal breathing, the above model and the consequent subdivision into partial-spectra can be very useful when the respiratory frequency is hardly recognized observing the spectral peaks or components of the variability signal. This can be due to irregular respiration which broadens the relevant component or to unfavorable signal-to-noise ratios, in cases of reduced variability, or to very slow breathing which pushes the respiratory component very close to the LF peak. In the last case, the model has a good performance

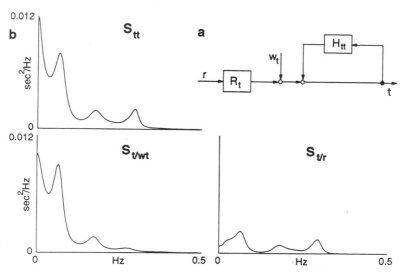

Figure 7. Spectral decomposition based on respiration exogenousness. a: ARX model adopted for the estimate; b: relevant spectral decomposition into a noncoherent (with respiration) and a coherent part (same subject of Figure 1).

when no real entrainment occurs, even if the LF and HF components appear to be fused in the spectral pattern. If entrainment[13] occurs and LF oscillation are phase-locked to respiration, it is impossible to perform any decomposition. Considering metronome breathing, the exogenous nature of respiration still holds; but the model is less useful as either a sharp respiratory peak is clearly identified and entrainment is more likely to occur when the sharp respiratory peak enters the LF band.

The exogenous nature of respiration is particularly useful when experiments with randomly controlled respiration are considered, in which a subject is trained to start a breath on a computerized trigger that occurs with a Poisson-like distribution.[7] So a wide-band spectral pattern of $S_{rr}(f)$ is obtained in order to optimize the estimate of the transfer function from 'r' to 't,' $H_{tr}(f)$, at all the frequencies of short-term variability. Saul et al[7] analyzed the pattern of $H_{tr}(f)$ in order to assess the sympatho-vagal balance in the sinus-node modulation: $H_{tr}(f)$ should present a tighter low pass-filtering action and a higher phase shift when the sympathetic drive is prevalent. This interpretation of $H_{tr}(f)$ is useful when the action of baroreceptive mechanisms can be neglected; ie, when respiratory arrhythmia is directly driven by respiration with no reflex interference with AP variability and resonances in AP control mechanisms.

RR-AP Respiration Interactions

Contemporaneous recordings of 't,' 's,' and 'r' can be analyzed by means of the multivariate model shown in Figure 8, which considers: the closed-loop interaction of 't' and 's'; the closed-loop regulation of 's' based on baroreceptive mechanisms; 'r' as exogenous input impinging both on 't' and 's'; and also spectral components introduced by other inputs (u_t and u_s), that are obtained as residuals after the identification of the previous interactions.[9]

Various indices can be computed using the parameters of the model identified from experimental data.[10] As illustrated above, index α_{cl} measures the effect of baroreceptive mechanisms on 't.' The genesis of LF oscillations is explored by considering the amplification of variability performed by an LF resonance peak in the closed-loop gain of 's' regulation, $G_{ss}(LF)=1/\{1-H_{ss}(LF)\}$, and also by evaluating the power of eventual LF components in the residuals u_t and u_s,

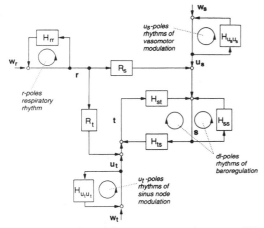

Figure 8. Model of the interactions between RR interval variability and SAP variability with respiration as exogenous signal. The parametric structure is evidenced together with the types of poles identified by the model.

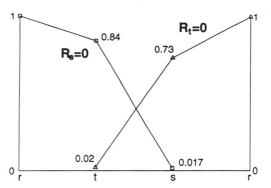

Figure 9. Analysis of the effects of respiration on the variability signals performed driving directly either the RR interval (R_s=0) or SAP (R_t=0). (same subject of Figure 1).

P_{ut}(LF) and P_{us}(LF) respectively. Further considerations about LF genesis are given below by means of spectral decomposition.

The mechanical action of 't' on 's' is evaluated by the one-beat-lag parameter of H_{st}(f), h_{st}(1); a negative value indicates that SAP is decreased by a long preceding RR interval, due to diastolic arterial depletion, while a positive value indicates a prevalence of the effect of a higher heart filling. The one-beat-lag parameter of H_{ss}(f), h_{ss}(1), is strongly affected by the arterial windkessel time constant, which partially maintains an SAP change in the next beat, but can be also influenced by fast neural mechanisms.

Direct respiratory arrhythmia is compared to reflex effects from respiratory SAP variability by means of a ratio between the variability of 't' due to 'r' introduced by R_t alone over that introduced by R_s. Figure 9 gives a pictorial representation of this procedure. The diagram from 'r' to 't' to 's' (labeled R_s=0) indicates the percent contribution of R_t to the respiratory variability of 't' and 's'; the diagram from 'r' to 's' to 't' (labeled R_t=0) is relevant to the contribution of R_s. In this example, a direct effect of 'r' on both 't' and 's' is evidenced.

As shown in Figure 8, the parametric structure given to the model is based on a loop of two dynamic adjustment models for 't' and 's' prediction and an autoregressive model for the analysis of 'r' spectral pattern. Dynamic adjustment models may contain an autoregression (eg, 's' to 's') and are fed by autoregressive noises (ie, u_t and u_s); so the poles of the multivariate model can be classified according to the functional parts in which they do appear. The figure displays only moving average blocks, which do not bear any pole, and therefore emphasizes the loops in which poles (and therefore resonances and spectral peaks) are created: the double-loop (dl-poles) structure of 's' and 't' interactions, and the autoregressive spectral factors of u_t (ut-poles), of u_s (us-poles), and of respiration (r-poles). So dl-poles describe spectral components related to resonances of closed-loop interactions, often an LF resonance of pressure regulation. Ut-poles are related to rhythmic components affecting the sinus node, which are detected at LF during particular experimental conditions and which are likely to be centrally driven.[10] Us-poles describe oscillations affecting AP but not caused by baroreceptive regulation and, therefore, can be related to vasomotor activity which may introduce components at LF or at lower frequencies.[11]

In this way, a more detailed spectral decomposition is obtained through the identification of the multivariate model. In fact, the model describes the spectrum of 't'

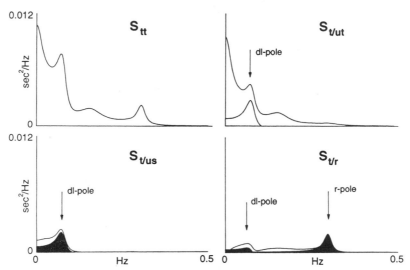

Figure 10. Spectral decomposition of RR interval variability into partial-spectra and into components relevant to the poles classified by the model in Figure 8. (same subject of Figure 1).

(or of 's') as the sum of three partial-spectra relevant to the three inputs, u_t, u_s, and 'r':

$$S_{tt}(f) = S_{t/ut}(f) + S_{t/us}(f) + S_{t/r}(f) =$$
$$|N_{tt}(f)|^2 \cdot \lambda_t^2 + |N_{ts}(f)|^2 \cdot \lambda_s^2 + |N_{tr}(f)|^2 \cdot \lambda_r^2.$$

$N_{tt}(f)$, $N_{ts}(f)$, $N_{tr}(f)$ are the whole transfer functions from the relevant white noises (w_t, w_s, and w_r respectively) to the variability series 't'; λ_t^2, λ_s^2, and λ_r^2 are the variances of the respective white noises. The above transfer functions can be easily computed from the model and are the elements of the transfer function matrix of the joint process description of the model.[11,23]

The three partial-spectra have the same form of ARMA spectra which can be decomposed through the residual method according to their poles. So a further spectral decomposition follows, that permits the labeling of the spectral components according to the relevant poles. All the three partial-spectra share dl-poles; therefore, dl-spectral components are subdivided according to the effects of the three inputs which can excite the resonance of regulation mechanisms. For example, in Figure 10, an LF reso-

nance of pressure control can be excited by a broad-band vasomotor activity (u_s) which by itself may not have any particular spectral peak (absence of u_s-poles in this case) but which is selectively enhanced by baroreceptive mechanisms. It can also be excited by 't' changes (u_t) and by the LF tail of the respiration spectrum. Each spectrum also contains the poles of the relevant input; ie, ut-poles, us-poles and r-poles respectively; eg, in experiments in which an LF ut-pole is detected, a peak in $S_{t/ut}(f)$ is enhanced, which is absent in the other partial-spectra; the relevant spectral components quantifies the effect of a rhythm conveyed by u_t, which can be related to a neural modulation of the sinus node. In other cases us-poles do enhance LF components in $S_{t/us}(f)$, which can be put in relation to the spontaneous rhythmicities of vasomotor activity.[11]

Acknowledgments: The authors are indebted to Professor A. Malliani and coworkers, Medicina Interna II, Ospedale 'L. Sacco,' Università, Milano, Italy and particularly to Dr. D. Lucini for providing us the presented data.

References

1. Sayers BMcA. Analysis of heart rate variability. Ergonomics 1973; 16:85-97.
2. Koepchen HP. History of studies and concepts of blood pressure waves. In: Miyakawa K, Polosa C, Koepchen HP (eds). Mechanisms of Blood Pressure Waves. Berlin, Germany: Springer Verlag, 1984; 3-23.
3. Askelrod A, Gordon D, Ubel FA, et al. Power spectrum analysis of heart rate fluctuations: a quantitative probe of beat-to-beat cardiovascular control. Science 1981; 213:220-222.
4. Pagani M, Lombardi F, Guzzetti S, et al. Power spectral analysis of heart rate and arterial pressure variability as a marker of sympatho-vagal interaction in man and in conscious dog. Circ Res 1986; 59:178-193.
5. De Boer RW, Karemaker JM, Strackee J. Relationships between short-term blood pressure fluctuations and heart-rate variability in resting subjects. Med Biol Eng Comput 1985; 23:352-364.
6. Baselli G, Cerutti S, Civardi S, et al. Spectral and cross-spectral analysis of heart rate and arterial blood pressure variability signals. Comp Biomed Res 1986; 19:520-534.
7. Saul JP, Berger RD, Chen MH, et al. Transfer function analysis of autonomic regulation. II. Respiratory sinus arrhythmia. Am J Physiol 1989; 256:H153-H161.
8. Baselli G, Cerutti S, Livraghi M, et al. Causal relationships between heart rate and arterial pressure variability signal. Med Biol Eng Comput 1988; 26:374-378.
9. Baselli G, Cerutti S, Civardi S, et al. Cardiovascular variability signals: towards the identification of a closed-loop model of the neural control mechanisms. IEEE Trans Biomed Eng 1988; BME-35:1033-1046.
10. Baselli G, Cerutti S, Badilini F, et al. A model for the assessment of heart period and arterial pressure variability interactions and of respiration influences. Med Biol Eng Comput 1994. In press.
11. Baselli G, Porta A, Ferrari G, et al. Multivariate identification and spectral decomposition for the assessment of cardiovascular control. In: Di Rienzo M, et al (eds). Computer Analysis of Blood Pressure and Heart Rate Signals. IOS Press, 1994. In press.
12. Pagani M, Lombardi F, Guzzetti S, et al. Power spectral analysis of heart rate and arterial pressure variability as a marker of sympatho-vagal interaction in man and in conscious dog. Circ Res 1986; 59:178-193.
13. Kitney RI, Linkens D, Selman A, et al. The interaction between heart rate and respiration. II. Nonlinear analysis based on computer modelling. Automedica 1982; 4:141-153.
14. Baselli G, Cerutti S, Civardi S, et al. Heart rate variability signal processing: a quantitative approach as an aid to diagnosis in cardiovascular pathologies. Int J Biomed Comput 1987; 20:51-70.
15. Smyth HS, Phil D, Sleight P, et al. Reflex regulation of arterial pressure during sleep in man, a quantitative method of assessing baroreflex sensitivity. Circ Res 1969; 24:109-121.
16. Steptoe A, Vögele C. Cardiac baroreflex function during postural change assessed using non-invasive spontaneous sequence analysis in young men. Cardiovasc Res 1990; 24:627-632.
17. Robbe H, Mulder L, Ruddel H, et al. Assessment of baroreceptor reflex sensitivity by means of spectral analysis. Hypertension 1987; 10:538-543.
18. Askelrod S, Gordon D, Mawed JB, et al. Hemodynamic regulation: investigation by spectral analysis. Am J Physiol 1985; 249:H867-H875.
19. Södeström T, Stoica T. System Identification. London, England: Prentice Hall, 1989.
20. Pagani M, Somers V, Furlan R, et al. Changes in autonomic regulation induced by physical training in mild hypertension. Hypertension 1988; 12:600-610.
21. Baselli G, Biancardi L, Porta A, et al. Multichannel parametric analysis of the coupling between respiration and cardiovascular variabilities. J Ambulat Monit 1992; 5:153-165.
22. Bianchi A, Bontempi B, Cerutti S, et al. Spectral analysis of heart rate variability and respiration in diabetic subjects. Med Biol Eng Comput 1990; 28:205-211.
23. Baselli G, Porta A, Ferrari G, et al. Multivariate ARMA spectral decomposition in the assessment of cardiovascular variabilities. IEEE Proc Comput Cardiol Conf; Sept. 1993; London, 731-734.

Chapter 12

Components of Heart Rate Variability:
Basic Studies

Solange Akselrod

Introduction

As expressed by the mere existence of this book, during the last decade more and more effort has been invested in understanding the fluctuations in cardiovascular parameters. The rationale of this interest is intuitively clear: the fluctuations result from the continuous interaction between the neural or humoral control of cardiovascular function and the intrinsic, as well as extrinsic, sources of noise. As such, they reflect the mechanisms of cardiovascular homeostasis, in conjunction with the possible mechanisms of perturbations. Homeostasis [1] in itself does not result in rigid constancy. Rather, it implies that the system is kept within specific limits, allowing small oscillations around optimal values. Even under steady state conditions, heart rate (HR) and blood pressure (BP) display spontaneous beat-to-beat and breath-to-breath fluctuations. These occur at very specific frequencies, closely related to the physiological functioning of the system. As early as 1733,

Hales noticed waves in HR and BP at the frequency of respiration (also described by Ludwig in 1847 and Hering in 1869), while low-frequency (LF) waves (0.05 Hz) were observed by Mayer (1876) in arterial BP, independent of respiration[2,3].

Thorough analysis of the fluctuations in instantaneous HR, BP or flow has since been able to provide direct insight into the physiology of the participating autonomic control branches.[4-8] An important by-product of such investigation can be the understanding of the autonomic impact of a wide variety of perturbations, such as a change in temperature, a deep breath, mental stress, or the transition from supine to standing position.[9-11] The enormous advantage of analyzing these fluctuations is that the information can be provided on-line, noninvasively and without interfering with the normal dynamic functioning of the control mechanisms.

Effectiveness of cardiovascular control is and has been traditionally expressed by a mean HR and a mean BP value, obviously

From: Malik M., Camm AJ (eds.): *Heart Rate Variability.* Armonk, NY. Futura Publishing Company, Inc., © 1995.

overlooking any information carried by the oscillations around this mean. In the past, in order to compensate for this deficiency whenever variability information was expected to be relevant, some simple time-domain analysis has often been performed. In its most basic form, it usually included the computation of the mean and the variance (or rms value) of a series of RR intervals[12,13] or an estimate of the maximal change relative to some control state,[14-16] or the count of the beats with a variation above a certain threshold.[17,18] Additional measures, like histograms or higher moments of the RR interval distribution, have been applied as well. However, these measures imply the loss of important information, such as the direct relation to the time axis or the frequency content of the variations. To overcome some of these shortcomings, more sophisticated ways of analysis have been adopted. An elegant example of a method borrowed from the time domain consists in cautious detection and counting of the occurrence of short (2 to 6 beats) and longer (above 10 beats) trains of consecutive RR intervals displaying a similar trend (all increasing or all decreasing).[19] However, the most extensively applied methods belong to the frequency domain and consist usually in carefully designed algorithms for the computation of power spectra (FFT or autoregressive) of HR or other cardiovascular parameters (Figure 1).[20,21]

Specific Insight Provided by Heart Rate Fluctuations

As a rule, the instantaneous HR has been chosen by researchers as the main cardiovascular candidate for analysis of fluctuations, being the most straightforward keyhole into cardiovascular control[9,10,22,23] and the most easily measured. Various methods, extensively described in the previous chapters, have been applied to quantitate the heart rate variability (HRV) and elucidate its origins.

The implementation of these methods for the investigation of HR fluctuations is aimed at highlighting the various limbs of autonomic cardiovascular control, and defining their dynamic response to intrinsic and extrinsic perturbations. It is important to mention that a similar approach to other hemodynamic signals, and in particular to blood pressure, has the ability to throw light on additional control mechanisms, such as those affecting vasomotor tone.

Spectral Analysis of Heart Rate Fluctuations

The frequency-domain approach (spectral analysis) has yielded the most important breakthrough in the amount and the specificity of the information that has been obtained from HRV (Figure 2). The initial studies have merely focused on the determination of the features of the typical HR

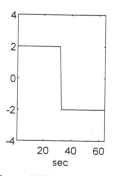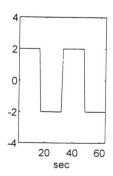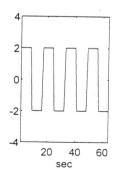

Figure 1. Three different series of instantaneous HR values, having the same number of values at low and high level, and thus the same histogram. However, their frequency content and thus the power spectrum of their fluctuations is totally different.

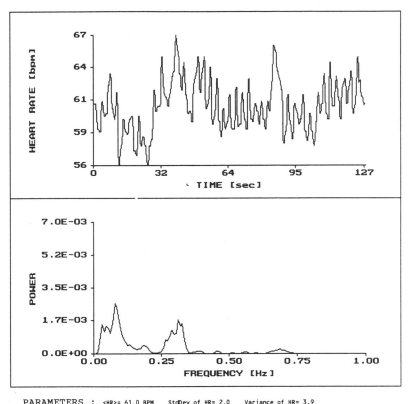

PARAMETERS : <HR>= 61.0 BPM   StdDev of HR= 2.0   Variance of HR= 3.9

Begin: 1000 End: 1130 Window: 0.25 Time scale: 1.00 Factors: 100.000;100.000

Figure 2. Typical HR time series and corresponding HR power spectrum for a healthy adult in supine position.

power spectrum and their physiological implications.[6-8,24,25] During the last few years the applicability of HR spectral analysis has gradually been extended from the fields of basic research to the clinical setup, as evidenced by the large number of clinical studies undertaken.[9,10,22,23]

However, before HR spectral analysis could be safely used as a diagnostic tool to detect or to quantitate abnormalities in cardiovascular control, a reliable knowledge of the standard pattern needed to be established. A variety of control mechanisms and noise sources take part in the creation of the HR fluctuations, providing sometimes independent, sometimes loosely interacting or closely linked contributions.[7,26-29] Figure 3 displays a simplified, schematic model of the main cardiovascular control branches and noise sources, which

is only a rough approximation of the complexity of this system.

A first step in understanding the contribution of the various participating branches and noise sources is to obtain a typical power spectrum of HR fluctuations. The next step is then to try and establish whether any specific physiological mechanism is reflected within a specific frequency and amplitude range. These two steps were actually the principal scope of the earlier research performed in the field of HRV. Only then could the crucial question be asked: what are the possible applications?

General Features of Heart Rate Power Spectrum

A typical HR time series and corresponding power spectrum obtained in a

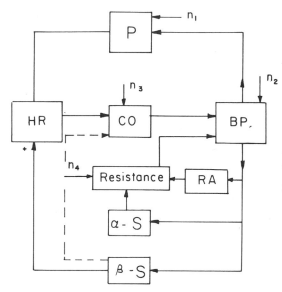

Figure 3. Schematic model of cardiovascular control. P: parasympathetic; S: sympathetic; RA: renin-angiotensin control; CO: cardiac output; the n_i's: various noise sources, the most important of which is the respiratory contribution to n_1 via neural and to n_2 via mechanical.

healthy adult is shown in Figure 2, for a 256-second trace. It is apparent that most of the power is concentrated in two frequency ranges: a high-frequency (HF) range, centered around the frequency of respiration (in adults usually between 0.2 to 0.4 Hz); and a lower frequency range, below 0.15 Hz. The latter has often been subdivided into an LF (below 0.09 Hz) and mid- (0.09 to 0.15 Hz) frequency range.

The HF peak is frequently called the respiratory peak and corresponds to the HR variations related to the respiratory cycle, or what is known as respiratory sinus arrhythmia. The mid-frequency and LF fluctuations are seldom characterized by two clear and independent peaks, and they usually merge into one common region of power. There is, therefore, no simple answer to the question as where to actually determine the cutoff frequency between both; it has usually been chosen as 0.09 or 0.1 Hz, occasionally 0.08 Hz.[6,11,30] Often only an LF range is taken into account and the mid-frequency range is neglected, having a lower power content. Sometimes a wider LF range is considered,

up to 0.12 or 0.15 Hz.[8,11,31,32] In studies based on autoregressive computation of the spectrum, the LF power of fluctuations is usually obtained from the peak located around 0.1 Hz and smoothly extending towards slightly higher frequencies.[10,11]

In general, since in most investigations the LF range is considered the range in which the sympathetic activity is reflected (as shown below), it is reasonable to choose its upper limit as the frequency at which sympathetic gain markedly decreases, around 0.1 Hz.[33] When considering particular mechanisms, such as the quantification of thermal effects, or postural changes or hemorrhage, one might gain sensitivity at being more specific about the frequency boundaries of LF and/or mid-frequency ranges.[11,30,34,35] Regarding the determination of the lower boundary of the LF range, the limiting and relevant parameter is the trace length chosen, since its reciprocal (usually multiplied by a safety factor of about 5), determines the minimal frequency above which spectral information is considered as reliable.

Significance of Spectral Content

The power distribution in two principal frequency ranges can be interpreted in view of the neural branches controlling or transferring the fluctuations, but also as a function of the various mechanisms creating the fluctuations and adding noise somewhere along the cardiovascular control system.

The general features shown in Figure 2 are true in all human subgroups: the young and older adults, children, neonates, and fetuses. The main differences appear in the total power, the relative power distribution among the LF to HF range, and the width and location of the respiratory peak.

For instance, as a function of age, adults display a gradual decrease in total power of fluctuations, while the ratio of LF to HF power remains essentially unchanged.[24,36-38] The increase in the LF to HF ratio observed with transition to standing position (or during tilt test), are blunted by age.[24,36,38] In children, from birth to adolescence, marked age-dependent change should be taken into account in the low to high balance, related to the respective development and predominance of sympathetic and vagal control.[39] Interesting spectral properties can be observed in neonates: their HR power spectrum may display a much wider respiratory peak, often ill defined, even though their respiratory power spectrum may show a clear and narrow peak corresponding to regular breathing.[40,41] Irregular or periodic breathing in neonates will obviously widen the respiratory peak and even add LF power (respiratory amplitude modulation) to the HR power spectrum.[42]

The basic features, as shown in Figure 2, are of course affected by health or disease. Indeed, the response of the autonomic system depends on the nature of the noise sources (eg, breathing pattern) or perturbations (eg, hemorrhage or change in position) and on the stability, developmental stage or integrity of the autonomic activity involved.[30,34,35,38,41] Thus, there are obvious indications to use the HR power spectrum as a tool to estimate dysfunction or maturation of autonomic control.[9,10,22,23,30,31,43-45]

It is amazing to realize that in the wide diversity of mammals investigated, essentially the same spectral pattern can be observed. Most of the basic studies were performed in dogs[6,7,24,28,38,46,47] and yielded HRV patterns similar to Figure 2, as did other studies in sheep, rabbits, cats[48,49] or rats.[50-56] As a general rule, however, the smaller the animal, the higher its HR and breathing rate. Again, the principal differences lay in the absolute power level and in the balance between LF to HF fluctuations, as well as in the respiratory rate and in the width of the respiratory peak.

This qualitative resemblance among species makes the HR power spectrum an ideal tool for the investigation of drug effects or disease characteristics in animal models.[9,10,22]

Vagal and Sympathetic Contribution

Since it is basic knowledge that the sinoatrial (SA) node is innervated by both sympathetic and parasympathetic nerve endings, a selective blockade of either of these branches should markedly affect the HR fluctuations and their power spectrum. On the other hand, selective enhancement of either of these branches should also be reflected in the HR power spectrum.

Specific blockade experiments have shown that a very short latency of HR response, within two to three beats, indicates a vagal rather than a sympathetic mechanism.[57,58] Rosenblueth and Simeone[57] have shown that slow HR fluctuations can be mediated by both sympathetic and parasympathetic control, while sympathetic activity is unable to mediate faster HR changes. Elaborate time-domain analysis may enable us to differentiate sympathetic from vagal control on this basis.[19] Spectral analysis, by definition, separates the components of a signal based on their frequency and should thus directly discriminate between the frequency ranges to which slower or faster mechanisms contribute. Vagal activity is then expected to express itself up to frequency ranges higher than the ones reached by sympathetic activity.

Estimate of Vagal Activity

Basic studies have determined that total vagal blockade could essentially eliminate the power of HR fluctuations in the HF range and strongly reduce the power in the LF range.[6,7,8] With gradual vagal blockade, the ratio of the LF to HF power also increases significantly, indicating a clear shift in the sympathovagal balance, towards sympathetic predominance.[10]

The Respiratory Peak as an Estimate of Vagal Activity

Later studies have shown that the respiratory peak can actually be considered as

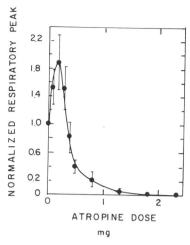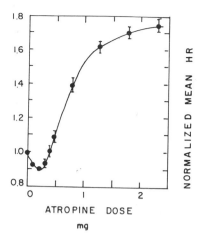

Figure 4. Bimodal dose-dependent effect of atropine on the respiratory peak of the HR power spectrum is averaged over a group of healthy adults. At very low doses, a small paradoxical increase of the respiratory peak is observed, followed by a marked dose-dependent decrease with gradual increase of the atropine dose. An almost mirror-image effect is observed on mean HR. Both respiratory peak and mean HR are normalized by their value at baseline for each subject and then averaged.

a quantitative measure of vagal control.[59,60] An example of the high sensitivity of this spectral estimate of vagal activity is given by a dose-response atropine study performed in human volunteers, who received stepwise increasing bolus doses of the vagal blocker atropine.[60,61]

A strong and gradual dose-dependent reduction of the respiratory peak (down by several orders of magnitude) in the HR power spectrum was observed as a function of the atropine dose, concomitant with an increase in mean HR (Figure 4). The well-known peripheral effect of vagal blockade achieved by atropine can thus be quantified in a dose-dependent way, by HR spectral analysis and, more specifically, by the respiratory peak. Yet, it is even more interesting to mention the small, but clear, paradoxical increase in the respiratory peak measured together with a slight decrease in mean HR, at very low doses of atropine (Figure 4). This observation can be ascribed to a central effect of the atropine, enhancing vagal output to the periphery,[62,63] which is masked at higher doses by the peripheral blockade.[60]

The ability to observe such a bimodal dose-response curve and to recognize this behavior as a pure dose-dependent change in vagal activity is a convincing proof to the sensitivity of the respiratory peak as a probe for vagal control. Changes in the respiratory peak can thus be used to quantitate the parasympathetic dose-dependent effect of cholinergic and anticholinergic agents, as well as to detect possible vagolytic and vagomimetic side effects of drugs.[60-62,64]

More generally, presuming the necessary precautions, the respiratory peak can be used as an estimate for vagal activity, a measure for the integrity of vagal control, and a detector of its possible malfunction.

Limitations Related to the Respiratory Peak

It is therefore extremely important to understand and comply with the limitations related to the estimation of vagal tone from respiratory HR fluctuations. Having seen how sensitive the HF part of the HR power spectrum is to the level of vagal blockade, one would be tempted to use the respiratory peak as a quantitative estimate of vagal activity. This is certainly valid when a comparison to some initial or baseline state can be made, in particular when considering changes in vagal tone in the same individual due to some intervention, or differences between carefully matched groups of subjects.

However, one should carefully take into consideration that the respiratory peak in the HR power spectrum is affected not only by vagal tone. Indeed, it is extremely sensitive to changes in breathing rate or in breath volume.[65-68]

This dependence is visualized in Figure 5, which displays how the respiratory peak changes as a function of breathing rate. In this example, we apply for the analysis of the HR fluctuations, a recently developed method, which we designed for the time-frequency analysis of nonstationary multi-component signals, allowing the spectral components to vary in time. We aimed this approach at solving the need to investigate signals with a time-dependent frequency content and in which the analysis of the transients may actually yield the most interesting information. Typical examples are the need to quantify tilt studies or to estimate the effects of ischemia.[69-72]

During the experiment for which typical results are presented in Figure 5, healthy volunteers were told to breathe according to computer generated sounds, the rate of which varied as a function of time. The respiratory frequency varied from 0.2 to 0.5 Hz, while each rate was kept constant for the duration of 1 minute. The resulting instantaneous HR signal obtained simultaneously with the time-varying breathing rate was then submitted to our algorithm for time-dependent spectral analysis. The resulting time-frequency distribution is shown in Figure 5A in a 3-D representation and in Figure 5B as a contour plot.

Since breathing rate was not constant, the respiratory peak in the HR power spectrum is expected to move around in a 3-D graph showing the true time-frequency distribution. In a regular HR power spectrum obtained by means of standard spectral analysis techniques, in case of a changing respiratory frequency (which is typical for infants), these variations would have been smeared out over the entire time trace, and would appear as a broadening of the respiratory peak. In the 3-D representation of the HR time-frequency distribution computed with our algorithm (Figure 5A), the respiratory peak progresses towards the higher frequencies as a function of time, according to the generated beeper frequency controlling the breathing rate. The corresponding time-dependent analysis of the respiration signal can be performed as well. One can then clearly observe the full agreement in the time dependence of the location of the respiratory peak in the HR, of the peak in respiration, and of the value of the computer generated frequency.

This mixed time-frequency approach can be used to unfold physiological information hidden behind the respiratory peak. For instance, it clearly demonstrates that the power of the respiratory peak decreases as its frequency increases. This behavior has been previously observed,[67] but is not always accounted for in HRV studies. It agrees with the results of broad-band respiration experiments which showed that the transfer function between respiration and HR decreases with frequency.[33,73-75]

By similar means, it can be shown that the respiratory peak is not only affected by breathing rate, but is clearly reduced as breathing volume decreases.[33,68] The main conclusion to keep in mind is that, when considering the respiratory peak as a measure of vagal control, one has to check carefully whether the breathing parameters have not changed before an estimate of vagal tone may be safely made.

A typical example as to the importance of the breathing parameters is the LF modulation of breathing volume (or breathing amplitude modulation), often observed in neonates.[41,42,76] This may contribute a significant amount of power in the LF range of the respiratory spectrum, which can also be transferred as power in the LF range of the HR power spectrum. Under such conditions, part of the LF power of the HRV may be contributed by respiration.

Whether the respiratory peak in the HR power spectrum is an absolute measure of vagal tone is therefore limited to situations in which breathing is carefully monitored and possible changes can be taken into con-

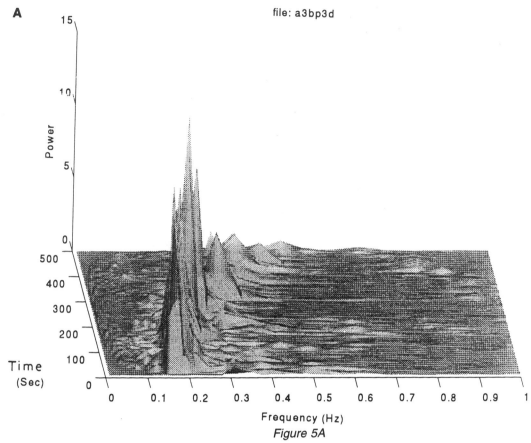

A

file: a3bp3d

Figure 5A

Figure 5A. 3-D plot. Results of time-frequency analysis of HR fluctuations for a healthy subject, breathing at a time-dependent rate.

sideration. An elegant way, though difficult to apply clinically, to overcome these limitations could be to compute the transfer function from instantaneous lung volume to HR under conditions of randomized breathing rate.[33,73-75] The amplitude of the transfer function above 0.1 or 0.15 Hz would provide a cleaner measure of vagal control, accounting for the entire frequency range of breathing. However, such strict breathing conditions (like random or fixed rate under calibrated volume measurement conditions) as opposed to spontaneous breathing, might have their own uncontrolled and individual effect on autonomic balance. They are in contradiction with the basic advantage of the HR spectral analysis, which is its ability to estimate autonomic control under noninvasive, nonperturbing conditions.

Estimate of Sympathetic Activity

The second neural input, directly impinging on the SA node, is the beta-sympathetic activity. Its contribution to the HR power spectrum is more difficult to separate. However, again under well-controlled conditions, a quantitative estimate of beta-sympathetic activity can be obtained.

In the initial dog studies, in which total vagal blockade was achieved with glycopyrrolate (and ascertained with acetylcholine), subsequent beta-sympathetic blockade eliminated the residual LF fluctuations. This double or combined blockade results in an almost metronome-like HR with a flat, nearly-zero power spectrum, displaying a minimal amount of power.[6,7,33] The negligible remainders are essentially a result of mechanical modulation due to respiration

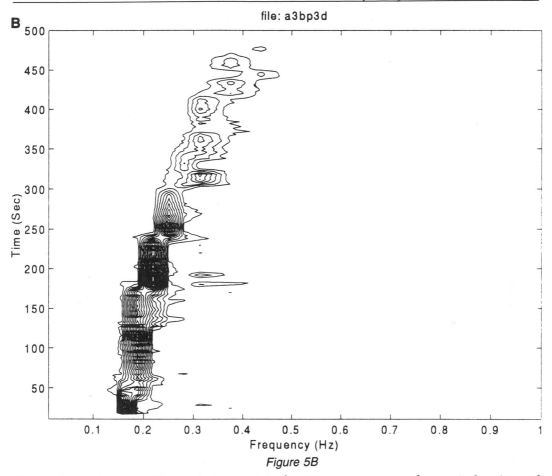

file: a3bp3d

Figure 5B

Figure 5B. Contour plot. The respiratory peak in the HR power spectrum changes its location and its power as a function of breathing rate.

causing some baseline wandering of the ECG signal or slightly affecting the shape of the ECG complex and thus influencing the detection of the R wave. A very small nonautonomic HR control mechanism has also been suggested, possibly related to the rate of change in lung volume.[33] Electrical noise or some residual modulation of the PR interval, if HRV is assessed from RR interval, may still cause some minor fluctuations in HR. However, following double blockade (vagal and beta-sympathetic) the HR power spectrum is several orders of magnitude below baseline. Patients with paced or transplanted hearts produce similar, relatively (to control) powerless HR power spectra.[7,77,78]

These findings thus confirm that the residual HR fluctuations after vagal block-

ade are of sympathetic origin. They are band limited to the LF range, in clear agreement with basic physiological investigations,[57] and with later transfer function studies.[33]

Beta-sympathetic activity on its own, as well as the specific effect of beta-sympathetic blockade, is much more difficult to display and quantitate in humans and in dogs, who can both be defined as mainly 'vagal' under resting conditions, even more so in supine position. The baseline beta-sympathetic tone is so low that the effect of its blockade may be minimal, and strongly dependent on the initial sympathetic tone.[7,8] In subjects who display exaggerated sympathetic activity, such as migraine patients, the LF HR fluctuations are on one hand much stronger than in healthy subjects; on the other hand, they can be markedly reduced by propranolol,[44,45] thus clearly proving their beta-sympathetic mediation. In the rat, a small and much more sympathetically controlled animal, beta-blockade considerably diminishes the LF fluctuations.[52]

The intrinsic difficulty in the independent measurement of sympathetic tone and the effect of beta-sympathetic blockade is the fact that LF fluctuations reflect combined sympathetic and vagal activity. Considering only the LF power, not much can be concluded about sympathetic tone. Only when specific additional knowledge about the HF power is available (for instance if it is unaffected by an intervention or affected in the opposite direction than the LF power), then one may infer that changes occurring in the LF band are of sympathetic origin.[9,10,22-24,44,45] Otherwise, sympathetic changes may be easily masked by vagal activity in the LF band.

Position has a marked effect on the HR power spectrum as displayed during transition from supine to standing position in a healthy human (Figure 6). Upon standing, one observes an increase in sympathovagal balance, as expressed by the ratio of LF to HF power. Clear changes can also be observed in the absolute values of both LF and HF power (Figure 6). The respiratory peak decreases, while the LF fluctuations are enhanced upon standing. In this case, it is easy to conclude upon a reduction in vagal tone accompanied by an increase in sympathetic tone, as expected to overcome the orthostatic hypotension.[10,24]

Since the position change has such a well-defined effect, it can be used as a perturbation to test the integrity of autonomic control. With age, the response becomes gradually blunted.[36-38] Disease can have a marked effect on the expected orthostatic autonomic changes. In subjects with familial dysautonomia, an impaired response to standing is observed[30]; in migraine patients, the increase in LF power is exaggerated.

Prolonged head-up tilt, or 'tilt test' has become widely applied as an aid to detecting reasons for unexplained syncope. In conjunction with spectral analysis of HR fluctuations during the various stages of the test, particularly after the transition in position and just before fainting, the tilt test can provide better understanding of autonomic function and possible imbalance in patients suffering from syncope.[38,69]

Hence, in general, beta-sympathetic activity is reflected within the LF band, yet a quantitative measure of its contribution to cardiovascular control requires great care. The existence of vagal activity in the same frequency band has to be taken into consideration.

Sympathovagal Balance as the Ratio of Low/High Frequency Power

The ratio of power in low/high frequency bands (L/H) can be used as a measure of sympathovagal balance.[10] It is probably a valid estimate under a wide range of physiological situations, particularly when the focus is placed on the changes in sympathovagal balance under various conditions.

It is extremely difficult to determine a mathematical expression for the dependence of the LF power on sympathetic and parasympathetic tone. The dependence seems more involved than a plain linear function and it is far from being just a multiplicative relationship. Therefore, the division of L/H will not provide an accurate measure, neither of the sympathetic tone, nor of the ratio of sympathetic to parasympathetic activity. However, even if the functional relationship is a complex combination of sympathetic and parasympathetic tone, the fact that the LF band includes both contributions, whereas the HF reflects only vagal tone, is a legitimate (qualitative) justification to consider L/H as an estimate of sympathovagal balance.

The L/H ratio may not only provide insight into the autonomic balance, but also provide an estimate of sympathetic activity, supposing an estimate of vagal tone is available, for instance, from the respiratory peak.

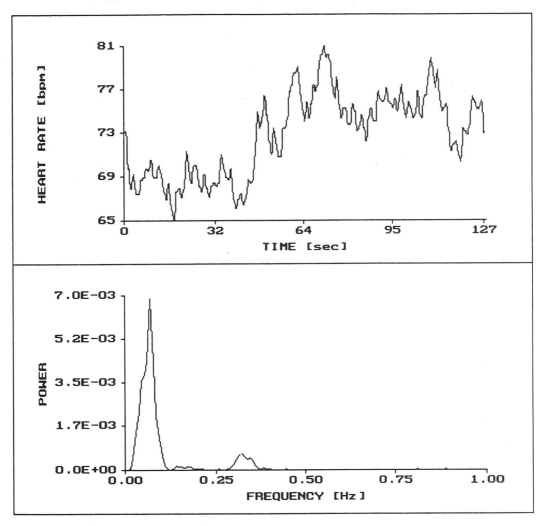

PARAMETERS : <HR>= 73.2 BPM   StdDev of HR= 3.9   Variance of HR=14.9

Begin: 1350 End: 1499 Window: 0.25 Time scale: 1.00 Factors: 100.000;100.000

Figure 6. Effect of standing on autonomic control, as displayed by HR time series and corresponding HR power spectrum, for the same subject as in Figure 2.

In addition, the L/H ratio offers the possibility to measure whether reciprocal versus nonreciprocal changes have occurred in sympathetic and parasympathetic activity.[79] Furthermore, it may throw light on a variety of situations, including complex clinical malfunctions, under which unbalanced or nonreciprocal changes in autonomic activity may occur.

Remarks Related to Estimate of Sympathetic and Vagal Tone

In summary, as the basic guideline for the independent estimate of vagal and beta-sympathetic activity, it is important to stress once again the most crucial conclusion from the basic blockade experiments. The fluctuations in beta-sympathetic tone are restricted to the LF range of the spectrum, having a longer response time than vagal control.[6,57] In the HF range, above 0.15 Hz in humans, only vagal activity contributes. Therefore, in humans, it is much easier to obtain a separate and quantitative estimate of vagal control than of sympathetic control, except under very specific conditions such as:

1. a marked enhancement in sympathetic tone, expressed by a clear increase in LF power concomitant with an unchanged or reduced HF peak; or
2. a reduction in LF peak (if initially high) while the respiratory peak is unchanged or increased.

In those cases, the changes in LF fluctuations can most probably be ascribed to changes in sympathetic activity. The first set of conditions is quite likely to happen, being a reciprocal change (eg, transition to standing, or, migraine patients relative to healthy controls). The second one, which requires a large drop in sympathetic activity, will rarely occur from normal supine conditions, since an increase in respiratory peak is usually related to enhanced vagal activity which will by itself contribute to the power in the LF band.

It is important to emphasize that experimental protocols or clinical evaluations can provide a wider insight into autonomic control if they are designed so that subjects are considered not only under baseline conditions, but also following autonomic changes elicited by a specific intervention.

Frequency Specificity of the Physiological Mechanisms Involved in Heart Rate Variability

When considering the typical human HR power spectrum, it can be subdivided according to the frequency specificity of the neural control systems mediating the fluctuations (sympathetic and parasympa-

thetic) as discussed above. It can also be subdivided according to the sources of the fluctuations.

Classical studies in HRV have distinguished mainly between three such sources.[4-6,80,81] As detailed extensively above, the HF band is very clearly the expression of an HR modulation by respiratory activity (see Figure 5). This modulation (see noise sources in Figure 3) can have a mechanical (via effects of respiration on venous filling, contractility, blood pressure) and/or a neural component,[23] both contributing to the amplitude of fluctuations with a varying weight at the same frequency, the respiration frequency.[82]

Again, the LF range is more complex. Around the frequency of 0.1 to 0.13 Hz (within the mid-frequency band), one observes the contribution due to baroreflex control.[5,80,81] This assumption is based on a variety of experimental evidence. One of the possible indications is the correspondence of this frequency with the time constant of the baroreflex loop. Another proof is the ability to enhance the power of HR fluctuations in this frequency band by inflating and deflating an aortic balloon at a rate nearby this baroreflex frequency, and thus causing entrainment of the natural frequency of the system.[81] An additional indication for the contribution of the baroreflex control in this frequency band is the buildup of a peak around 0.1 Hz in standing position.[30,83]

At the lower end of the LF range is the frequency band where vasomotor and thermal control express themselves.[84-86] Different studies have pointed both towards slightly different frequency bands, usually below 0.1 Hz.[87] Basic experiments affecting vasomotor tone have markedly influenced the fluctuations in this LF band, in particular in the BP signal and then reflexively in the HR signal; it would seem that alpha-sympathetic effect on vasculature acts in a slightly higher frequency band than renin-angiotensin vasomotor control.[55,56] In experiments where, intermittently and at a constant rate, a warm or cold stimulus was applied to a subject, the power of HR fluctuations has been markedly enhanced in the corresponding frequency band. It thus seems that the mechanism of thermal regulation can also be entrained, provided the frequency of the hot/cold stimulus is near enough to the natural frequency of thermal control.[5,80,81] A constant temperature stimulus, such as a change in ambient temperature, has been shown to affect the power spectra of a variety of cardiovascular parameters, HR, BP and even blood flow velocity.[87]

Various Control Systems Affecting Heart Rate Variability Indirectly

Up to now, we have only considered the two control systems innervating the SA node: the vagal and beta-sympathetic branches, which directly modulate the heart rate. Due to the complexity of the cardiovascular control system (Figure 2 is only a very simplified version of it), it is clear that other control limbs and various noise sources may have a marked, though indirect effect on HR fluctuations.

Interventions which alter arterial resistance, such as alpha-sympathetic or renin-angiotensin blockade, directly influence blood pressure and its fluctuations, and then reflexively affect HR and its fluctuations.[6,7,55,56] Transition from supine to standing position have an immediate and direct effect on HR, aimed at avoiding a drop in BP. However, posture affects BP control via alpha-sympathetic activation, which then indirectly reverberates on HR via the baroreflex control.

Migraine patients are a typical example of how direct and indirect pharmacological interventions can modify HR fluctuations. Indeed, they display enhanced LF fluctuations, possibly due to vasomotor instability (when exacerbated, also responsible for migraine attacks), which can be strongly affected by several independent interventions.[44,45,88] Their LF power is reduced to normal level, either by beta-blockade (directly affecting the gain of the feedback loop

at the site of the SA node), or by calcium (Ca)-blockade affecting vasomotor tone and its fluctuations (representing the main noise source to the feedback loop). Furthermore, the LF fluctuations in migraine subjects are strongly enhanced by transition to standing position, much more so than in control subjects, while Ca-blockade eliminates this exaggerated response. It is clear that Ca-blockade does not impinge on the SA node, and still it reduces HR fluctuations.[88]

These are only a few among the numerous examples to illustrate that not only interventions affecting vagal or beta-sympathetic tone have an effect on HR fluctuations. It is enough to change the spectral content of one of the noise sources to affect the HR power spectrum, ie, a variation in breathing activity will modify the HF fluctuations, a change in arterial resistance or in vessel wall rigidity may affect LF fluctuations.[56,89] Any change in one of the specific parameters directly affecting BP, flow or cardiac output will immediately impinge on the pattern of the HR power spectrum, eg, a change in blood volume such as under hemorrhage,[34,35,56] or a change in peripheral resistance[50,55,56] may markedly affect LF fluctuations.

It is also extremely important to realize that even if only a single autonomic neural branch is active within a specific frequency band, the power of HR fluctuations in that frequency band is not necessarily proportional to the mean level of neural activity. The power of HR fluctuations within that frequency band is mainly a reflection of the variations in the corresponding neural activity. The exact relation between the level of neural fluctuations and the mean level of neural activity is far from being known. However, usually the assumption is made that the level of fluctuations in neural activity is linearly related to the mean level, which is probably true near mid-level of activity, not at zero level and not at saturation. Even so, the power of HR fluctuations will have a complex dependence on mean level of that specific neural tone, on its relationship to its own fluctuations, on its interaction with other neural branches (even with those acting at other frequencies) and the combination of their effect on the SA nodal cells.[23,32]

The greatest care should be taken to consider HR fluctuations and the information conveyed by their power spectrum within the framework of all the control mechanisms and noise sources affecting cardiovascular control.

References

1. Cannon WB. Organization for physiological homeostasis. Physiol Rev 1929; 9:399-431.
2. Hales S. Haemastaticks. In: Hales S (ed). Statistical Essays. London, England: Innys and Manby, 1735; (II)1-86.
3. Miyakawa K, Koepchen HP, Polosa C. Mechanisms of blood pressure waves. Tokyo, Japan: Japan Sci Soc Press/ Berlin, Germany: Springer-Verlag, 1984.
4. Sayers BMcA. Analysis of heart rate variability. Ergonomics 1973; 16:17-32.
5. Hyndman BW, Kitney RI, Sayers BMcA. Spontaneous rhythms in physiologic control systems. Nature 1971; 233:339-341.
6. Akselrod S, Gordon D, Ubel FA, et al. Power spectrum analysis of heart rate fluctuations: a quantitative probe of beat-to-beat cardiovascular control. Science 1981; 213:220-222.
7. Akselrod S, Gordon D, Madwed JB, et al. Hemodynamic regulation: investigation by spectral analysis. Am J Physiol 1985; 249:H867-H875.
8. Pomeranz B, Macaulay RJB, Caudill MA, et al. Assessment of autonomic function in man by heart rate analysis. Am J Physiol 1985; 248:H151-H153.
9. Appel ML, Berger RD, Saul JP, et al. Beat-to beat variability in cardiovascular variables: noise or music ? J Am Coll Cardiol 1989; 14:1139-1148.
10. Malliani A, Pagani M, Lombardi F, et al. Cardiovascular neural regulation explored in the frequency domain. Circulation 1991; 84:482-492.
11. Jaffe RS, Fung DL, Behrman KH. Optimal frequency ranges for extracting information on autonomic activity from the heart rate spectrogram. J Auton Nerv Syst 1993; 46:37-46.
12. Pfeifer M, Cook D, Brodsky J, et al. Quantitative evaluation of cardiac parasympathetic neuropathy in normal and diabetic men. Diabetes 1982; 31:339-345.
13. Hayano J, Sakakibara Y, Yamada A, et al. Accuracy of assessment of cardiac vagal tone by heart rate variability in normal subjects. Am J Cardiol 1991; 67:199-204.
14. Eckberg DL. Parasympathetic cardiovascular control in human disease: a critical review of methods and results. Am J Physiol 1980; 239:H581-593.
15. Smith SA. Reduced sinus arrhythmia in diabetic autonomic neuropathy: diagnostic value of an age-related normal range. BMJ 1982; 285:1599-1601.
16. Arnold RW, Dyer JA, Gould AB, et al. Sensitivity to vasovagal maneuvers in normal children and adults. Mayo Clin Proc 1991; 66:797-804.
17. Ewing DJ, Neilson JMM, Shapiro CM, et al. Twenty-four hour heart-rate variability: effects of posture, sleep, and time of the day in healthy controls and comparison with bedside tests of autonomic function in diabetic patients. Br Heart J 1991; 65:239-244.
18. Nolan J, Flapan AD, Capewell S, et al. Decreased cardiac parasympathetic activity in chronic heart failure and its relation to left ventricular function. Br Heart J 1992; 67:482-485.
19. Coumel Ph, Hermida JS, Wennerblom B, et al. Heart rate variability in myocardial hypertrophy and heart failure and the effects of beta blocking therapy. A non-spectral analysis of heart rate oscillations. Eur Heart J 1991; 12:412-422.
20. Berger R, Akselrod S, Gordon D, et al. An efficient algorithm for spectral analysis of heart rate variability. IEEE Trans Biomed Eng 1986; 33:900-904.
21. Baselli G, Cerutti S, Civardi S, et al. Heart rate variability signal processing: a quantitative approach as an aid to diagnosis in cardiovascular pathologies. Int J Biomed Comput 1987; 20:51-70.
22. Akselrod S. Spectral analysis of fluctuations in cardiovascular parameters: a quantitative tool for the investigations of autonomic control. Trends Pharmacol Sci 1988; 9:6-10.
23. van Bolhuis HH, Bootsma M, Swenne CA. Is analyse van de hartritmvariabiliteit klinish toepasbaar? Ned Tijdschr Cardiol 1993; 7:333-345.
24. Pagani M, Lombardi F, Guzzetti S, et al. Power spectral analysis of heart rate and arterial pressure as a marker of sympatho-vagal interaction in man and conscious dog. Circulation 1986; 59:178-193.

25. DeBoer RW, Karemaker JM, Strackee J. Relationships between short term blood pressure fluctuations and heart rate variability in resting subjects. I. A spectral analysis approach. Med Biol Eng Comput 1985; 23:352-358.

26. Akselrod S, Wasserman G, Oz O, et al. BP fluctuations in the normotensive versus the hypertensive cardiovascular system: simulations and experiment. IEEE Comp in Cardiol 1992; 92:199-202.

27. DeBoer RW, Karemaker JM, Strackee J. Relationships betweeen short term blood pressure fluctuations and heart rate variability in resting subjects. II. A simple model. Med Biol Eng Comput 1985; 23:359-364.

28. Madwed JB, Albrecht P, Mark RG, et al. Low-frequency oscillations in arterial blood pressure and heart rate: a simple computer model. Am J Physiol 1989; 25:H1573-H1579.

29. Baselli G, Cerutti S, Civardi S, et al. Cardiovascular variability signals: towards the identification of a closed-loop model of the neural control system. IEEE Trans Biomed Eng 1988; 35:1033-1046.

30. Maayan C, Axelrod FB, Akselrod S, et al. Evaluation of autonomic dysautonomia by power spectral analysis. J Auton Nerv Syst 1987; 21:51-58.

31. Weise F, Heydenreich F. A non-invasive approach to cardiac autonomic neuropathy in patients with diabetes mellitus. Clin Physiol 1990; 10:137-145.

32. Saul JP, Rea RF, Eckberg DL, et al. Heart rate and muscle sympathetic nerve variability during reflex changes of autonomic activity. Am J Physiol 1991; 258: H713-H721.

33. Saul JP, Berger RD, Albrecht P, et al. Transfer function analysis of the circulation: unique insights into cardiovascular regulation. Am J Physiol 1991; 261:H1231-H1245.

34. Madwed JB, Sands KEF, Saul JP, et al. Spectral analysis of beat-to-beat variability in HR and ABP during hemorrhage and aortic constriction. In: Lown B, Malliani A, Prosdocimi M (eds). Neural Mechanisms and Cardiovascular Disease. Fidia Research Series. Padova, Italy: Liviana Press 5, 1986; 291-301.

35. Oz O, Eliash S, Cohen S, et al. The effect of changes in blood volume on low frequency blood pressure fluctuations in spontaneously hypertensive rats. IEEE Comp in Cardiol 1989; 89:61-64.

36. Shannon DC, Carley DW, Benson H. Aging of modulation of heart rate. Am J Physiol 1987; 253:H874-H877.

37. Waddington JL, MacCulloch, Sambrooks JE. Resting heart rate variability in man declines with age. Experientia 1979; 35:1197-1198.

38. Lipsitz LA, Mietus J, Moody GB, et al. Spectral characteristics of heart rate variability before and during postural tilt. Circulation 1990; 81:1803-1810.

39. Perry JC, Garson MD. Diagnosis and treatment of arrhythmias. Adv Pediatr 1989; 36:177-200.

40. Hirsch M, Karin J, Shechter B, et al. Detection of fetal breathing activity in real time by means of spectral analysis of fetal heart rate analysis. 2nd World Congress on Perinatal Medicine; 1993; Rome, Italy.

41. Chatow U, Davidson S, Reichman BL, et al. The development and maturation of the autonomic nervous system in premature and full-term infants using spectral analysis of heart rate fluctuations. In press.

42. Giddens DP, Kitney RI. Neonatal heart rate variability and its relation to respiration. J Theor Biol 1985; 113:759-780.

43. Lishner M, Akselrod S, Mor-Avi V, et al. Spectral analysis of heart rate fluctuations: a non-invasive method for the early diagnosis of diabetic neuropathy. J Auton Nerv Syst 1987; 19:119-125.

44. Appel S, Kuritzki A, Zahavi I, et al. Evidence for the instability of the autonomic nervous system in patients with migraine headache. Headache 1992; 32:10-17.

45. Ziegelman M, Kuritzki A, Appel S, et al. Propranolol in the prophylaxis of migraine. Evaluation by spectral analysis of beat-to-beat heart rate fluctuations. Headache 1992; 32:169-174.

46. Rimoldi O, Pierini S, Ferrari A, et al. Analysis of short-term oscillations of R-R and arterial pressure in conscious dogs. Am J Physiol 1990; 258:H967-H976.

47. Brown DR, Randall DC, Knapp CF, et al. Stability of the heart rate power spectrum over time in the conscious dog. FASEB J 1989; 3:1644-1650.

48. Chess GF, Tam RMK, Calaresu FR. Influence of cardiac inputs on rhythmic variations of heart period in the cat. Am J Physiol 1975; 228:775-780.

49. Montano N, Lombardi F, Gnecchi-Ruscone TG, et al. Spectral analysis of sympathetic discharge, R-R intervals and systolic arterial pressure variabilities in decerebrate cats. J Auton Nerv Syst 1992; 40:21-32.

50. Akselrod S, Eliash S, Oz O, et al. Hemodynamic regulation in the spontaneously hypertensive rat: investigation by spectral analysis. Am J Physiol 1987; 253:H176-H183.

51. Cerutti C, Gustin MP, Paultre CZ, et al. Autonomic nervous system and cardiovascular variability in rats: a spectral analysis approach. Am J Physiol 1991; 261:H1292-H1299.

52. Japundzic N, Grichois ML, Zitoun P, et al. Spectral analysis of blood pressure and heart

rate in conscious rats: effects of autonomic blockers. J Auton Nerv Syst 1990; 30:91-100.

53. Persson PB, Stauss H, Chung O, et al. Spectrum analysis of sympathetic nerve activity and blood pressure in conscious rats. Am J Physiol 1992; 263:H1348-H1355.

54. Rubini R, Porta A, Baselli G, et al. Power spectrum analysis of cardiovascular variability monitored by telemetry in conscious unrestrained rats. J Auton Nerv Syst 1993; 45:181-190.

55. Eliash S, Oz O, Cohen S, et al. The role of renin-angiotensin and alpha-control in the regulation of blood pressure in a normotensive versus a hypertensive system. IEEE Comp in Cardiol 1990; 89:155-158.

56. Akselrod S, Oz O, Eliash S. Neural and humoral factors in regulation of blood pressure, in the investigation of essential hypertension. In: Di Rienzo M, Mancia G, et al (eds). Blood Pressure and Heart Rate Variability. Amsterdam, Holland: IOS Press, 1993.

57. Rosenblueth A, Simeone FA.. The interrelations of vagal and accelerator effects on the cardiac rate. Am J Physiol 1936; 110:42-55.

58. Eckberg DL. Nonlinearities of the human carotid baroreceptor-cardiac reflex. Circ Res 1980; 47:208-216.

59. Katona PG, Jih F. Respiratory sinus arrhythmia: noninvasive measure of parasympathetic cardiac control. J Appl Physiol 1975; 39:801-805.

60. Alcalay M, Izraeli S, Wallach R, et al. Paradoxical pharmacodynamic effect of atrpine on parasympathetic control: a study by spectral analysis of heart rate fluctuations. Clin Pharmacol Ther 1992; 52:518-527.

61. Izraeli S, Alcalay M, Benjamini Y, et al. Modulation of the dose-dependent effects of atropine by low-dose pyridostigmine: quantification by spectral analysis of heart rate fluctuations in healthy human beings. Pharmacol Biochem Behav 1991; 39:613-617.

62. Vibyral T, Bryg RJ, Maddes ME, et al. Transdermal scopolamine increases heart rate variability by selective parasympathetic stimulation. IEEE Comp in Cardiol 1989; 49.

63. Katona PG, Lipson D, Dauchot PJ. Opposing central and peripheral effects of atropine on parasympathetic control. Am J Physiol 1977; 232:H146-H157.

64. Alcalay M, Izraeli S, Wallach-Kapon R, et al. Pharmacological modulation of vagal cardiac control measured by heart rate power spectrum: a possible bioequivalent probe. Neurosci Biobehav Rev 1991; 15:51-55.

65. Anrep GV, Pascual W, Rossler R. Respiratory variations of the heart rate. I. The reflex mechanism of the respiratory arrhythmia. Proc R Soc Lond B Biol Sci 1936; 119:191-217.

66. Angelone A, Coulter NA. Respiratory and sinus arrhythmia: a frequency dependent phenomena. J Appl Physiol 1964; 19:479-482.

67. Hirsh JB, Bishop B. Respiratory sinus arrhythmia in humans. How breathing pattern modulates heart rate. Am J Physiol 1981; 241:H620-H629.

68. Brown TE, Beightol LA, Koh J, et al. Important influence of respiration on human R-R interval power spectra is largely ignored. J Appl Physiol 1993; 75:2310-2317.

69. Baharav A, Mimouni M, Sagie T, et al. The role of the autonomic nervous system in the pathogenesis of vasovagal syncope. Clin Auton Res 1993; 3:261-269.

70. Bianchi AM, Mainardi L, Ptrucci MG, et al. Time-variant power spectrum analysis for the detection of transient episodes in HRV signals. IEEE Trans Biomed Eng 1993; 40:136-144.

71. Marchesi C, Venturi M, Pola S, et al. Sequential estimation of the power spectrum for the analysis of variability of non-stationary cardiovascular signals. Proc IEEE 1991; 13:578-579.

72. Novak P, Novak V. Time-frequency mapping of the heart rate, blood pressure and respiratory signals. Med Biol Eng Comput 1993; 31:103-110.

73. Berger RD, Saul JP, Cohen RJ. Assessment of autonomic response by broad band respiration. IEEE Trans Biomed Eng 1989; BME-36:1061-1065.

74. Berger RD, Saul JP, Cohen RJ. Transfer function analysis of autonomic regulation. I. The canine atrial rate response. Am J Physiol 1989; 256:H142-H152.

75. Saul JP, Berger RD, Chen MH, et al. Transfer function analysis of autonomic regulation. II. Respiratory sinus arrhythmia. Am J Physiol 1989; 256:H153-H161.

76. Priess G, Iscoe S, Polosa C. Analysis of periodic breathing pattern associated with Mayer waves. Am J Physiol 1975; 228:768-774.

77. Sands KEF, Appel ML, Lilly LS, et al. Assessment of heart rate variability in human cardiac transplants recipients using power spectrum analysis. Circulation 1989; 79:76-82.

78. Bernardi L, Keller F, Sanders M, et al. Respiratory sinus arrhythmia in the denervated human heart. J Appl Physiol 1989; 67:1447-1455.

79. Kollai M, Koizumi K. Reciprocal and non-reciprocal action of the vagal and sympathetic nerves innervating the heart. J Auton Nerv Syst 1979; 1:33-52.

80. Hyndman BW. The role of rhythms in homeostasis. Kybernetik 1974; 15:227-236.

81. Kitney RI, Rompelman O. The Study of Heart Rate Variability. Oxford, England: Clarendon Press, 1980.
82. Laude D, Goldman M, Escourrou P, et al. Effect of breathing pattern on blood pressure and heart rate oscillations in humans. Clin Exp Pharmacol Physiol 1993; 20:619-626.
83. Weise F, Baltrush K, Heydenreich F. Effect of low dose atropine on heart rate fluctuations during orthostatic load: a spectral analysis. J Auton Nerv Syst 1989; 26:223-230.
84. Burton AC. The range and variability of the blood flow in the human fingers and the vasomotor regulation of body temperature. Am J Physiol 1939; 127:437-453.
85. Kitney RI. An analysis of the nonlinear behaviour of the human thermal vasomotor control system. J Theor Biol 1974; 52:231-248.
86. de Trafford JC, Khan O, Lafferty K, et al. Thermal entrainment methods for studying Raynaud's phenomenon. J Biomed Eng 1988; 10:101-104.
87. Lossius K, Eriksen M, Walloe L. Thermoregulatory fluctuations in heart rate and blood pressure in humans: effect of cooling and parasympathetic blockade. J Auton Nerv Syst 1994; 47:245-254.
88. Zigelman M, Appel S, Davidovitch S, et al. The effect of verapamil Ca antagonist on autonomic imbalance in migraine- evaluation by spectral analysis of beat-to-beat heart rate fluctuations. In press.
89. Akselrod S, Wasserman G, Oz O, et al. BP fluctuations in the normotensive versus the hypertensive cardiovascular system: simulation and experiment. IEEE Comp in Cardiol 1991; 91:701-704.

Chapter 13

Reproducibility of Heart Rate Variability Measurement

Josef Kautzner

Heart rate variability (HRV) has substantial potential in both physiological studies and clinical investigations.[1-9] However, spontaneous variation of HRV parameters in time may have deleterious effects on its value. Therefore, practical utility of HRV assessment is related to reproducibility of HRV parameters over time.

Assessment of Reproducibility

Because of diverse statistical and data analytical methods, it is relatively difficult to compare the results of the studies currently available. Therefore, a brief outline of data analysis will be discussed here.

In some studies, Pearson's product-moment correlation coefficients were used to estimate the reproducibility of HRV data over time. However, this approach is in principle not suitable for assessment of reproducibility of measurement of any kind. It should be emphasized that high correlation does not reflect negligible differences of one recording from other, but rather that values from one subject resemble more previous values from the same subject than those from others. Furthermore, correlation depends on the quantitative range of the values in the sample, being greater for higher range.

To combat the problem, other techniques representing measurement error have been advised. Repeatability of measurement can be easily assessed by the plotting of differences between two values against their mean for each subject. Calculation of the mean and standard deviation of the differences then allows the assessment of whether 95% of differences is less than two standard deviations. This is the basis for a coefficient of repeatability.[10,11] The reproducibility may be also assessed using coefficient of variation which is the standard deviation divided by the mean and usually expressed in percent. As the value of this parameter depends on both the standard deviation and the mean, it can be applied when the standard deviation is proportional to the mean.[11]

From: Malik M., Camm AJ (eds.): *Heart Rate Variability*. Armonk, NY. Futura Publishing Company, Inc., © 1995.

Other researchers use more sophisticated statistical techniques such as intraclass correlation coefficient to evaluate the strength of the association between the two measurements.[12,13] This method may be considered as a measure of intrasubject reproducibility, being the fraction of person-to-person variance of observed measurements due to the variance of steady state values. However, whether these statistics offer any advantage over simpler and more easily interpretable methods remains questionable.

Normal Subjects

At present, there is a paucity of data about the reproducibility of various HRV parameters over time in normal subjects. To estimate short-term reproducibility of HRV, Huikuri et al[14] analyzed the mean ±SD of 5-minute RR intervals (SDNN index) both over two consecutive 24-hour periods and 1 week apart in a group of healthy adults (mean age: 31.3 years, range: 20 to 40 years). Although day-to-day reproducibility could have been compared with 1-week reproducibility in a substantial proportion of individuals (16 and 18, respectively), the authors grouped all data together and found mean SDNN index value 68 ±16 milliseconds with interindividual coefficient of variation of 24%. The mean intraindividual coefficient of variation for 24-hour average HRV between repeated recordings was 7%±6%. Using published data, it is possible to recalculate the mean intraindividual coefficient of variation separately for 2 consecutive days and for a period of 1 week. Then, the day-to-day variation tends to be lower (coefficient of variation: 4.2%±2.9%) as compared to the 7-day period (coefficient of variation: 7.3%±7.36%). In addition, the study showed characteristic circadian rhythm of HRV with significant intraindividual variation in hour-to-hour HRV reaching its maximum during 3 hours before waking (Figure 1).

Van Hoogenhuyze et al[15] compared broader spectrum of time-domain parameters (SDANN, SDNN index and so-called CV or coefficient of variation for 5-minute SD values, which is obtained by dividing the SD value for each 5-minute period by the mean RR interval for that period) in 33 normal subjects of comparable age (mean: 34 years, 19 males). Despite a close correlation between HRV values from two successive 24-hour recordings (Pearson's correlation coefficients ranging from 0.87 to 0.95), considerable individual day-to-day variation was revealed (from 0.2% to 46% for the SDANN and 0.4% to 25.9% for SDNN index to 0% to 16% for CV values). Mean values of day-to-day differences were relatively low (12.3%±11.7% for SDANN, 7.8%±6.9% for SDNN index and 5.7±4.3 for CV parameter). Interestingly, a significant correlation between mean RR interval and SDANN or SDNN index was found (0.64 and 0.54, respectively), while CV values showed no such relationship. Furthermore, mean heart rate (HR) was significantly higher in women (mean RR interval 748.8±69.4 versus 862.9±77.9, $p < 0.01$) and conversely, HRV parameters were significantly lower than in men (SDANN 123.6±27.2 versus 162.5±49.8 milliseconds, $p < 0.013$ and SDNN 65.3±16.1 versus 82.7±25.8 milliseconds, $p < 0.034$). CV values did not differ for the two groups.

Similarly, Hohnloser et al[16] showed good reproducibility of group HRV data obtained in 17 healthy subjects (mean age: 24±2.5 years) on days 2,7, and 28. Correlation coefficients for several time-domain (SDNN, rMSSD, and pNN50) and frequency-domain measurements varied between 0.546 and 0.863. However, when comparing data of individual patients, significant percent differences between repeated measurements of HRV parameters were revealed. This variation was higher for estimates of short-term components of HRV (23.5%±14.6% for pNN50, 18.5%±12.6% for rMSSD) compared to SDNN (10.7%±6.8%).

Although previously mentioned studies demonstrated good overall reproducibility of HRV parameters in normal middle-aged subjects, they unanimously showed

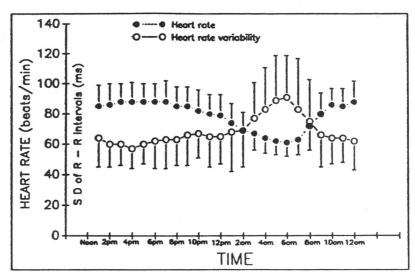

Figure 1. The circadian pattern of HRV and HR in a group of healthy young adults (mean ±SD). Reproduced with permission from Huikuri et al.[14]

that considerable day-to-day variations may occur. In this respect, rather different results have been reported by Kleiger et al[12] for their group of 14 normal subjects, aged 25 to 55 years. The whole spectrum of time-domain (SDNN, SDNN index, pNN50, and rMSSD) and frequency-domain (total power and both low- and high-frequency power components) HRV parameters were studied in order to assess their reproducibility between baseline and placebo (ie, when receiving placebo therapy) 24-hour electrocardiogram (ECG) recordings performed 3 to 65 days apart. Surprisingly, the mean and standard deviations of all HRV measures were virtually identical between placebo and baseline measurements and within the studied time range. For most of the measured variables, the intraclass correlation coefficient, which was used as a measure of individual variability, exceeded 0.84. However, for SDNN parameter, the value of intraclass coefficient was 0.7, while for pNN50 reached 0.9. Furthermore, no difference was found in reproducibility of recordings obtained within 18 days and those performed later.

In summary, currently available data suggest adequate short-term (within days up to 1 month) stability of HRV measures derived from 24-hour ambulatory monitoring in normal subjects. However, it appears that significant intraindividual variation of HRV parameters may occur between two recordings. This may be more pronounced in some HRV indices but relevant data are contradictory. Furthermore, the reproducibility of HRV assessment may be influenced by differences in mean HR between different recording periods. This should be taken into consideration especially when groups and individuals are compared. Finally, little information is known about gender differences in HRV, and reported differences in reproducibility between men and women appear to be related to differences in HR.

Patients with Cardiovascular Diseases

Taking good reproducibility of HRV parameters in normal subjects into consideration, even less day-to-day variation might be expected in clinically stable patients with cardiac disease and depressed HRV. This was shown by Van Hoogenhuyze et al[15] for 22 stable congestive heart failure outpatients with a history of previous myocardial infarction (mean age: 59

years, 18 males). In comparison with a previously mentioned group of 33 younger normals, they demonstrated similar group reproducibility of selected time-domain HRV parameters, and more importantly, less day-to-day variation of HRV values in the range associated with increased risk of mortality (ie, SDANN <50 milliseconds and SDNN index <30 milliseconds). They also revealed that day-to-day variation of one specific HRV measure does not always parallel that for other measures. This may reflect differences in spectral content which is covered by individual time-domain measures.

In another study from Washington University and Columbia College of Physicians and Surgeons, Bigger et al[17] found remarkable stability of HRV measures in two samples of postmyocardial infarction patients. They examined 40 pairs of 24-hour ECG recordings obtained both from the Cardiac Arrhythmia Pilot Study (CAPS) and from the Electrophysiologic Study Versus Electrocardiographic Monitoring (ESVEM) trial. CAPS patients consisted of intermediate risk patients with asymptomatic but prognostically significant ventricular arrhythmias, while the ESVEM population was comprised of high-risk patients with a history of spontaneous malignant ventricular arrhythmias. Despite significant differences between both groups in clinical variables, ie, lower ejection fraction and higher number of ventricular premature beats or runs of nonsustained ventricular tachycardia in the ESVEM population, and higher proportion of those receiving beta-blockers among CAPS patients (50% versus 18%), stability of frequency-domain HRV measures was excellent for measurements in both groups. For the ESVEM group, all intraclass correlation coefficients exceeded 0.85, indicating reproducibility even better than for the above mentioned group of 14 healthy volunteers.[12] For the CAPS group, intraclass correlation coefficients were in the similar range as in normal individuals, ie, >0.79. Interestingly, intraclass correlation coefficient for ultra-low frequency power was apparently higher in both patient populations (0.79 in CAPS and 0.86 in ESVEM) than in normal population (0.54).

Recently, we have performed a study of day-to-day reproducibility of commonly used time-domain HRV measures early after myocardial infarction (ie, the first recording started on day 4 to 5 after hospital admission).[18] The study population consisted of 33 clinically stable patients (mean age: 54.6±10.8 years, 28 males). QRS complexes were labeled using a commercial analyzer (Marquette Laser Holter 8000) and all artifactual RR intervals were visualized and carefully edited. HRV analysis was performed using an in-house software. Statistical analysis of reproducibility of individual HRV indices was based on comparsion of the absolute values of relative errors, that is values R.E. = $|A\text{-}B|/[(A+B)/2]$, where A and B represent the value of the same parameter measured on day 1 and 2, respectively. The mean of the absolute values of relative errors for all of the time-domain indices except of the pNN50 parameter demonstrated good reproducibility, ranging from 11%±13% for SDNN index to 18%±19% for triangular interpolation method (Figure 2). The values for SDANN and SDNN index are comparable with day-to-day differences quoted by Van Hoogenhuyze et al[15] in their group of patients with coronary heart disease and stable congestive heart failure (16%±14% versus 13.8%±13.5% and 11%±13% versus 8.5%±7.3% respectively). However, statistical comparison of relative errors showed that the pNN50 measure was significantly less reproducible (Figures 3A-B) compared to other HRV measures (mean value of relative error: 45%±45%). A similar feature was found by Hohnloser et al[16] in normal subjects (average value of day-to-day percent difference: 23.5±14.6) but was not apparent in a group of 22 patients with either atypical chest pain and normal coronary arteries or previous myocardial infarction (here the value 19.2%±19.2% was fully comparable with values for other HRV measures such as 18.4±13.7 for SDNN.

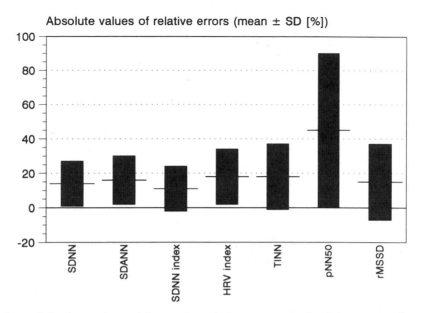

Figure 2. Mean of absolute values of day-to-day relative errors calculated for commonly used time-domain HRV indices in a population of survivors of the acute phase of myocardial infarction (mean values ±SD).

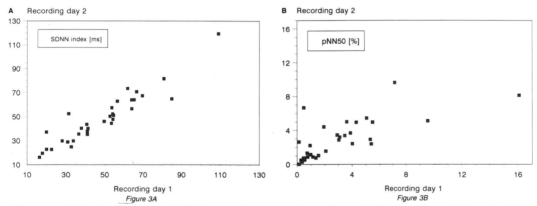

Figures 3A-B. An example of differences between the values of SDNN index (A) and pNN50 parameter (B) obtained from consecutive 24-hour recordings during early convalescent phase of myocardial infarction.

In summary, HRV measures appear to be stable not only in normal subjects, but also in various subsets of patients with previous myocardial infarction. In fact, clinically stable patients with lower HRV values presented with much less day-to-day variation in HRV indices. The reproducibility of pNN50 parameter seems to be controversial and the rMSSD estimate of short-term components of HRV might be preferable. Otherwise, the stability of HRV measures allows their use for risk stratification studies, even relatively early after acute phase of myocardial infarction. However, the potential influence of various factors such as the aging, gender, different physical and mental activity and medication needs further investigations.

Patients with Other Diseases

Of the broad spectrum of noncardiological diseases, HRV appears to be useful especially for early diagnosis of diabetic neuropathy and in monitoring of its progression. Therefore, the reproducibility of HRV assessment is again an issue of primary interest. Contrary to predicting arrhythmic events in patients with cardiovascular diseases, diabetic neuropathy can be assessed using simple bedside maneuvers or frequency-domain analysis carried out during steady state conditions. This is possible because diabetic neuropathy is characterized by widespread neuronal degeneration and thus, by well-defined autonomic dysfunction.

Nolan et al[19] evaluated short- and long-term reproducibility of pNN50 parameter from repeated ambulatory ECGs in 28 diabetics at an interval of 29 ± 11 days and in 18 diabetics at an interval of 195 ± 24 days. Both intraclass correlation coefficients and coefficients of repeatability showed better reproducibility in the first group (0.91 versus 0.86 for intraclass coefficients and 0.614 versus 0.870 for coefficients of repeatability). The short-term reproducibility was comparable to those of 19 normal subjects and 74 patients with documented cardiac disease. Thus, together with reproducibility data from normal subjects, HRV assessment appears to be able to detect even smaller variations in cardiac parasympathetic activity due to natural progression of diabetic neuropathy or due to the therapeutic intervention.

Conclusion

As the most valuable prognostic information has been achieved by processing 24-hour ECG recordings, a great number of possible disturbances to HRV measures is to be expected. Despite multiple physiological inputs such as mental activity, day/night cycles, different patterns of physical activity and/or ventilation, and other factors like aging or gender, the variation between repeated measurements of HRV seems to be low. In any case, the reproducibility of HRV indices is far superior to those of other variables that are also known to predict mortality in survivors of myocardial infarction, such as ventricular ectopy or episodes of silent ischemia. Thus, HRV might be preferable for risk stratification studies and for evaluation of the efficacy of various interventions.

References

1. Kleiger RE, Miller JP, Bigger JT Jr, et al. Decreased heart rate variability and its association with increased mortality after acute myocardial infarction. Am J Cardiol 1987; 59:256-262.
2. Martin GJ, Magid NM, Myers G, et al. Heart rate variability and sudden death secondary to coronary artery disease during ambulatory electrocardiographic monitoring. Am J Cardiol 1987; 60:86-89.
3. Lombardi F, Sandrone G, Pernpruner S, et al. Heart rate variability as an index of sympathovagal interaction after acute myocardial infarction. Am J Cardiol 1987; 60:1239-1245.
4. Cripps TR, Malik M, Farrell TG, et al. Prognostic value of reduced heart rate variability after myocardial infarction: clinical evaluation of a new analysis method. Br Heart J 1991; 65:14-19.
5. Bigger JT Jr, Fleiss JL, Steinmann RC, et al. Frequency domain measures of heart period variability and mortality after myocardial infarction. Circulation 1992; 85:164-171.
6. Smith SA. Reduced sinus arrhythmia in diabetic autonomic neuropathy: diagnostic value of an age-related normal range. BMJ 1982; 285:1599-1601.
7. Ewing DJ, Neilson JMM, Shapiro JA, et al. Twenty-four hour heart rate variability: effects of posture, sleep and time of day in healthy controls and comparison with bedside tests of autonomic function in diabetic patients. Br Heart J 1991; 65:239-244.
8. Malpas SC, Maling TJB. Heart rate variability and cardiac autonomic function in diabetes. Diabetes 1990; 39:1177-1181.
9. Kuroiwa Y, Wada T, Tohgi H. Measurement of blood pressure and heart-rate variation while resting supine and standing for the evaluation of autonomic dysfunction. J Neurol 1987; 235:65-68.
10. Bland JM, Altman DG. Statistical methods for assessing agreement between two meth-

ods of clinical measurement. Lancet 1986; i:307-310.

11. Bland JM. An Introduction to Medical Statistics. Oxford, England: Oxford University Press, 1987; 276–296.

12. Kleiger RE, Bigger JT, Bosner MS, et al. Stability over time of variables measuring heart rate variability in normal subjects. Am J Cardiol 1991; 68:626-630.

13. Shrout PE, Fleiss JL. Intraclass correlations: uses in assessing rater reliability. Psychol Bull 1979; 86:420-428.

14. Huikuri HV, Kessler KM, Terracall E, et al. Reproducibility and circadian rhythm of heart rate variability in healthy subjects. Am J Cardiol 1990; 65:391-393.

15. Van Hoogenhuyze D, Weinstein N, Martin GJ, et al. Reproducibility and relation to mean heart rate of heart rate variability in normal subjects and in patients with congestive heart failure secondary to coronary artery disease. Am J Cardiol 1991; 68:1668-1676.

16. Hohnloser SH, Klingenheben T, Zabel M, et al. Intraindividual reproducibility of heart rate variability. PACE 1992; 15:2211-2214.

17. Bigger JT Jr, Fleiss JL, Rolnitzky LM, et al. Stability over time of heart period variability in patients with previous myocardial infarction and ventricular arrhythmias. Am J Cardiol 1992; 69:718-723.

18. Kautzner J, Hnatkova K, Staunton A, et al. Day to day reproducibility of time domain measures of heart rate variability in survivors of the acute phase of myocardial infarction. In press.

19. Nolan J, Flapan AD, Goodfield NE, et al. Reproducibility of time domain measurement of cardiac parasympathetic activity from ambulatory electrocardiograms. J Am Coll Cardiol 1993 ; 21:158A.

Chapter 14

Association of Heart Rate Variability Components with Physiological Regulatory Mechanisms

Alberto Malliani

Introduction

The obvious reason for the growing interest in the study of cardiovascular variability has to be found in the hope that this approach might underscore unprecedented tools to explore neural regulatory mechanisms. In this context, the paper by Akselrod and coworkers [1] was the first to propose the general hypothesis that the power spectrum analysis of heart rate (HR) fluctuations might furnish a quantitative probe of beat-to-beat cardiovascular control. The regulatory components taken into consideration were the sympathetic, parasympathetic and renin-angiotensin systems.

Since our initial studies,[2] we thought that this approach was unlikely to be a field for serendipity and, accordingly, all our work has been coupled to a precise physiological hypothesis.

Our previous endeavour had been to demonstrate that excitatory and inhibitory cardiovascular reflexes interact normally, even in those reflex responses such as baroreflex, often attributed to a single reflex mechanism.[3] Whatever may be the complexity of this interaction among multiple and, in part, opposing reflex mechanisms likely to accompany most hemodynamic events occurring in closed-loop conditions,[4] their actions should still converge into relatively simple consequences such as an increase or decrease in HR. The conceptualization of the neural control of HR, on the other hand, cannot escape from the traditional scheme of a reciprocal organization characterizing the sympathetic and vagal modulations of sinus node pacemaker activity. In terms of direct findings, for instance, we had observed[5] that the activity of sympathetic or vagal efferent nerve fibers, isolated from the same cardiac nerve directed to the heart, was reflexly influenced in an opposite direction by the same stimulus, such as an increase in arterial pressure (AP) or an elec-

From: Malik M., Camm AJ (eds.): *Heart Rate Variability*. Armonk, NY. Futura Publishing Company, Inc., © 1995.

trical stimulation of an appropriate afferent pathway. Thus, a baroreceptor stimulation increased the vagal and at the same time reduced the sympathetic efferent activity, suggesting a synergistic interaction likely to promote a bradycardia response.

In short, when we proposed [2,6] that the power spectrum analysis of heart rate variability (HRV) could furnish a tool to explore the sympatho-vagal interaction in experimental and clinical conditions, we were thinking of a balance which, rather than a vague concept, was instead the net output of a highly complex black box.

In the following part of this article, I shall summarize the evidence which supports the following conclusions:

1. the respiratory rhythm of heart period variability, defined as the high-frequency (HF) spectral component, is a marker of vagal modulation;
2. the rhythm corresponding to vasomotor waves and present in heart period and AP variabilities, defined as the low-frequency (LF) component, is a marker of sympathetic modulation; and
3. a reciprocal relationship exists between these two rhythms that is similar to that characterizing the sympatho-vagal balance.[7]

Methodological Considerations

Two major oscillatory components are usually detectable in RR variability (Figure 1), one of which, synchronous with respiration, is described as HF (about 0.25 Hz and varying with respiration) while the other, corresponding to the slow waves of AP[8,9] is described as LF (about 0.1 Hz). However, the center frequency of the LF component can also vary considerably (from 0.04 to 0.13 Hz).[7,10]

In addition, the component below 0.03 Hz and with a center frequency around 0 Hz contributes substantially to total power as it can represent its 40% to 50% in resting conditions[6] and up to 80% to 85% during standard Holter recordings.[10] This compo-

nent contains noise, slow trends, and possibly very slow oscillations and therefore, to be adequately analyzed, requires longer series of data and different algorithms.[11] However, there are peculiar circumstances, such as markedly periodic breathing,[12] in which clear oscillatory components are also detectable with the usual spectral methodology in this frequency range. Therefore, this part of the spectrum can either be defined as a DC component,[6,7] a term which emphasizes the contribution of the nonrhythmical variations, or as a very low-frequency (VLF) component,[10,13] which rather alludes to the possibility that it might also contain some hidden rhythmicity.[14]

The sum of these various components of RR variability—that is, total power—corresponds, in the time domain, to the variance (which is measured in milliseconds[2]) or to standard deviation (which, being the square root value of variance, is measured in milliseconds). Intuitively, the absolute power (still in milliseconds[2]) of a given spectral component cannot provide consistent information as to its relative contribution with respect to the total power, although all components are strongly correlated with total power. Thus, some form of normalization appears essential to permit an appreciation of the distribution of power across the frequency axis.

Normalized Units

Since our initial studies[6] we have proposed the use of normalized units: a crucial point is that in our methodology the normalization of LF and HF components is effected after subtracting from total power the VLF component, a procedure that substantially reduces the confounding effect of noise. Normalized units are obtained with the following relationships:

$$P(nu) = \frac{P(ms)^2}{\sigma^2(ms)^2 - P_{VLF}(ms)^2} * 100$$

where P represents the power of either LF or HF components, in (nu) or (millisec-

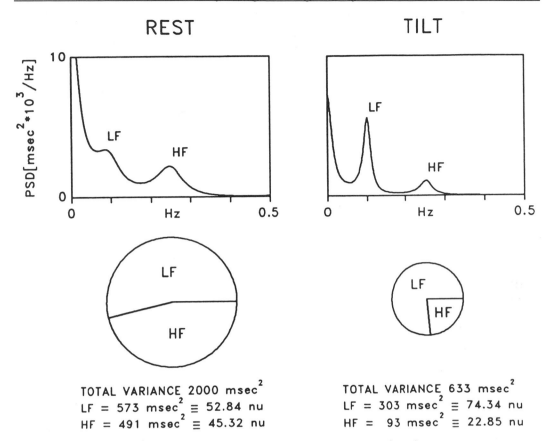

Figure 1. Example of spectral analysis of RR interval variability in a healthy subject examined at rest and during a passive tilt. At rest there are two major components (LF and HF) of similar power, whereas during tilting the LF component predominates. In this case the total variance during tilting is markedly reduced so both LF and HF powers seem to be diminished when expressed in absolute units. The use of normalized units (nu) clearly indicates the altered relation between the two spectral components induced by tilting. The pie charts show this relative distribution together with the absolute power of the two components (represented by the area). From Malliani et al.[13]

onds^2), σ^2 represents total power, and P_{VLF} indicates the power of the VLF component (Figure 1).

In the absence of a computation of normalized units, the ratio LF:HF can also provide information on the state of the sympatho-vagal balance.[6,7]

Early Indentification of Spectral Components and the Rationale for the New Approach

Sayers and his coworkers,[15,16] employing the Fast Fourier Transform algorithm, reported the existence of three peaks in RR variability of human subjects, respec-

tively, around 0.25, 0.10, and 0.03 Hz, each corresponding to a predetermined frequency band. Akselrod et al[1] confirmed, in conscious dogs, the existence of the same spectral peaks being the two of lower frequency centered at about 0.12 and 0.04 Hz. The mid-frequency peak (0.10 to 0.12 Hz) was considered, by all these authors, to be related to the frequency response of the baroreflex; while the frequency of 0.03 to 0.04 Hz was related to thermoregulatory activity[16] and to renin-angiotensin system.[1] These proposals seem to require a profound revision on the basis of actual knowledge. De-Boer and his coworkers[17,18] were among the first to appreciate that the short-term spectral components were linked to two main disturbances, represented by respiration and vasomotion. By showing the correspondent high coherence existing between heart period and AP variability spectra, they consistently favored the view of only two main frequency components.

At the same time, the use of autoregressive algorithms[6,7,10,13] which can automatically furnish the number, amplitude, and center frequency of the oscillatory components without requiring a priori decisions, clearly indicated that two, not three short-term rhythmical components were hidden in the normal RR and AP variability signals. Cross-spectra with high coherence [19] and physiological considerations[7] were surely the crucial elements for this revision; in addition, when the center frequency of the LF component was followed for the 24-hour period[10] or during various experimental conditions,[20] it was evident that it could oscillate from about 0.04 to 0.13 Hz.

The reason for reiterating these points, that should now almost be taken for granted, is that some authors[21-23] explicitly maintain the position of arbitrarily subdividing the LF region with a cut at 0.07 to 0.075 Hz. In this way two simultaneous confounding effects are obtained:

1. the rhythmical activity associated to vasomotion, the so-called mid-frequency, is deprived of the lower end of its Gaussian distribution; and
2. this amputated but significant power is now added to DC or VLF components.

Obviously, some results obtained in these studies[21,23] contrast with those collected with a more physiological procedure.

Animal Studies

An experimental observation which cannot be disregarded for its basic relevance stems from the simultaneous and direct recordings of sympathetic and vagal efferent impulse activities. In the example of Figure 2, the spectral analysis of RR, sympathetic and vagal variabilities reveals corresponding LF and HF components with a predominance of LF in the sympathetic discharge and of HF in the vagal activity. This fact indicates the difficulties that might arise in attributing one rhythm to one specific neural pathway.[7]

Conversely, a relatively simple solution to the problem of the genesis of short-term fluctuations was searched for in the consideration that the time delay of parasympathetic transmission is considerably shorter than that of sympathetic transmission and that, accordingly, only the parasympathetic nervous system appeared capable of mediating the HF rhythmicity.[1] This proposal was reinforced with the transfer function analysis based on a linearity hypothesis.[24]

However, this proposal does not consider the fact that sympathetic and vagal activities interact continuously at central and peripheral levels, in presynaptic and postsynaptic transmission. Therefore, considering the complexity of interactions and nonlinearity, an approach based on multifarious observations of *what* occurs rather than *how* it might occur appears more realistic.

An example might easily clarify the distinction: an electroencephalogram can monitor the sleep-wakefulness cycle, the deterioration of consciousness, the effects of drugs, the presence of abnormal processes like epilepsy—and yet we do not know, in most of these cases, the respective role played by the reticular, diencephalic, or cortical structures in the genesis of a given rhythm. Thus, a rhythm, being a flexible and dynamic property of neural networks, should neither be restricted to one specific neural pathway to convey a functional significance nor should its genesis be completely known before we might use it as a convenient marker.

The conscious dog is characterized, in quiet resting conditions, by a marked preva-

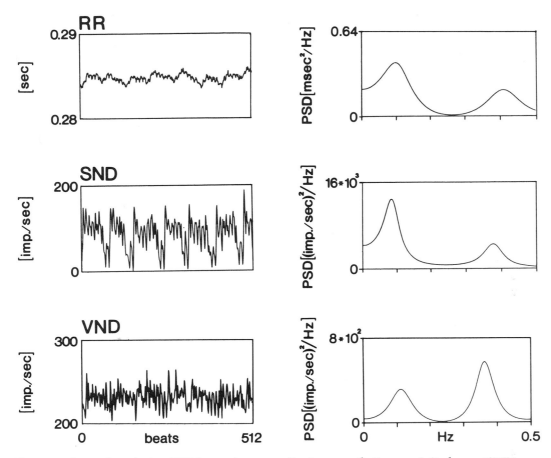

Figure 2. Spectral analysis of RR interval, preganglionic sympathetic neural discharge (SND) recorded from third left thoracic sympathetic ramus communicans, and efferent vagal neural discharge (VND) simultaneously recorded from left cervical vagus in an artificially ventilated decerebrate cat. Time series of the three signals are illustrated on left panels, whereas their autospectra are represented on right panels. A predominant LF characterizes RR and SND autospectra, whereas a greater respiratory HF component is present in VND variability. PSD: power spectral density. From Malliani et al.[7]

lence of the HF component.[20,25] This finding seems to reflect its well-known high vagal tone (Figure 3). Rimoldi et al[20] reported that a small LF component was always present in systolic arterial pressure (SAP) variability but in only 50% of the cases in RR variability. However, whenever sympathetic excitation occurred, a significant shift of power toward LF was observed. In the dog, sympathetic excitation is usually accompanied by a marked reduction of variance or total power of RR variability; the use of normalized units or LF/HF ratio is therefore mandatory to appreciate the redistribution of power. In the case of Figure 3, sympathetic excitation was obtained:

1. with baroreceptor unloading during nitroglycerin infusion;
2. during physical exercise leading to an increased AP, as a likely consequence of an enhancement in central command and peripheral excitatory reflexes[26]; and
3. during coronary artery transient occlusion, as a likely consequence of a cardiocardiac sympathetic excit-

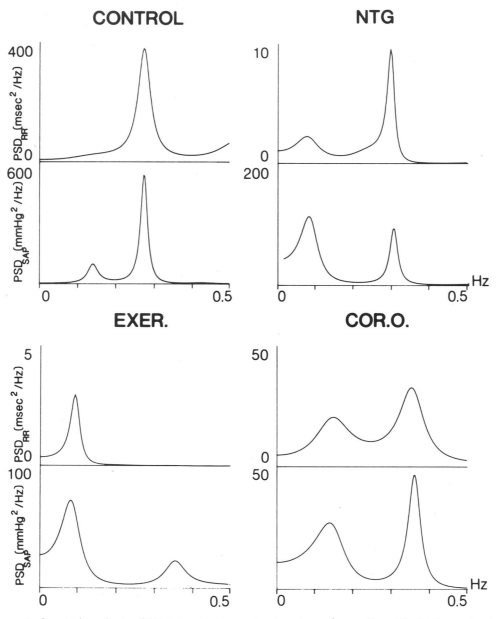

Figure 3. Spectral analysis of RR interval (upper tracings in each panel) and SAP (lower tracings in each panel) variabilities in conscious dogs at rest (CONTROL) and during experimental maneuvers leading to a sympathetic predominance (ie, nitriglycerin infusion (NTG), treadmill exercise (EXER.), and transient acute coronary artery occlusion (COR.O.). Note at control the presence of a single major HF component in the RR interval autospectrum; in SAP, a smaller LF component is also evident. During sympathetic activation, spectral distribution is altered in favor of LF; simultaneously, a drastic reduction in RR variance occurs (notice different scales on ordinates). PSD, power spectral density. From Malliani et al.[7]

atory reflex,[27,28] in absence of significant AP changes.[20]

Therefore, LF component should not be considered a specific reflection of a baroreflex compensatory response,[24] but rather a general marker of sympathetic excitation, regardless of its mechanism.

Interventions on Neural Mechanisms

Subtractive reasoning is always tempting; it has been a traditional approach in neurosciences to guess about the functions of a given structure by observing the effects of its ablation. Benefits and pitfalls have often had to struggle, before a different perspective could disclose a further complexity.

In the study by Akselrod et al,[1] the spectrum reported in their Figure 1 had a large part of its power distributed below the respiratory frequency, indicating an animal likely to be excited. After muscarinic receptor blockade, the remaining power was all concentrated in the extreme low part of the spectrum. Combined beta-adrenergic and muscarinic blockade led to a metronome-like heartbeat. Their conclusion was that the parasympathetic nervous system mediates fluctuations corresponding to HF and mid-frequency peaks, whereas both sympathetic and parasympathetic systems mediate the LF oscillation.

In the experiments by Rimoldi et al[20] muscarinic receptor blockade drastically reduced RR variance, but all the remaining power, in control conditions and during baroreceptor unloading, was concentrated in the LF region. In this case, however, the conclusion was drawn that, independently of total power, the drastic prevalence of the LF over HF component (in nu) was indicating the unbalanced sympathetic predominance induced by the drug. After chronic bilateral stellectomy producing cardiac sympathetic denervation, baroreceptor unloading no longer induced an increase in the LF component of RR variability. On the contrary, the increase in the LF component of SAP variability was still present. It was inferred that in RR variability HF was mainly a marker of vagal mechanisms, whereas the sympathetic outflow appeared essential to the LF increase. Furthermore, the importance of neural mechanisms in mediating LF and HF components of RR variability and LF of SAP variability was proven by their disappearance during ganglionic transmission blockade obtained with intravenous infusion of trimethaphan.

Subsequently, in acute experiments on decerebrate cats,[29] reflex sympathetic excitations induced an increase in the LF component of variability spectra of both RR interval and impulse activity of cardiac sympathetic nerves, while the HF components were simultaneously reduced. In contrast, reflex sympathetic inhibitions were accompanied by a decrease in LF components of both variability signals, while the HF components were simultaneously increased. Finally, a significant and positive correlation was found between changes in the sympathetic efferent discharge and the amplitude of LF component of either RR interval or sympathetic discharge variabilities.

Human Physiological Studies

The total power of RR interval variability has been interpreted as a selective index of cardiac parasympathetic tone[30,31]: although the sympathetic excitation that leads to tachycardia is often accompanied by a reduction in variance, there are numerous physiological and pathophysiological conditions in which the sympatho-vagal balance can shift without significant changes in heart period and total power.[6,7,32]

This balance can instead be assessed with remarkable accuracy by the relation between LF and HF components in nu or by the LF/HF ratio.

In the power spectrum of a normal adult in resting conditions the power of LF is greater than that of HF, with an LF/HF ratio of usually more than 1.[6,7] However, in adolescents this ratio can be less than 1. In a group of healthy controls and élite athletes (while detrained) with a mean age of 16 years, the LF/HF ratio was, respectively, 0.78 and 0.50.[33] As to the effects of active training, the reader should refer to the chapter by Pagani et al in this book.[34]

Effects of Maneuvers Enhancing Sympathetic Drive

In all cases, adults or adolescents, passive tilt or, more simply, standing up is invariably accompanied by an increase in the LF and a decrease in the HF component of RR variability.[2,6,7,35,36] The LF/HF ratio is greatly enhanced to values as great as 20 in young subjects.

In a just completed study,[37] we investigated the capability of power spectrum analysis of HRV to assess the changes in sympatho-vagal balance during graded orthostatic tilt. In our hypothesis, the sympathetic excitation and the vagal withdrawal characterizing the orthostatic position were conceived as the endpoint in a continuum of intermediate changes paralleling the progression of the stimulus. Healthy volunteers were thus subjected to a series of passive head-up tilt steps randomly chosen among the following angles: 15°, 30°, 45°, 60°, and 90°.

As already reported,[6,7,38] age was significantly correlated to variance and to the absolute values in milliseconds^2 of LF and HF components. The tilt angle was tightly correlated to both LF and HF expresses in nu, and to the LF/HF ratio (r = 0.78; -0.72; 0.68, respectively).

Hence, on similar very high probability grounds, this study appears to legitimize a sort of circling conclusion. On one side, the hypothesis that sympathetic excitation and vagal withdrawal progress in a continuum seems reinforced, and on the other side, the conclusion seems supported a fortiori that this methodology, without artificially separating the influence of either neural outflow,

can reveal with unprecedented efficacy some aspects of neural regulation.

On the other hand, lower levels of correlation were found with HF in milliseconds^2 and RR interval. Conversely, no correlation was present between tilt angle and either variance or LF in milliseconds.[2]

We have repetitively stressed[39] that physiological interventions which increase or decrease total power can induce discordant changes in LF absolute power. In the case of tilting, variance and, thus, absolute value of LF tend to decrease, while LF in nu increases, owing to the concentration of power towards the LF region. Vice versa, concerning the HF component, the changes in variance and in HF absolute values are concordant and therefore the absolute value of HF also correlate with tilt angle.

Other maneuvers are also quite effective in enhancing sympathetic drive, such as mental or physical stress for which we again refer to the chapter by Pagani et al.[34]

Effects of Maneuvers Enhancing Vagal Drive

Controlled respiration at frequencies within the resting physiological range[40] provides a convenient tool to enhance the vagal modulation of heart period, probably also achieved through the synchronization of all respiratory components. In concrete terms, the power of the HF component becomes predominant at rest during metronome breathing; in one study[6] the LF/HF ratio was significantly reduced from 2.5 to 0.7. Furthermore, during controlled respiration, increases in the LF component and LF/HF ratio observed with tilt were markedly blunted in regard to those obtained during spontaneous respiration.[6] If the frequency of controlled breathing is decreased enough to approach LF rhythm, the two components merge into one more powerful oscillation.[7,40] In general, all of the studies that have been performed under controlled respiration in the broad range of 0.20 to 0.30 Hz were likely to be characterized by a sympatho-vagal balance shifted in favor of the vagal component.

In general, it is worthwhile to consider that in the oriental tradition the control of respiration mastered to its furthest possibilities was associated to the intention of suppressing what we would consider a sympathetic drive.

Rotational stimulation represents another maneuver capable of inducing a prevalence of HF component (Lucini et al, unpublished data).

Continuous 24-Hour Analysis of the RR Interval

Initial observations[41] with spectral analysis clearly indicated the possibility of assessing the circadian oscillations of the sympathovagal balance. When LF was analyzed in nu over the 24-hour period[7,10,42-44] it displayed a clear circadian pattern (Figure 4) with a marked nocturnal decrease corresponding to the well-known reduction of sympathetic activity. These changes were mirrored by simultaneous increases in HF component, as an expression of the enhanced vagal activity accompanying the largest portion of sleep. The LF component could instead appear unchanged, or even increased during the night,[45] if expressed in absolute units, in parallel with the nocturnal rise of variance leading to the unwarranted conclusion that '24 hour LF power is primarily parasympathetically and not sympathetically mediated.'[45] But, as we have already questioned,[39] 'at which point and on which grounds quantity (ie, length of data) would invert quality (ie, shifting from sympathetic into parasympathetic modulation)?'

Furthermore, the circadian oscillation of the LF component that we have described was not observed in a study[21] in which this component was subdivided into two predetermined bands of interest, as already mentioned, and the heart period was derived from ambulatory pressure recordings performed with a system of narrow frequency response.

Interestingly, the circadian LF oscillation was lost in patients with essential hypertension[42], in diabetic patients with or without autonomic neuropathy,[43] and markedly blunted in patients 4 weeks after myocardial infarction.[44]

Finally, continuous 24-hour analysis of SAP variability[10] indicated that the LF component of SAP variability, obtained from ambulant subjects with a high-fidelity recording system, increased abruptly upon awakening, while the patients were still in bed, and remained elevated throughout the day. Physical activity induced further increases in the LF component of SAP variability, which underwent a marked reduction during the night.

From the simultaneous analysis of RR interval and SAP variability, an index was obtained[46-48] capable of assessing the gain of the baroreflex mechanism. This index reached maximal values during the night and minimal ones during the day, as expected, but also underwent minute-to-minute changes around its average value.[48] This last point indicates the danger implicit in assigning one particular value for baroreflex slope in each individual in a given condition, a word of caution already clearly expressed by DeBoer and coworkers.[18]

Pharmacological Blockades and Neural Lesions

The observations by Selman et al[49] documented that atropine administration was capable of practically abolishing the respiratory component of RR variability. This findings was corroborated by the study of Pomeranz et al.[35] On the basis of these studies[1,20] as well as animal studies, the relation between vagal activity and HF component of RR variability has become generally accepted.

However, there has been disagreement in the literature regarding the interpretation of the LF component. In the same study by Pomeranz et al,[35] intravenous administration of atropine in supine patients under con-

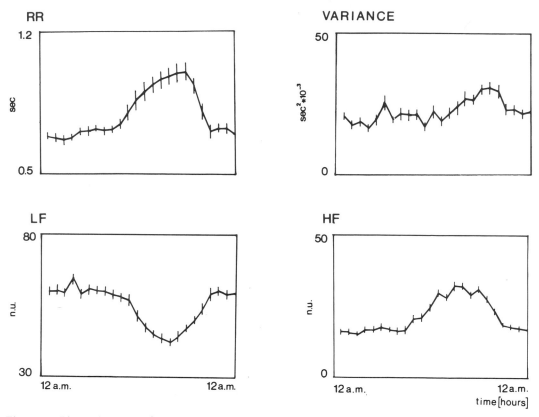

Figure 4. Plots of average hourly values of RR interval, of its variance (in absolute units), and of LF and HF components (in nu) during 24 hours in a group of nonhospitalized subjects free to move. From Furlan et al.[10]

trolled respiration was also capable of reducing the LF component by 84%; it was concluded that, in this position, the LF component is mediated entirely by the parasympathetic system. However, calculations of LF/HF ratio from their average published data suggest that this ratio (~0.5, ie, a value very close to the ~0.7 found by Pagani et al[6] with autoregressive algorithms in subjects under controlled respiration) was increased by muscarinic receptor blockade to ~1, thus indicating a shift in power distribution in favor of LF. In short, in our opinion, the data by Pomeranz et al[35] could be interpreted in a quite different manner: in conditions of vagal predominance induced by metronome breathing, atropine induces a sympathetic predominance as revealed by the LF/HF ratio. Obviously these data would have probably been clearer if the subjects were breath-

ing spontaneously and if spectral components were evaluated in normalized units.

In view of the significant correlation between total power and the absolute power of spectral components, the importance of using normalized units, or the LF/HF ratio, to assess changes in the frequency distribution of spectral power applies not only to conditions characterized by large abatements of total power such as exercise or muscarinic receptor blockade, but also to conditions accompanied by increases in total variance such as happens with beta-adrenergic blockade.

In fact, Pagani et al[6] reported that the increase in variance observed after beta-adrenergic blockade is characterized by a spectral distribution shifted in favor of HF, as assessed by normalized units and by the

LF/HF ratio. This is in accordance with the interpretation that LF is a marker of sympathetic modulation of the sinoatrial (SA) node and that interventions that are known to reduce sympathetic activity produce a shift in power distribution in favor of the HF component. Cook et al,[50] using data obtained from spectra averaged over 24 hours, reported, as expected, that beta-adrenergic blockade enhances the absolute power of the LF band. These data were surprisingly interpreted as an indication that LF was a marker of vagal tone. However, also in this case, the use of LF/HF ratio clearly captures the shift in power distribution towards HF, known to attend beta-adrenergic blockade. Indeed, these authors[50] found a value of LF/HF of 2.5 at control and of 1.6 during beta-adrenergic blockade, as already reported.[6]

In terms of subtractive reasoning, the papers by Inoue and coworkers[51,52] were of crucial importance. These authors reported that the LF component was absent in the RR variability spectrum of six quadriplegic patients[51] and in the SAP variability spectrum of seven similar patients.[52] The interpretation of these findings was that the absence of an LF component in RR and SAP variability spectra was likely to depend upon the interruption at the spinal level of those pathways connecting supraspinal centers, where these rhythms were considered to originate, with spinal sympathetic outflow.

However, the reality turned out to be more complex. In a very recent study we examined the heart period and AP variabilities in 15 chronic, neurologically complete, quadriplegic patients during control conditions, head-up tilt and controlled respiration.[53] In seven of these patients, no LF component was present in resting conditions, in RR and SAP variabilities, thus confirming the data by Inoue et al.[51,52] Vice versa, in six quadriplegic patients an LF component was clearly detectable in the spectrum of both variability signals, although it was reduced in absolute and normalized units if compared with control subjects. In the two remaining patients, an LF component was present in the spectrum of RR variability only. During tilt, in three of the four patients that presented an adequate HR response (ie, a tachycardia of at least 10%) a paradoxical LF response was found in that this component became no longer detectable in either spectra. Furthermore, the six patients who presented an LF component in both RR and SAP variabilities maintained it during controlled respiration. Finally, in five patients, two recording sessions were performed with a lapse of about 6 months between them. During the second recording, the LF component of RR variability appeared markedly increased in three of the four patients in whom this component was already detectable, and became evident in the remaining patient. The LF component of SAP variability spectrum underwent similar changes. Variance also tended to increase during the second recording although changes were not significant.

These findings could be explained by two opposite hypotheses. First, the LF component could be mediated at rest by vagal mechanisms, according to the hypothesis of Pomeranz et al,[35] and its disappearance during tilt, as well as the tachycardia response, could reflect a vagal withdrawal. However, within this hypothesis it is surprising that LF was not present in all patients studied a few months after the lesion, when vagal tone seems to predominate[54]; on the contrary, it appeared to increase with time, as revealed by the repeated recordings. Furthermore, this hypothesis of a prevalent vagal genesis does not explain the presence of an LF component in SAP variability. As to the two quadriplegic patients who were characterized by an LF component only in the RR variability spectrum, it might be worthwhile to mention that, in dogs, alpha-adrenergic receptor blockade, drastically reducing the LF component of SAP variability, leaves unaffected the LF component of RR variability.[26] Thus, the LF component present in RR variability spectrum cannot only represent a compensatory HR baroreflex response to vasomotor waves as suggested by Appel et al.[24]

Second, vice versa, the LF component in RR and SAP variabilities could signal the development of a spinal rhythmicity, increasing with time and influencing the various levels of sympathetic outflow distributed to the heart and peripheral vessels. However, the puzzling finding within this second hypothesis corresponds to the LF decrease or disappearance with tilt. Our satellite hypothesis is the following: the reductions in venous return and cardiac dimensions that accompany a tilting maneuver are likely to decrease the discharge of the cardiovascular thoracic sympathetic afferent fibers[28] and thereby the reflex activity of the sympathetic outflow. On the contrary, controlled respiration in quadriplegic patients might provide a way to activate simultaneously vagal pulmonary afferents and those cardiovascular vagal and sympathetic afferent fibers highly sensitive to volume changes. Hence, both vagovagal and sympatho-sympathetic circuits might be excited, each with its prevailing rhythm, with no possibility for a reciprocal relationship due to the interruption of neural linking pathways. And, in fact, some quadriplegic patients[53] developed or maintained unchanged an LF component in RR and SAP variability spectra during controlled respiration, while normal subjects are usually characterized by a reduction of LF component under these conditions.[6]

Another study on eight quadriplegic patients under controlled respiration by Koh and coworkers[55] has also just reported the existence of an LF component in RR and SAP variability spectra. From published data it is impossible to appreciate whether all patients were similar in this respect and which were the exact values of this finding. However, the crucial point, in the authors' opinion, was that a phenylephrine infusion could increase the absolute power of both LF and HF component (as described by one of their figures) and that such increases were abolished by atropine. The authors concluded[55] that LF was vagally mediated in response to a baroreflex. I personally consider this conclusion totally unwarranted for the following reasons:

First, had this mechanism been the basic one, one should have expected this response (and tested the hypothesis) in control subjects. At an inspection of the published data it appears that their control subjects, who already had an increased vagal tone (due to controlled respiration), further increased the HF predominance during phenylephrine infusion (ie, the baroreceptor stimulation shifted the sympatho-vagal balance towards the expected vagal predominance). Second, it does not explain why at least half of the patients do not present an LF component.[51-53] Third, it provides for the LF component of AP variability an explanation (in addition to that of a spinal rhythmicity) quite difficult to accept, ie, that of a coordinated vascular smooth muscle activity (which would be more likely to be chaotic and poorly detectable in the absence of the coordinating function exerted by the sympathetic modulation). On the other hand, if a spinal rhythmicity had to cause an LF component in AP variability, for which discriminating reason should it not produce a similar oscillation in RR variability? As to the effects of atropine (although no data were provided concerning the distribution of the residual power), it is likely that a further subtracting intervention in a model already deprived of a normal interaction might produce other consequences than those simply postulated.

In conclusion, a view which is based on the already demonstrated existence of a spinal rhythmicity[56] and on the reflexogenic function of sympathetic afferents[28] seems at least more concerned about the complexity of neural organization and less dependent from a nowadays obsolete conception of the baroreflex as the unique mechanism for neural cardiovascular regulation.

The Interpretation of Rhythms

Never has a tool been a benefit independently from how it was used. The stimulating question by Appel et al[24] whether beat-to-beat cardiovascular variability generates noise or music, has probably not been sufficiently appreciated. Indeed, music does not rely principally on decibels (ie, absolute power) but on notes (ie, frequencies) and on their relationship (including relative intensity), although some power is needed for the existence of notes. In such a context it is surprising that some authors[57] active in the field, can state that the 'most straight-forward way' of measuring the LF power is the 'area under the power spectral density curve.' It might be straightforward but, taken alone, does not decodify what goes on. They also added that in our approach 'the reciprocal change in low frequency power (in nu) and high frequency power (in nu) is defined a priori by their mathematical relation, not by physiologic data or theory'.[57] We believe that the opposite is true: we moved from a simple theory and we think that we have found a way to prove it.

The interaction between opposite mechanisms appears as a general rule in biology.[4,7,28] A simple flexor-extensor movement around one joint involves *both* agonistic and antagonistic muscles and millions of neurons, but can be schematized in a reciprocal relationship just like the sympathovagal interaction on sinus node pacemaker activity. The normalization procedure (or the LF/HF ratio) is a simple tool to compare the relative power of the two main short-term cardiovascular rhythms (one needs information on both flexor and extensor muscles to understand the control of the joint).

Both these rhythms and a large part of variance are likely to arise from a continuous interaction.[7] Two examples might be worthwhile. First, in the acute phases after the lesion, quadriplegic patients can have a lower than normal variance[51,53] (and Guzzetti et al, unpublished data) in the presence of an intact vagal circuitry and, often, of a resting bradycardia. Second, Pruett and coworkers[58] have recently reported that in patients undergoing spinal anesthesia, when the spread of spinal block reached the highest thoracic segments (above T_3), a remarkable abatement of vari-

ance and of both spectral components occurred. Both types of observation, therefore, suggest that variance cannot be considered as a pure effect of vagal activity but reflects a more complex interaction, although maneuvers abating vagal tone can drastically reduce variance. Thus, subtractive reasoning does not necessarily lead to bidirectional conclusions.

Which might be the function of these rhythms? For a worker, to dare to propose a hypothesis it should be legitimate. In the case of LF component, the hypothesis emerges more explicitly: vasomotion appears necessary at least as a sort of jogging for the vessels (to keep them in shape and ready to respond). Similar rhythmic frequencies probably characterize the vascular smooth muscle machinery and the neural mechanisms which modulate it. In this way the vasomotor activity from a chaotic process becomes a rhythm.

On the other hand, respiration influences in a rhythmic way most of cardiovascular and respiratory afferents; it is conceivable that the neural outputs redistributed back to respiratory and cardiovascular sites maintain the same rhythmicity, again to avoid the predominance of chaotic interactions (which, still, are likely to occur).

The nub of this view is that two main rhythms, one marker of excitation and one of quiet, would be organized in a reciprocal manner as it was hypothesized by Hess[59] for the two general behaviors that he ascribed to the integration by diencephalic structures. Thus the spectral methodology could underscore the state of this balance, both at central and peripheral levels, according to a closed-loop conception.[4,7] Our subsequent hypothesis (Montano et al, unpublished data) is that different populations of central neurons, independently of their specific function, receive this information. In brief, a necessary synchronization also becomes a neural code.

We believe that so far, abundant and different observations have always reinforced the hypothesis that in the presence of an adequate variability and stationarity the state of sympatho-vagal balance is well reflected by the power in nu of the LF and HF components of RR interval variability.[7,13,37] Adopting the opposite view[57] of using only absolute values, variance becomes the only independent measurement, while spectral components provide scanty additional information and are almost a redundancy.[39]

Each investigator should try what the best use for this tool might be, but if by chance the normalized methodology should reflect what is likely to occur (as in our hands) it might be wise to accept its soundness. This could be in line with an era which, at the frontier, has substituted possibility for certainty.

References

1. Akselrod S, Gordon D, Ubel FA, et al. Power spectrum analysis of HR fluctuations. A quantitative probe of beat to beat cardiovascular control. Science 1981; 213:220-222.
2. Brovelli M, Baselli G, Cerutti S, et al. Computerized analysis for an experimental validation of neurophysiological models of heart rate control. Comp Cardiol 1983; 205-208.
3. Gnecchi Ruscone T, Lombardi F, Malfatto G, et al. Attenuation of baroreceptive mechanisms by cardiovascular sympathetic afferent fibers. Am J Physiol 1987; 253:787-791.
4. Malliani A, Pagani M, Lombardi F. Positive feedback reflexes. In: Zanchetti A, Tarazi RC (eds). Handbook of Hypertension, Volume 8. Pathophysiology of Hypertension. Amsterdam, Holland: Elsevier Science Publishing Co. Inc., 1986; 69-81.
5. Schwartz PJ, Pagani M, Lombardi F, et al. A cardiocardiac sympatho-vagal reflex in the cat. Circ Res 1973; 32:215-220.
6. Pagani M, Lombardi F, Guzzetti S, et al. Power spectral analysis of heart rate and arterial pressure variabilities as a marker of sympathovagal interaction in man and conscious dog. Circ Res 1986; 59:178-193.
7. Malliani A, Pagani M, Lombardi F, et al. Cardiovascular neural regulation explored in the frequency domain. Circulation 1991; 84:482-492.
8. Mayer S. Studien zur Physiologie des Herzens und der Blutgefässe: 5 Abhandlung: Uber spontane Blutdruckschwankungen. Sber Akad Wiss Wien 1876; 74:281-307.
9. Koepchen HP. History of studies and concepts of blood pressure waves. In: Miyakawa K, Koepchen HP, Polosa C (eds). Mechanism of Blood Pressure Waves. Tokyo, Japan: Japan Science Society Press/Berlin, Germany: Springer-Verlag, 1984; 3-23.
10. Furlan R, Guzzetti S, Crivellaro W, et al. Continuous 24-h assessment of the neural regulation of systemic arterial pressure and R-R variabilities in ambulant subjects. Circulation 1990; 81:537-547.
11. Cerutti S, Bianchi A, Mainardi L. Spectral analysis of heart rate variability signal. In: Malik M, Camm AJ (eds). Heart Rate Variability, 1994. In press.
12. Saul JP, Arai Y, Berger RD, et al. Assessment of autonomic regulation in chronic congestive heart failure by heart rate spectral analysis. Am J Cardiol 1988; 61:1292-1299.
13. Malliani A, Lombardi F, Pagani M. Power spectrum analysis of heart rate variability: a tool to explore neural regulatory mechanisms. Br Heart J 1994; 71:1-2.
14. Persson PB, Ehmke H, Kohler WW, et al. Identification of major slow blood pressure oscillations in conscious dogs. Am J Physiol 1990; 259:H1050-H1055.
15. Sayers BMcA. Analysis of heart rate variability. Ergonomics 1973; 16:17-32.
16. Kitney RI, Rompelman O. The Study of Heart Rate Variability. Oxford, England: Clarendon Press, 1980.
17. DeBoer RW, Karemaker JM, VanMontfrans GA. Determination of baroreflex sensitivity by spectral analysis of spontaneous blood-pressure and heart-rate fluctuations in man. In: Lown B, Malliani A, Prosdocimi M (eds). Neural Mechanisms and Cardiovascular Disease. Padova, Italy: Liviana Press, 1986; 303-315.
18. DeBoer RW, Karemaker JM, Strackee J. Hemodynamic fluctuations and baroreflex sensitivity in humans: a beat-to-beat model. Am J Physiol 1987; 253:680-689.
19. Baselli G, Cerutti S, Civardi S, et al. Spectral and cross-spectral analysis of heart rate and arterial blood pressure variability signals. Comput Biomed Res 1986; 19:520-534.
20. Rimoldi O, Pierini S, Ferrari A, et al. Analysis of short-term oscillations of R-R and arterial pressure in conscious dogs. Am J Physiol 1990; 258:H967-H976.
21. Parati G, Castiglion P, Di Rienzo M, et al. Sequential spectral analysis of 24-hour blood pressure and pulse interval in humans. Hypertension 1990; 16:414-421.

22. Mathias JM, Mullen TJ, Perrott MH, et al. Heart rate variability: principles and measurement. ACC Curr J Rev 1993; 10-12.

23. Takalo R, Korhonen I, Turjanmaa V, et al. Short-term variability of blood pressure and heart rate in borderline and mildly hypertensive subjects. Hypertension 1994; 23:18-24.

24. Appel ML, Berger RD, Saul JP, et al. Beat to beat variability in cardiovascular variables: noise or music? J Am Coll Cardiol 1989; 14:1139-1148.

25. Randall DC, Brown DR, Raisch RM, et al. SA nodal parasympathectomy delineates autonomic control of heart rate power spectrum. Am J Physiol 1991; 260:H985-H988.

26. Rimoldi O, Furlan R, Pagani MR, et al. Analysis of neural mechanisms accompanying different intensities of dynamic exercise. Chest 1992; 101:226S-230S.

27. Malliani A, Schwartz PJ, Zanchetti A. A sympathetic reflex elicited by experimental coronary occlusion. Am J Physiol 1969; 217:703-709.

28. Malliani A. Cardiovascular sympathetic afferent fibers. Rev Physiol Biochem Pharmacol 1982; 94:11-74.

29. Montano N, Lombardi F, Gnecchi Ruscone T, et al. Spectral analysis of sympathetic discharge, R-R interval and systolic arterial pressure in decerebrate cats. J Autonom Nerv Syst 1992; 40:21-32.

30. Ewing DJ, Neilson JMM, Travis P. New method for assessing cardiac parasympathetic activity using 24 hour electrocardiograms. Br Heart J 1984; 52:396-402.

31. Kleiger RE, Miller JP, Bigger JT, et al. Decreased heart rate variability and its association with increased mortality after acute myocardial infarction. Am J Cardiol 1987; 59:256-262.

32. Vybiral T, Bryg RJ, Maddens ME, et al. Effect of passive tilt on sympathetic and parasympathetic components of heart rate variability in normal subjects. Am J Cardiol 1989; 63:1117-1120.

33. Furlan R, Piazza S, Dell'Orto S, et al. Early and late effects of exercise and athletic training on neural mechanisms controlling heart rate. Cardiovasc Res 1993; 27:482-488.

34. Pagani M, Lucini D, Rimoldi O, et al. Effects of physical and mental exercise on heart rate variability. In: Malik M, Camm AJ (eds). Heart Rate Variability, 1994. In press.

35. Pomeranz B, Macaulay RJB, Caudill MA, et al. Assessment of autonomic function in humans by heart rate spectral analysis. Am J Physiol 1985; 248:H151-H153.

36. Fallen EL, Kamath MV, Ghista DN. Power spectrum of heart rate variability: a non-invasive test of integrated neurocardiac function. Clin Invest Med 1988; 2:331-340.

37. Montano N, Gnecchi Ruscone T, Porta A, et al. Power spectrum analysis of heart rate variability to assess the changes in sympatho-vagal balance during graded orthostatic tilt. Circulation 1994. 90:1826-1831.

38. Lipsitz LA, Mietus J, Moody GB, et al. Spectral characteristics of heart rate variability before and during postural tilt. Circulation 1990; 81:1803-1810.

39. Pagani M, Lombardi F, Malliani A. Heart rate variability: disagreement on the markers of sympathetic and parasympathetic activities. J Am Coll Cardiol 1993; 22:951-954.

40. Kitney R, Linkens D, Selman A, et al. The interaction between heart rate and respiration. II. Nonlinear analysis based on computer modelling. Automedica 1982; 4:141-153.

41. Pagani M, Furlan R, Dell'Orto S, et al. Simultaneous analysis of beat by beat systemic arterial pressure and heart rate variabilities in ambulatory patients. J Hypertens 1985; 3:S83-S85.

42. Guzzetti S, Dassi S, Pecis M, et al. Altered pattern of circadian neural control of heart period in mild hypertension. J Hypertens 1991; 9:831-838.

43. Bernardi L, Ricordi L, Lazzari P, et al. Impaired circadian modulation of sympathovagal activity in diabetes. Circulation 1992; 86:1443-1452.

44. Lombardi F, Sandrone G, Mortara A, et al. Circadian variation of spectral indices of heart rate variability after myocardial infarction. Am Heart J 1992; 123:1521-1529.

45. Goldsmith RL, Bigger JT Jr, Steinman RC, et al. Comparison of 24-hour parasympathetic activity in endurance-trained and untrained young men. J Am Coll Cardiol 1992; 20:552-558.

46. Cerutti S, Baselli G, Civardi S, et al. Spectral analysis of heart rate and arterial blood pressure variability signals for physiological and clinical purposes. Comput Cardiol 1987;435-438.

47. Robbe HWJ, Mulder LJM, Rüddel H, et al. Assessment of baroreceptor reflex sensitivity by means of spectral analysis. Hypertension 1987; 10:538-543.

48. Pagani M, Somers V, Furlan R, et al. Changes in autonomic regulation induced by physical training in mild hypertension. Hypertension 1988; 12:600-610.

49. Selman A, McDonald A, Kitney R, et al. The interaction between heart rate and respiration. I. Experimental studies in man. Automedica 1982; 4:131-139.

50. Cook JR, Bigger JT, Kleiger RE, et al. Effect of atenolol and diltiazem on heart rate variability in normal persons. J Am Coll Cardiol 1991; 17:480-484.

51. Inoue K, Miyake S, Kumashiro M, et al. Power spectral analysis of heart rate variability in traumatic quadriplegic humans. Am J Physiol 1990; 260:H1722-H1726.

52. Inoue K, Miyake S, Kumashiro M, et al. Power spectral analysis of blood pressure variability in traumatic quadriplegic humans. Am J Physiol 1991; 260:H842-H847.

53. Guzzetti S, Cogliati C, Broggi C, et al. Influences of neural mechanisms on heart period and arterial pressure variabilities in quadriplegic patients. Am J Physiol 1994; 34. In press.

54. Mathias CJ, Frankel HL. Cardiovascular control in spinal man. Annu Rev Physiol 1988; 50:577-592.

55. Koh J, Brown TE, Beightol LA, et al. Human autonomic rhythms: vagal cardiac mechanisms in tetraplegic subjects. J Physiol 1994; 474:483-495.

56. Fernandes de Molina A, Perl ER. Sympathetic activity and the systemic circulation in the spinal cat. J Physiol 1965; 181:82-102.

57. Goldsmith RL, Bloomfield D, Rottman J, et al. Heart rate variability: disagreement on the markers of sympathetic and parasympathetic activities. J Am Coll Cardiol 1993; 22:951-954.

58. Pruett JK, Yodlowski EH, Introna RPS, et al. The influence of spinal anesthetics on heart rate variations. Pharmacol (Life Sci Adv) 1991; 10:51-55.

59. Hess WR. The Functional Organization of the Diencephalon. New York, New York: Grune & Stratton Inc., 1957.

Chapter 15

Baroreflex Sensitivity and Heart Rate Variability in the Assessment of the Autonomic Status

Maria Teresa La Rovere, Andrea Mortara, Gian Domenico Pinna, Luciano Bernardi

Heart rate (HR) and its variability comprise the cardiovascular response to broadly defined stimuli, these stimuli being physical, psychological or enviromental. Since the cardiovascular system is a 'pressure' controlled system, factors that alter blood pressure (BP) will primarily govern fluctuations in HR. Several biological sensors in the vessels and in the heart respond to changes in BP and/or volume. The arterial baroreflex is of special interest in that it responds rapidly to the abrupt transients of arterial pressure (AP) that occur in daily life so as to maintain circulatory homeostasis. The purpose of this chapter is to describe baroreceptor physiology and some methods used for assessing baroreceptor activity, then to analyze the role of arterial baroreceptors in the modulation of heart rate variability (HRV), and finally to discuss some possible clinical correlations between baroreflex sensitivity (BRS) and HRV.

Arterial Baroreceptors

The mechanisms of arterial baroreflex control in humans have been extensively reviewed previously.[1,2] Arterial baroreflex afferents originate in the carotid sinus and aortic arch. Mechanoreceptors located in these areas change their rate of firing with change in AP (ie, the higher the pressure, the greater the firing rate and the lower the pressure, the smaller the number of impulses sent to the nervous system per unit time). The afferent impulses from the baroreceptors (which travel along the glossopharyngeal and vagal nerves) are conducted to the so-called cardioinhibitory and vasomotor centers in the medulla oblongata (and other parts of the central nervous system) where they modulate the parasympathetic outflow to the heart and the sympathetic nervous system outflow to the heart and the blood vessels. Therefore, barorecep-

From: Malik M., Camm AJ (eds.): *Heart Rate Variability.* Armonk, NY. Futura Publishing Company, Inc., © 1995.

tors control HR, vasoconstriction, venoconstriction and cardiac contractility in order to regulate arterial BP.

Reflex cardiac sympathetic responses are slower than parasympathetic responses.[3-5] The control of HR by the vagus develops with almost no time lag and can provide virtually instantaneous regulation, whereas changes in HR and in the systemic vascular resistance are produced by the efferent sympathetic activity with a few seconds delay and make it appear that these cannot function when extremely rapid adaptation must occur.[6] The reflex cardiac response to baroreceptor stimulation is probably more complex, involving effects on stroke volume and cardiac output mediated by the efferent vagus.[7,8]

Inherently tonic activity normally is present in the sympathetic outflow from the brain stem; the pressor center constantly discharges impulses which tend to maintain some degree of constriction in the blood vessels and increase HR. This activity is increased by sinoaortic deafferentation. The arterial baroreceptors thus have a continual depressor action. The fact that sinoaortic denervation almost abolishes vagal tone indicates that the so-called cardioinhibitory center is not tonically active unless played upon (as it usually is) by afferent nerves.

Baroreflexes not only operate on a dynamic basis to control abrupt changes in AP but are also operating continuously in the steady state condition. As a consequence, the baroreceptor activity can be investigated either by the application of a variety of mechanical or pharmacological manipulations that cause abrupt changes sensed by the BP receptors, or by analyzing the spontaneous fluctuations of the AP in steady state conditions. Arterial baroreflex response patterns are modulated by the simultaneous interplay on the medullary centers of the afferent inputs from the multiple reflexogenic areas in the heart and in the vessels. Alterations of respiration, cardiac mechanoreceptors, chemoreceptors and cardiopulmonary receptors, and exercise and posture continu-

ously modify central responsiveness to incoming baroreceptor information and lead to reflex interactions of great complexity and diversity. Humoral substances such as vasopressin, angiotensin II and epinephrine may also modify baroreflex responses by acting at peripheral (afferent or efferent) or central level. The enormous complexity of baroreflex interactions has been recently extensively reviewed.[9]

Pertaining to the subject of this chapter, respiration, has to be underlined as one of the most important mechanisms for modulation of arterial baroreflex control of HR. During inspiration, mechanoreceptors in the lung are stimulated and activate the lung inflation reflex. Inspiration reduces baroreceptor stimulation of vagal motonuclei and vagal efferent firing, as demostrated by Katona et al,[10] with direct recording of vagus nerve activity in anesthetized dogs. Evidence in humans has been provided by the greater extent of reflex RR interval lengthening during expiration than during inspiration, in response to a pressure rise caused by angiotensin administration[11] or neck suction.[12] Respiratory gating of vagal baroreflex responses in normal human subjects is influenced by the frequency of breathing and tidal volume. Respiratory sinus arrhythmia is preserved at breathing rates of 3, 6, and 12 breaths/minute, while it is abolished at breathing rates of 24 breaths/minute.[13] In normal subjects, the effects of tidal volume on sinus arrhythmia are smaller in that a 50% increase in tidal volume induces only a 15% increase in respiratory sinus arrhythmia.[14]

Methods for Assessment of Baroreceptor Activity

Human baroreflex studies are subject to the limitations imposed by studying a complex integrated physiological system, but despite this, several quantitative approches have been developed for evaluating BRS: pharmacological elevations or reductions of AP; neck suction or pressure; and analyses of spontaneous fluctuations of AP and RR interval. All of these methods are limited by either theoretical or practical considerations.

Vasoactive Drugs

The most widely used method for studying baroreflex control of HR was devised in the 1960s by the Oxford group.[11] The concept of the technique is to study the reflex HR response to physiological activation or deactivation of the baroreceptors obtained by drug-induced changes in AP. Originally these investigators measured the reflex bradycardia during BP rise induced by intravenous injection of small boluses of angiotensin. The use of angiotensin as a pressor agent was subsequently replaced by the use of phenylephrine, a pure alpha-adrenoreceptor stimulant, devoid of direct effects on cardiac contractility and the central nervous system.[15,16] With phenylephrine, doses of 50 to 150 μg are used to increase systolic AP by 20 to 30 mm Hg above baseline value. A linear correlation is found when prolongations of successive RR intervals after the injection are plotted as function of preceding systolic pressure changes. The slope of this regression line (expressed as milliseconds of increase in RR interval per mm Hg rise in pressure) allows a quantification of the sensitivity of the arterial baroreflex control of HR. Several injections are generally repeated at few minutes interval and the corresponding slopes are averaged in order to reduce measurement variability between tests. This variability is mainly due to rate of injection, steepness of AP increase, and selection of the analysis time window. The final slope is usually obtained by at least three slopes with the greater correlation coefficients. In normal subjects[11] and hypertensive patients,[17] BRS is directly related to the baseline RR interval values. This finding has not been observed in postinfarction patients.[18] Similar linear relationships can be obtained by the measurement of the RR interval shortening following reduction in BP induced by a vasodilator

agent (ie, nitroglycerin, sodium nitroprussiate). The fact that the baroreflex slopes obtained by increasing AP are significantly higher than those obtained by decreasing pressure, to a similar extent, would suggest that responses to rising and falling AP are asymmetrical in humans.[19] Vasoactive drugs provide a physiological perturbation of the baroreflex system since all the arterial baroreceptor areas are stimulated (activated or deactivated) in the same direction. Moreover, the subject is unaware of the stimulus, thus avoiding the influence of emotional factors which, by activating sympathetic activity, could reduce HR response (see below). Therefore, in the presence of similar physiological and laboratory conditions and in the absence of pharmacological interventions, baroreflex responses have been found to be highly reproducible in healthy subjects.[20] Reproducible baroreflex responses have also been documented in coronary patients who were studied 1 month and 12 months after an acute myocardial infarction.[21]

While, with the Oxford method, a ramp increase of AP is produced and the associated dynamic changes in RR interval are analyzed, in the Korner's method,[22] reflex RR interval lengthening is assessed at different steady levels of BP increase, which are maintained for 10 to 15 minutes by phenylephrine infusion. The time required for the infusion limits the use of this procedure in the clinical setting.

Several theoretical objections have been stated to the use of vasoactive drugs. One of these is related to the direct effect of vasoactive drugs on BP and cardiovascular resistance which prevent evaluation of baroreflex control of AP. Other objections include the simultaneous activation of reflexes from the cardiopulmonary region, and changes in baroreceptor transduction due to the contraction of smooth muscle fibers in the arterial wall. However, these considerations do not seem to be of great practical importance for the doses of drugs used in clinical practice. The most important practical limitation with the ramp method of baroreflex testing is the need of a beat-to-beat AP measurement, thus initially requiring an invasive approach. The development of a device for noninavsive recording of BP (FINAPRES from FINger Arterial PRESsure) has now enabled a widespread use of the Oxford technique. The FINAPRES is based on servo-plethysmomanometry, employing the volume-clamp technique.[23,24] The accuracy of BP measurement of FINAPRES has been documented during the Valsalva maneuver, sustained handgrip, postural changes and vasoactive interventions.[25,26] These studies on small groups of subjects, have shown that the brachial-to-finger pressures differ only quantitatively, but the pattern of BP changes is similar. Validation on a larger population of post-myocardial infarction patients is currently taking place as part of an ongoing prospective study of the prognostic value of HRV and BRS. Preliminary data on 246 BRS tests performed using BP values from both invasive and noninvasive measurement have demonstrated a strong correlation (Pearson correlation coefficient = 0.94) between the two approaches.[27] Noninvasive measurement of AP strongly reinforces the practical ease of baroreflex testing by the vasoactive drug technique.

Baroreflex function has been widely explored with the phenylephrine ramp method both in physiological conditions and disease processes. Circadian variations in BRS have been reported,[28] and an increase in BRS during sleep has been observed.[11] The increase in baroreflex gain during sleep, though not entirely reproducible, has been related to a reset of the baroreflex by the reduction in BP.[29] These findings are well in line with the increase in the vagal-related high-frequency (HF) component of the HR power spectra during night time.[30] On the other hand, physical exercise[31,32] and mental arousal[33] are associated with a reduction in baroreflex control of HR while the BP control is left relatively unaffected.[34] The impairment of baroreflex control of sinus node function during exercise is directly related to the intensity of exercise; it is not known whether lower baroreflex responses are due to true reductions of baroreflex gain or reflect a resetting to operate at higher BP and HR levels.

There is an inverse relationship between age and BRS[20] probably caused by a loss of compliance of the arterial wall,[35] though a central impairment has also been suggested.[36]

Arterial baroreflex control is abnormal in patients with cardiovascular diseases[37] and tends to involve reciprocal changes of sympathetic and parasympathetic activity. Baroreflex malfunction may participate in the maintenance or evolution of the pathological process. The location of the defect underlying baroreflex abnormalities in patients with cardiovascular disease is generally poorly understood in that one or more of the afferent, central, efferent or end-organ components may be involved. A growing mass of evidence points to prognostic implication of impaired baroreflex function. The first observation relating prognosis to BRS was provided by Billman et al[38] who showed that, in the period after a myocardial infarction, dogs with diminished baroreflex slopes were much more likely to develop ventricular fibrillation than dogs with steep slopes. Subsequent studies in patients after their first myocardial infarction confirmed that a depressed BRS is associated with an increased risk of sudden death (Figure 1).[18,39] The mechanism by which BRS is reduced after myocardial infarction is not completely known, but it is likely to involve a derangement of the afferent information from the heart which impairs the baroreceptor reflex,[40] or by increased circulating angiotensin which depresses the baroreflex centrally.[41]

Neck Chamber Technique

The neck chamber technique allows local activation or deactivation of carotid baroreceptors by application of measurable positive and negative pneumatic pressures to the neck region. The first model of neck

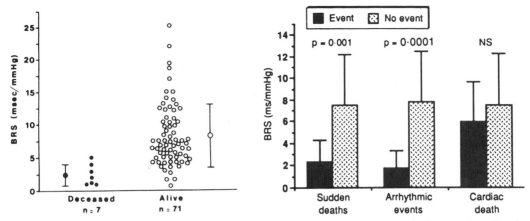

Figure 1. Relation between depressed BRS and adverse events after myocardial infarction. On the left: plot showing the relation between BRS and cardiovascular mortality (four deaths were sudden and three were due to heart failure) in a group of 78 patients with a recent myocardial infarction. It is worthy to note that deceased patients have a markedly depressed BRS as compared to survivors and four of them are in the extreme lower end of the distribution of BRS for the entire population. Updated and modified with permission from La Rovere et al.[18] On the right: column graph (mean±SD) of BRS according to the clinical events in 122 patients after a recent myocardial infarction. BRS slope was significantly reduced in patients suffering sudden death and arrhythmic events (including sudden death and ventricular fibrillation), but it was not significantly lower when all cardiovascular deaths were considered. Modified with permission from Farrell et al.[39]

chamber was described in 1957 by Ernsting and Parry.[42] Among the different types subsequently developed, the one proposed by Eckberg[43] (a lead collar which encircles only the anterior and lateral aspects of the neck and can be molded to suit the neck of each individual subject) and the one proposed by Ludbrook[44] (which completely surrounds the neck) have been more extensively used. An increase in neck chamber pressure is sensed by the baroreceptor as a decrease in BP and, thus, activate a double response which determines vagal withdrawal to the heart and sympathetic activation to the arterial vessels. Conversely, a decrease in neck chamber pressure results in reflex reduction of BP and HR.

Neck suction is more easy to use than pressure and is well tolerated by the subject. In addition, the suction can be administered with special patterns (ie, fluctuating) so that both relative activation and deactivation of the carotid baroreceptor can be observed. For these reasons, neck suction is presently the preferred stimulus (Figure 2).

Two distinctive features of the neck chamber technique need to be emphasized:

1. the stimulus is, to a great extent, 'pure' that is, is confined to the baroreceptor areas. This is a quite important advantage with respect to other maneuvers which can be used to study the baroreceptor activity. For example, the changes in baroreceptor activity induced by the Valsalva maneuver occur through important changes in intrathoracic pressure, venous return, pulmonary and systemic pressures, inotropism and left/right ventricular wall stress,[45,46] so that separating the autonomic from the mechanical effects is extremely complex; and

2. unlike the vasoactive drugs, neck stimulation, due to its specific and confined action, allows observation of the response on both the heart and the circulation.

There are several limitations of the neck chamber technique. The technique is complex to use and the collection of data is time-consuming. Furthermore, neck chambers are not comfortable to wear, and the sub-

IMPULSIVE AND SINUSOIDAL NECK SUCTION STIMULATIONS

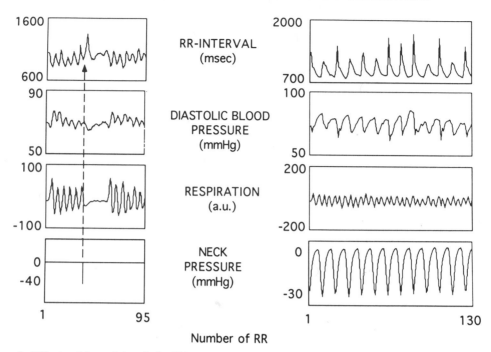

Number of RR

Figure 2. Effects of impulsive (left: 600 ms to 40 mm Hg pulse) and sinusoidal (right: 0 to -30 mm Hg, 0.1 Hz) neck suction on RR interval and diastolic BP in a normal subject. Respiration is held at end-expiration during impulsive, whereas is maintained at 15 breaths per minute (ie, 0.25 Hz) during sinusoidal neck suction. Notice the sudden bradycardia and hypotension immediately following the impulsive suction, and the profound modulation of both RR interval and diastolic BP induced by the 0.1 Hz sinusoidal neck suction.

jects, aware of the stimulus applied, may have some emotional reaction. The hypothesis that the aortic baroreflex, not directly stimulated, may interfere with the response at the carotid level, appears mainly theoretical; since the HR response occurs within the same or the next heart period, while the BP response is more gradual (within the next one or two heart periods) this may not be a limitation when the immediate HR changes are evaluated.

There are conflicting data on the reproducibility of human responses to baroreceptor stimulation by the neck chamber technique, probably depending on different methodologies.[47,48] As with the vasoactive drugs, an asymmetry in the control of the circulation by activation or deactivation of the carotid baroreceptor has been shown.[48]

The Valsalva Maneuver

Valsalva's maneuver has been the most widely used test of human autonomic function; the test is nonpharmacological and can be used to obtain quantitative information about the integrity of responses to elevations and reductions of AP mediated by both the sympathetic and parasympathetic systems. Responses to this test have been studied extensively in normal subjects and patients with cardiovascular disease.

Autonomic reflexes are produced by abrupt transient voluntary elevations of intrathoracic and intra-abdominal pressures provoked by straining. The method is widely variable in that straining may be initiated after a maximal inspiration, after a 'full' inspiration, or at the end of a normal inspiration. The duration of straining may vary from 10 to 40 seconds; mouth pressure may be raised to more than 40 mm Hg.

Hamilton et al[49] proposed that responses to the maneuver can be divided into four phases:

1. a brief transient rise in BP and reduction in HR immediately after the onset of straining.

   The BP rise during phase 1 of the Valsalva maneuver appears to depend mainly upon mechanical factors due to the compressive effect on the aorta of the increased intrathoracic and intra-abdominal pressures and to the increase in stroke volume. The HR reduction is neurally and vagally mediated, because it is virtually absent in transplanted human hearts[50] and prevented by atropine.[51] The RR interval lengthening probably results exclusively from increased afferent traffic from carotid baroreceptor, since it is likely that during this phase afferent traffic from aortic baroreceptors decreases;

2. a fall, and then a recovery, in BP and an increase in HR during the continuation of straining.

   During phase 2, the continuation of straining impedes venous return and leads to a reduced stroke volume and cardiac output. As a consequence, pressures in all baroreceptive areas fall and increase in HR and sympathetic vasoconstrictor tone are reflexly mediated by baroreceptor inhibition. The increase in peripheral vascular resistance leads to a return toward control levels of AP;

3. a brief further reduction in AP and increase in HR at release of straining, which results from the decrease in intrathoracic pressure; and

4. a sustained overshoot of BP and a concomitant reduction in HR. During phase 4, venous inflow and stroke volume return toward normal values and AP returns to, and

then rises above, control values because of the reflex vasoconstriction (partly mediated by reduced activity of cardiopulmonary receptors). Blood pressure elevation, by activating sinoaortic baroreceptors, leads to bradycardia.

Notwithstanding its apparent simplicity, the Valsalva maneuver is a very complex test that involves several populations of autonomic receptors (arterial and cardiopulmonary baroreceptors and possibly chemoreceptors). As previously outlined, the detailed Valsalva method used is heterogenous and therefore both the results obtained and the interindividual reproducibility are widely variable, particularly when normal subjects and patients with cardiac disease are compared.

Several groups have used phase 4 of the Valsalva maneuver to assess BRS,[52-54] showing a high correlation between baroreflex slopes derived from the bolus phenylephrine method and those obtained by analyzing the overshoot bradycardia of the Valsalva maneuver (Figure 3).

Analysis of Spontaneous Baroreflex Sensitivity

Nonperturbational measures of BRS can be obtained by analyzing the normal spontaneous fluctuations in AP and pulse-interval normally observed in conscious animals and humans. Two basic approaches have been proposed and validated, one based on 'time-domain' and one based on 'frequency-domain' measurements.

With the 'time-domain' approach, a computer program automatically identifies those sequences of three or more consecutive heartbeats characterized by a progressive increase in systolic BP and a progressive lenghthening in RR or pulse-interval, or characterized by a progressive reduction in systolic BP and a progressive shortening in RR or pulse-interval. The threshold value for including beat-to-beat systolic BP and

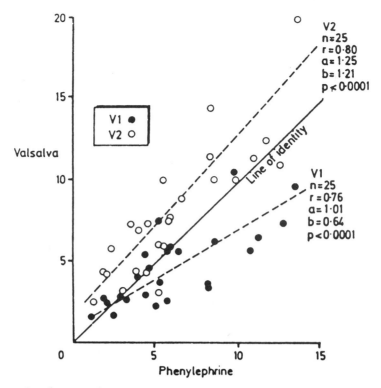

Figure 3. Scatter plot showing the relation between BRS assessed by phenylephrine method and by Valsalva maneuver (ms/mm Hg). *V1* applies to analyses using all of phase IV. *V2* applies to analyses using the BP overshoot only. Note that, although the Pearson correlation coefficient is above 0.75, the use of all phase IV tends to underestimate BRS, while the use of the systolic BP overshoot alone overestimates it. Reprinted with permission from Smith et al.[53]

pulse-interval changes in a sequence are set at 1 mm Hg and 6 milliseconds, respectively. Similarly to what is done when vasoactive drugs are injected, information on the sensitivity of baroreflex control of HR can be obtained by computing the slope of the regression line between changes in systolic BP and the following changes in RR or pulse-interval.[26]

The 'frequency-domain' approach uses the spectral analysis of simultaneously obtained sequences of RR interval and BP. The idea is that each spontaneous oscillation in BP elicits an oscillation of similar frequency in the RR interval by effect of the arterial baroreflex activity. Hence, the baroreflex gain is obtained by dividing the amplitude of RR oscillation by the amplitude of the same oscillation in the BP. The function that describes this gain at each oscillatory frequency is the modulus of the so-called

transfer function between systolic pressure and RR interval. Usually this function is computed in two major bands: that centered around 0.1 Hz, called low frequency (LF), and that around the respiratory frequency called HF band. Some authors indicate the two gains as 'alfa LF' and 'alfa HF'.[55] Under the assumption that the transfer from systolic pressure to RR interval is linear, alfa LF and alfa HF can be simply computed by the square root of the ratio between the spectral component of the RR spectrum and that of the systolic pressure spectrum in the LF and HF band, respectively. In order to be confident that the assumption of linearity holds, the coherence function between pressure and RR interval is computed first. The function attains a value between zero and unity and provides a measure of the amount of linear relationship between the variability of the two signals at each frequency. This measure is comparable to the correlation coefficient in linear regression analysis in time domain, except that it is computed at each frequency of the spectrum. A coherence >0.5 is commonly required for modulus function computation. Mean values of BRS, as assessed by this method and by the phenylephrine method, have been found to be similar[55,56] even if the Pearson correlation coefficient resulted moderate (r=0.6, p<0.001)[55] and high (r=0.9, p<0.001)[56].

Baroreflex Activity and Heart Rate Variability

It is well established that HR is the result of a balance between sympathetic and parasympathetic sinus-atrial node innervation. Both divisions of the autonomic nervous system are antagonist in their effect and exhibit complex interactions. As said above, the sympathetic and parasympathetic systems differ substantially in their response speed as a consequence of the different dynamics of acetylcholine and noradrenaline on the depolarization pattern of the sinus-atrial node cells. This results in a fast vagal (within a single beat), but a much slower sympathetic control of HR.[57]

The sympatho-vagal interaction to the sinus-atrial node represents only one of the efferent pathways of the more complex cardiovascular regulatory system involving different receptors in the vessels and in the heart, afferent fibers, and the central nervous system. Arterial baroreceptors play a central role in the dynamic control not only of HR but also of HRV.

Recently, the simultaneous noninvasive analysis of respiration, HR and BP oscillations has given new insight in the comprehension of the respiratory and vasomotor related variability.[58-60] This technique allowed the development of several theoretical models of short-term cardiovascular regulation. Some of these models describe the cardiovascular variables such as HR, systolic and diastolic pressure as signals continuously varying in time and sampled at equally spaced intervals,[60] while other models follow a beat-to-beat approach where the respiratory signal is sampled every cardiac beat.[59,61]

Chapter 11 (Baselli's chapter) focuses on these models. Some of them will be summarized in the following.

DeBoer Model[61]

This is a beat-to-beat model of the cardiovascular system designed to study the spontaneous short-term variability in arterial BP and HR in humans at rest. The model assumes that respiratory sinus arrhythmia is caused by an initial direct mechanical respiratory modulation of pulse pressure (by stroke volume variations) which is subsequently converted into fluctuations of HR via baroreflex activation and deactivation. Owing to the frequency dependent relationship between systolic pressure and RR interval variability, at normal respiratory frequencies (>0.2 Hz), only the vagal part of the baroreflex remains effective, suggesting that respiratory sinus arrhythmia is parasympathetically mediated. The 10-second rhythm in HR and BP (oscillation around 0.1 Hz) is described as a resonance phenomenon due to the delay in the sympathetic feed-back loops of the baroreflex system.

Baselli Model[59]

This is a closed-loop, beat-to-beat model of the cardiovascular system based on autoregressive identification pathways involving feedforward (representing the cardiac and arterial effects on systolic pressure due to variations of interval length) and feedback (representing the baroreflex effect on HR). A second closed-loop describes the lumped cardiovascular effects on systolic AP not depending on HR (peripheral resistance, venous return, contractility). This method estimates the relative contribution of centrally and mechanically induced respiratory fluctuations of BP and HRV. No distinction is made in this model between sympathetic and parasympathetic transfer characteristics to the sinus-atrial node. It is suggested that respiration affects AP more directly than HR, while a resonance in the pressure-pressure feedback seems to be responsible for the 10-second rhythm.

Saul Model[60]

The only effector mechanism included in this model of cardiovascular control is the HR reflex with a clear distinction between vagal and sympathetic efferent pathways to the sinoatrial node. The transfer between each of the two limbs and HR is modeled as a single-pole low-pass filter with a time constant which depends on the posture (supine or upright); the sympathetic transfer is placed in series with a delay of 1.7 seconds, as calculated in experimental studies. Baroreceptors are modeled as a constant gain in series with a time delay of 0.3 seconds. As a consequence, the total baroreceptor-HR reflex has a vagal delay of 0.3 seconds and a sympathetic delay of 2.0 seconds.

In this model, the respiration enters the baroreflex-HR closed loop at two sites:

1. centrally, with a direct effect on HR through sympathetic and vagal activity; and
2. mechanically, as a result of the coupling between respiration and the vasculature (through modulation of ventricular filling), in such a way that changes in BP are more related to respiratory flow rather than to lung volume.

Below 0.25 Hz, both the autonomic and mechanical effects seem to influence BP significantly, while above 0.25 Hz the mechanical influence of respiration is probably predominant. In this model the baroreflex does not control peripheral resistance, venous return, or cardiac contractility and does not show resonating properties around 0.1 Hz.

All these theoretical models seem to suggest that baroreflex activity is the major determinant of HRV, both in the HF and LF spectral bands. Respiration modulates arterial BP by inducing intrathoracic pressure changes which modify the venous return and, consequently, the stroke volume. At normal respiratory frequencies (>0.2 Hz) respiratory sinus arrhythmia is thus mainly caused by the baroreflex response to respiratory BP changes. Respiration usually produces an oscillation at a frequency between 0.20 to 0.40 Hz (HF band) of both systolic and diastolic AP. Via baroreflex stimulation, this oscillation is suddenly transmitted to the sinus-atrial node by the fast vagal efferent pathway (delay <0.5 seconds). This is well represented in the spectrum of systolic, diastolic pressure and HRV by a peak centered at the respiratory frequency and by a nearly zero phase lag at the same frequency, in the phase spectrum of systolic pressure versus RR interval.[61]

Closed-loop models of cardiovascular regulation which include the baroreflex control of peripheral resistance, clearly demonstrate that LF oscillations of HR around 0.1 Hz may result from a resonance of the negative feed-back reflex mechanisms involving sympathetic neurons, sinoaortic baroreceptors and peripheral vasculature. On the basis of animal studies, a time delay of about 3.0 seconds is usually assumed for total peripheral resistance response to changes in baroreceptor activity. The existence of a concomitant time delay in the systemic AP response is crucial for producing the 10-second BP oscillations[62]; the baroreceptor discharge reduction caused by a fall in AP produces an excitation of the sympathetic nervous system, which in turn causes a delayed rise of AP. The higher pressure results in an increased baroreceptor activity and inhibition of sympathetic drive, but pressure increase will continue until the delayed relaxation of smooth muscle occurs. Then, pressure falls, baroreceptor activity again decreases and the cycle continues. As a consequence, LF HR oscillations mainly represent a delayed compensatory response to BP fluctuations mediated by the baroreflex. Evidence to support this speculation has been provided in anesthetized dogs by observing that atrial pacing does not cause a decrease of LF BP fluctuations.[58]

The explanation, so far, reported of LF HR and BP oscillations is usually referred to as the 'peripheral' hypothesis. According to the 'central' hypothesis, on the other hand, arterial BP oscillations are the result of a rhythmicity of sympathetic neural activity which may be produced and maintained entirely within the central nervous system.[63] In this case the afferent periodic signal from pressoreceptors might have an additional 'synchronizing' influence upon the central oscillator.

Since sympathetic modulation is fundamental in the generation of the 10-second rhythm, the conjecture that LF oscillations around 0.1 Hz are related to sympathetic activity seems to be justified. However, in the variability of HR, the vagal efferent activity contributes to LF oscillations as well, being involved in the baroreceptor response to fluctuations of AP. These simple considerations can explain why atropine abolishes most of the LF as well as the HF component of HR power spectrum.[64]

Moreover, the notion that LF power cannot be considered merely as an index of sympathetic activity is also confirmed by the paradox observed in two conditions—severe heart failure and strenuous exercise—which are accompanied by sympathetic arousal and vagal withdrawl, but the power in the LF band has been found markedly reduced.[65,66] Such a finding seems related to a reduced modulation of the HR via a depressed baroreflex activity.

To investigate the role of the carotid baroreceptors in the genesis of the LF oscillation, a study has been recently performed with stimulation of the baroreceptors by neck suction in a group of healthy volunteers.[67] Ten short (600 milliseconds) and abrupt (-40mm Hg) stimulations of the carotid baroreceptors were performed and averaged in each subject. Following the stimulus, the period of the reflex fluctuations in the RR interval, BP and skin circulation was then measured. If the LF fluctuations in BP are indeed due to baroreceptor-sympathetic

feedback loops, a sudden perturbation of the system by a transient change in BP should cause the following chain of events:

1. the fast vagal response;
2. the slow sympathetic response;
3. the effect of the responses as a new wave which activate, again, the vagal and sympathetic system.

In order to remove the complex influence of continuous changes in venous return induced by respiration, the transient perturbation was administered during apnea. It was found that a <1-second selective stimulation of the arterial baroreceptors generates a damped oscillation in the cardiovascular variables (RR interval, systolic and diastolic AP) at a frequency near 0.1 Hz. It was also observed that the slow oscillation was initiated in the BP and was damped as subjects maintained the apnea (ie, did not further perturb the cardiovascular system in a rhythmic way), suggesting that it was the result of a baroreflex stimulus and not the result of a central rhythm.

Following this first experience, we carried out a preliminary study by stimulating the carotid baroreceptors via a servo-controlled neck chamber that can provoke a periodic neck suction at one of two frequencies: 0.1 Hz and 0.2 Hz. Respiratory rate was mantained at 15 breaths per minute (0.25 Hz). By using this technique it was possible to see the effect of a pure baroreceptor stimuli on LF and HF power of HR and BP variability distinct from the power related to respiration. The studies were performed in normals and in two heart failure patients with preserved or markedly reduced baroreflex control. We observed that, similarly to the spontaneous fluctuations, the LF peak in either HR and BP variability was present or generated only if the baroreflex control of the autonomic outflow was relatively intact and if the rate of stimulation was slow enough (around 0.1 Hz) for the sympathetic efferent system to be able to respond (Figure 4). These preliminary data suggest that

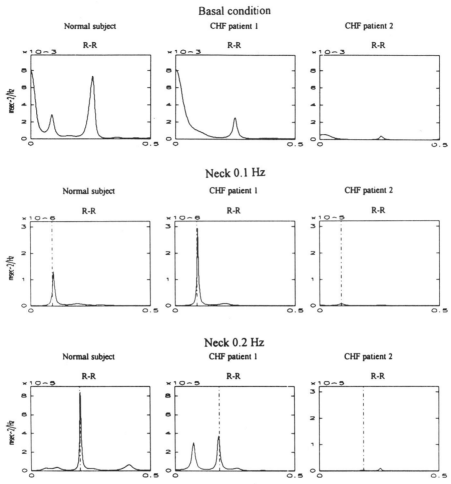

Figure 4. From the top to the bottom: power spectral density of the tachogram in basal condition, and during sinusoidal neck suction at 0.1 and 0.2 Hz; tests are performed during controlled respiration (0.25 Hz), in a normal subject and in two congestive heart failure (CHF) patients with preserved (patient 1) or markedly reduced (patient 2) BRS. Magnitude of RR variability decreases from the normal subject to patients, and between patients with advancing baroreflex dysfunction. Note that sinusoidal neck suction at both 0.1 and 0.2 Hz generates a well-defined peak only in the normal subject and in patient 1 (with preserved baroreflex control), while in patient 2, this peak seems negligible.

power spectral analysis of cardiocirculatory variables is greatly influenced by the activity of the arterial baroreflex.

Correlations Among Baroreceptor Sensitivity and Measures of Heart Rate Variability

Given the importance of an intact baroreflex function in modulating vagal and sympathetic activity, it would be logical to find a correlation between quantitative measures of autonomic control, ie, correlation between BRS and HRV.

This issue had been addressed for the first time in the late 1980s.[68] Baroreflex sensitivity, as assessed by the phenylephrine method, and four Holter measurements of HRV were compared in 32 patients after myocardial infarction. Among the most used HRV parameters, three time-domain indices and the HF power of the HR power spectrum were considered for analysis. In this study, the LF power was not included

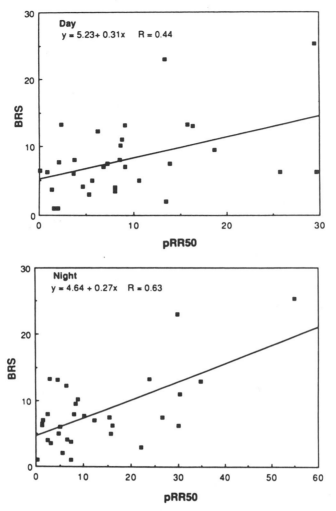

Figure 5. Correlation between BRS in ms/mm Hg and the percent of successive normal RR intervals differing >50 ms (pRR50) plotted separately for day and night. Note that although correlation is stronger at night than during the day, it results <0.70, suggesting that baroreceptor slope and Holter measures are not redundant measures of vagal activity. Modified and reprinted with permission from Bigger et al.[68]

in the analysis, since the highest correlation was expected between a marker of vagal reflexes (BRS) and measures of vagal tone (time-domain parameters, HF power). Although significant (p <0.01), the correlation was rather weak, since it did not exceed 0.63 (Figure 5). It was concluded that the two methodologies are not redundant and that reflex changes during abrupt perturbations (as explored by a pharmacological intervention) or during steady state conditions (as assessed by Holter measurements of HRV) represent different aspects of the autonomic

control of the heart which are not completely interchangeable.

The same issue has been reassessed in patients with severe congestive heart failure in whom baroreflex abnormalities are associated with increased sympathetic activity. In a group of 114 subjects BRS and all spectral components of HRV were significantly related, but with the highest correlation obtained between BRS and the LF component of 0.70 (p <0.0001).[69]

Recently Honloser et al[70] compared the potential predictive value of BRS and HRV in postmyocardial infarction patients who had experienced at least one episode of ventricular fibrillation or sustained ventricular tachycardia, and in a matched control group without tachyarrhythmic events. They observed that postmyocardial infarction patients who develop life threatening ventricular tachyarrhythmias differ strikingly in terms of BRS, but not in terms of HRV. The authors suggest that, if it is assumed that a considerable portion of life-threatening arrhythmias in postmyocardial infarction patients may be related to a reflex increase in sympathetic activity caused by a transient ischemic episode, a further amount of acetylcholine release (via vagal reflex activation) over that released by tonic activity should be necessary to counteract this arrhythmogenic influence of sympathetic overactivity. On this basis, one might speculate that those individuals more prone to fatal arrhythmias and cardiac arrest would be identified more easily by the assessment of BRS (which explores the capability of the reflex to release acetylcholine), then by the analysis of HRV (which explores the tonic release of acetylcholine).[70]

Conclusions

Baroreflex modulation of HR and BP contributes significantly to circulatory control in health and disease. An intact baroreflex control of the autonomic outflow seems to be important to the generation of power in both LF and HF bands of HR and BP power spectrum variability.

However, BRS and measures of HRV are only partly related in the assessment of the autonomic function and the available data suggest a different role of the two methodologies in clinical practice.

A prospective multicenter clinical trial was undertaken in 1991 with the goal to provide a definite answer about the prognostic implications of BRS and HRV. ATRAMI (Atonomic Tone and Reflexes After Myocardial Infarction) has enrolled 1200 patients with a recent myocardial infarction in over 25 centers in Europe, the United States and Japan, and the follow-up will be completed by the end of 1994.

References

1. Brown AM. Receptors under pressure: an update on baroreceptors. Circ Res 1980; 46:1-10.
2. Mancia G, Mark AL. Arterial baroreflexes in humans. In: Shepherd JT, Abboud FM (eds). Handbook of Physiology. Section 3: The Cardiovascular System. Bethesda, Md: American Physiological Society, 1983; 755-793.
3. Coleman TG. Arterial baroreflex control of heart rate in the conscious rat. Am J Physiol (Heart Circ Physiol 7) 1980; 238:H515-H520.
4. Thames MD, Kontos HA. Mechanisms of baroreceptor-induced changes in heart rate. Am J Physiol 1970; 218:251-256.
5. Wang SC, Borison HL. An analysis of the carotid sinus cardiovascular reflex mechanism. Am J Physiol 1947; 150:712-721.
6. Borst C. Circulatory Effects of Electrical Stimulation of the Carotid Sinus Nerve in Man. Amsterdam, Holland: University of Amsterdam, 1979. PhD Thesis.
7. Vatner FS, Higgins CB, Franklin O, et al. Extent of carotid sinus regulation of the myocardial contractile state in conscious dogs. J Clin Invest 1972; 51:985-990.
8. Casadei B, Meyer TE, Coats AJS, et al. Baroreflex control of stroke volume in man: an effect mediated by the vagus. J Physiol 1992; 448:539-550.
9. Eckberg DL, Sleight P. Human Baroreflexes in Health and Disease. Oxford, England: Clarendon Press, 1992; 153-215.
10. Katona PG, Poitras JW, Barnett GO, et al: Cardiac vagal efferent activity and heart period in the carotid sinus reflex. Am J Physiol 1970; 218:1030-1037.
11. Smyth HS, Sleight P, Pickering GW. Reflex regulation of arterial pressure during sleep in man: a quantitative method of assessing baroreflex sensitivity. Circ Res 1969; 24:109-121.
12. Eckberg DL, Nerhed C, Wallin BG. Respiratory modulation of muscle sympathetic activity and vagal cardiac outflow in man. J Physiol 1985; 365:181-196.

13. Eckberg DL. Parasympathetic cardiovascular control in human disease: a critical review of methods and results. Am J Physiol 1980; 239:H581-H593.
14. Eckberg DL. Human sinus arrhythmia as an index of vagal cardiac outflow. J Appl Physiol 1983; 54:961-966.
15. Koch-Weser J. Nature of inotropic action of angiotensin on ventricular myocardium. Circ Res 1965; 16:230-237.
16. Scroop GC, Whelan RF. A central vasomotor action of angiotensin in man. Clin Sci 1966; 30:70-90.
17. Bristow JD, Honour AJ, Pickering JW, et al. Diminished baroreflex sensitivity in high blood pressure. Circulation 1969; 39:48-54.
18. La Rovere MT, Specchia G, Mortara A, at al. Baroreflex sensitivity, clinical correlates and cardiovascular mortality among patients with a first myocardial infarction. A prospective study. Circulation 1988; 78:816-824.
19. Pickering TG, Gribbin B, Sleight P. Comparison of the reflex heart rate response to rising and falling arterial pressure in man. Cardiovasc Res 1972; 6:277-283.
20. Gribbin B, Pickering TG, Sleight P, et al. Effect of age and blood pressure on baroreflex sensitivity in man. Circ Res 1971; 29:424-431.
21. La Rovere MT, Mortara A, Cobelli F, et al. Baroreflex sensitivity improvement after physical training in post-myocardial infarction patients. Eur Heart J 1989; 10(suppl):126. Abstract.
22. Korner PI, West MJ, Shaw J, et al. 'Steady state' properties of the baroreceptor-heart rate reflex in essential hypertension in man. Clin Exp Pharmacol Physiol 1974; 1:65-76.
23. Penaz J, Voight A, Teichmann W. Beitrag zur fortlaufenden indirekten Blutdruckmessung. Zschr Inn Med 1976; 31:1030-1033.
24. Molhoek GP, Wesseling KH, Settles JJ, et al. Evaluation of the Penaz servo-plethysmomanometer for continuous, non-invasive measurement of finger blood pressure. Basic Res Cardiol 1984; 79:598-609.
25. Imholz BPM, van Montfrans GA, Settels JJ, et al. Continuous non-invasive blood pressure monitoring: reliability of FINAPRES device during the Valsalva manoeuvre. Cardiovasc Res 1988; 22:390-397.
26. Parati G, Casadei R, Groppelli A, et al. Comparison of finger and intra-arterial blood pressure monitoring at rest and during laboratory testing. Hypertension 1989; 13:647-655.
27. La Rovere MT, Mortara A, Bigger JT Jr, et al. Reliability of non-invasive measurement of baroreflex sensitivity after myocardial infarction. ATRAMI, an international

28. multicenter prospective study. Eur Heart J 1993; 14(suppl):253. Abstract.
29. Hossman V, Fitzgerald GA, Dollery CT. Circadian rhythm of baroreflex reactivity and adrenergic vascular response. Cardiovasc Res 1980; 14:125-129.
30. Bristow JD, Honour AJ, Pickering TG, et al. Cardiovascular and respiratory changes during sleep in normal and hypertensive subjects. Cardiovasc Res 1969; 3:476-485.
31. Furlan R, Guzzetti S, Crivellaro W, et al. Continuous 24-hour assessment of the neural regulation of systemic arterial pressure and RR variabilities in ambulant subjects. Circulation 1990; 81:537-547.
32. Pickering TG, Gribbin B, Petersen ES, et al. Comparison of the effect of exercise and posture on the baroreflex in man. Cardiovasc Res 1971; 5:582-586.
33. Bristow JD, Brown EB Jr, Cunningham DJC, et al. Effect of bicycling on the baroreflex regulation of pulse interval. Circ Res 1971; 28:582-592.
34. Sleight P, Fox P, Lopez R, et al. The effect of mental arithmetic on blood pressure variability and baroreflex sensitivity in man. Clin Sci 1978; 55:381S-382S.
35. Sherrer U, Pryor SL, Bertocci LA, et al. Arterial baroreceptor buffering of sympathetic activation during exercise-induced elevation of arterial pressure. J Clin Invest 1990; 86:1855-1861.
36. Gozna ER, Marble AE, Shaw A, et al. Age-related changes in the mechanics of the aorta and pulmonary artery of man. J Appl Physiol 1974; 36:407-411.
37. Ma S, Chapleau MW, Abboud FM. Defect in central mediation of the baroreflex with aging. FASEB J 1992; 6:A951.
38. Eckberg DL, Drabinsky M, Braunwald E. Defective parasympathetic control in patients with heart disease. N Engl J Med 1971; 285:877-883.
39. Billman GE, Schwartz PJ, Stone HL. Baroreceptor reflex control of heart rate: a predictor of sudden cardiac death. Circulation 1982; 66:874-880.
40. Farrell TG, Odemuyiwa O, Bashir Y, et al. Prognostic value of baroreflex sensitivity testing after acute myocardial infarction. Br Heart J 1992; 67:129-137.
41. Thorn P. Vagal reflexes elicited by left ventricular C-fibers during myocardial ischemia in cats. In: Schwartz PJ, Brown AM, Malliani A, et al (eds). Neural Mechanisms in Cardiac Arrhythmias. New York, NY: Raven Press, 1978; 179-190.
42. Scroop GC, Whelan RF. A central vasomotor action of angiotensin in man. Clin Sci 1966; 30:79-90.

42. Ernsting J, Parry DJ. Some observations on the effects of stimulating the stretch receptor in the carotid artery of man. J Physiol 1957; 137:45P-46P.

43. Eckberg DL, Cavanaugh MS, Mark AL, et al. A simplified neck suction device for activation of carotid baroreceptors. J Lab Clin Med 1975; 85:167-173.

44. Ludbrook J, Mancia G, Ferrari A, et al. The variable-pressure neck-chamber method for studying the carotid baroreflex in man. Clin Sci 1978; 55:189-194.

45. Bernardi L, Saviolo R, Spodick DH. Do hemodynamic responses to the Valsalva manoeuvre reflect myocardial dysfunction? Chest 1989; 95:986-991.

46. Buda AJ, Pinsky MR, Ingles NB, et al. Effect of intrathoracic pressure on left ventricular performance. N Engl J Med 1979; 301:453-459.

47. Eckberg DL. Adaptation of the human carotid baroreceptor cardiac reflex. J Physiol (London) 1977; 269:579-589.

48. Mancia G, Ferrari A, Gregorini L, et al. Circulatory reflexes from carotid and extracarotid baroreceptor areas in man. Circ Res 1977; 41:309-315.

49. Hamilton WF, Woodbury RA, Harper HT Jr. Physiologic relationships between intrathoracic intraspinal and arterial pressures. JAMA 1936; 107:853-856.

50. Bernardi L, Keller F, Sanders M, et al. Respiratory sinus arrhythmia in the denervated human heart. J Appl Physiol 1989; 67:1447-1455.

51. Leon DF, Shaver JA, Leonard JJ. Reflex heart rate control in man. Am Heart J 1970; 80:729-739.

52. Palmero HA, Caeiro TF, Iosa DJ, et al. Baroceptor reflex sensitivity index derived from phase 4 of the Valsalva maneuver. Hypertension 1981; 3(suppl II):134-137.

53. Smith SA, Stallard TJ, Salih MM, et al. Can sinoaortic baroreceptor heart rate reflex be determined from phase IV of the Valsalva manoeuvre? Cardiovasc Res 1987; 21:422-427.

54. Trimarco B, Volpe M, Ricciardelli B, et al. Valsalva maneuver in the assessment of baroreflex responsiveness in borderline hypertensives. Cardiology 1983; 70:6-14.

55. Pagani M, Somers V, Furlan R, et al. Changes in autonomic regulation induced by physical training in mild hypertension. Hypertension 1988; 12:600-610.

56. Robbe HWJ, Mulder LJM, Ruddel H, et al. Assessment of baroreceptor reflex sensitivity by means of spectral analysis. Hypertension 1987; 10:538-543.

57. Hech HH. Comparative physiological and morphological aspects of the pacemaker tissue. Ann NY Acad Sci 1965; 127:49-83.

58. Akselrod S, Gordon D, Madwed JB, et al. Hemodynamic regulation: investigation by spectral analysis. Am J Physiol 1985; 249:867-875.

59. Baselli G, Cerutti S, Civardi S, et al. Cardiovascular variability signals: toward the identification of a closed-loop model of the neural control mechanisms. IEEE Trans Biomed Eng 1988; 35:1033-1046.

60. Saul JP, Berger RD, Albrecht P, et al. Transfer function analysis of the circulation: unique insights into cardiovascular regulation. Am J Physiol (Heart Circ Physiol 30) 1991; 261:H153-H161.

61. DeBoer RW, Karemaker JM, Strakee J. Hemodynamic fluctuations and baroreflex sensitivity in humans: a beat to beat model. Am J Physiol 1987; 253:680-689.

62. Madwed JB, Albrecht P, Mark RG, et al. Low-frequency oscillations in arterial pressure and heart rate: a simple computer model. Am J Physiol 1989; 256:H1573-H1579.

63. Polosa C. Central nervous system origin of some type of Mayer waves. In: Miyakawa K, Koepchen HP, Polosa C (eds). Mechanisms of Blood Pressure Waves. Berlin, Germany: Springer-Verlag/ Tokyo, Japan: Japan Sci. Soc. Press, 1984; 277-292.

64. Pomeranz B, Macaulay RJB, Caudill MA, et al. Assessment of autonomic function in humans by heart rate spectral analysis. Am J Physiol (Heart Circ Physiol 17) 1985; 248:H151-H153.

65. Mortara A, La Rovere MT, Signorini MG, et al. Can power spectral analysis of heart rate variability identify a high risk subgroup of congestive heart failure patients with excessive sympathetic activation? A pilot study before and after heart transplantation. Br Heart J 1994; 71:422-430.

66. Bernardi L, Salvucci F, Suardi R, et al. Evidence of an intrinsic mechanism regulating the heart rate variability in the transplanted and in the intact heart during submaximal dynamic exercise. Cardiovasc Res 1990; 24:969-981.

67. Bernardi L, Leuzzi S, Piepoli M, et al. Evidence that low frequency (LF) variavility of the RR interval power spectrum analysis (PSA) in humans is generated by the arterial baroreflex. XXXII Congr International Union of Physiological Sciences. Glasgow, August 1-6, 1993; 173/25P.

68. Bigger JT Jr, La Rovere MT, Steinman RC, et al. Comparison of baroreflex sensitivity and heart period variability after myocardial in-

farction. J Am Coll Cardiol 1989; 14:1511-1518.

69. Mortara A, La Rovere MT, Pantaleo P, et al. Relationship between baroreceptor sensitivity and sympathetic oscillations of heart rate variability in congestive heart failure. Eur Heart J 1994; 15(suppl):442. Abstract.

70. Honloser SH, Klingenheben T, van de Loo A, et al. Reflexes versus tonic vagal activity as a prognostic parameter in patients with sustained ventricular tachycardia or ventricular fibrillation. Circulation 1994; 89:1068-1073.

Chapter 16

Heart Rate and Heart Rate Variability

Philippe Coumel, Pierre Maison-Blanche, Didier Catuli

Summary

The relationships between heart rate (HR) and heart rate variability (HRV) are not simple. Both depend on the autonomic nervous system (ANS) so that they are not independent variables, and technically the quantification of HRV is influenced by the HR level. The complexity of these relationships is not sufficient a reason to ignore HR when studying HRV, as it is so frequently the case in the literature.

The HR and various normalized and non-normalized indices of HRV using spectral and nonspectral methods were studied in 24-hour recordings of a very homogeneous cohort of 17 healthy males aged 20 years. The HR-HRV relationships were evaluated by considering the same data in two different ways: looking at the 24 mean hourly values provides information on the circadian behavior of the indices, whereas looking at the average 24-hour individual data allows to approach the direct incidence of the RR interval on HRV evaluation. The correlations between HR and HRV are clearly weaker when considered through individuals than over time: that they can come close to one in the latter case does not mean that measuring HRV is just another way to evaluate HR, but that normal physiology supposes a harmonious behavior of the various indices.

A much greater attention paid to the impairment of the HR-HRV correlations in diseased hearts should allow to progress more efficaciously than just looking at the decrease of the flexibility of the ANS balance.

Introduction

The interest of clinicians for the ANS has generated a number of studies devoted to the evaluation of its balance through the HRV. A certain confusion has then been introduced for those who are not familiar with the ANS physiology, as well as the numerous possible technical approaches. Some of

This study was supported in part by grants from Institut National de la Santé et de la Recherche Médicale (1992) and Fédération Française de Cardiologie (1992).

From: Malik M., Camm AJ (eds.): *Heart Rate Variability*. Armonk, NY. Futura Publishing Company, Inc., © 1995.

them globally address the HRV (eg, the standard deviation techniques) in the time domain, without trying to discern any peculiar type of modulation. Others (eg, the cycle differences greater than 50 milliseconds, 'NN50') purposefully concentrate on vagal modulations. In the frequency domain, the reference method is the spectral analysis, with several technical variants. Neither method should be preferred, and they all have their technical and theoretical advantages and limitations. Simply, one must realize that they are more or less adapted to exploring various facets of the complex problems related to the ANS, its physiological and pathological variations.

Curiously, a common characteristic of the majority of studies in the literature is not to consider the relationships between the cardiac frequency and its variations, the HR and the HRV, as if they were totally different matters. In essence, HRV results from the modulation of the supposedly constant intrinsic HR (HRo) by the sympatho-vagal balance. If HRV is supposed to provide information on the vago-sympathetic interplay, in the clinical situation HRo is not known and HR is just another marker of the sympatho-vagal balance. As such, even if the information contained in HR are complex since by definition they are hybrid, they must be considered. They may be either redundant or complementary, more or less relevant, but ignoring HR when studying HRV is not acceptable because these two variables are not independent. In this chapter, the emphasis will be put on the various technical problems and physiological significance of the relationships between HR and HRV.

Material and Methods

Study Population

For the purpose of the present study, we used a variety of technical approaches of HRV in a very homogeneous cohort. The objective was to eliminate, as much as possible, the identified biases in the ANS physiology, eg, age, sex, activity, and heart disease; but the unavoidable consequence is that our observations apply exclusively to young, healthy males. The study group consisted of 17 volunteers accomplishing their military service, which explains their uniform age (20 years, ranging from 19 to 22). They all had a normal heart at clinical, electrocardiogram (ECG) and echocardiographic examination. All underwent a 24-hour Holter recording while having a routine daily activity with a homogeneous timetable in terms of awake and sleeping hours, meals, due to the particular conditions of their daily life. All these subjects otherwise underwent a number of tests exploring various aspects of the ANS physiology (exercise, tilt test, Valsalva maneuver, etc.), but none of these tests were carried out on the day of Holter recording, which was left free.

Methods

Recordings were performed with Marquette 8000 recorders. They were analyzed on the Elatec system, which digitizes two channels at a 200-Hz sampling rate, and stores the raw data on a 400 MB hard disk. The processor used for that study rates at a speed of 50 MHz. The RR series (beat labels and RR interval values in milliseconds) extracted from the raw data by the detection and classifications algorithms are also stored for further analysis.

The selection of RR intervals was carefully done. All HRV parameters were computed from normal-to-normal RR values (QRS complexes of sinus origin). Prior to any HRV calculation, the 24-hour RR series were validated to eliminate artifacts, under-detections and overdetections. This goal was achieved by reviewing procedures including beat classification, and elimination of arrhythmic events (validated ventricular and supraventricular beats of nonsinus origin were ignored, and the corresponding periods were linearly interpolated). For each procedure, manual corrections such as beat label changes, deletion or insertion were incorporated in the RR series.

Spectral analysis was computed over periods of 256 seconds (frequency resolution of 1/256 Hz = 0.004 Hz). It was not performed if more than 20% of the beats in the 256 seconds window were not normal. As a 50% overlapping function was applied on the 256 seconds buffer, the analysis was computed every 128 seconds, and the spectra were averaged: for instance, a 1-hour spectrum was obtained from 24 individual spectra. The 256 seconds tachograms were sampled at a 4-Hz frequency to obtain equidistant sampling, mean RR interval value was substracted and the signal was multiplied by a Hanning window to reduce the leakage error. The overlapping at 50% and the use of a Hanning window are the most common preprocessing methods already published. Finally, the power spectral density of the preprocessed signal was computed and the results were expressed in milliseconds^2 per Hz. The area under the spectral density curve between two limits was integrated, and expressed in milliseconds.^{2} Two spectral bands were systematically calculated: the low-frequency (LF) band between 0.04 and 0.15 Hz, and the high-frequency (HF) band between 0.15 and 0.40 Hz. The normalization procedure can be done in two different ways. One consists of dividing the power of the LF component (%LF) by the total variance diminished by the power of the very low frequencies (below 0.03 Hz). The other is to consider the ratio of the two components LF/HF.

The time-domain parameters are those currently used in the literature, with the exception of the method of triangular interpolation of the frequency distribution of RR interval duration.[1] We did not have the algorithms for so doing, and this method is particularly adapted to situations in which an attentive validation of the events cannot be routinely performed. Again, a filter eliminated the supraventricular and ventricular arrhythmias, usually limited to isolated extrasystoles and their compensatory pause. The NN50 is the number of differences between adjacent normal RR intervals that are greater than 50 milliseconds, and the pNN50 is the normalized value in terms of percentage of the total number of beats per time unit. Both NN50 and pNN50 calculations were achieved only on a triplet N-N-N of normal QRS complexes, which is not the case for the SDNN (standard deviation of all normal RR intervals in the 24-hour period). Other time-domain indices like the rMSSD (root mean square of successive differences), the SDANN index (standard deviation of the average normal RR intervals for 5-minute segments), the SDNN index (mean of the standard deviation of all normal RR intervals for 5-minute segments) were obtained, and will not be discussed because it is established[2] and we verifed again that they were largely redundant with the other parameters already selected.

Our peak-valley method of 'oscillations' has been described in detail[3] and will be briefly recalled. The digitized ECG data are transferred to a personal computer (AST 486) and processed by the ATREC II system. The principle is to detect in time series of RR intervals, various types of HR fluctuations: decreasing or increasing RR intervals form shorter and longer HR oscillations. The algorithm looks for a sequence of acceleration or slowing over a preselected number of 2 to 4, 8 to 15 consecutive RR intervals, encompassed by an opposite trend. Scanning the sequences of 2, 3, 4, etc. and up to 30 cardiac cycles as the central sequence showed the various patterns known in the frequency domain. With this method the HF peak corresponds to central sequences over 2 to 4 cycles, forming the class of 'shorter' oscillations (SO). The central sequences of 8 to 15 cycles forming 'longer' oscillations (LO) correspond to other bands of the spectrum. Quantitation is done through the product (in ms/min) of the number of oscillations of either type times their amplitude (the difference in milliseconds between the longest and the shortest cycle of the sequence). It is important to note that the oscillation wavelength is thus defined in terms of number of beats rather than in time units.

This evaluation of the HRV can further distinguish between the amplitude of the HR oscillations, their number, and their symmetry, but these aspects will not be detailed. The ratio LO/SO, by analogy with the spectral analysis, was used for normalization.

Notwithstanding the method used, all the values were considered on an hourly basis. The average recording duration was 23.1 hours. Daytime period included the 8 hours between 11:00 am, and 7:00 pm, night period the 4 hours between 1:00 am, and 5:00 am. Particular attention was paid to examining the subjects either individually or as a group, and the hourly data of HR and HRV will be presented in two different ways: the mean daily values of each of the 17 individuals, or each of the 24 hourly values of the circadian period obtained by averaging the corresponding hour in all subjects. The results are expressed as the mean ±SD. The coefficient of variance represents the SD/mean.

Results

Studying the relationships between HR and HRV over the 24-hour period supposes that one examines the behavior of ANS indices as a function of the HR in the context of which they were obtained. Plotting either the 24 mean hourly HR values or the aver-

age 24-hour HR versus another parameter gives in fact two different informations. The actual HR results from the modulation of HRo by the ANS, but the way the latter correlates with the former depends on the time scale (Tables 1 and 2).

Hourly Means of Heart Rate Over 24 Hours and Individual Mean 24-Hour Heart Rate

In the upper panel of Figure 1, the data from the 17 patients were averaged on an hourly basis, so that the typical S-shaped curve of the circadian HR is displayed. In this representation, the trend of HR (73.9±11.2 bpm, range: 58 to 87, coefficient of variance: 15.1) can be regarded as one of the many indices of the ANS balance. HR levels depend on the subjects' activity that are time related, and very similar from subject to subject so that the standard deviation of every hour (mean: 13.2) represents interindividual differences which are remarkably stable (SD = 2.8). In fact, hourly HR values form timers, as lower frequencies are recorded at night and higher values at daytime. In contrast, the lower panel of Figure 1 represents the mean 24-hour HR in each of the 17 individuals. As expected, the mean values slightly differ (73.6±9.3 bpm, range: 59 to 92, coefficient of variance: 12.6) because they were not ob-

Table 1
Correlations of Hourly Data

	LF/HF	LO/SO	%LF	pNN50	NN50	.00	.00	.00	.00
HR	.93	.90	.51	.98	.41	.82	.92	.87	.97
LF/HF	1	.94	.30	.93	.48	.67	.88	.87	.91
LO/SO		1	.28	.88	.47	.68	.82	.86	.88
%LF			1	.55	.17	.73	.50	.16	.45
pNN50				1	.49	.86	.94	.83	.94
NN50					1	.37	.47	.38	.39
LF						1	.87	.59	.76
HF							1	.75	.87
LO								1	.88
SO									1

"r" values in hourly data (n = 24)
.00 = NS   .00 = P<.05   *.00* = p<.01   **.00** = p<.001

Table 2
Correlations of Individual Data

	LF/HF	LO/SO	%LF	pNN50	NN50	LF	HF	LO	SO
HR	.58	.68	.09	.87	.46	.46	.38	.49	.79
LF/HF	1	.59	.31	**.70**	.04	.23	.50	.27	*.63*
LO/SO		1	.37	.50	.06	.03	.15	**.72**	**.80**
%LF			1	.07	.16	**.70**	.45	.22	.11
pNN50				1	.42	.69	.63	.26	.73
NN50					1	.43	.11	.16	.18
LF						1	**.81**	.13	.30
HF							1	.16	.41
LO								1	.53
SO									1

"r" values in individuals (n = 17)
.00 = NS   .00 = P<.05   *.00* = p<.01   **.00** = p<.001

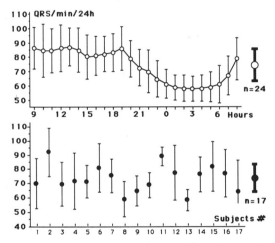

Figure 1. Hourly means of HR of the cohort, and 24-hour HR in the 17 subjects. The typically S-shaped pattern of circadian rhythm (with two peaks at meal hours) results from averaging the hourly data of the 17 subjects. It explains why in the upper panel the 24 standard deviations are homogeneous from hour to hour, whereas in the lower panel the 24-hour data of the individuals are variable from subject to subject.

tained in the same way: in this representation the circadian influences are not apparent and are simply reflected by the individual standard deviations.

One must realize that in the two panels of the figure, the same data concerning the same parameter were used, but the significance of HR is ambivalent: clock time in the whole group, or the combination of HRo and mean 24-hour ANS balance in a given

subject. The correlations between HR and any HRV index must be interpreted accordingly. This preliminary remark should be kept in mind at each and every step in the following results.

Heart Rate and the Standard Deviation of the RR Intervals SDNN

The SDNN is known as a very global index of HRV: it is easy to obtain provided the data are of good quality. Even in this homogeneous group of young healthy men, the interindividual differences are important (164 milliseconds ±61, range: 45 to 257). The SDNN is correlated with the day-to-night ratio of HR (1.49±0.18, r = 0.46).

Heart Rate and the Normalized Indices of Heart Rate Variability

Various indices have been proposed to express the ANS balance, characterized by a daytime sympathetic predominance which alternates with a vagal predominance at night, and the trivial image of this alternance is given by the HR trend and its day/night ratio. Any index fitting with this curve is supposed to adequately reflect the ANS modulation. This is the case for the LF/HF ratio of the spectrum (Figure 2), as well as the ratio of LO/SO of our peak-

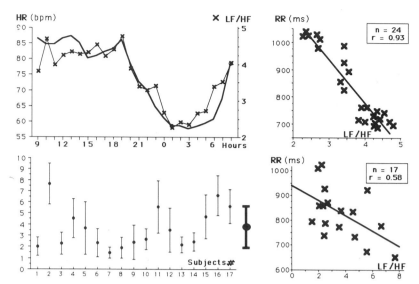

Figure 2. Normalized index of the spectrum. In the left upper panel the LF/HF ratio is displayed on an hourly basis, so that each value represents 17 individual data. The corresponding hourly HR is also figured as a continuous line: both parameters closely match and the scatterplots in the right upper panel confirm the strong correlation (vertical axis in RR interval values rather than HR). The left lower panel displays the 17 individual LF/HF ratios, so that the standard deviations represent the 24 hourly values in every subject. The correlation with RR is weaker.

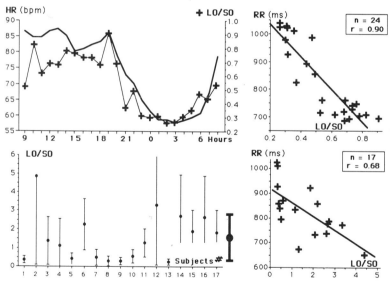

Figure 3. Normalized index of the nonspectral method. The representation is the same as in Figure 2, and the patterns are almost identical: a strong correlation exists between the hourly mean HR and LO/SO ratio (upper panels), whereas the values are much more variable when considered in individuals.

valley method (Figure 3). The correlations between the hourly HR and these indices are excellent (r = 0.93 for LF/HF, r = 0.90 for LO/SO, Table 1). They are poor (r = 0.51) for the %LF. These excellent correlations apply to the mean values of the entire cohort. They are lower if the circadian period is considered in each individual (r = 0.62±0.19 for L/H, r = 0.72±0.17 for LO/SO, r = 0.44±0.22 for %LF).

Rather than a direct relationship between HR and HRV, these values express the common correlation between these indices on the one hand, and clock time on the other. The environment conditions the alternating sympathetic and vagal predominance in all individuals. Both HR and HRV reflect this state, so that their circadian variations are consistent although not equal: the values of the day-to-night ratios in the 17 individuals are 1.49±0.18 for HR, 2±.69 for L/H, 2.9±1.6 for LO/SO. Correlating the HR and a marker of the ANS balance has a different meaning on a time basis or on a patient basis: in Figures 2 and 3 and Tables 1 and 2, the different correlation coefficients (0.93 versus 0.58 for LF/HF, 0.90 versus 0.68 for LO/SO) express the differences between the respective impacts of time and cardiac cycle on these ratios.

Heart Rate and the Specific Indices of Heart Rate Variability

The preceding normalized indices were supposed to represent an image of the balance between the vagal and sympathetic tones, but the real aim of HRV studies is to obtain specific information on each of the two limbs of the ANS. That the HF band of the spectrum or the SO of the peak-valley method are vagally mediated is firmly established. The situation concerning the other indices is less clear. The LF component contains a mixture of information, but the proportion of respective vagal and sympathetic influences is undetermined, and this may also apply to LO.

Heart Rate and the Cycle-to-Cycle Differences (NN50 and pNN50)

The NN50 is recognized as a very specific index of vagal tone. However, its dependence on the HR is so evident that two modes of normalization are routinely preferred: the pNN50 and its variant the 'NN 6.25' (in which the 'jumps' correspond to cycle-to-cycle differences above 6.25% of the preceding cycle). Linking the evaluation of one variable to the other obviously does not contribute to clarify the specific relationships between the two.

Expressing the pNN50 on an hourly basis makes the correlation with RR almost equal to 1 (Figure 4 and Table 1), whereas the absolute number of NN50 has a very poor Pearson coefficient (r = 0.41). The phenomenon is similar in individuals in whom the coefficients of correlation with HR are 0.87 for pNN50 and 0.46 for NN50 (Figure 4, Table 2). The identical behavior of the evaluations per hour or per individual may suggest that measuring the pNN50 looks after all no more than measuring the HR itself in these normal subjects.

Heart Rate and the Spectral Analysis

The striking phenomenon shown in Figure 5 is the obvious parallelism in the behavior of the LF and HF over the 24-hour period: both increase at night, and the real problem is to determine if they increase because of the clock hour or because the RR interval lengthens. From the comparison of the correlation coefficients on the circadian period or in individuals (lower part of Figure 5, Tables 1 and 2) the correlation is twice as good with time than with RR (around 0.87 versus around 0.42). The latter suggests some independence between HR and the spectral evaluation of HRV, because the correlation hardly reaches the p = 0.05 level of significance. On the other hand, the parallel behavior of spectral components raises some concern about their specificity.

Heart Rate and the Heart Rate Oscillations

The circadian pattern of LO and SO in Figure 6 looks strikingly different from that of LF and HF, and somewhat more in keeping with what one would logically expect: the LO are higher at daytime, whereas the SO increase at night. However, there is a strong correlation of these variables with the HR as such: if the correlations with the time-related

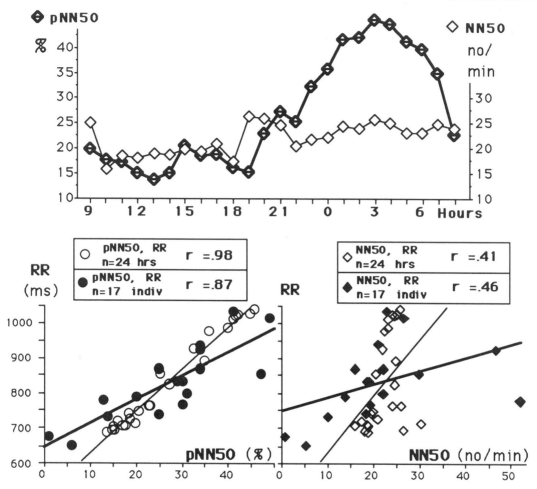

Figure 4. Normalized and non-normalized cycle-to-cycle differences greater than 50 milliseconds. In the upper panel the mean hourly values of pNN50 (in percentage of the number of beats, left scale) and NN50 (in number per minutes, right scale) are displayed over the 24-hour period. The correlations of these two variables with RR are shown in the lower left and right panels, respectively: the symbols (circles for pNN50, diamonds for NN50) are open for the 24 mean hourly values, and solid for the 17 mean 24-hour individual values. Normalizing the NN50 on an hourly basis makes the correlation almost equal to 1.

data are as good as for the spectral components (r = 0.97 for SO and 0.87 for LO), the correlations with the HR of individuals are greater (r = 0.79 for SO and 0.49 for LO).

Discussion

The reasons why the relationships between HR and HRV are scarcely studied in the literature are not clear to us. For instance, in an article especially devoted to looking at the correlations between the various indices of HRV[2] 11 of them were exten-

sively scrutinized but the HR was not alluded to. Actually, with some noticeable exceptions[4-7] few studies deal with the problem, and among them some form basic landmarks.[8-11]

There are two very different categories among the studies dealing with HRV: those using brief recording sessions, as opposed to long-term ambulatory recordings. Although they address the same phenomenon, they have major differences. Brief recording sessions give the opportunity to monitor or even control important parame-

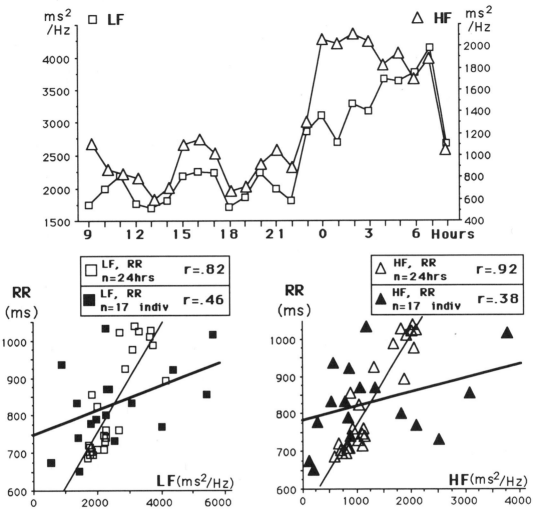

Figure 5. Circadian behavior of spectral components. The mean hourly values of LF and HF (in ms^2/ Hz) are displayed over 24 hours. Both LF (squares, left scale) and HF (triangles, right scale) increase at night, the latter more markedly than the former. The correlations with RR shown in the lower panels are much stronger for the hourly data (open symbols) than for the individual data (solid symbols).

ters like the respiratory rate and the tidal volume,[12] as well as the blood pressure[13]: then the strict methods of physiological research are applied, and recently the attention was called on the fact that controlled conditions were far from being observed in the literature.[12] Long-term ambulatory recording is usually preferred in the clinical conditions, and the abundance of the data is supposed to compensate for the lack of precision concerning the recording conditions. We concentrated our study on the latter approach.

The Physiological Determinants of Heart Rate and Heart Rate Variability

The HR varies according to the influence of the ANS on the intrinsic HRo, and in theory the latter can be determined only when the former is completely blocked by drugs. HRo is a constant, which decreases with age, and differs from patient to patient: in a homogeneous cohort aged 20 years like ours, its average value calculated from the Jose and Collison[14] studies is allegedly 106/ min (HRo = 118-[age * 0.56]). To interpret

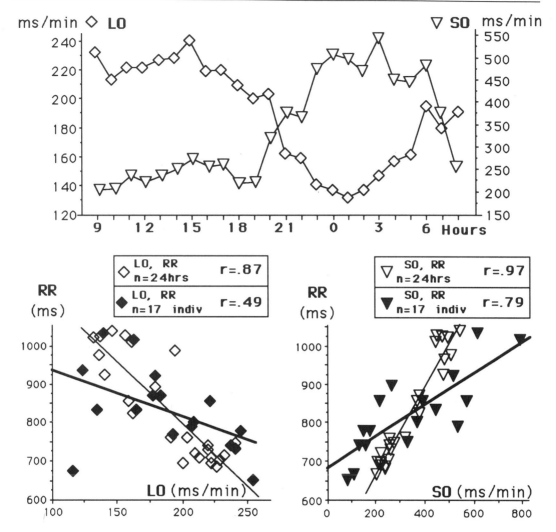

Figure 6. Circadian behavior of nonspectral data. The mean hourly values of LO (diamonds, left scale in ms/min) and SO (triangles, right scale) have a strikingly opposite behavior that looks consistent with the type of ANS activity they are supposed to represent: LO are higher at daytime, whereas SO are higher at night. In the lower panels the correlations of hourly data (open symbols) and individual data (solid symbols) with RR are comparable with what is observed in the frequency domain.

the actual HR variations over the 24-hour period, Rosenblueth[8] proposed the formula 'HR = HRo * m * n' in which 'm' and 'n' represent the sympathetics (Σ) and the vagus (X). For the purpose of the following discussion, this formula can be written more conveniently: HR = HRo * (Σ/X). That the mean sympatho-vagal balance (Σ/X) is constant in a given individual, although it may differ from subject to subject, is intuitively

as evident as the constancy of HRo. Not only is this intuitive, but another possibility would be hard to imagine if the preceding formula is correct, simply because it was consistently verifed that the actual mean 24-hour HR is indeed reproducible from day to day in individuals.[15,16]

We may thus consider the expression (Σ/X) as the average level at which the ANS balance is set, and the best image we can

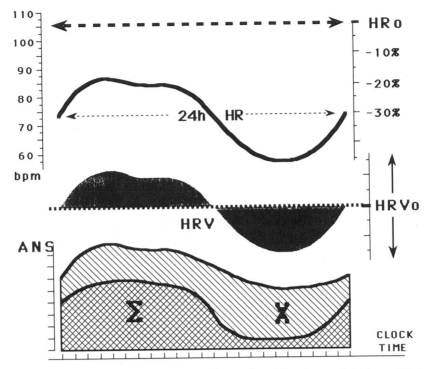

Figure 7. Schematic diagram of HR and HRV relationships. The observed 24-hour HR is supposed to result from the product of intrinsic HR (HRo) times the average basic ANS influence (HRVo): the permanently tonic vagal influence accounts for the 30% lower value of mean 24-hour HR with respect to HRo. The circadian variations of HR are due to the changing sympathovagal balance over time, and the lower diagram figures what may be the respective amounts of sympathetic (Σ) and vagal (X) tones. The fact that the former predominates at daytime and the latter at night is compatible with a greater level of both at daytime compared to night.

have of it probably is formed by the normalized indices using spectral as well as nonspectral techniques. Therefore, one may think of an intrinsic HRV (HRVo) as it is done for HRo. Actually, the day-to-day values of HRV indices are quite reproducible,[15,16] which is in keeping with theory. The diagram of Figure 7 is just a visual expression of the formula HR = HRo * HRVo, and if we apply the formula to our own data it is quite clear that the mean 24-hour HR of the whole group of 17 patients (73.9 bpm) is 30% lower than the HRo. This implies the tonic predominance of the vagal tone over the sympathetic tone all over the circadian period, which is not in contradiction with the notion of an alternating *relative* predominance of either limb at daytime or at night. It suffices to realize that the vagal drive is

less predominant over the sympathetic drive at daytime than it is at night.

The circadian changes of HR as well as HRV reflect the impact of the ANS on HRo, and its flexibility with respect to a constant mean level of sympatho-vagal balance. Then studying the relationships between HR and HRV may give some insight on both HRo and HRVo, using HR and HRV as tools serving differently according to whether they are considered on a subject or an hourly basis. Normal individuals have a common circadian behavior, but the mean 24-hour levels of HRo and HRVo largely differ from individual to individual, as well as the ANS flexibility. In other words, the mean 24-hour HR corresponds to the product HRo * HRVo, whereas time-related HRV changes (as well as HR, a further index of HRV) reflect the circadian flexibility of the ANS.

Physiological and Statistical Significance of the Heart Rate-Heart Rate Variability Correlations

The Problem of Normalized Indices

In theory, the data concerning the circadian variations of the ANS balance should make it possible to resolve the equation: HR = HRo * HRVo. This would be easy if there were basically no correlations between HR and HRV in the individual data, because it would be licit to consider HR and HRV as independent variables. If HRo and HRVo are constants, indeed they should be independent. But these correlations do exist, although they are obviously weaker (Table 2) than for the hourly data (Table 1) so that the interindividual correlations must reflect a sort of technical bias which is the impact of the RR value on the measurement of its variations. The same type of problem exists in the relationships between the respiratory rate and its impact on the power of the RR interval. It concerns LF as well as HF,[12] and it is usually overlooked, as is overlooked the impact of HR on the measurement of HRV indices.

One is tempted to eliminate the proper role of HR by using various normalizations of HRV. The risk is to normalize for HR in a uniform way, whereas the significance of HR is changing. Occasionally, it is interesting to recall that the problem of considering percentages or absolute values was, in Katona's opinion,[10] at the origin of the different interpretations proposed by Rosenblueth[8] on the one hand, Warner[11] on the other, based on similar models. The former interpreted the results as implying no interaction between sympathetic and vagal effects, whereas the latter concluded that the interaction did exist.

Despite their relative weakness, many individual HR-HRV correlations presented in Table 2 are indeed significant. This concerns normalized (LF/HF, LO/SO, pNN50)

and non-normalized specific indices (LF, SO, LO). These correlations in individuals could be used to adequately normalize the 24-hour data. For instance, the actual values of any HRV variable throughout the 24 hours, notwithstanding the HR level, can be mathematically derived from the characteristics of slope and intercept of this variable in a homogeneous group of patients. If such an approach cannot resolve the difficult problem of evaluating the ANS state in a given patient at a precise moment, at least it would allow to compare groups.

We had this approach when we studied three groups of patients[3] who were not different in terms of age, but who had either a normal heart, or a left ventricular hypertrophy, or a congestive heart failure. The significant correlations between HR and HRV allowed to use the analysis of covariance, a much more powerful test than the analysis of variance, because it takes advantage of the correlation between the covariables, HR in this case. In this study it was clear that two phenomena characterized an increasing impairment of the ANS physiology:

1. the loss of HRV is largely emphasized in the literature, but not the specific change of the sympathetic predominance which was present only in patients with left ventricular hypertrophy; and

2. more interestingly, a loss of the correlations between HR and HRV was found as the hemodynamic state deteriorated, a trend which reflects the impaired state of the ANS in these conditions. The value of the Pearson coefficients of correlation between HR and the LO/SO ratio were 0.92 in normals, 0.76 and 0.69 in the groups without or with heart failure, respectively. In other words, with the progression of the disease, the patients are clearly losing one of the main characteristics of the HR-HRV relationships which

reflects the physiological harmony of the ANS functions.

Finally, we were surprised not to find good performances of a largely used index which is the %LF. This probably relates with the fundamental differences between Holter uncontrolled data, and well-controlled brief recording sessions in which specific conditions of the ANS changes are explored. Bootsma et al[6] used %LF and its relation to HR during incremental head-up tilt (from 0° to 80°) in 21 young healthy males (age: 25.3±4.1): the HR increased from 61±9.1 bpm to 85.9±18.3, while %LF increased from 45.8±16.7 to 79.8±13.8, with correlation coefficients of 0.80±0.13. By extrapolating the individual linear LF-HR relation, these authors calculated the theoretical value at which all vagally mediated fluctuations were supposed to disappear; the mean of these extrapolated HR was 105±27 bpm, a value which looks slower than the estimated HRo probably because the latter is supposed to be free of any autonomic influence rather than an exclusive sympathetic influence.

Behavior of the Indices of Heart Rate Variability: Mutual Correlations and Specificity

The nonspecific indices of HRV have the obvious interest of reflecting the overall flexibility of the ANS, and they are robust. This applies to the SDNN and many derived indices.[1] The variance is just equal to the area under the power spectrum, and estimates of the HR variance (or the SD which is its square root) depend on the record length: the longer the record, the greater the estimated variance as more LF power is included. The 24-hour SDNN reflects primarily the VLF power, not the peaks above 0.01 Hz.[17] Its robustness compensates for its poor specificity, and the HR flexibility reflected by this type of indices explains why they are reliable as prognostic indices in cardiopathies.[18,19]

Bigger et al[2] showed that SDNN correlates strongly (r ≥0.9) with SDANN, ultra LF, VLF and LF, which is not surprising because these components represent more than 90% of the total power. That pNN50 correlates with rMSSD and overall with HF and SO further confirms that they are all indices of the vagal activity, but they all correlate also well, if not always strongly with the SDNN. In fact, all the indices of vagal activity strongly correlate between themselves and with the HR when the hourly data are considered (Table 1). This does not mean that they are redundant. It is logical, after all, to find a harmony in the ANS when looking at its behavior in young healthy people in whom it is supposed to work normally. This can be found on a short-term basis in strictly controlled conditions,[6,12,20] as well as in Holter recordings. Rather than the absolute values of the parameters, the strength of the correlations constitute characteristics of normality.

The analysis of the components of the normalized indices yield expected results for those which are supposed to depend on the vagus, but curious patterns for the others. This illustrates some controversies in the literature[21] and the ambiguity is reinforced by our observations. Schematically, if the increase of vagal indices is expected at night, one is surprised to see that the 'sympathetic' indices just do the same: that LF contains a mixture of vagal and sympathetic information was stated from the beginning,[5] but it was implicitly thought that even if the exact proportion was undetermined, at least it was constant. Further studies suggested that there were greater sympathetic than vagal influences.[20] The consistency of the results in the literature about the circadian behavior of LF is striking with a single exception,[22] the reasons of which are unclear. Not only the LF increases at night like any component of the spectrum, but Murakawa's findings[7] are in keeping with ours. This author studied logLF, logHF and log(LF/HF) in 23 subjects, and correlated these variables taken at daytime and at night for three levels of HR (60, 70 and 80/minute). The relationship between log(LF/HF) and HR was not consistent, but the correlation between diurnal and nocturnal logHF value was significant at all three rates whereas the diurnal log (LF/HF) was correlated with the nocturnal value only at 70/min.

We were surprised to see that the behavior of the LO looked different. In fact, Figures 5 and 6 are not so different in the sense that what is important is not the isolated behavior of either parameter, but its relation with the other. Indeed the vagal influences predominate in the LF, but they are less predominant than in the HF component. The data found in a study[23] which was the occasion of an active debate[21] illustrate this situation in which specific and normalized indices are only apparently conflicting; looking at the data in this study, the HF power was 4.2 times greater, and the LF was 2.8 times greater in trained people compared to controls, which may be interpreted as the evidence of a reduced influence of the vagus on LF. This is confirmed by the behavior of LF in terms of day/night ratio compared to HF: 1.4 versus 2.4. This is the very reason why the LF/HF and LO/SO finally yield identical information. They are both strongly correlated with HR overtime (Table 1) to the point that it may appear useless to look at something else other than the HR. However, these indices are much less correlated among individuals (Table 2), and their sensitivity is reflected in the coefficient of variance: 15 for the HR, 21 for the LF/HF ratio, 37 for the LO/SO.

Even though these numbers are in favor of a greater sensitivity of nonspectral approaches, the debate is not closed. Spectral analysis is largely used but suffers from technical limitations that are not necessarily familiar to its users. It may not be applicable in all situations: ideally it requires very precise conditions of stationarity of the HR, symmetry of its variations and the total absence of artifacts, all conditions which make it better adapted to short-term recording sessions than to 24-hour observations. Even for short recording sessions, a major drawback to spectrum analysis also is that it provides only the global properties of relatively long time series of several minutes. However, autonomic regulation of the cardiovascular system can change rapidly in response to demand.[24] If the power spectra were taken at very short intervals, eg, 5 to 10 seconds, then one should begin to see the changes over time. But for these very short time series, the statistical properties of the spectra degrade seriously. Other techniques like complex demodulation[25] are able to provide time-local descriptions of HRV necessary to characterize such changing autonomic regulation, and to approach specifically the role of the amplitude of the spectrum, which is ignored in the conventional Fast Fourier Transform analysis.

Conclusion

The role of HR in the evaluation of HRV cannot be ignored any longer, as is so often the case in the literature devoted to the ANS. The primary reason simply is that HR forms indeed probably the best index of the ANS balance, and the easiest to measure. A second important reason is that the evaluation of all other indices is influenced by this parameter, so that it must be taken into account. A third reason probably is even more important in essence: the strong correlations between HR and HRV do have a physiological significance. The evidence of these correlations should not support the simplistic conclusion that after all looking at HRV is just a complex way to measure HR because the information is redundant. One should be prepared to verify that undisturbed cardiac physiology tends to a perfect harmony between HRV and HR. This harmony deteriorates everytime an alteration of the cardiovascular system occurs. The loss of the physiological correlations, rather than being neglected or even ignored, should be looked for; it is a sign in itself as well as a way to make a better usage of the complex tool formed by HRV.

References

1. Malik M, Farrell T, Cripps T, et al. Heart rate variability in relation to prognosis after myocardial infarction: selection of optimal processing techniques. Eur Heart J 1989; 10:1060-1074.

2. Bigger JT Jr, Fleiss JL, Steinman RC, et al. Correlations among time and frequency domain measures of heart period variability two weeks after acute myocardial infarction. Am J Cardiol 1992; 69:891-898.

3. Coumel P, Hermida JS, Wennerblöm B, et al. Heart rate variability in myocardial hypertrophy and heart failure, and the effects of beta-blocking therapy. A nonspectral analysis of heart rate oscillations. Eur Heart J 1991; 12:412-422.

4. Ewing DJ, Neilson JMM, Travis P. New method for assessing cardiac parasympathetic activity using 24-hour electrocardiograms. Br Heart J 1982; 52:396-402.

5. Akselrod S, Gordon D, Ubel FA, et al. Power spectrum analysis of heart rate fluctuations: a quantitative probe of beat-to-beat cardiovascular control. Science 1981; 213:220-222.

6. Bootsma M, Swenne CA, VanBolhuis HH, et al. Heart rate and heart rate variability as indexes of the sympathovagal balance. Am J Physiol. 1994; 266:H1565-H1571.

7. Murakawa Y, Ajiki K, Usui M, et al. Parasympathetic activity is a major modulator of the circadian variability of heart rate in healthy subjects and in patients with coronary artery disease or diabetes mellitus. Am Heart J 1993; 126:108-114.

8. Rosenblueth A, Simeone FA. The interrelations of vagal and accelerator effects on the cardiac rate. Am J Physiol 1934; 110:42-45.

9. Levy MN, DeGeest H, Zieske H. Effects of respiratory center activity on the heart. Circ Res 1966; 18:67-78.

10. Katona PG, Jih F. Respiratory sinus arrhythmia: a noninvasive measure of parasympathetic cardiac control. J Appl Physiol 1975; 39:801-805.

11. Warner HR, Russell RO. Effect of combined sympathetic and vagal stimulation on heart rate in the dog. Circ Res 1969; 24:567-573.

12. Brown TE, Beightol LA, Koh J, et al. Important influence of respiration on human RR interval spectra is largely ignored. J Appl Physiol 1993; 75(5):2310-2317.

13. Furlan F, Guzzetti F, Crivellaro W, et al. Continuous 24-hour assessment of the neural regulation of systemic arterial pressure and RR variabilities in ambulant subjects. Circulation 1990; 81:537-547.

14. Jose AD, Collison D. The normal range and determinants of the intrinsic heart rate in man. Cardiovasc Res 1970; 4:160-167.

15. Van Hoogenhuyze D, Weinstein N, Martin GJ, et al. Reproducibility and relation to mean heart rate of heart rate variability in normal subjects and in patients with congestive heart failure secondary to coronary heart disease. Am J Cardiol 1991; 68:1668-1676.

16. Huikuri HV, Kessler KM, Terracall E, et al. Reproducibility and circadian rhythm of heart rate variability in healthy subjects. Am J Cardiol 1990; 65:391-393.

17. Apple ML, Berger RD, Saul JP, et al. Beat to beat variability in cardiovascular variables: noise or music? J Am Coll Cardiol 1989; 14:1139-1148.

18. Kleiger RE, Miller JP, Bigger JT Jr, et al. Decreased heart rate variability and its association with increased mortality after acute myocardial infarction. Am J Cardiol 1987; 59:256-262.

19. Farrell TG, Bashir Y, Cripps T, et al. Risk stratification for arrhythmic events in postinfarction patients based on heart rate variability, ambulatory electrocardiographic variables and the signal-averaged electrocardiogram. J Am Coll Cardiol 1991; 18:687-697.

20. Pagani M, Lombardi F, Guzzette S, et al. Power spectral analysis of heart rate and arterial pressure variability as a marker of sympatho-vagal interaction in man and conscious dog. Circ Res 1986; 59:178-193.

21. Pagani M, Lombardi F, Malliani A. Heart rate variability: disagreement on the markers of sympathetic and parasympathetic activities. Letter to the editor. JACC 1993; 22:951-954.

22. Chakko CS, Mulingtapang RF, Huikuri HV, et al. Alterations in heart rate variability and its circadian rhythm in hypertensive patients with left ventricular hypertrophy free of coronary artery disease. Am Heart J 1993; 126:1364-1372.

23. Rochelle L, Goldsmith J, Bigger JT Jr, et al. Comparison of 24-hour parasympathetic activity in endurance-trained and untrained young men. J Am Coll Cardiol 1992; 20:552-558.

24. Levy NL, Yang T, Wallik DW. Assessment of beat-by-beat control of heart rate by the autonomic nervous system: molecular biology techniques are necessary, but not sufficient. J Cardiovasc Electrophysiol 1993; 4:183-193.

25. Shin SJ, Tapp WN, Reisman SS, et al. Assessment of autonomic regulation of heart rate variability by the method of complex demodulation. IEEE Trans Biomed Eng 1989; 36:274-283.

Chapter 17

Heart Rate Variability and Sympatho-Vagal Interaction after Myocardial Infarction

Federico Lombardi, Giulia Sandrone

The presence of alterations in autonomic control of cardiac function has long been considered in patients surviving an acute myocardial infarction. Experimental evidence available since the last century indicated that ligation of a coronary artery was associated with changes in heart rate (HR), arterial pressure (AP) and ventricular function, as well as with the occurrence of rhythm disorders.[1] The importance of neural factors in determining the type of response to acute coronary artery occlusion was also well recognized. Initially,[2] vagally mediated depressor reflexes were consistently observed to be a result of the activation of afferent vagal nerve fibers leading to an excitation of vagal and inhibition of sympathetic outflows directed to the heart.[3] Subsequently, it was proved that myocardial ischemia could also be accompanied by excitatory sympathetic reflexes mediated by the activation of afferent cardiac sympathetic fibers.[3,4] While the vagally mediated depressor reflexes were readily accepted in view of their finalistic purpose of reducing

cardiac work during ischemia, the existence of excitatory and, apparently, purposeless and even dangerous sympathetic reflexes was negated for a number of years.[3]

Experimental observations appear to provide adequate insights to explain the different hemodynamic pictures which occur in the acute phase of a myocardial infarction. The whole spectrum ranging from hypotension and bradycardia to hypertension and tachycardia could be considered the result of the complex interaction of the direct depressive effect of acute ischemia on ventricular function with the multiple neural reflexes elicited from the different reflexogenic areas.[3,5]

The tight relation between the autonomic nervous system and susceptibility to ventricular fibrillation was also demonstrated experimentally.[6] Sympathetic hyperactivity was found to alter cardiac electrical properties and to favor the occurrence of malignant ventricular arrhythmias, whereas vagal activation exerted a protective and antifibrillatory effect.[6-9]

From: Malik M., Camm AJ (eds.): *Heart Rate Variability*. Armonk, NY. Futura Publishing Company, Inc., © 1995.

Within this context, the first clinical attempt to correlate the hemodynamic profile of patients during the acute phase of myocardial infarction to a specific autonomic pattern was provided by the study of Webb et al[10]. These authors reported that within 60 minutes from the onset of symptoms related to an acute myocardial infarction, the hemodynamic profile varied importantly in relation to the site of the infarction. Inferior wall infarcts were more often associated with sinus bradycardia, transient hypotension, or atrioventricular (AV) block (which indicated an increase of parasympathetic activity), whereas anterior wall infarcts were more often associated with sinus tachycardia or transient hypertension (suggesting a sympathetic activation). Moreover, the presence of an 'autonomic disturbance' as reflected by changes in HR and systolic arterial pressure (SAP) coincided with the highest incidence of life-threatening arrhythmias.

Even less defined was the information concerning the persistence of alterations in neural control mechanisms during the post-acute phase of myocardial infarction, despite the critical role of adrenergic mechanisms in favoring the occurrence of malignant ventricular arrhythmias and highest incidence of arrhythmic deaths observed in the first few months after the acute event.[11] The presence of an impaired vagal control of heart period, which could lead to a sympathetic predominance, was initially suggested[12] by the observation of an abnormal HR response to Valsalva maneuver. Additional evidence, however, was only recently provided by several authors[13-15] who reported a reduced slowing of HR in response to phenylephrine administration in most postmyocardial infarction patients.

It is therefore understandable why a new impetus to the study of the alterations of autonomic control mechanisms has originated from the possibility of applying, to the majority of patients after a myocardial infarction, a noninvasive approach based on the analysis of heart rate variability (HRV).

In the present article, we shall concentrate on the description of the changes in sympatho-vagal interaction as they can be reflected by the changes in HRV in experimental and clinical conditions such as coronary artery occlusion and the acute and postacute phase of a myocardial infarction. A few methodological aspects will be also initially considered.

Assessment of Sympatho-Vagal Interaction by Time- and Frequency-Domain Analysis of Heart Rate Variability

Few considerations (for further details see the chapter by Malliani in this book[16]) may facilitate the interpretation of the large amount of data collected in experimental animals and in patients surviving an acute myocardial infarction.

It is generally accepted that changes of sympatho-vagal balance toward a sympathetic or a vagal predominance are associated with, respectively, an increase or a reduction of HR. The shortening or lengthening of the heart period determine consensual changes in HRV. Hence, tachycardia and bradycardia are associated with, respectively, a reduction or an increase in SD or variance of RR intervals. Thus, several authors[17-19] proposed to use measures of the total variability as indices of parasympathetic tone. While this assumption may retain some validity when analyzing recordings performed during controlled resting conditions, the biological interpretation of time measures of HRV appears more complex when considering 24-hour Holter recordings. In fact, spectral analysis, by determining the contribution of each oscillatory component to total variance, has indicated that respiration related high-frequency (HF) component accounts for up to 40% of total power only in resting conditions, during controlled respiration,[20] whereas it accounts for less than 5% when considering ambulatory monitoring. This may well explain why contrasting interpretations have been provided by different groups who evaluated the presence of alterations in neural control mechanisms according to the results of the analysis of HRV performed on short-term or 24-hour periods.

An additional point which deserves a few comments is the interpretation of individual spectral components. While the HF respiration-related component is generally considered a measure of vagal modulation of heart period,[20-23] the interpretation of low-frequency (LF) component appears more complex.[20,23] This is largely dependent upon two apparently contrasting findings: whereas a marked increase in LF can be observed when sympathetic excitation occurs in absence of significant tachycardia, no change or even a reduction in the power of this component are instead detectable when sympathetic excitation is associated with a significant reduction in heart period and in total power.[23] Moreover, when considering different subjects, differences in total variance determine consensual variations in the absolute power of each spectral component and limit the possibility of appreciating differences in the power of individual components between groups.

To override this limitation, which becomes even more important when considering 24-hour recordings, we have proposed [20,23] to express the power of LF and HF spectral components in terms of normalized units. The normalization procedure minimizes the direct effects due to variations in total power and emphasizes the changes in the amplitude of LF and HF components in terms of the reciprocal relation which appear to characterize the pattern of discharge of sympathetic and vagal outflows directed to the heart. This neural interaction, which, in our opinion, is appropriately reflected by changes in LF and HF components expressed in normalized units, is also emphasized by considering the changes in LF/HF ratio. Nevertheless, it is, however, important to reiterate that a rhythm cannot be equated to a specific neural circuit as both LF and HF rhythms can be simultaneously detected in the pattern of discharge of both sympathetic and vagal fibers directed to the heart.[23]

Experimental Coronary Artery Occlusion

As previously indicated, ligation of a coronary artery is accompanied by the simultaneous activation of excitatory and inhibitory reflex mechanisms.[2-5] It was therefore of interest to evaluate[24] whether the changes in spectral components were adequate to signal the changes in sympathetic and vagal regulatory activities directed to the heart during a brief coronary artery occlusion. In conscious dogs (Figure 1), transient occlusion of a distal branch of either the left circumflex or anterior descending coronary artery was associated with an increase in sinus rate and with a drastic reduction of total variance, whereas mean AP remained unchanged. Spectral analysis of HRV revealed that in comparison to the control period, coronary artery occlusion was characterized by a marked increase, in normalized units, of LF and by a significant reduction of HF component. All these changes were consistent with an increased sympathetic and a reduced vagal activity directed to the heart which, in absence of significant changes in AP, were likely to be the results of excitatory reflexes originating from the heart.[3-5] In the example illustrated in Figure 1, the presence of an excitatory sympathetic response was also reflected by the appearance of a predominant LF component in SAP variability which was not detectable in control conditions.

In an animal model of cardiac sudden death, Hull et al[25] examined the prognostic value of time-domain measures of HRV, measured before and after an experimental myocardial infarction, in relation to the susceptibility to ventricular fibrillation during a brief coronary artery occlusion performed in the final part of an exercise stress test. These authors observed[25] that after myocardial infarction, a diminished HRV characterized susceptible dogs compared to the

CORONARY ARTERY OCCLUSION

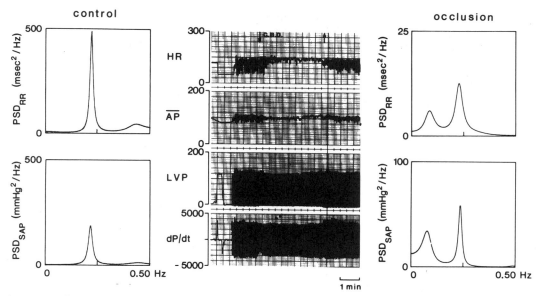

Figure 1. Effects of transient coronary artery occlusion on the autospectra of RR interval (top) and SAP (lower panels) variabilities. Analog recordings of HR, mean AP, left ventricular pressure (LVP) and dP/dt are also illustrated. The occlusion period is defined by the arrows. In control conditions only a respiration-related HF component is present in the autospectra of both variability signals. During the occlusion period the decrease in HF is associated with the appearance of a well-recognizable LF component. From Rimoldi et al.[24]

resistant ones, whereas a similar SD of RR intervals was measured in both groups of animals in the control study. Thus, a reduced HRV was highly predictive of risk for sudden death in infarcted animals, whereas this parameter appeared useless when identifying resistant or susceptible dogs before a myocardial infarction. This latter finding has to be taken into consideration when attributing a clinical value to a reduced HRV in patients without a previous myocardial infarction.[26]

Acute Myocardial Infarction

It was the merit of Wolf et al[27] to report for the first time that patients with preserved sinus arrhythmias had a lower in-hospital mortality than patients without sinus arrhythmias. A higher incidence of inferior myocardial infarction, as well as slower HRs at the time of in-hospital admission, also characterized patients with sinus ar-

rhythmias. All the above findings were considered to be suggestive of a preserved vagal tone.

The association between the localization of the infarction and a specific autonomic pattern was also confirmed by a subsequent study[28] which reported a diminished count of abrupt changes in adjacent cardiac cycles in patients with an anterior myocardial infarction studied within 24 hours from the onset of symptoms. This finding was interpreted as a sign of a diminished parasympathetic activity directed to the heart.[28]

In an ongoing study[29] in 26 patients recorded within 6 hours from the onset of symptoms related to an acute myocardial infarction, spectral analysis of HRV revealed that LF (63±3 nu) was largely predominant over HF (19±2). The presence of a sympathetic excitation and of a reduced vagal tone was also indicated by the high value of the LF/HF ratio (6±1). Signs of sympathetic excitation were also evident in patients with an inferior myocardial infarction, thus indicating that the vagal predominance, which according to Pantridge's group[10] should characterize the hyperacute phase of an inferior myocardial infarction, was soon followed by signs of sympathetic hyperactivity. The beneficial effects of beta-blocker administration in the acute phase of myocardial infarction, independently of its localization, provides a confirmatory support to these experimental findings.

Our experience[29] regarding a small group of patients who presented an episode of ventricular fibrillation during the early phase of myocardial infarction, indicates, in addition, that an increase in LF/HF ratio is usually observed in the minutes preceding the arrhythmic event; although in a few cases a sudden and marked reduction in RR variance represented the only major finding.

Finally, it is worth noting that a similar reduction in the time-domain measures of HRV was reported in patients with either an anterior or an inferior myocardial infarction when they were studied within 2 to 3 days from the acute event.[30] Of interest was the finding that a reduced 24-hour SD of RR interval, which was interpreted as a sign of an altered modulation of heart period, was strongly related to indices of the extent and clinical severity of the infarction.[30]

By analyzing HRV with spectral techniques 4 days after the acute event, Kamath and Fallen[31] were able to observe a marked predominance of LF component and a reduced HF during the daytime, whereas during the night HF increased. The changes in spectral indices which were blunted in patients treated with beta-blockers indicated a shift of sympatho-vagal balance toward a sympathetic excitation and a reduced vagal tone. Also in this study,[31] the observed changes in spectral indices of sympathetic and vagal modulation were not related to the site of the infarction.

Postacute Phase of Myocardial Infarction

Patients after the acute phase of myocardial infarction represent the largest population in whom HRV has been extensively studied to obtain information on the clinical outcome and to evaluate the alteration in autonomic control of heart period.

As already mentioned in this book, Kleiger et al[18] reported in a large group of patients, that a reduced 24-hour SD of normal RR intervals measured on Holter recordings performed 11 ± 3 days after an acute myocardial infarction, had the strongest univariate correlation with mortality. These authors explained their findings, hypothesizing that a decreased HRV correlates with increased sympathetic or decreased vagal tone which could predispose to ventricular fibrillation.[18]

The subsequent analysis[19] of the causes in differences in HRV seemed to support this hypothesis. High-risk patients were characterized by faster HRs during daytime and nighttime and minor differences in day-night mean HR, as well as by a diminished number of abrupt changes in adjacent cardiac cycles. All the above factors which concurred to determine a reduced HRV were considered to reflect the effects of an increased sympathetic and a reduced vagal activity directed to the sinus node. In the same year, we published a study[32] in which we analyzed, with spectral techniques, HRV of a smaller group of patients 2 weeks after myocardial infarction during controlled resting conditions (Figure 2) and 90° head-up tilt. In comparison to a group of age-matched control subjects, postmyocardial infarction patients were characterized by a predominant LF and a smaller HF and by a significantly greater LF/HF ratio. Hence, spectral analysis indicated in this group of patients surviving an acute myocardial infarction, signs of sympathetic excitation and of a reduced vagal tone. The alterations of neural control of heart period were also reflected by the lack of response of the spectral indices of sympathetic and vagal modula-

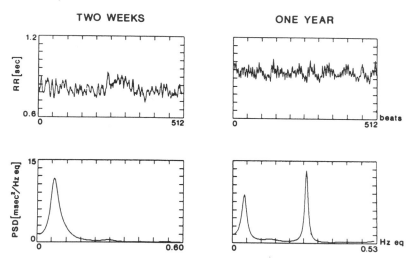

Figure 2. Spectral analysis of RR variability in a patient 2 weeks (left) and 1 year (right panel) after a myocardial infarction. A predominant LF and a smaller HF indicating a sympathetic excitation and a reduced vagal tone are present at the time of discharge. At 1 year two clearly identifiable LF and HF components are evident. From Lombardi et al.[32]

tion and by the LF/HF ratio to a sympathetic stimulus such as 90° tilt. In the same study,[32] we reported three patients who died suddenly within 3 months of the acute event. They were characterized by a markedly reduced RR variance (231±63 milliseconds[2]) and by a different energy distribution in the spectrum. The most relevant part of the power was distributed below 0.03 Hz, the residual absolute power of LF and HF was minimal (Figure 3) and only by introducing a normalization procedure was it possible to detect that the respiration related HF component was predominant over LF. It is our opinion that in high-risk patients with a complicated myocardial infarction, a diminished responsiveness of sinus node to neural inputs or a saturating effect[33] of a persistent and sustained discharge of sympathetic fibers directed to the heart may account for the marked reduction in HRV and, in particular, for the quite complete suppression of the two main rhythmical oscillations which are detected in normal hearts.

This also seems to be the case when considering the results of spectral analysis performed on 24-hour Holter recordings where noise, slow trends and very low-frequency (VLF) oscillations contribute to that part of the spectrum below 0.03 Hz, which,

as known, account for 85% to 90% of total power. The recent observations of Bigger et al[34,35] who reported an increased mortality in postmyocardial infarction patients with a reduced power in all frequency bands including LF, seem to confirm our hypothesis.

Time- and frequency-domain analysis of HRV has also been used to obtain information on the time-course of changes in sympatho-vagal interaction after myocardial infarction. An increase in 24 SD of RR interval or in RR variance to values approximating to 50% to 90% of that observed in age-matched normal subjects has been reported by several authors[30,32,36,37] in the first few months after the acute event. Within the same period, we also observed[32] a normalization of spectral indices of sympathetic and vagal modulation (Figure 2) and of LF/HF ratio. In these patients, the recovery of a more physiological balance between sympathetic and vagal control activities was also reflected by a normal response of spectral indices to a sympathetic stimulus such as 90° head-up tilt. Of interest was the observation[37] that the time-course of changes in LF and HF components and in LF/HF ratio towards normal values were present in patients in whom areas of efferent sympathetic denervation were persistently detected by

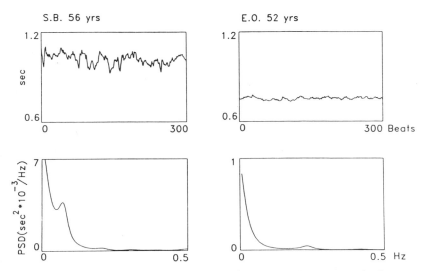

Figure 3. Spectral analysis of HRV in two patients characterized, respectively, by a normal (left) and a markedly reduced (right panels) RR variance. In the first patient (S.B.) a predominant LF is well detectable, whereas in the second one (E.O.), in addition to a VLF component, only a small respiration related HF is evident.

means of I-123 MIBG scintigraphy. The presence of a nonhomogenous electrophysiological response of cardiac cells to an increased sympathetic drive to the heart, which is suggested by these experimental findings, might contribute to explain the increase in arrhythmic mortality observed in the first few months after an acute myocardial infarction.

The presence of alterations in neural control mechanisms was also reflected by the 24-hour pattern of variation of mean RR interval and of time- and frequency-domain measures of HRV observed in postmyocardial infarction patients. As previously indicated, a diminished day-night difference in cardiac cycle duration was consistently reported in these patients and interpreted as a consequence of an impaired parasympathetic modulation of heart period.[19] A decreased pattern of variation of SD of RR intervals or of RR variance was also observed in high-risk patients. This latter finding, which could partially be related to the prevailing tachycardia, suggests the presence of a more severe alteration of neural regulatory mechanisms in these high-risk patients.[38]

By analyzing with spectral techniques Holter recordings of a group of 20 patients

4 weeks after an uncomplicated myocardial infarction and with an ejection fraction greater than 40%, we compared[39] the circadian variation of spectral indices of sympathetic and vagal modulation with those of a group of age-matched control subjects. As previously reported,[40] normal subjects were characterized by the predominance of LF component during the daily hours and of HF during the night, which reflected the expected 24-hour pattern of variation of sympatho-vagal balance. An elevation of LF (64 ± 3 versus 56 ± 2 nu) throughout the entire recording period and a smaller HF (23 ± 2 versus 32 ± 2 nu) during the night differentiated postmyocardial infarction patients from controls and indicated the presence of a persistent sympathetic activation. The alteration of sympatho-vagal balance toward a sympathetic predominance and a diminished vagal tone was also reflected by the attenuation of the nocturnal decrease in LF component and by the smaller increase in HF during the same period. It is important to reiterate that, as a result of the significant reduction in total variance, the absolute power of LF and HF was markedly reduced throughout the 24-hour period in postmyocardial infarction patients. However, the

sympathetic predominance and the reduced vagal tone characterizing these patients were also indicated by the greater values of the LF/HF ratio calculated in either absolute or normalized units.[39]

The possibility of using the analysis of HRV in order to study the effects of pharmacological and nonpharmacological interventions on sympathetic and vagal neural regulatory activities has been suggested by a few recent reports.[41-44]

The administration of atenolol or metoprolol to a group of patients 4 weeks after an uncomplicated myocardial infarction[41] was associated with important changes in time- and frequency-domain measures of HRV. The expected bradycardia was accompanied by an increase in 24-hour RR variance. Spectral analysis revealed that this effect was largely due to an increase of the power in the frequency range between 0 and 0.03 Hz which corresponded to the VLF range. This finding appears of particular interest when considering that, despite the incomplete understanding of the underlying physiological mechanisms, a decrease in the power of the VLF component was highly predictive of increased mortality and of augmented arrhythmic risk after a myocardial infarction.[34,35] The possibility of a link between the beneficial effects of beta-blockers and the observed increase in total variance and, in particular, in the VLF component appears attractive and deserves further investigation.

In agreement with our previous observations,[20] the antiadrenergic effects of beta-blockers was reflected by the reduction of LF component and by the increase in HF in comparison to what was observed before drug administration.[41] As a result, there was a reverting of the altered circadian pattern of spectral indices of sympathetic and vagal modulation which characterized these patients (Figure 4). Of clinical interest was the observation that beta-blocker administration markedly attenuated the early morning increase of LF component and of LF/HF ratio. The possibility that this pharmacological intervention could limit the unpredict-

able consequences of the surge in sympathetic activity that characterize this period of the day, may represent one of the mechanisms by which these drugs exert their protective effects.

The effects of pharmacological parasympathetic stimulation induced by low-dose transdermal scopolamine, have been recently evaluated by analyzing HRV in patients after myocardial infarction. Vybiral et al[42] reported that 24-hour application of scopolamine was associated with a marked augment in the time-domain measures of HRV. These changes were considered to reflect a more effective parasympathetic modulation of heart period. A similar interpretation was provided by De Ferrari et al[43] to explain the observed changes in the time- and frequency-domain measures of HRV induced by short-time application of scopolamine. These authors also reported a significant decrease in LF/HF ratio, as well as an increase in baroreceptor reflex sensitivity; both findings were considered to reflect the vagomimetic action of this drug.

Finally, spectral analysis of HRV seems to be adequate to evaluate the effects of short-term exercise training on the autonomic modulation of heart period. In a preliminary study[44] carried out on 22 patients with a first and recent myocardial infarction, we analyzed the response of spectral indices of sympathetic and vagal modulation to a sympathetic stimulus (90° head-up tilt) before and after 4 weeks of physical training. A control group of patients not assigned to a training program was also considered. At entry, in both groups, spectral analysis was characterized by a predominant LF and a smaller HF component. This pattern was consistent with a shift of sympatho-vagal balance towards a sympathetic excitation and a reduced vagal tone as previously reported in most postmyocardial infarction patients.[32,37,39] Tilt did not determine additional significant changes in spectral components. Physical training induced, as expected, a significant increase in exercise duration and in the anaerobic threshold in trained patients, whereas no

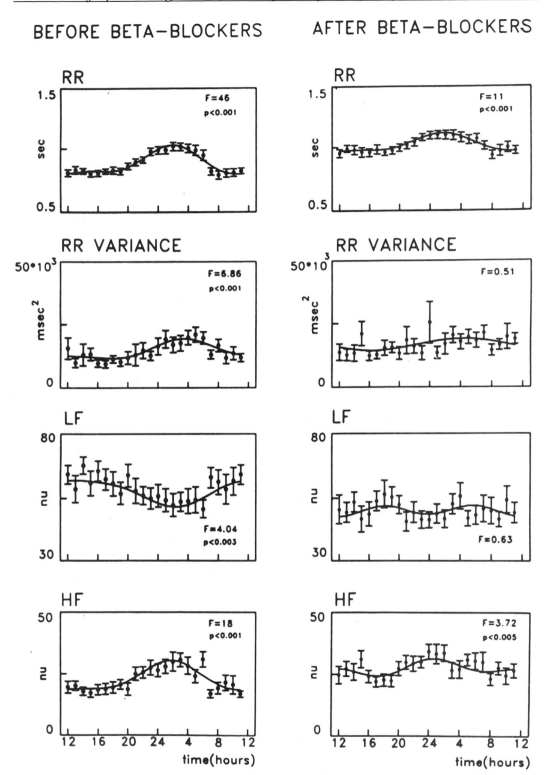

Figure 4. Effects of beta-blocker administration on the 24-hour pattern of variations of RR interval, RR variance, LF and HF spectral components of HRV in patients after myocardial infarction. From Sandrone et al.[41]

changes were observed in the untrained group. After physical training, however, tilt produced a significant increase in LF (from 69±5 to 84±3 nu) component and a decrease in HF (from 19±4 to 7±1 nu) component while no changes were detectable in untrained patients. These data, which must be considered taking into account the normalization of the response of spectral indices to head-up tilt observed only about 12 months after the acute event,[32] seem to suggest that physical training might contribute to accelerate the restoration of a more physiological sympatho-vagal balance and responsiveness of spectral indices to a sympathetic stimulus.

Closing Remarks

Time- and frequency-domain analysis of HRV is a safe and noninvasive technique which offers the possibility of evaluating the alteration of neural regulatory activity in patients after myocardial infarction.

Even if the importance of neural mechanisms in conditioning the prognosis of post-myocardial infarction patients is well-established, the definition of the 'autonomic profile' remains an attractive prospective for most of the patients. The possibility of identifying, with a 5-minute recording, the presence of an autonomic imbalance with either a marked sympathetic or vagal over-activity, might facilitate therapeutic interventions in the hyperacute phase of myocardial infarction. Furthermore, the presence of shift of sympatho-vagal balance towards an increased sympathetic and a diminished vagal tone may facilitate the identification of patients who could take advantage of beta-blocker therapy after hospital discharge.

Future research has to be directed to investigate the neural and non-neural mechanisms responsible for the drastic reduction in HRV observed in high-risk patients, and to analyze whether the changes in RR variance and spectral components induced by different interventions are indeed associated with changes in the clinical outcome of these patients.

References

1. Porter WT. On the result of ligation of the coronary arteries. J Physiol 1894; 15:121-128.
2. Costatin LR. Extracardiac factors contributing to hypotension during coronary occlusion. Am J Cardiol 1963; 11:205-217.
3. Bishop VS, Malliani A, Thorèn P. Cardiac mechanoreceptors. In: Shepherd JT, Abboud FM, Geiger SR (eds). Handbook of Physiology, Section 2, Volume III. The Cardiovascular System, Peripheral Circulation and Organ Blood Flow. Bethesda, Md: American Physiological Society, 1983; 497-555.
4. Malliani A, Schwartz PJ, Zanchetti A. A sympathetic reflex elicited by experimental coronary occlusion. Am J Physiol 1969; 217:703-709.
5. Lombardi F, Casalone C, Della Bella P, et al. Global versus regional myocardial ischaemia: differences in cardiovascular and sympathetic responses in cats. Cardiovasc Res 1984; 18:14-23.
6. Lown B, Verrier RL. Neural activity and ventricular fibrillation. N Engl J Med 1976; 294:1165-1172.
7. Lombardi F, Verrier RL, Lown B. Relationship between sympathetic neural activity, coronary dynamics and vulnerability to ventricular fibrillation during myocardial ischemia and reperfusion. Am Heart J 1983; 105:958-965.
8. Malliani A, Schwartz PJ, Zanchetti A. Neural mechanisms in life-threatening arrhythmias. Am Heart J 1980; 200:705-715.
9. Schwartz PJ, La Rovere MT, Vanoli E. Autonomic nervous system and sudden cardiac death. Circulation 1992; 85:77-91.
10. Webb SW, Adgey AAJ, Pantridge JF. Autonomic disturbance at onset of acute myocardial infarction. Br Med J 1972; 3:89-92.
11. Podrid PJ, Fuchs T, Candinas R. Role of the sympathetic nervous system in the genesis of ventricular arrhythmias. Circulation 1990; I:103-113.
12. Ryan C, Hollenberg M, Harvey DB, et al. Impaired parasympathetic responses in patients after myocardial infarction. Am J Cardiol 1976; 37:1013-1018.
13. Schwartz PJ, Zaza A, Pala M, et al. Baroreflex sensitivity and its evolution during the first

year after a myocardial infarction. Am J Cardiol 1987; 60:1239-1245.

14. La Rovere MT, Specchia G, Mortara A, et al. Baroreflex sensitivity, clinical correlates and cardiovascular mortality among patients with a first myocardial infarction: a prospective study. Circulation 1988; 78:816-824.

15. Farrell TG, Paul V, Cripps TR, et al. Baroreflex sensitivity and electrophysiological correlates in patients after acute myocardial infarction. Circulation 1991; 83:945-952.

16. Malliani A. Association of heart rate variability components with physiologic regulatory mechanisms. In: Malik M, Camm AJ (eds). Heart Rate Variability. Armonk, NY: Futura Publishing Co., 1994. In press.

17. Ewing DJ, Neilson JMM, Travis P. New method for assessing cardiac parasympathetic activity using 24-hour electrocardiograms. Br Heart J 1984; 52:321-327.

18. Kleiger RE, Miller JP, Bigger JT Jr, et al. Decreased heart rate variability and its association with increased mortality after acute myocardial infarction. Am J Cardiol 1987; 59:256-262.

19. Bigger JT Jr, Kleiger RE, Fleiss JL, et al. Components of heart rate variability measured during healing of acute myocardial infarction. Am J Cardiol 1988; 61:208-215.

20. Pagani M, Lombardi F, Guzzetti S, et al. Power spectral analysis of heart rate and arterial pressure variabilities as a marker of sympathovagal interaction in man and conscious dog. Circ Res 1986; 59:178-193.

21. Kitney RI, Rompelman O. The Study of Heart Rate Variability. Oxford, England: Clarendon Press, 1980.

22. Akselrod S, Gordon D, Ubel FA, et al. Power spectrum analysis of heart rate fluctuations: a quantitative probe of beat-to-beat cardiovascular control. Science 1981; 213:220-222.

23. Malliani A, Pagani M, Lombardi F, et al. Cardiovascular neural regulation explored in the frequency domain. Circulation 1991; 84:482-492.

24. Rimoldi O, Pierini S, Ferrari A, et al. Analysis of short term oscillations of RR and arterial pressure in conscious dogs. Am J Physiol 1990; 258:H967-H976.

25. Hull S, Evans AR, Vanoli E, et al. Heart rate variability before and after myocardial infarction in conscious dogs at high and low risk of sudden death. J Am Coll Cardiol 1990; 16:978-985.

26. Lombardi F, Torzillo D, Sandrone G, et al. Beta-blocking effect of propafenone based on spectral analysis of heart rate variability. Am J Cardiol 1992; 70:1220-1228.

27. Wolf MM, Varigos GA, Hunt D, et al. Sinus arrhythmia in acute myocardial infarction. 1978; 2:52-53.

28. McAreavey D, Neilson JMM, Ewing DJ, et al. Cardiac parasympathetic activity during the early hours of acute myocardial infarction. Br Heart J 1989; 62:165-170.

29. Malliani A, Lombardi F, Pagani M, et al. Power spectral analysis of cardiovascular variability in patients at risk for sudden cardiac death. J Cardiovasc Electrophysiol 1994; 5:274-286.

30. Casolo GC, Stroder P, Signorini C, et al. Heart rate variability during the acute phase of myocardial infarction. Circulation 1992; 85:2073-2079.

31. Kamath MV, Fallen EL. Diurnal variations of neurocardiac rhythms in acute myocardial infarction. Am J Cardiol 1991; 68:155-160.

32. Lombardi F, Sandrone G, Pernpruner S, et al. Heart rate variability as an index of sympathovagal interaction after acute myocardial infarction. Am J Cardiol 1987; 60:1239-1245.

33. Malik M, Camm AJ. Components of heart rate variability—what they really mean and what we really measure. Am J Cardiol 1993; 72:821-822.

34. Bigger JT Jr, Fleiss JL, Steinman RC, et al. Frequency domain measures of heart period variability and mortality after myocardial infarction. Circulation 1992; 85:164-171.

35. Bigger JT Jr, Fleiss JL, Rolnitzky LM, et al. Frequency domain measures of heart period variability to assess risk late after myocardial infarction. J Am Coll Cardiol 1993; 21:729-736.

36. Bigger JT Jr, Fleiss JL, Rolnitzky LM, et al. Time course of recovery of heart period variability after myocardial infarction. J Am Coll Cardiol 1991; 18:1643-1649.

37. Spinnler MT, Lombardi F, Moretti C, et al. Evidence of functional alterations in sympathetic activity after myocardial infarction. Eur Heart J 1993; 14:1334-1343.

38. Malik M, Farrell T, Camm AJ. Circadian rhythm of heart rate variability after acute myocardial infarction and its influence on the prognostic value of heart rate variability. Am J Cardiol 1990; 66:1049-1054.

39. Lombardi F, Sandrone G, Mortara A, et al. Circadian variation of spectral indices of heart rate variability after myocardial infarction. Am Heart J 1992; 123:1521-1529.

40. Furlan R, Guzzetti S, Crivellaro W, et al. Continuous 24-hour assessment of the neural regulation of systemic arterial pressure and RR variabilities in ambulant subjects. Circulation 1990; 81:537-547.

41. Sandrone G, Mortara A, Torzillo D, et al. Effects of beta-blockers (atenolol or metoprolol) on heart rate variability after acute myocardial infarction. Am J Cardiol 1994. In press.

42. Vybiral T, Glaeser DH, Morris G, et al. Effects of low dose transdermal scopolamine on heart rate variability in acute myocardial infarction. J Am Coll Cardiol 1993; 22:1320-1326.

43. De Ferrari GM, Mantica M, Vanoli E, et al. Scopolamine increases vagal tone and vagal reflexes in patients after myocardial infarction. J Am Coll Cardiol 1993; 22:1327-1334.

44. La Rovere MT, Mortara A, Sandrone G, et al. Autonomic nervous system adaptations to short-term exercise testing. Chest 1992; 101:299s-303s.

Chapter 18

Effect of Age on Heart Rate Variability

Olusola Odemuyiwa

Heart rate variability (HRV) increases with gestational age and during early postnatal life,[1] but a decline in autonomic function is already detectable between the ages of 5 and 10 years.[2,3] In adults, differences in HRV between age groups were reported by Schlomka nearly 60 years ago,[4] but the study was criticized because the respiratory frequency and pattern were not standardized. Nevertheless, the findings were confirmed by Hellman and Stacey,[5] who studied subjects during metronomc respiration and corrected for age-related differences in tidal volume. Several other studies have since shown that HRV changes with age, but the magnitude and course of this change depends on the age range studied, the experimental conditions, and the method used for assessing HRV.

O'Brien et al[6] studied the influence of age on HRV in 310 healthy subjects aged 18 to 85 years. There were at least 50 subjects in each decade from 20 to 70 years. Heart rate (HR) was recorded at rest, during a single deep breath, during and after a Valsalva maneuver in the supine or semirecumbent position and then during standing for 60 seconds. The following indices of HRV in the time domain were derived: HR difference (the difference between the maximum and the minimum HR during the maneuver), HR ratio (the ratio of the maximum to the minimum HR during each maneuver), the standard deviation of the HR and the ratio of the RR intervals on the 15th and 30th beats after standing. There was a nonlinear decline in HRV with age. This decline appeared steeper in the younger than in the older subjects. Multiple correlation analysis showed that age accounted for between 15% and 33% of the variation in HRV. Similar findings have been reported by Ingall et al[7] in a study of 76 healthy subjects aged between 5 and 85 years, and recently by Bruggermann et al.[8]

Pagani and colleagues[9] found that the ratio of low-frequency (LF) to high-frequency (HF) spectral components of HRV did not change with age and suggested, therefore, that aging is associated with a new equilibrium between sympathetic and parasympathetic activity. However, their findings were derived from a narrow age range and other workers have shown that

From: Malik M., Camm AJ (eds.): *Heart Rate Variability*. Armonk, NY. Futura Publishing Company, Inc., © 1995.

components of HRV change with age at different rates. Shannon et al[10] measured HRV in the supine and standing positions in 33 male subjects aged between 9 and 62 years. LF power declined linearly across the whole age range, but HF power declined significantly only between the ages of 9 and 30 years. They also found that the age-related decline in LF power was greater in the erect than in the supine position. This was because a reflex increase in LF power on standing was seen only in subjects aged under 30 years. Hirsch and Bishop[11] also showed that respiratory sinus arrhythmia measured during metronomic respiration and at constant tidal volumes declined rapidly between the ages of 22 and 35 years and then showed no further decrease up to the age of 78 years. A larger study[2] examined the influence of age on time- and frequency-domain indices of HRV in the supine and standing positions and during spontaneous and metronomic respiration. The time-domain (standard deviation of RR intervals) and the frequency-domain (area under the curve from 0.04 Hz to 0.32 Hz) indices decreased in a linear fashion with increasing age ($p<0.0001$) in both positions during spontaneous and metronomic breathing. However, the influence of age on the ratio of LF to HF content varied with posture: this ratio was higher in the younger subjects during metronomic respiration in the supine and standing positions and during spontaneous respiration in the standing, but not the supine position. Younger subjects showed a greater activation of LF fluctuations and a more marked reduction in HF fluctuations when they stood up. Lipsitz et al[12] reported similar findings using 60° head-up tilt in 12 healthy, young (18 to 35 years) and 10 healthy, old (71 to 94 years) subjects. In this study, (Figures 1 and 2) an increase in LF bands during upright tilt was seen only in the young group and there was no change in HF band during upright tilt in any age group. However, the angle of tilt was lower and the mean age of the subjects was higher than in previous reports. Other workers[13,14] have reported a relatively greater decline in the so-called nonrespiratory components of HRV with increasing age, but these studies were carried out only during spontaneous respiration.

Age has a less marked influence on HRV after myocardial infarction. In a study of 808 postinfarction patients, Kleiger et al[15] found a weak inverse correlation ($r = -0.2$) between HRV and age; other workers[16-18] have reported similar findings. This is probably because factors such as the size of infarction are more important determinants of autonomic balance (see Chapter 19). Nevertheless, the proportion of patients with markedly depressed HRV early after myocardial infarction is higher in older (aged >60 years) than in younger patients, and the predictive value of HRV for sudden death declines with increasing age. Sudden arrhythmic deaths also appear to be more common in younger patients. While the causes of these findings are not well understood, they have implications for risk stratification based on HRV. If the influence of age on the relationship between HRV and sudden arrhythmic death is overlooked, a significant number of older patients may receive inappropriate treatment or several young patients at high risk of sudden death may be missed.[19] Risk stratification can be refined by defining age-corrected normal values for HRV after infarction or by using different variables for predicting events in different age groups.

Pfeffer and colleagues[20] have shown that the decline in HRV with age, or, more accurately, differences in HRV between age groups, is mainly due to a decline in parasympathetic function. The relative importance to these findings of changes in integratory central neural activity, in afferent and efferent parasympathetic pathway responsiveness and in sinus node function is unknown.

The trajectory of decline in HRV with age may be modified by regular exercise. In one study at least, the age-related decline in HRV may have been due to differences between age groups in the number of

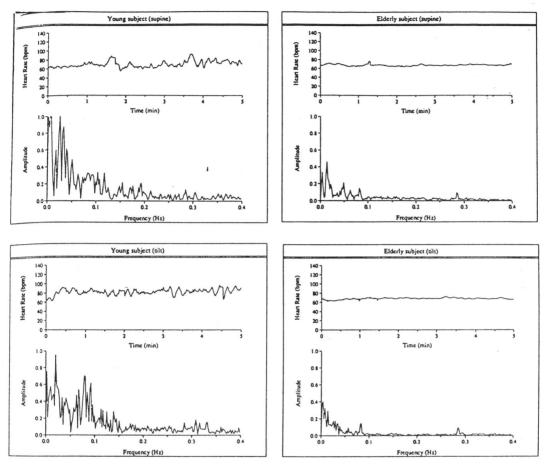

Figure 1. HR time series (top panel) and frequency spectra in one young and one old subject in supine and tilt positions. The young subject shows a greater fluctuation in HR and an increase in the LF component (0.06 Hz to 0.10 Hz) during tilt. Courtesy of LA Lipsitz.[12]

subjects engaged in regular exercise. In the study reported by Hellman and Stacey,[5] for example, 10 of the 16 subjects aged between 21 and 43 years, and only 1 of the 8 aged between 44 and 65 took part in regular exercise: and none of the younger, but 5 of the older group were either overweight or had a history of heart disease.

On the other hand, in a similar study,[11] the 37-year-old and the 78-year-old male subjects who undertook regular exercise both had the same value of respiratory sinus arrhythmia. Studies in underfed rodents[21,22] also provide evidence that age-related changes in autonomic function can be modi-

fied. If these reports are confirmed and a presumed immutable age-related decline in HRV is reversible or preventable, would population-based changes in the decline of HRV with age, however these were achieved, reduce arrhythmic events after myocardial infarction,[23] reduce the duration of ischemic events in patients with coronary lesions,[24] or increase the incidence of vaso-vagal attacks[12]? Would subjects at a high risk of developing cardiac disease need to be screened for autonomic dysfunction? The study of the aging process and of the relationship between age and HRV may provide answers to these questions.

Spectral Reserve Loss with Age

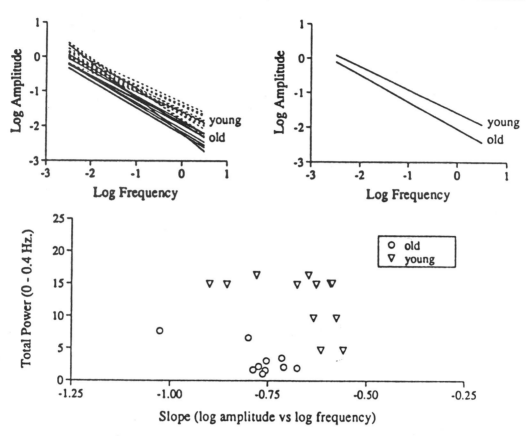

Figure 2. Log amplitude versus log frequency plots in i) individual young and old subjects and ii) average regression lines for young and old subjects. Older subjects have relatively reduced amplitude at all frequencies and steeper slopes indicating relatively greater attenuation of HF HRV. Courtesy of LA Lipsitz.[12]

References

1. Van Ravenswaaij CM, Hopman JC, Kollee LA, et al. Influences on heart rate variability on spontaneously breathing preterm infants. Early Hum Dev 1991; 27:187-205.

2. Schwartz JB, Gibb WJ, Tran T. Aging effects on heart rate variability. J Gerontol 1991; 46:M99-M106.

3. Finley JP, Nugent ST, Hellenbrand W. Heart rate variability in children. Spectral analysis of developmental changes between 5 and 24 years. Can J Physiol Pharmacol 1987; 65:2048-2052.

4. Schlomka G. Untersuchungen uber die physiologische unregelmassigkeit des Herschlages. Z Kreislaufforsch 1937; 29:510-524.

5. Hellman JB, Stacey RW. Variation of respiratory sinus arrhythmia with age. J Appl Physiol 1976; 41:734-738.

6. O'Brien IAD, O'Hare P, Corrall RJM. Heart rate variability in healthy subjects: effects of age and the derivation of normal ranges for tests of autonomic function. Br Heart J 1985; 55:348-354.

7. Ingall TJ, Mcleod J, O'Brien PC. The effect of ageing on autonomic nervous system function. Aust N Z J Med 1990; 20:570-577.

8. Bruggermann T, Andresen D, Voller H, et al. Heart rate variability from ambulatory ECG recordings in a normal population. Eur Heart J 1992; 13:1984. Abstract.

9. Pagani M, Lombardi F, Guzzetti S, et al. Power spectral analysis of heart rate and ar-

terial pressure variabilities as a marker of sympatho-vagal interaction in man and conscious dog. Circ Res 1986; 59:178-193.

10. Shannon DC, Carley DW, Benson H. Aging of modulation of heart rate. Am J Physiol 1987; 253:H874-877.

11. Hirsch JA, Bishop B. Respiratory sinus arrhythmia in humans: how breathing pattern modulates heart rate. Am J Physiol 1981; 241:H620-H629.

12. Lipsitz LA, Mietus J, Moody GB, et al. Spectral characteristics of heart rate variability before and during postural tilt: relations to aging and risk of syncope. Circulation 1990; 81:1803-1810.

13. Jennings JR, Mack ME. Does aging differentially reduce heart rate variability related to respiration? Exp Aging Res 1984; 10:19-23.

14. Simpson DM, Wicks R. Spectral analysis of heart rate indicates reduced baroreceptor-related heart rate variability in elderly persons. J Gerontol 1988; 43:M21-M24.

15. Kleiger RE, Miller JP, Bigger JT, et al. Decreased heart rate variability and its association with increased mortality after acute myocardial infarction. Am J Cardiol 1987; 59:256-262.

16. Odemuyiwa O, Farrell T, Malik M, et al. Effect of age on the electrophysiological and autonomic correlates of sudden death after myocardial infarction. PACE 1991; 14:2049-2053.

17. Casolo GC, Stroder P, Signorini C, et al. Heart rate variability during the acute phase of myocardial infarction. Circulation 1992; 85:2073-2079.

18. Hermosillo AG, Dorado M, Casanova JM, et al. Influence of infarct-related artery patency on the indexes of parasympathetic activity and prevalence of late potentials in survivors of acute myocardial infarction. J Am Coll Cardiol 1993; 22:695-706.

19. Odemuyiwa O, Farrell TG, Malik M, et al. Influence of age on the relation between heart rate variability, left ventricular ejection fraction, frequency of ventricular extrasystoles, and sudden death after myocardial infarction. Br Heart J 1992; 67:387-391.

20. Pfeffer MA, Weinberg CR, Cook D, et al. Differential changes of autonomic nervous system function with age in man. Am J Med 1983; 75:249-258.

21. Vanhoutte PM. Aging and vascular responsiveness. J Cardiovasc Pharmacol 1988; 12(suppl 8):S11-S18.

22. Masoro EJ. Food restriction in rodents: an evaluation of its role in the study of aging. J Gerontol 1988; 43:B59-64.

23. Farrell TG, Bashir Y, Cripps T, et al. Risk stratification for arrhythmic events in postinfarction patients based on heart rate variability, ambulatory electrocardiographic variables and the signal-averaged electrocardiogram. J Am Coll Cardiol 1991; 18:687-697.

24. Trimarco B, Chierchia S, Lembo G, et al. Prolonged duration of myocardial ischaemia in patients with coronary heart disease and impaired cardiopulmonary baroreceptor sensitivity. Circulation 1990; 81:1792-1802.

Chapter 19

The Relationship between Ventricular Function and Heart Rate Variability

Olusola Odemuyiwa

In animals there is a direct correlation between myocardial damage, the subsequent hemodynamic deterioration, and the adrenergic response.[1] In humans, however, the relationship between heart rate variability (HRV) and the most widely used index of ventricular function, the ejection fraction is more complex and depends on the population studied. Rich et al[2] found no significant correlation between the left ventricular ejection fraction and HRV in 112 patients who had elective coronary angiography, but the mean ejection fraction in the study was 65% and only 15 patients had an ejection fraction of under 50%. However, there is disagreement over the effect of ventricular function on HRV even in patients with poor ventricular function, because hemodynamic variables and neurohormonal activity vary so widely, even in patients with the same ejection fraction.[3] Nolan and colleagues[4] found a significant linear correlation between HRV and the ejection fraction (r = 0.49, p<0.05) in 60 patients with ischemic heart disease. The ejection fractions ranged from 5% to 35% and the mean ejection fraction was 18%. Kienzle et al,[3] however, found no correlation between HRV and the ejection fraction in 23 patients with idiopathic dilated cardiomyopathy. The age range of the patients and the mean and range of ejection fractions were 21% and 8% to 34%, respectively, similar to those in the other study,[4] but most oral medication was discontinued for more than 4 half-lives and diuretics for 12 hours before the study. The results may therefore have been influenced by changes in hemodynamics, neurohormonal activity and even the ejection fraction after treatment was discontinued.

The relationship between HRV and the ejection fraction may also depend on the method of assessment of HRV. Stein et al[5] computed the resting-resting ejection fraction and time- and frequency-domain indices of high-frequency (HF), low-frequency (LF), and ultra LF HRV in 38 patients with nonischemic causes of chronic severe mitral regurgitation. Of these, only the standard deviation of the 5-minute mean RR intervals

From: Malik M., Camm AJ (eds.): *Heart Rate Variability*. Armonk, NY. Futura Publishing Company, Inc., © 1995.

Table 1

Probable Determinants of the Relationship between
Ventricular Function and Heart Rate Variability

a) Low Heart Rate Variability and Poor Ventricular Function

Extensive infarction
Heart failure
Occluded infarct artery

b) Low Heart Rate Variability and Normal Ventricular Function

Site of infarction
Diuretics
Oral inotropes
Anxiety
Valvar regurgitation

c) Poor Ventricular Function and Normal Heart Rate Variability

Angiotensin converting enzyme inhibitors
Scopolamine
Beta-blockers

d) Normal Ventricular Function and Heart Rate Variability

Small infarction
Combination of factors from b and c

e) Other Influences

Method of measuring heart rate variability
Time since infarction or damage
Age of patients and hemodynamic state before myocardial infarction

(SDANN), a measure of ultra LF HRV, correlated with left (r = 0.49, p = 0.002) or right ventricular ejection fraction (r = 0.43, p = 0.007). Whether these results apply to patients with other causes of left ventricular dysfunction is unknown.

HRV appears to be related to the size of acute myocardial infarction: it is higher in patients who received thrombolytic therapy than in patients who did not, is inversely related to peak CK-MB value (r= -0.54) and is higher in non-Q-wave infarction than in Q-wave infarction.[6] According to Kleiger et al[7] and other workers, however (Figure 1), there is only a weak correlation (r = 0.2 to r = 0.4) between HRV and the ejection fraction early after myocardial infarction.[6,8] Kleiger and colleagues[7] also found that HRV did not correlate either with pulmonary congestion on the chest X-ray or with anterior wall motion abnormalities on radionuclide angiography; whereas others have shown that patients in Killip Class 2-4 have lower HRV than those in Killip 1 , and that HRV is

significantly reduced in postinfarction patients with signs or symptoms of heart failure.[6,9] Differences in contractility of the non-infarcted myocardium, in ventricular size and shape, in autonomic nerve innervation and damage, the use of vasodilators, beta-blockers or diuretics as well as anxiety, the severity of associated coronary lesions and the patency of the infarct-related artery may explain these findings. In some patients, a normal ejection fraction may be maintained by reflex, but potentially deleterious increases in sympathetic drive, explaining the poor correlation between the ejection fraction and HRV in postinfarction patients who die suddenly soon after infarction.[10] Other factors which may influence the relationship between the ejection fraction and HRV after infarction include hemodynamic and autonomic function before infarction and the time elapsed since infarction.

Compared to patients with poor left ventricular function and a patent infarct-related artery, patients with poor left ven-

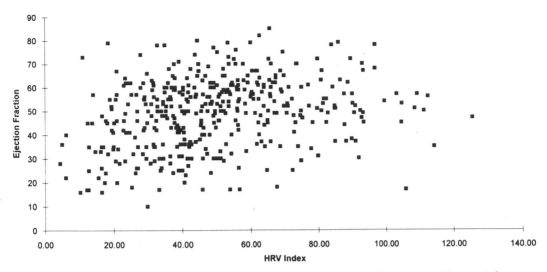

Figure 1. Scatter diagram from the Post Infarction Survey Programme St. George's Hospital showing the relationship between the ejection fraction and HRV in 433 survivors of a first myocardial infarction (r = 0.25 overall and r = 0.19 in the 227 patients treated with streptokinase).

tricular function and an occluded infarct-related artery appear to be at an increased risk of sudden death. This risk appears to be reduced by beta-blocker therapy.[11,12] Since reduced HRV is a marker for an increased risk of sudden death, the protective benefit of a patent infarct-related artery may be modulated through an effect on autonomic function. Two recent reports appear to support this hypothesis. The first study found that in patients with an ejection fraction <40%, HRV was lower in patients with an occluded infarct-related artery than in those with a patent infarct-related artery. There was no difference in mean ejection fractions between the two groups of patients.[13] These findings need to be confirmed in prospective studies. A similar study by Hermosillo and colleagues showed that HRV was higher in patients with a patent infarct-related artery, but whether the ejection fraction was also higher in these patients was not examined.[14]

Cardiac autonomic innervation is neither symmetrical nor uniform, and shows transmural differences.[15] In cats, coronary occlusion evokes cardiovascular reflexes which strongly reflect these differences.[16,17]

In humans, however, the infarct site does not appear to have an independent effect on the relationship between the ejection fraction and HRV.[6] Therefore, there is no consistent relationship between the ejection fraction and HRV probably because the extent to which the ejection fraction reflects ventricular dysfunction and correlates with hemodynamic and neurohumoral changes is particularly sensitive to the population studied and the experimental conditions. Nevertheless, the indices may be seen as complementary indices of ventricular function, particularly early after myocardial infarction and in patients in chronic heart failure. The effect of treatment on these indices and on the relationship between them may explain the improvement in prognosis when patients in chronic heart failure are treated with angiotensin converting enzyme inhibitors[18] and the relatively high mortality associated with oral inotrope therapy in these patients.[19] Drugs which produce an improvement in both the ejection fraction and HRV may be safer than those which cause an increase in the ejection fraction at the expense of a decline in HRV.

References

1. Karlsberg RP, Penkoske PA, Cryer PE, et al. Rapid activation of the sympathetic nervous system following coronary occlusions: relationship to infarct size, site and haemodynamic impact. Cardiovasc Res 1979; 13:523-529.

2. Rich MW, Saini JS, Kleiger RE, et al. Correlation of heart rate variability with clinical and angiographic variables and late mortality after coronary angiography. Am J Cardiol 1988; 62:714-717.

3. Kienzle MG, Ferguson DW, Birkett CL, et al. Clinical, hemodynamic and sympathetic neural correlates of heart rate variability in congestive heart failure. Am J Cardiol 1992; 69:761-767.

4. Nolan J, Flapan AD, Capewell S, et al. Decreased cardiac parasympathetic activity in chronic heart failure and its relation to left ventricular function. Br Heart J 1992; 67(6):482-485.

5. Stein KM, Borer JS, Hochreiter C, et al. Prognostic value and physiological correlates of heart rate variability in chronic severe mitral regurgitation. Circulation 1993; 88(1):127-135.

6. Casolo GC, Stroder P, Signorini C, et al. Heart rate variability during the acute phase of myocardial infarction. Circulation 1992; 85:2073-2079.

7. Kleiger RE, Miller JP, Bigger JT, et al. Decreased heart rate variability and its association with increased mortality after acute myocardial infarction. Am J Cardiol 1987; 59:256-262.

8. Farrell TG, Bashir Y, Cripps T, et al. Risk stratification for arrhythmic events in post-infarction patients based on heart rate variability, ambulatory electrocardiographic variables and the signal-averaged electrocardiogram. J Am Coll Cardiol 1991; 18:687-697.

9. Lombardi F, Sandrone G, Pernpruner S, et al. Heart rate variability as an index of sympathovagal interaction after acute myocardial infarction. Am J Cardiol 1987; 60:1239-1245.

10. Odemuyiwa O, Malik M, Farrell TG, et al. A comparison of the predictive characteristics of heart rate variability and left ventricular ejection fraction for all-cause mortality, arrhythmic events and sudden death after acute myocardial infarction. Am J Cardiol 1991; 64:434-439.

11. Cigarroa RG, Lange RA, Hillis LD. Prognosis after acute myocardial infarction in patients with and without residual anterograde coronary blood flow. Am J Cardiol 1989; 64:155-160.

12. Glamann DB, Lange RA, Hillis LD. Beneficial effect of long-term beta blockade after acute myocardial infarction in patients without anterograde flow in the infarct artery. Am J Cardiol 1991; 68:150-154.

13. Odemuyiwa O, Jordaan P, Malik M, et al. Autonomic correlates of late infarct artery patency after first myocardial infarction. Am Heart J 1993; 125:1597-1600.

14. Hermosillo AG, Dorado M, Casanova JM, et al. Influence of infarct-related artery patency on the indexes of parasympathetic activity and prevalence of late potentials in survivors of acute myocardial infarction. J Am Coll Cardiol 1993; 22:695-706.

15. Zipes DP. Influence of myocardial ischaemia and infarction on autonomic innervation of heart. Circulation 1990; 82:1095-1105.

16. Corr PB, Pearle DL, Hinton JR, et al. Site of myocardial infarction. A determinant of the cardiovascular changes induced in the cat by coronary occlusion. Circ Res 1976; 39:840-847.

17. Thames MD, Klopfenstein HS, Abboud FM, et al. Preferential distribution of inhibitory cardiac receptors with vagal afferents to the inferoposterior wall of the left ventricle activated during coronary occlusion in the dog. Circ Res 1978; 43:512-519.

18. Flapan AD, Nolan J, Neilson JM, et al. Effect of captopril on cardiac parasympathetic activity in chronic cardiac failure secondary to coronary artery disease. Am J Cardiol 1992; 69(5):532-535.

19. Feldman AM, Bristow MR, Parmley WW, et al. Effects of Vesnarinone on morbidity and mortality in patients with heart failure. N Engl J Med 1993; 329:149-155.

Chapter 20

Effects of Physical and Mental Exercise on Heart Rate Variability

Massimo Pagani, Daniela Lucini, Ornella Rimoldi, Raffaello Furlan, Simona Piazza, Luca Biancardi

Introduction

In humans and in conscious animals, organized behavior involving either physical or mental activity, initiates complex adjustments in circulatory control, that aim at an appropriate matching with the new peripheral demands and are mediated mostly by the autonomic nervous system.

It is well recognized that the disparate patterns of increased heart rate (HR), myocardial contractility, cardiac output, arterial pressure (AP) and appropriate peripheral blood flow distribution depend upon an autonomic control shifted towards sympathetic predominance [1,2] in a dynamic interaction with the changing humoral milieu. However, the exact details and reciprocal timing of the changes in sympathetic and vagal activity are still a matter for investigation. For instance, it is debated whether changes in either autonomic branch occur simultaneously or are out of phase. Recent studies in conscious animals indicate that during exercise, sympathetic excitation occurs very early, and can be already clearly observed during the initial phase of activity.[3] On the contrary, the majority of available studies in humans maintain that initially, with light levels of activity, the autonomic response is characterized by vagal withdrawal, which is only later followed by sympathetic arousal, when exercise reaches higher intensity levels.[4-6] However, clinical studies on autonomic control may be limited, as they frequently use intermittent determinations, and do not address simultaneously both sympathetic and vagal mechanisms. Furthermore, sympathetic activity is assessed with procedures such as the determination of plasma catecholamines[7] or recordings of the electrical activity of sympathetic nerve fibers from peripheral nerves[8] to the muscles or to the skin which are invasive, and might thus add a variable amount of physiological 'noise,' as a consequence of fear or pain. Finally, these measures, in view of the discrete nature of effer-

From: Malik M., Camm AJ (eds.): *Heart Rate Variability*. Armonk, NY. Futura Publishing Company, Inc., © 1995.

ent sympathetic innervation, might only partially represent cardiac control.[9]

The capacity of mental factors to modify bodily functions and well-being has attracted attention since ancient times. For instance, in classic Greece, alteration in the regularity of chest motion, which either *jumped* or *trembled*, were considered forerunners of various emotional levels.[10] About 30 years ago, Goldie and Green [11] reported that alterations in the respiratory pattern were indeed early and sensitive indicators of changes in the level of arousal.

A more detailed study of the relationship between plains of arousal and cardiovascular control mechanisms in behaving animals and individuals required several methodological advancements.[12] The possibility to assess the activity of the autonomic nervous system at a distance, continuously and not intermittently, and without disturbing the experimental subject was a preliminary methodological step. Additionally, the experimental context and its theoretical model, usually addressed with the ill-defined concept of stress, required a better characterization. The major drawback of traditional approaches derived from the fundamental circular nature of the quantitative assessment of the stress levels, which is based upon the subject's self-appraisal.[13]

In this chapter, we address the changes in heart rate variability (HRV) occurring in response to either physical or mental activity, considering separately acute responses from long-term effects. Following the model of a sympatho-vagal (Figure 1) balance in cardiovascular control,[14,15] we shall focus on autoregressive spectral analysis of RR interval variability as a means to obtain noninvasively quantitative indices of underlying changes in autonomic control of the sinoatrial (SA) node (see chapter 14).[16] Briefly, with the approach used in our laboratory, and utilizing normalized units, the low frequency (LF) component of RR interval variability (LFRR) provides a marker of sympathetic modulation of the SA node: conversely, the high-frequency (HF), respiratory-related component (HFRR) is a marker of vagal activity; finally, the LF/HF ratio is a convenient synthetic index of the changes in the sympatho-vagal balance. Since a multivariate approach is frequently helpful to clarify the complex modifications occurring in response to either physical or mental tasks, we will outline, as well, key findings obtained with the simultaneous analysis of systolic arterial pressure (SAP) and of respiration.[17] We shall summarize above all experimental results obtained in our laboratory where we employ various types of standardized physical or mental stimuli, which will henceforth be indicated as *physical* or *mental exercises*.

Methodology

Since initial studies,[18] we followed the main hypothesis that a model of neurovisceral control of the circulation based on the concept of sympatho-vagal balance, coupled with a quantitative assessment of the spontaneous oscillatory components hidden in the cardiovascular variability signals, would provide quantitative markers of the attendant sympathetic and vagal modulatory activity.[14-16] Compared with other techniques used to explore autonomic control, spectral analysis of heart period variability is unique since it provides an opportunity to examine continuously the reciprocal changes in sympathetic and vagal modulation, not only at rest but also in dynamic conditions. The use of radiotelemetric techniques to obtain the electrocardiogram (ECG) and respiratory signals at a distance with minimal disturbance to the subject also permits the monitoring of extreme situations, such as running in the field [1] or human space missions.[19]

In dynamic conditions, the values of hemodynamic parameters are greatly different from those observed at rest. Hence, the analogue to digital acquisition, mathematical manipulation of data, and subsequent interpretation of results of spectral analysis require specific considerations. It is a rule of thumb to increase the frequency

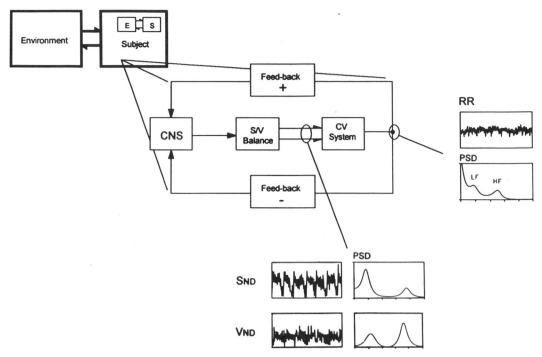

Figure 1. Schematic outline of the circular relationship between *environment* and *subject* (top left), as can be used to model the effects of real life stimuli on neural control of the circulation. The presence of a subjective representation of the relationship within the *subject* is alluded to by the small inset. The blown up schema (center) refers to the presence of both positive and negative feedback circuits in cardiovascular neural control mechanisms. The continuous dynamic balance between sympathetic and vagal control activities (S/V balance) determines beat-by-beat end-organ performance. In both sympathetic (SND) and vagal (VND) nerve traffic (center bottom) spectral analysis discloses the presence of simultaneous LF and HF components, paralleling the occurrence of two major similar components in the RR variability signal (far right), which provide quantitative information on the state of the sympatho-vagal balance. Modified from Pagani et al[12] and Malliani et al.[15]

of the acquisition process whenever the pulse interval is reduced, in order to minimize the variance of the subsequent determination of the RR interval variability series. In our laboratory we observed that an acquisition rate of 300 samples/seconds per channel is adequate at rest, and twice that frequency is usually sufficient in the case of high HRs, around 120 to 130 beats per minute. Increasing the acquisition rate enhances the accuracy of the determination of the fiducial point, ie, the peak of the R wave, which may be further refined by the additional procedure of parabolic interpolation, leading to a better signal to noise ratio. This improvement may prove crucial in conditions, such as with submaximal treadmill exercise in man, when RR interval variance

may be reduced from control resting values of about 2000 to as little as 40 millisecond,[2] and only less than 50% of this variability is concentrated in the LF and HF components.[20] On the contrary, AP variability increases during exercise (from values of about 30 mm Hg^2 at rest to about 100 mm Hg^2 during exercise[21]). Consequently, the accuracy in the determination of absolute values, in this specific instance, may not be as critical. In dynamic conditions, it is crucial to avoid motion artifacts, and the frequency distortion typical of fluid filled catheters in order to perform adequately subsequent spectral analysis. For this reason in man, when undergoing submaximal treadmill exercise, we employ a high-fidelity system based on a # 3 Millar microtip

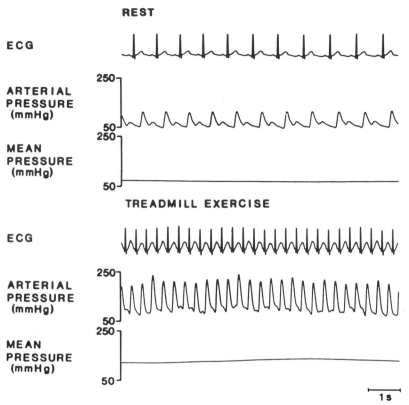

Figure 2. Example of high-fidelity systemic AP recording obtained with a #3 Micro tip Millar transducer previously inserted percutaneously through the radial artery. Notice the absence of artifacts even during strenuous treadmill exercise (Bruce protocol, stage 4). Reproduced with permission from Furlan et al.[23]

transducer, which provides clean AP signals up to the stage 4 of Bruce protocol (Figure 2).[22,23]

The use of high-fidelity techniques is also critical in the study of dynamic exercise in conscious dogs.[24] In this case a solid state pressure gauge is implanted chronically in the left ventricular cavity. From the left ventricular pressure signal a threshold algorithm computes the beat-by-beat series of interdiastolic time intervals (Figure 3). The differences with the ECG derived interval series is small and can be disregarded in the subsequent computation. On the contrary, a more considerable error in the computation is added when using the intersystolic series to obtain the tachogram.

Considering, in more detail, specific aspects of physical and mental exercise, it is important to point out that these two conditions are not completely different in nature,

but they are to some extent intertwined. Obviously, the stress of physical exercise, such as running, involves, massively, the musculoskeletal system, but an activated central drive is also present.[25] On the other hand, mental calculations or stressful interviews, typical examples of mental exercise, entail a moderate level of muscular engagement as well. The respiratory pattern is altered both during physical and mental exercise, although in a quite different manner.[26] Studies should also consider the gradual nature of the changes from resting to exercise conditions. In our laboratory we have conveniently reduced this complexity by defining, somehow arbitrarily, standardized experimental conditions.

To this end, in addressing the autonomic effects of **physical exercise** we consider:

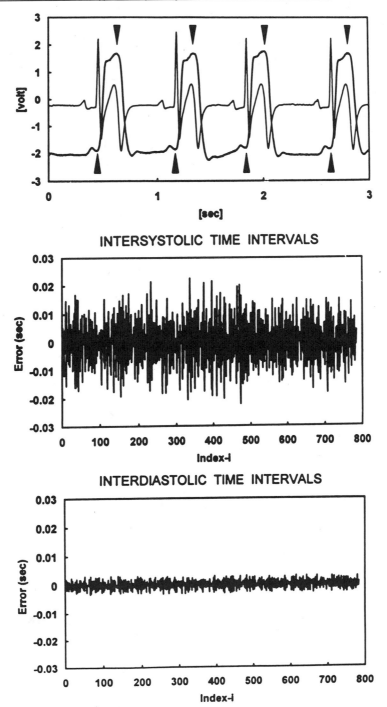

Figure 3. Example of the technique employed to obtain the pulse-interval series, ie, tachogram, from the left ventricle pressure (LVP) in conscious dogs. The top panel depicts the simultaneously recorded ECG and LVP signals. The mid panel displays the beat-by-beat difference between the ECG derived tachogram and the interval series obtained from LVP, using peak systolic values as fiducial points: notice the large values of this error. On the contrary, the error is trivial when the intervals are computed taking the end-diastolic values as fiducial points (bottom panel).

1. the amount of muscular involvement, ie, small or large muscular masses[27];
2. the type of physical activity, ie, tonic or phasic[27];
3. the subject's position, ie, recumbent or upright[14,15];
4. the frequency, intensity, and duration of the physical task [28];
5. the short- and long-term aftereffects[29,30]; and
6. the adequacy and limitations of the technique.[22,31,32]

Likewise, to address the neurovisceral effects of **mental exercise**[33] it is important:

1. to consider separately subjective (ie, self-report) from objective (ie, measurable) components of behavior[12];
2. to define explicitly and from an operational point of view the context and the environment,[13] the type of task,[34] ie, silent or talking,[35] or the additional involvement of a factor of human confrontation,[36] as it happens during interviews[35] or with mental arithmetic[12,37]; and
3. to address the time resolution and the sensitivity of the technique employed, as well as any potential direct influence upon the study subject.[12]

Physical Exercise

Small Muscular Masses

Dynamic or static handgrip represents a simple, convenient type of exercise involving only a small fraction of muscular masses, while still inducing sizeable changes in cardiovascular performance. As an additional advantage, this type of exercise can be performed also with the subjects lying motionless in bed. Electroneurographic recordings obtained from nerves directed to peripheral muscles or to the skin provided clear-cut evidence that handgrip induces a marked increase in sympathetic traffic simultaneously with an increase in AP and a slight tachycardia.[8,38] Data indicated that the local release of metabolites is an important contributory factor to this efferent sympathetic excitation. Typically, this excitation appeared shortly after the initiation of exercise, and gradually increased in parallel with the effort intensity.

Spectral analysis of heart period variability could provide a methodological advantage, as it furnishes a simultaneous assessment of both sympathetic and vagal control mechanisms directly modulating the SA node. Additionally, the use of multivariate approaches provides indices of the changes in sympathetic efferent vasomotor activity (as assessed by the power of the LF component of SAP variability[15]) and of the baroreflex control of HR (as assessed by the frequency-domain index α).[39] With the available algorithms, requiring a stationary period of several hundred beats length (at least about 200 to 300 beats) for analysis, it is possible to obtain consistent results from the majority of subjects with 3- to 5-minute recordings of static, or dynamic (which is less demanding) handgrip at 25% to 30% of maximum effort. It is not customary to obtain adequate data with efforts of greater intensity.

An example of the time- and frequency-domain effects of both dynamic and static handgrip, performed at 25% of maximum effort, is depicted in Figures 4A-B.[40] It is apparent that the static stimulus is more effective than the dynamic one in inducing a slight reduction in RR interval and a clear increase in AP. Respiration, as well, appears more evidently stimulated in the former case. Data from an ongoing study (n = 60, age 31±1 years, Lucini et al, unpublished data) indicate that overall RR interval and its variance do not increase significantly during both dynamic and static handgrip. Spectral analysis shows an increase in LF_{RR} (from 53±2 to 66±2 normalized units, [nu]) and LF_{SAP} (from 5.2±0.6 to 8.7\$±1.0 mm Hg^2) which is well apparent with the static

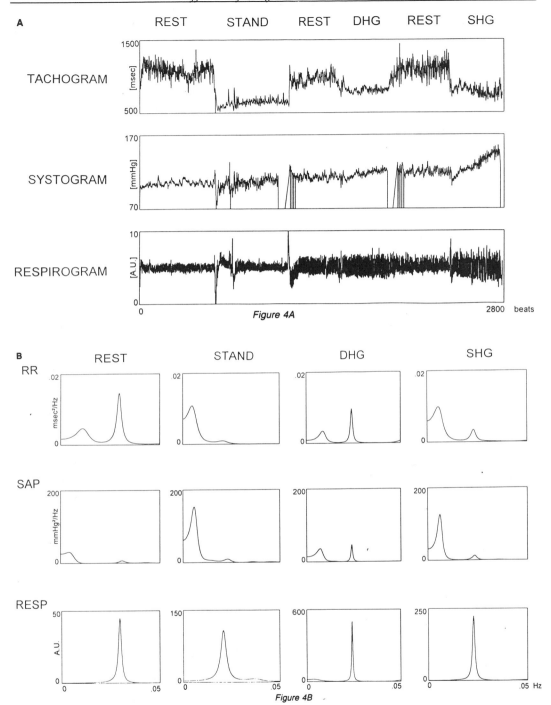

Figures 4A-B. Example of the effects of standing up (STAND), and of dynamic (DHG) and static (SHG) handgrip at 25% of maximal effort on time series of RR interval (TACHOGRAM), SAP (SYSTOGRAM) variability, and of respiration (RESPIROGRAM) in a young healthy volunteer (part A). Part B represents the corresponding spectra: notice the clear predominance of the LF component in the tachogram and systogram spectra during STAND and SHG. A respiratory activation is apparent during both DHG and SHG (notice the change in scale).

stimulus. These changes parallel the known attendant augmention of sympathetic activity.[8,38] Of interest is the simultaneous reduction in the HFRR component, a finding which suggests that vagal modulation is reduced as well during this type of moderate physical exercise. To infer the attendant neural adjustments, the interpretation of the results should consider the engagement of other control mechanisms, such as the likely increase in baroreceptor reflex buffer activity induced by the augmented pressure load (SAP rose from 116 ± 1 to 136 ± 2 mm Hg).[41] The illustration also depicts the condition of standing, which provides a comparison with an experimental stimulus, leading to a marked shift of the autonomic balance towards sympathetic predominance.[14,15] We collected preliminary data in patients indicating that the changes in spectral markers of neural control of the heart period produced by handgrip may be blunted in disparate clinical conditions, such as in arterial hypertension[42] or during the convalescence from a prior myocardial infarction.[35]

Large Muscular Masses

The stress of dynamic physical exercise, either on a bicycle or on a treadmill, is routinely employed in clinical practice to detect the presence of myocardial ischemia, or to assess cardiac functional reserve capacity. Usually incremental standardized protocols are followed, until a specific target HR response or clinically relevant endpoints are reached. During exercise the circulatory system is stimulated to near maximum[1-6] by means of increased sympathetic and reduced vagal activity. Dynamic exercise is usually performed in the upright position on a treadmill,[20] or sitting up in the case of a bicycle ergometer.[43-46] Both conditions, even before the initiation of the exercise, are characterized by an autonomic balance already shifted towards sympathetic predominance,[15,47] an observation which should be taken into account when defining the control pre-exercise state.[20,43,46]

With intense physical exercise, HR rises up to 200 bpm, a rate which is associated to a marked abatement of RR variance, thus the absolute power (in milliseconds^2) of spectral components appears also drastically reduced (see Table 1). During high-intensity exercise there is an increase of non-stationarity and nonlinearity in the RR variability signal (see Methodology) which further handicaps the subsequent analysis, and specific algorithms have been proposed for these extreme conditions, such as Coarse Graining Spectral Analysis.[31]

Figures 5A-B clearly highlights the key features of RR variability during treadmill exercise[20]: a drastic reduction in total power, which is evident as soon as stage 2 of Bruce protocol, (see also Table 1). With increasing effort, however, the reduced variance approaches the limit of resolution of the system. The autospectrum detects the presence of very small HF components. These have been considered evidence of non-neural influences on RR interval variability spectra.[45]

The simultaneous assessment, with high-fidelity techniques of SAP variability indicates, at variance with RR interval, an increase in total power during exercise.[20,21] In keeping with the known enhancement of sympathetic drive, there is also a clear increase of the LF component as compared with clinostatic rest, both at the initial[20,21] and final stages of exercise.[48] The presence of two HF components in SAP variability spectra is apparent at stage 4 of the Bruce protocol (Figure 5). The simultaneous analysis of respiration and of step frequency (not shown in the illustration) indicates that these two non-neural phenomena are transferred, as well, as individual peaks in the variability signal.

During the higher levels of exercise there is a marked engagement of respiration, with an increasing frequency and depth of ventilation (from 12.5 ± 1.2 to 61.5 ± 3.4 L/min in a study by Bernardi et al).[45] Additionally, exercising muscles shift towards anaerobic metabolism and lactate production.[49] These additional confunding factors, as well as previous considerations,

Table 1
Changes in Time and Frequency Domain Measures of RR Interval Variability

Variable	Orthostatic Position[a]	Physical Exercise[b] Light	Heavy	Mental Exercise[c]
RR	↓	↓↓	↓↓	↓
σ^2	~	↓↓	↓↓↓	~
VLF%	~	↑	↑↑	~
LF msec^2	~↑	↓↓	↓↓↓ (?)	↑
LF nu	↑↑	↑↑	↓↓ (?)	↑↑
HF msec^2	↓	↓↓	↓↓↓ (?)	↓
HF nu	↓↓	↓↓	↓↓ (?)	↓↓
LF/HF	↑↑	↑↑	~ (?)	↑↑

a) data from passive tilt[14] or active standing[47]; b) data from humans[20] and conscious dogs[20,41]; c) data from.[35,37] (?) During heavy dynamic exercise the extreme reduction of variance might render the process of spectral analysis inappropriate or meaningless.

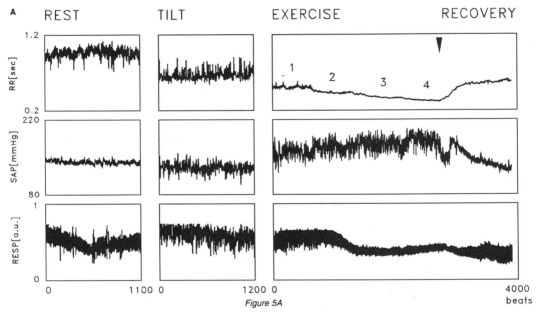

Figure 5A

indicate that at the moment, available models and algorithms cannot be used confidently to infer from the RR variability signals the state of the sympatho-vagal balance during maximal exercise, and that they are adequate only with light and moderate levels of physical activity.

Given the incremental nature of the complex changes induced by dynamic exercise on cardiovascular variabilities and on respiration, a different approach would be to focus only on small as opposed to high levels of intensity such as with simple walking.[50] This experimental approach would

lead to an increase in sympathetic (and decrease in vagal) drive in absence of the confounders indicated above. Additionally, the gravity factor should also be explicitly addressed, as the upright posture, before exercise already shifts the spectral powers towards the LF component.

We are currently investigating the effects of mild incremental levels of exercise, performed in the recumbent position, using a bicycle ergometer, since this avoids the confounding effect of the simultaneous engagement of gravitational mechanisms. Figure 6 depicts an example of the effects of

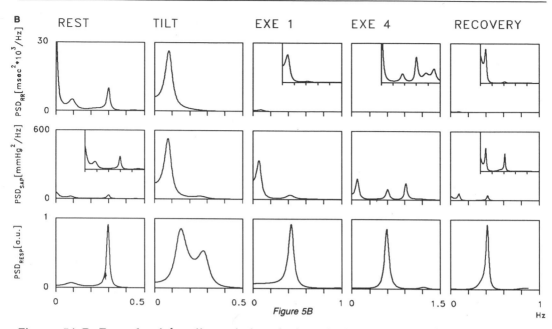

Figures 5A-B. Example of the effects of tilt and of treadmill exercise, at light (EXE1, stage 2 of Bruce protocol) and heavy loads (EXE4, stage 4 of Bruce protocol) on the time series of RR interval, SAP and of respiration (RESP). AP was obtained with a high-fidelity approach, using a #3 Micro tip Millar transducer, advanced through the radial artery (part A). The corresponding autospectra are depicted in part B. Note the marked reduction of total power of RR interval variability with exercise and recovery (magnified insets are shown: x30 at EXE 1; x3000 at EXE 4; x100 at Recovery). However, during EXE1 a clear LF predominance is apparent, as well as during recovery. During intense exercise (EXE4), the variability signal is almost abolished, and the autospectra shows only HF components, of very small amplitude. Conversely, the autospectra of SAP demonstrate during tilt and during EXE1 and EXE4 a predominant LF component. In this latter case, however, two additional HF peaks are apparent: one is synchronous with respiration, and the one with the highest center frequency corresponds to the step frequency. (Magnified insets, at both Rest and Recovery, are x6).

mild levels of incremental exercise (up to 75 W) on RR interval variability. A shift in spectral powers towards a marked LF predominance is apparent, since the initial very low level of 25 W. This finding, in accordance with prior experimental investigations,[3] indicates an early, as opposed to late, increase in sympathetic activity, which, importantly, is simultaneous to a reduction in vagal activity. An attendant stimulation of respiration is also indicated by the simultaneous quantitative analysis of respiratory movements.[51]

The experimental examination of the effects of exercise on heart period variability in conscious dogs confirms the induction of a marked prevalence of LF component also in this model.[20,41] Analysis of SAP variability discloses, along with a prevailing LF com-

ponent, the presence of mechanical disturbances at the respiratory frequency. At 4 km/h of run a clear component, at a frequency higher than respiration is apparent, which is likely to underscore the mechanical effects of running (Figures 7A-B), as it happens in man (see Figure 5).[48]

In summary, with the exclusion of heavy levels of exercise both in man and dogs, and duly considering the attendant engagement of other factors such as gravity and baroreflex mechanisms, it appears that the use of spectral analysis of RR interval variability and of nu permits the exploration of the simultaneous changes in sympathetic and vagal balance induced by mild levels of exercise.

On the contrary, the use of preselected bands of interest and absolute units to as-

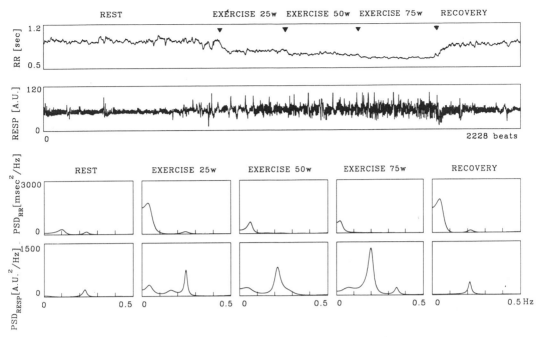

Figure 6. Example of the effects on RR interval variability and on respiration, of stepwise bicycle exercise, performed in the recumbent position, at moderate intensity (approximately 30% of max theoretical effort for age and sex).

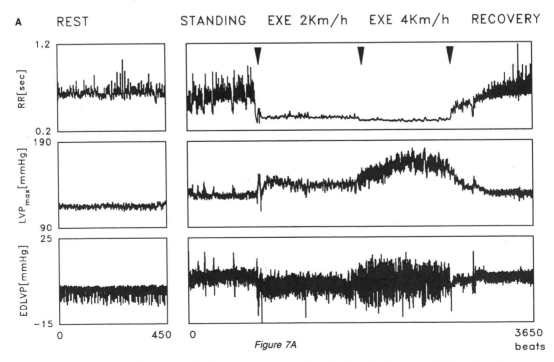

sess spectral powers[44] are not adequate to infer cardiac control.[15] It might also be added that the use of multiparametric approaches, with the simultaneous recording and analysis of other variability signals such as AP and respiration, permits a more complete assessment of the exercise-induced changes in cardiovascular control mecha-

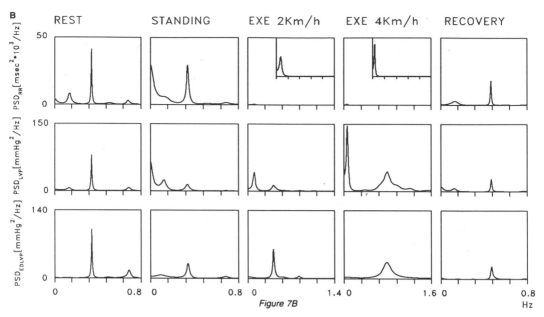

Figures 7A-B. Example of the effects of standing and treadmill exercise (2 and 4 km/h, 0° incline) on time series of RR interval, left ventricle systolic pressure (LVP max, from an implanted solid state pressure gauge) variability and of respiration (assessed by end diastolic LVP) (part A). The corresponding autospectra (PSD) are depicted in part B. Notice the magnified insets in the PSDRR during EXE (ordinate scale, x50). A largely prevailing LF component in both RR and LVP autospectra is evident during exercise. Conversely, a major HF component is shown at rest, owing to the prevailing vagal tone present in this condition in the conscious dog.

nisms, such as the profound reduction in the gain of baroreflex mechanisms.[39]

Aftereffects of Exercise

Hemodynamic studies have clearly delineated that after intense physical exercise of sufficient intensity, the return to control, pre-exercise levels is not immediate, but requires a sizeable amount of time. During this period cardiac function might remain above normal.[29,52]

We have recently addressed[30] this issue in healthy, otherwise sedentary young volunteers subjected to maximal exercise. The shift of the sympatho-vagal balance towards sympathetic predominance induced by this stimulus remained well evident at 1 hour after cessation of the effort, and required more than 24 hours to subside (Figure 8). The presence of enhanced LF/HF ratio shortly after exercise (8 minutes) has also been repeated by Arai et al.[44]

Long-term adaptation to repetitive exercise is more complex to study, since it results from a mix of several factors: biochemical, structural, metabolic, humoral and neural.[30] Additional modulatory influences derive from genetic components, the age of the subject, the intensity of the exercise training routine, and the simultaneous presence of short time after effects from the previous day's activity.

Thus, in athletes examined during their 1-month period of yearly rest,[30] spectral analysis of RR variability demonstrated, along with the expected training bradycardia, a prevailing HF component. This finding was in keeping with the known potentiation of vagal mechanisms induced by long-term athletic training.[53]

Surprisingly, during the yearly season of activity and competition, we observed a paradoxical prevalence of LF[30] in resting heart period variability spectra. We have ascribed this finding to a sympathetic over-

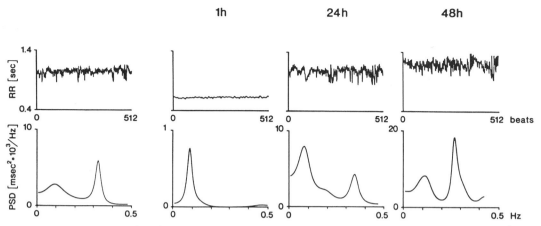

Figure 8. Example of the changes in RR interval variability (upper panels) and corresponding autospectra (lower panels) at control (left) and following a session of maximal dynamic exercise in a control subject. Time after cessation of exercise is indicated at the top. Changes in the total power during different experimental conditions are reflected by the different ordinate scales in the autospectra. At 24 hours after the interruption of exercise, the spectral profile is characterized by predominance of the LF component, while the mean RR interval has returned to control value. Only after 48 hours postexercise does the autospectrum reach a pattern similar to control conditions. Reproduced with permission from Furlan et al.[30]

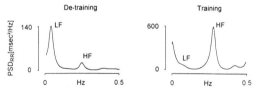

Figure 9. Effect of aerobic training on RR interval variability spectra in a patient with congestive heart failure. Notice the power shift towards HF in the trained state, indicating a vagal predominance. Modified from Coats et al.[55]

activity resulting from the aftereffects of the previous day's heavy routine of training on cardiac control mechanisms.

Long-term physical training could lead to beneficial changes of hemodynamics and control mechanisms, which might be of clinical relevance, eg, lowering AP in essential hypertension,[39] increasing baroreflex gain in subjects with ischemic heart disease[54] and improving exercise tolerance together with increasing vagal drive in congestive heart failure[55] (Figure 9). In a study on mild hypertensive subjects[39] who underwent a 6-month aerobic training program, we observed at rest, together with a slight reduction in AP,

a reduction in normalized LF_{RR} and an increase in HF_{RR} powers. Additionally, we found an increase in the baroreflex slope and in the index α, a frequency-domain index of baroreflex gain. Therefore, the complex autonomic adjustments induced by long-term physical training can be quantitatively assessed with monovariate and multivariate spectral analysis of cardiovascular variability in the clinical setting.

Mental Exercise

Experimental investigations on the effects of behavioral and mental factors on heart period variability can be traced to the initial studies employing spectral analysis of RR variability.[56] The use of a simple Fast Fourier Transform (FFT) approach, the subdivision of the spectrum in preselected bands without a normalization procedure,[14-16] and the attention, frequently, only to HRV signals, led to inconsistent results.[57] In particular, the capacity of the spectral analytical approach to detect the increase in sympathetic activity produced by mental activity was questioned.[58]

In our laboratory we have developed a specific approach as part of an integrated, ongoing research on the influence of mental factors on cardiovascular physiopathology.[12]

The methodology is based upon a continuous radiotelemetry of ECG and respiratory signals.[51] The subsequent use of spectral analysis of RR variability[14-16] allows the quantification of the changing dynamics of the sympatho-vagal balance. Furthermore, with this method respiratory activity can also be assessed in terms of amplitude, frequency and nonlinear dynamics.[12] Finally, specific and explicit attention to the context allowed us to avoid the issue of autoreferenciality.[13]

In fact, the subjective components of emotionally charged behaviors or situations are simply not considered, while they are substituted by the quantitative relationship between changes in environmental variables and physiological parameters (Figure 1). In doing so, visceral components and their control mechanisms, become, themselves, behavior.[59]

In order to minimize the emotional impact of the instrumentation on the subjects, recordings are performed in a laboratory which has the appearance of a normal office with no medical instrumentation in sight. A one-way mirror, and a closed-circuit TV allow continuous observation of the experimental room.

As shown in the example of Figure 10A-B referring to a human subject,[12] routinely we record ECG and respiration (by radiotelemetry) and noninvasive AP (with a Finapres device).

Usually we consider two tasks: the IKT and mental arithmetic (Figure 10). The IKT is a reaction time task, developed and tested in the University of Giessen,[34] which entails the use of a computer device, set to maintain the error rate of the subjects at 50%. The IKT is performed by leaving the subject alone. The mental arithmetic task consists of having the subject perform a sequential subtraction of a one- or two-digit number

from a four-digit number (usually 7 or 17 from 1001) as fast as possible.[37] One investigator is present, pressing the subject to increase his pace of computation. Thus, mental arithmetic entails the additional factor of human confrontation.[36]

With the IKT, we consistently observed an increase in AP, a slight tachycardia, and a modest shift of the spectral distribution towards the LF component which was clear only in healthy controls. Mental arithmetic induced more marked changes, that were apparent both in controls and patients.[60]

As reported in the example of Figure 10, mental arithmetic causes a clear shift of the spectral balance towards a predominance of the LF component. This finding, which indicates an enhanced sympathetic modulation and reduced vagal drive to the SA node, can be assessed continously throughout the study period using a recursive algorithm (Figure 11).[61] Simultaneously [22,23] using high-fidelity AP recordings, a large increase in the LF component could also be noticed, together with a reduction of the frequency-domain index of baroreflex gain (α).[37]

Since during these laboratory stimuli the study subjects remain essentially motionless, noninvasive AP variability signals, obtained with the Finapres technique (Figure 10), are usually adequate for subsequent spectral analysis, and provide results similar to those obtained with an invasive high-fidelity approach.[37]

The importance of the environment, particularly when perceived as potentially hostile, was addressed in a series of experiments on conscious dogs.[37] When the animals were first brought to the experimental laboratory, which was new to them, and hence they were subjected to a kind of stressful environment, a quite large LF component was present both in RR interval and SAP variability signals (Figure 12). Vice versa, when the animals had become fully acquainted with the laboratory environment and personnel, the autospectra of both RR interval and SAP variabilities indicated the presence of a largely prevailing HF component. It is noteworthy to recall that during

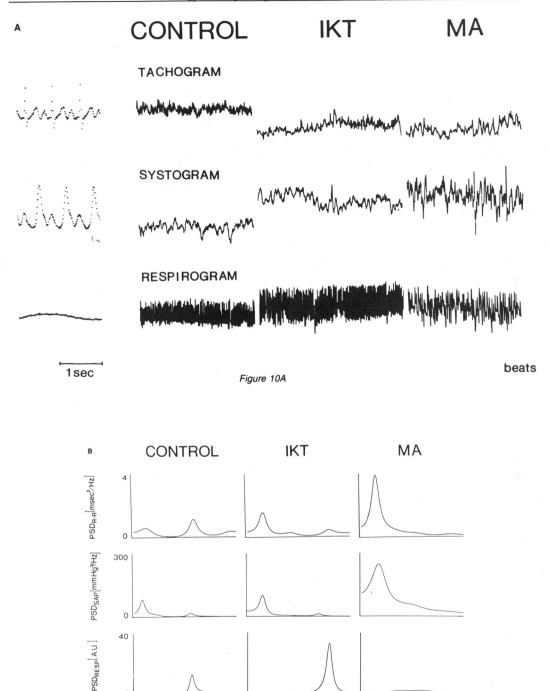

Figures 10A-B. Example of the continuous signal acquisition of ECG, AP (by Finapres) and respiration (by piezoelectric belt) (left panels). The relevant time series (tachogram, systogram and respirogram) are represented in the right panels, for the conditions of CONTROL, IKT, and mental arithmetic (MA). The respective autospectra are represented in part B. Notice the clear increase of the LF component with MA. During this latter the respiratory autospectrum becomes flat and broadened, as a consequence of the altered respiratory pattern present during talking. Reproduced with permission from Pagani et al.[12]

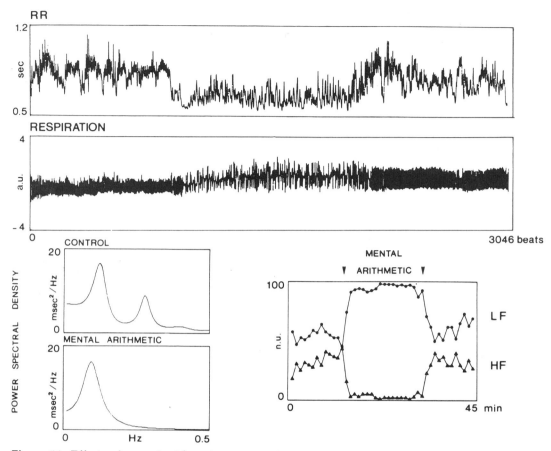

Figure 11. Effects of mental arithmetic on spectral analysis of RR variability. Top panels represent the continuous series of RR intervals (top tracing) and of respiration (bottom tracing). Note the reduction of RR interval values during mental arithmetic. The bottom part of the figure depicts (left panels) the autospectra of RR interval variability at control (top) and during mental arithmetic (bottom). The right panel shows a continuous representation of the power of the LF and HF components of RR variability during control, mental arithmetic and recovery. Reproduced with permission from Pagani et al.[61]

the stressful condition the respiratory pattern was markedly altered and characterized by a clear tachypnea.

We have also been exploring the sympathetic responsiveness to mental stimuli in pathophysiological conditions. We have observed a reduced responsiveness to mental challenges in both hypertensive subjects[60] and patients that were recovering from a recent (about 3-weeks old) acute myocardial infarction.[35] A blunting of the effects of mental stress on RR variability spectra has also been observed in the aged.[62] These results, therefore, extend to mental stimuli the reduced responsiveness of the

sympatho-vagal balance previously observed for physical stimuli in the same clinical conditions.[15] Signs of reduced vagal modulation of the SA node, correlated to enhanced pressor responses to mental challenges, were reported in coronary artery patients.[63] This observation provides additional support to the proposed link between stress,[64] autonomic cardiac control and coronary pathophysiology.

Long-Term Effects

The importance of subjective components in defining clinical outcomes of treat-

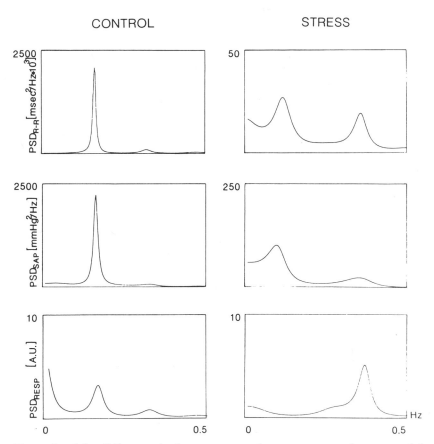

Figure 12. Example of the difference in the autospectra between a control nonstressful condition, and a condition characterized by situational stress in a conscious dog. Notice the presence of a single major respiratory component in the control condition, and the appearance of a large LF component, in the autospectra of both RR and SAP variability in the stressful condition. Reproduced with permission from Pagani et al.[37]

ment, the interest in nonpharmacological approaches, the possibility that mental factors might be instrumental not only in acute but also in chronic cardiovascular events justify attention to long-term effects of mental exercise and stress. The latter may be important in the context of a chronically elevated sympathetic overactivity as a contributory component to long-term conditions such as atherosclerosis[65] or hypertension.[66]

Following these lines, and employing spectral analysis we have addressed the hypothesis that a prevailing sympathetic activity might be present in essential hypertension.

In a study[67] comparing hypertensive patients with normotensive age matched controls, it was found that in RR variability

under resting conditions, LF was greater and HF smaller in hypertensive patients, suggesting an enhanced sympathetic activity and a reduced vagal activity. In hypertensive patients, passive tilt produced smaller increases in LF and decreases in HF than in normotensive controls. Furthermore, the values of LF at rest and the altered effects of tilt on LF and HF were significantly correlated with the degree of the hypertensive state, suggesting a continuum distribution.

When RR variability was studied throughout the 24-hour period[68] with the use of Holter recordings, patients with essential hypertension were characterized by the loss of the circadian rhythmicity of the LF component (Figure 13), whereas a small

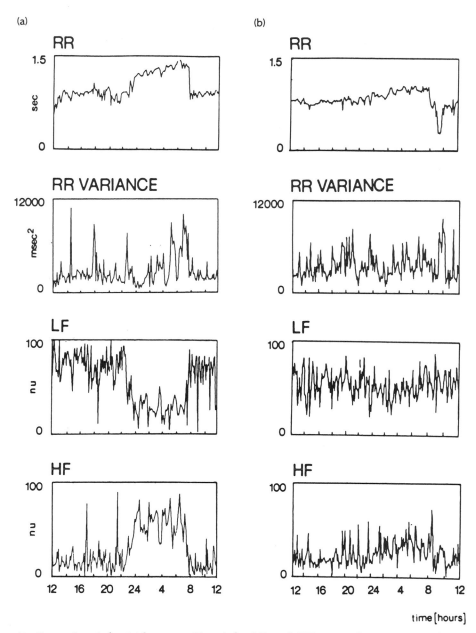

Figure 13. Example of the 24-hour profile of the LF and HF spectral components from Holter recordings in a normotensive (left) and hypertensive (right) ambulant subject. Notice that a clear circadian variation in both LF and HF components (in nu) is present only in the normotensive subject. Reproduced with permission from Guzzetti et al.[68]

nocturnal increase in HF was still detectable. In a study[39] in which both RR and SAP variability were simultaneously assessed, providing the frequency-domain index α of baroreflex gain, we observed that α underwent a clear day-night rhythmicity, with minimal values during the day. The index α

appeared reduced in hypertensive patients examined at rest. A subsequent study[47] indicated that the index α is negatively modulated by physiological increase in sympathetic drive produced by standing up, and it is increased by chronic beta-adrenergic receptor blockade.

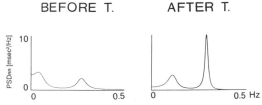

Figure 14. Example of the changes in the spectral profile of RR variability in a young healthy subject, examined at rest before (left) and after (right) a 3-month period of relaxation training (T). Notice the shift towards the HF component of the spectral power induced by training.

It appears that frequency-domain analysis provides a means to quantify in hypertensive patients the disturbance of neural control of the circulation that is characterized by enhanced sympathetic drive and reduced gain of buffer negative feed-back mechanisms. This approach could be coupled to more traditional investigations to address the long-term effects of behavioral factors both in the initiation[69] and in the treatment[70] of cardiovascular diseases. We addressed this possibility with a study (Lucini et al, unpublished data) aimed at verifying if the long-term mental exercise with specific training routines, could beneficially influence autonomic responsiveness to mental challenges. In a group of 13 healthy volunteers we found that a 3-month period of relaxation training leads to reduction at rest of LF component of RR interval variability (Figure 14). Additionally, the increase of the LF component produced by mental arithmetic appeared blunted after relaxation training, a finding which suggests a reduced sympathetic responsiveness. An additional, still little explored area of study, is the link between specific behavioral patterns and given profiles of neural control of the circulation. For in-

stance, subjects with type A personality have been reported to be characterized by signs of predominant sympathetic activity.[71] We have also observed (Pagani et al[72]) that subjects with unexplained fatigue (ie, Chronic Fatigue Syndrome) are characterized by a prevailing LF component at rest, in absence of any laboratory evidence of organic or psychiatric disease.

Conclusion

We have examined various aspects of spectral analysis of RR interval variability, alone or combined with AP variability, considering low and high intensities and different modalities of muscular exercise, both in man and in conscious dogs. Available evidence indicates that with appropriate algorithms, this approach can be used to study the changes in neural control of the circulation occurring with light intensity of effort.

As to mental factors, in the past few years a series of experimental and clinical studies have indicated that spectral analysis of RR variability, in view of its totally noninvasive nature, could be ideally suited to address the complex relationship[72] between the functional state of cardiovascular innervation, cardiovascular responses to behavioral stimuli, and initiation and maintenance of cardiovascular diseases.

This computer approach, by quantifying functional correlates of therapeutic approaches, could provide a convenient means to assess more objectively the clinical usefulness of nonpharmacological regimens, such as long-term training routines, that are based on a combination of both physical and mental exercise and aim at more balanced autonomic cardiac control.

References

1. Vatner SF, Pagani M. Cardiovascular adjustments to exercise: hemodynamics and mechanisms. Prog Cardiovasc Dis 1976; 19:91-108.
2. Mitchell JH, Kaufman MP, Iwamoto GA. The exercise pressor reflex: its cardiovascular effects, afferent mechanisms, and central pathways. Annu Rev Physiol 1983; 45:229-242.
3. Di Carlo SE, Bishop VS. Onset of exercise shifts operating point of arterial baroreflex to higher pressures. Am J Physiol 1992; 262(Heart Circ Physiol 31):H303-H307.
4. Robinson BF, Epstein SE, Beiser GD, et al. Control of heart rate by the autonomic nervous system. Studies in man on the

interrelation between baroreceptor mechanisms and exercise. Circ Res 1966; 19:400-411.

5. Christensen NJ. Sympathetic nervous activity during exercise. Annu Rev Physiol 1983; 45:139-153.

6. Shepherd JT. Circulatory response to exercise in health. Circulation 1987; 76(suppl VI):VI-3.

7. Cousineau D, Ferguson RJ, De Champlain J, et al. Catecholamines in coronary sinus during exercise in man before and after training. J Appl Physiol 1977; 43(5):801-806.

8. Mark AL, Victor RG, Nerhed C, et al. Microneurographic studies of the mechanisms of sympathetic nerve responses to static exercise in humans. Circ Res 1985; 57:461-469.

9. Meredith IT, Friberg P, Jennings GL, et al. Exercise training lowers resting renal but not cardiac sympathetic activity in humans. Hypertension 1991; 18:575-582.

10. Kurath H. The Semantic Sources of the Words for the Emotions in Sanskrit, Greek, Latin, and the Germanic Languages. Menasha, Wis: George Banta Publishing Company, 1921.

11. Goldie L, Green JM. Changes in mode of respiration as an indication of level of awareness. Nature 1961; 189:581-582.

12. Pagani M, Lucini D, De Bernardi F, et al. Mental stress. J Ambulat Monit 1992; 5:235-244.

13. Lazarus RS, Delongis A, Folkman S, et al. Stress and adaptational outcomes. Am Psychol 1985; 40:770-779.

14. Pagani M, Lombardi F, Guzzetti S, et al. Power spectral analysis of heart rate and arterial pressure variabilities as a marker of sympathovagal interaction in man and conscious dog. Circ Res 1986; 59:178-193.

15. Malliani A, Pagani M, Lombardi F, et al. Advances research series: cardiovascular neural regulation explored in the frequency domain. Circulation 1991; 84:482-492.

16. Malliani A. Association of heart rate variability components with physiological regulatory mechanisms. In press.

17. Baselli G, Cerutti S, Civardi S, et al. Cardiovascular variability signals: towards the identification of a closed-loop model of the neural control mechanisms. IEEE Trans Biomed Eng 1988; 35:1033-1046.

18. Brovelli M, Baselli G, Cerutti S, et al. Computerized Analysis for an Experimental Validation of Neurophysiological Models of Heart Rate Control. Computers in Cardiology. Silver Spring, Md: IEEE Computer Society Press, 1983; 205-208.

19. Pagani M. Autonomic adaptation to stress, exercise and space environment. JANS 1993; 43(suppl):S19.

20. Rimoldi O, Furlan R, Pagani MR, et al. Analysis of neural mechanisms accompanying different intensities of dynamic exercise. Chest 1992; 101:226S-230S.

21. Furlan R, Dell'Orto S, Crivellaro W, et al. Effects of tilt and treadmill exercise on short term variability in sytolic arterial pressure in hypertensive men. J Hypertens 1987; 5(suppl 5):S423-S425.

22. Pagani M, Furlan R, Dell'Orto S, et al. Continuous recording of direct height fidelity arterial pressure and electrocardiogram in unrestricted subjects. Cardiovasc Res 1986; 20:384-388.

23. Furlan R, Pagani M, Dell'Orto S, et al. Continuous 24-hour ambulatory recording of systemic and right ventricular pressures. J Ambulat Monit 1993; 6:47-54.

24. Rimoldi O, Pagani MR, Piazza S, et al. Assessement of beat-by-beat respiratory influence on cardiovascular parameters. J Ambulat Monit 1992; 5:56-77.

25. Hajduczok G, Hade JS, Mark AL, et al. Central command increases sympathetic nerve activity during spontaneous locomotion in cats. Circ Res 1991; 69:66-75.

26. Cerutti S, Emdin M, Marchesi C, et al. Workshop on continuous monitoring of respiration: methodological aspects and pathophysiological relevance. J Ambulat Monit 1992; 5:1-264.

27. Balady GJ. Types of exercise. Arm-leg and static-dynamic. Cardiol Clin 1993; 11:297-307.

28. Jones JH. Limits to maximal performance. Annu Rev Physiol 1993; 55:547-569.

29. Coats AJ, Conway J, Isea JE, et al. Systemic and forearm vascular resistance changes after upright bicycle exercise in man. J Physiol 1989; 413:289-298.

30. Furlan R, Piazza S, Dell'Orto S, et al. After effects of exercise and athletic training on neural mechanisms controlling heart period. Cardiovasc Res 1993; 27:482-488.

31. Yamamoto Y, Hughson RL, Peterson JC. Autonomic control of heart rate during exercise studied by heart rate variability spectral analysis. J Appl Physiol 1991; 71:1136-1142.

32. Furlan R, Piazza S, Dell'Orto S, et al. Effects of respiratory activity on heart rate and blood pressure variabilities during physical exercise. J Ambulat Monit 1992; 5:87-94.

33. Herd JA. Cardiovascular response to stress. Physiol Rev 1991; 71:305-330.

34. Kuhman W, Lachnit H, Vaitl D. The quantification of experimental load: methodological and empirical issues. In: Steptoe A, Ruddel

H, Neus H (eds). Clinical and Methodological Issues in Cardiovascular Psychophysiology. Berlin, Germany: Springer-Verlag, 1985; 45-52.

35. Pagani M, Mazzuero G, Ferrari A, et al. Sympathovagal interaction during mental stress. A study using spectral analysis of heart rate variability in healthy control subjects and patients with a prior myocardial infarction. Circulation 1991; 83(suppl II):II-43-II-51.

36. Rozanski A, Bairey CN, Krantz DS, et al. Mental stress and the induction of silent myocardial ischemia in patients with coronary artery disease. N Engl J Med 1988; 318:1005-1012.

37. Pagani M, Rimoldi O, Pizzinelli P, et al. Assessment of the neural control of the circulation during psychological stress. JANS 1991; 35:33-42.

38. Victor RG, Seals DR. Reflex stimulation of sympathetic outflow during rhythmic exercise in humans. Am J Physiol 1989; 257(Heart Cir Physiol 26):H2017-2024.

39. Pagani M, Somers V, Furlan R, et al. Changes in autonomic regulation induced by physical training in mild hypertension. Hypertension 1988; 12:600-610.

40. Pagani M, Iellamo F, Pizzinelli P, et al. Adaptational changes in the neural control of cardiorespiratory function in a confined environment: the CNEC # 3 experiment. Proceedings of EXEMSI 1992. In press.

41. Rimoldi O, Pagani MR, Piazza S, et al. Restraining effects of captopril on sympathetic excitatory responses in conscious dogs. A spectral analysis approach. In press.

42. Lucini D, Pagani M, Malliani A. Chronic atenolol blunts the vasomotor sympathetic drive accompanying light dynamic exercise. Eur Heart J 1993; 14(suppl):ii-iv. Abstract.

43. Perini E, Orizio C, Baselli G, et al. The influence of exercise intensity on the power spectrum of heart rate variability. Eur J Appl Physiol 1990; 61:143-148.

44. Arai Y, Saul JP, Albrecht P, et al. Modulation of cardiac autonomic activity during and immediately after exercise. Am J Physiol 1989; 256:H132-H141.

45. Bernardi L, Salvucci F, Suardi P, et al. Evidence for an intrinsic mechanism regulating heart rate variability in transplanted and the intact heart during submaximal dynamic exercise? Cardiovasc Res 1990; 24:969-981.

46. Dixon EM, Kamath MV, McCartney N, et al. Neural regulation of heart rate variability in endurance athletes and sedentary controls. Cardiovasc Res 1992; 26:713-719.

47. Lucini D, Pagani M, Mela GS, et al. Sympathetic restraint of baroreflex control of heart period in normotensive and hypertensive subjects. Clin Sci 1994. In press.

48. Piazza S, Furlan R, Dell'Orto S, et al. Oscillazioni ritmiche della variabilità della pressione arteriosa sistolica durante esercizio fisico al treadmill. X congresso Nazionale Società Italiana Ipertensione arteriosa. Lido di Venezia 23-24 Sett. 1993.

49. Wasserman K, Beaver WL, Whipp B. Gas exchange theory and lactic acidosis (anaerobic) threshold. Circulation 1990; 81(suppl II):II-14-II-30.

50. Furlan R, Guzzetti S, Crivellaro W, et al. Continuous 24 hour assessment of the neural regulation of systemic arterial pressure and R-R variabilities in ambulant subjects. Circulation 1990; 81:537-547.

51. Pizzinelli P, Lucini D, Bertoni L, et al. Chronic obstructive pulmonary disease. J Ambulat Monit 1992; 5:203-210.

52. Casiglia E, Palatini P, Bongiovi S, et al. Haemodynamics of recovery after strenuous exercise in physically trained hypertensive and normotensive subjects. Clin Sci 1994; 86:27-34.

53. Blomqvist CG. Cardiovascular adaptations to physical training. Annu Rev Physiol 1983; 45:169-189.

54. La Rovere MT, Specchia G, Mortara A, et al. Baroreflex sensitivity, clinical correlates, and cardiovascular mortality among patients with a first myocardial infarction. Circulation 1988; 78:816-824.

55. Coats AJS, Adamopoulos S, Radaelli A, et al. Controlled trial of physical training in chronic heart failure. Exercise performance, hemodynamics, ventilation, and autonomic function. Circulation 1992; 85:2119-2131.

56. Sayers McA B. Analysis of heart rate variability. Ergonomics 1973; 16:17-32.

57. Hyndman BW, Gregory JR. Spectral analysis of sinus arrhythmia during mental loading. Ergonomics 1975; 18:255-270.

58. Langewitz W, Ruddel H. Spectral analysis of heart rate variability under mental stress. J Hypertens 1989; 7(suppl 6):S32-S33.

59. Engel BT, Talan MI. Cardiovascular responses as behavior. Circulation 1991; 83(suppl II):II-9-II-13.

60. Lucini D, Pizzinelli P, Casati R, et al. Maintained pressor and reduced cardiac sympathetic responses to mental stimuli in essential hypertension. In: van Zwiten PA (ed). Central and Peripheral Sympathetic Mechanisms in Hypertension: Pathophysiological and Therapeutics Aspect. Focus on Urapidil. Royal Society of Medicine Services International Congress and Symposium Series, 1992; 196:5-12.

61. Pagani M, Furlan R, Pizzinelli P, et al. Spectral analysis of R-R and arterial pressure variabilities to assess sympathovagal interaction during mental stress in humans. J Hypertens 1989; 7(suppl 7):S14-S15.

62. Moriguchi A, Otsuka A, Mikami H, et al. Disparate cardiovascular responses to passive tilt and mental stress in young and elderly normotensives. J Hypertens 1991; 9(suppl 6):S74-S75.

63. Jiang W, Hayano J, Coleman ER, et al. Relation of cardiovascular responses to mental stress and cardiac vagal activity in coronary artery disease. Am J Cardiol 1993; 72:551-554.

64. Dimsdale JE. A new mechanism linking stress to coronary pathophysiology? Circulation 1991; 84:2201-2202.

65. Kaplan JR, Petterson K, Manuck SB, et al. Role of sympathoadrenal medullary activation in the initiation and progression of atherosclerosis. Circulation 1991; 84(suppl VI):VI-23-VI-32.

66. Malliani A, Pagani M, Lombardi F, et al. Spectral analysis to assess increased sympathetic tone in arterial hypertension. Hypertension 1991; 17(suppl II):36-42.

67. Guzzetti S, Piccaluga E, Casati R, et al. Sympathetic predominance in essential hypertension: a study employing spectral analysis of heart rate variability. J Hypertens 1988; 6:711-717.

68. Guzzetti S, Dassi S, Pecis M, et al. Altered pattern of circadian neural control of heart rate period in mild hypertension. J Hypertens 1991; 9:831-838.

69. Schnall PL, Pieper C, Schwartz JE, et al. The relationship between job strain, workplace diastolic blood pressure, and left ventricular mass index. JAMA 1990; 263:1929-1935.

70. Van Dixhoorn J. Relaxation Therapy in Cardiac Rehabilitation. Rotterdam, Netherlands: Erasmus Universiteit, 1990. Thesis.

71. Kamada T, Miyake S, Kumashiro M, et al. Power spectral analysis of heart rate variability in type As and type Bs during mental workload. Psychosom Med 1992; 54:462-470.

72. Pagani M, Lucini D, Mola GS, et al. Sympathetic overactivity in subjects complaining of unexplained fatigue. Clin Sci 1994; 87:655-661.

73. Lown B, Malliani A, Prosdocini M. Neural mechanisms and cardiovascular disease. Fidia Research Series, Volume 5. Padove, Italy: Liviana Press, 1986.

Chapter 21

Heart Rate Response to Provocative Maneuvers

Dietrich Andresen, T. Brüggemann, S. Behrens, C. Ehlers

Introduction

Autonomic nervous dysfunction is under discussion as a risk factor with regard to increased cardiovascular mortality.[1-4] For a measurement of these dysfunctions, the analysis of heart rate variability (HRV) was proposed. Frequently, HRV is measured from a continuous 24-hour long-term electrocardiogram (ECG) registration. Here, time-domain analysis[5] is applied, as well as frequency-domain analysis[6,7] (see also chapters 3-5).

Another possibility in diagnosing an autonomous nervous dysfunction is to carry out provocative maneuvers by means of so-called "cardiovascular reflex tests." This chapter deals with the pathophysiological fundamentals, the methodological performance, and finally, the possible clinical relevance of these tests in the frame of risk stratification in patients following acute myocardial infarction. Application of a test in the clinical everyday routine has to meet the following fundamental requirements:

1. a procedure which is easily carried out and puts little stress on the patient and on the operator;
2. a standardized examination protocol;
3. easily reproduced results; and
4. a clear delimitation of normal and pathological results.

Several tests have been proposed for examination of an autonomic dysfunction (Table 1). However, only some of them present scientifically valid data combined with the clinical experience to meet the above mentioned requirements. Only the following tests will be dealt with below in more detail: Valsalva maneuver, deep breath test, heart rate (HR) response to standing, and baroreflex sensitivity (BRS) test.

Valsalva Maneuver

For many years, the Valsalva maneuver has been used as a functional test of the

From: Malik M., Camm AJ (eds.): *Heart Rate Variability*. Armonk, NY. Futura Publishing Company, Inc., © 1995.

Table 1

Cardiovascular Reflex Tests That Have Been Suggested Testing for Autonomic
Nervous Dysfunction

Valsalva Maneuver[8]
Deep Breath Test[31]
Heart Rate Response to Standing[21]
Baroreflex Sensitivity[28]
Heart Rate Response to Mental Stress[34]
Heart Rate Response to Coughing[39]
Cold Face Test[40]

---

autonomic nervous system.[8] It is used in testing the afferent, central and efferent baroreflex paths.[9]

The test is usually carried out in a sitting position. A mouthpiece is connected by a tube to a manometer. The test person is asked to blow into the mouthpiece in order to build up a total pressure of over 40 mm Hg over 15 seconds. The course of this test is normally separated into four phases[10]: phase I entails the beginning of the strain during which time an abrupt rise of the systolic and diasystolic blood pressure (BP) as well as a decrease in HR occurs. The fast rise of the BP is due exclusively to mechanical reasons (compression of the aorta and volume dislocation into the periphery, as well as a rise of the left-ventricular HR volume).[11,12] The decreasing HR in this initial phase is the parasympathetic answer to the rising BP. Keeping the strain of expiration (phase II) results in a reduction of the venal backflow into the right atrium with a decrease of the left-ventricular HR volume and a consecutive decrease of the arterial BP. This drop in BP leads, by reflex action, to increased peripheral sympathetic activity,[13] as well as to a rise in the plasma-noradrenalin level[14] resulting in vasoconstriction and tachycardia. Phase III begins at the end of straining and is the mirror image of phase I. Due to the abrupt fall of intrathoracic strain, especially the capacity of the pulmonary-venous system is momentarily increased, thus causing a passing decrease of the cardiac output by backflow and a brief increase of the HR (about 4 seconds). In phase IV an overflow increase of the BP results from an increased cardiac output together with still present total peripheral resistance. The rise of BP in phase IV stimulates the baroreceptors, which induce a bradycardia as a parasympathetic answer. This reflecting bradycardia can be abolished by Atropin.[15] In the overall complex reflection event in the Valsalva maneuver, the parasympathetic, as well as the sympathetic nervous system is therefore included, while the HR response is mainly of vagal origin. A point in its favor is the fact that a change of the HR may be stopped by Atropin, but not by β-blockers.[16]

During the Valsalva maneuver, the HR is continuously measured and a so-called "valsalvia ratio" (VR) is calculated from the relation of the longest RR interval after strain, to the shortest RR interval during strain. A ratio of ≥1.2 is accepted as normal value. Naturally, the test would only be completed by an additional recording of the BP, but gauging the BP is methodically much more intensive even if it has been carried out noninvasively, so that reasons of practicability limit the procedure only to determine the HR.

Problems of Evaluation

As simple as conducting this test appears, the more difficult it is to interpret its results. Since the HR response correlates stronger with phase II than with phase IV,[17] the test may still be normal, despite a moderate bradycardia in phase IV. An indirect, moderately graded injury of the parasympathetic system with maintained sympathetic function would thus remain unrecognized by this test. Also, the evaluation of the test results in patients with congestive heart failure must be seen critically. In these conditions an increased pulmonary BP maintains left ventricular filling during phase II. Therefore, there might be no occurrence of tachycardia during phase II and no reflective bradycardia during phase IV.

The Deep Breath Test

A test which can also be carried out very easily and which has been clinically tried and tested many times, is the "deep breath test." In a normal person, short-term HR variabilities are considerably influenced by breathing. Inspiration leads to a rise, and expiration to a fall of the HR (Figure 1). This HR response to deep breath is exclusively parasympathetically related. Propanolol, as well as alpha-adrenergetic blockers, do not have any influence on the test, while Atropin completely suppresses the HR response. An investigation by Ewing et al on patients with cardiac transplants[18] was able

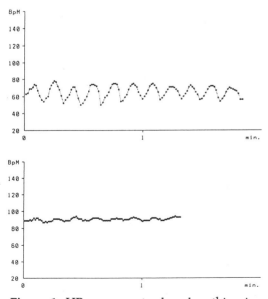

Figure 1. HR response to deep breathing in a normal subject (upper panel) and in a patient who died from sudden death following myocardial infarction (lower panel).

to show that humoral factors failed to influence the test.

The test is carried out in a sitting position. The patients are asked to breathe regularly in and out, six times for 5 seconds each, following the lead of a light bulb chain in a lamp column. During this phase (1 minute), an ECG is continuously recorded at 25 mm/s and single RR intervals are calculated on the computer. For each of the six breathing phases, the shortest RR interval is measured each time during inspiration, and the longest RR interval during expiration. The shortest and the longest mean RR interval is calculated, from which the maximal and minimal HR is subsequently determined. The difference between these two frequencies is a measure for the HRV.

Watkins et al have examined 54 normal persons. None of these persons exhibited an inspiration/expiration difference of ≥9 heartbeats/min, while 84% from a group of diabetics with autonomous neuropathy exhibited differences of ≤9 bpm.[19]

Problems of Evaluation

This test may be methodologically easy to carry out. Also, contrary to the Valsalva maneuver, the findings present no greater difficulties of interpretation, since the test is exclusively vagally related. Not quite standardized however, is the definition of a "normal result." In this case, a significant age relation was noted. A further disadvantage is that an increased sympathetic activity may weaken the cardiovagal reflex response.[20] In order to take these interferences into account, Ewing et al pragmatically evaluated a difference of ≤10 bpm to be pathologic, 10 to 14 beats as borderline cases, and over 15 bpm as normal, which they considered also to be age-independent.[18]

Heart Rate Response to Standing

When a person rises from a reclining position, an initial increase of heart frequency occurs and, while standing erectly, a relative decrease of the HR occurs.[21] The biggest rise of frequency is reached after the 15th beat, the most expressed relative bradycardia after the 30th beat. This change of frequency is mainly parasympathetically ruled, however, the influence of beta-blockers speaks for an additional sympathetic entity of influence.[22]

This test is also carried out in an easy way. The test person is asked to get up from the lying position and to stand upright free and still for 2 minutes. During the whole test phase an ECG is recorded and the transition from the lying to the upright position is marked. The relation 30:15 is defined as reading parameter.[18] This is the relation of the longest RR interval (30th beat) with the shortest RR interval (15th beat) after getting into the upright position.

Problems of Evaluation

This test, as the other two, is easily carried out, and the result of the measurement is determined without any difficulty. The evaluation is, however, incomparably more difficult than in the deep breath test, since the HRV is determined in a very complex manner by entities of sympathetic influence.

Baroreflex Sensitivity

The baroreflex is an important short-term regulator controlling the BP. As soon as the systemic BP falls, baroreflectors are activated.[23-25] This leads to an increase of the HR and to a normalization of the BP.[26,27] The BRS test uses inverted mechanisms,[28] namely, a decreasing HR due to a defined increase of the arterial BP.

The implementation is extensively described by Schwartz et al.[28] In reclining position, a venous sodium chloride infusion is made first, followed by a 30-minute stabilizing phase, and the basic BP and HR is determined. After this, a gradually increased infusion of Phenylephrine (maximal Phenylephrine dose: 120 μg/min) is ad-

ministered until the maximal increase of the mean BP by 30 mm Hg is reached. An ECG recording is taken each time the rising BP shows a plateau. The changes of the BP together with the change of the HR are plotted and linear regression analysis is calculated. The degree of the increase of the regression line is defined (ms/mm Hg) as the BRS.[28]

Clinical Importance of the Cardiovascular Reflex Tests

Data on the clinical importance of cardiovascular reflex tests in patients with basic cardiac diseases is limited. Above all, the testing procedures in patients with diabetes mellitus and other diseases of the autonomic nervous system (ANS)[29-31] have been evaluated. Only recently have initial investigations been published concerning the clinical relevance of reflex tests for patients in a state of postmyocardial infarction as well. The estimate that the testing procedures may be pathological, not just in cases of an autonomic neuropathy, but in patients, eg, after myocardial infarction as well, is based on the idea that the scarring of the heart will lead to an imbalance between sympathetic and parasympathetic innervation.[32] Once this imbalance leads to a dominating sympathetic tone with a simultaneously reduced vagal tone, the conditions for an increased electric instability are obvious.[1,33,34]

Schwartz et al have been the first to report on differing BRS in patients with postmyocardial infarction in comparison to a group of normal persons.[28] The mean BRS in myocardial infarction patients was significantly lower (8 ms/mm Hg) than in normal persons (12 ms/mm Hg). If overlaps were found between both groups, no BRS of ≤7 ms/mm Hg in any of the normal persons was observed, meanwhile, this was noted in 14/32 of the postinfarction patients (44%). In this context, it is interesting that in many myocardial infarction patients, a far reaching normalization of the BRS occurred during the further follow-up. A finding suggests remodeling in the postinfarction phase. The same group (La Rovere et al) also published a prospective study on 78 patients with postmyocardial infarction, wherein a significantly higher mortality was found in patients with a BRS of <3.0 ms/mm Hg, compared to those with a BRS ≥3.0 ms/mm Hg.[35] In the meantime, small investigations on the prognostic value of BRS on patients with coronary heart disease are also available.[36-38] In a recently published study by Hohnloser et al,[37] the authors were able to show that postinfarction patients, who had experienced an arrhythmic event (ventricular tachycardia/ventricular fibrillation) during the follow-up, had a significantly lower BRS than a carefully matched control group. And finally, the results of an ongoing multicenter study (ATRAMI), which integrates the tests on BRS into an overall risk stratification in postinfarction patients are eagerly awaited. From this study, a definite answer on the predictive value of this method in postinfarction patients can be discerned. So far, little clinical attention has been granted to the other noninvasive cardiovascular reflex tests. In a still ongoing prospective study, we have examined the predictive value of the Valsalva maneuver and of the deep breath test for the prognosis of postinfarction patients.

Method

Ninety-seven patients (28 women, 69 men) of a mean age of 63±12 years have been included. Five to 8 days after the acute event, a Valsalva maneuver test and a deep breath test were performed. The procedure of the test was in accordance with the method given above. A Valsalva ratio ≤1.1 was defined as pathological Valsalva maneuver test. An HR difference between inspiration and expiration ≤8 beats was defined as pathological deep breath test. The tests were each carried out in the morning between 8 and 12 o'clock. After their discharge, the patients were observed during an overall follow-up of 2 years.

Results

Twenty-three patients had an abnormal Valsalva maneuver; 38 patients, an abnormal deep breath test. Both an abnormal Valsalva maneuver and abnormal deep breath test were observed in 17 patients. Six patients had an abnormal Valsalva maneuver only, and 21 patients exclusively an abnormal deep breath test.

Table 2 lists the clinical differences between the patients with abnormal test results and those with normal findings. Pa-

Table 2

	VM/DB Abnormal	VM/DB Normal	p-Value
Age (years)	67 ± 12.3	61 ± 11.7	0.03
Female (%)	27	30	n.s.
Smokers (%)	63	55	n.s.
Hypertension (%)	59	42	0.04
Diabetes (%)	30	19	0.06
Previous MI (%)	16	15	n.s.
>20 VPB (holter) (%)	18	17	n.s.
EF ≤ 40% (%)	38	29	n.s
Thrombolysis (%)	66	77	n.s.
Ant. infarction (%)	45	45	n.s.

Clinical characteristics of 97 pts. with acute myocardial infarction according to the test-results (VM = Valsalva Maneuvers, DB = Deep Breath Test, VPB = ventricular premature beats during predischarge 24-h longterm-ECG, EF = Left ventricular ejection fraction).

tients with a pathological stress test showed no differences with regard to their left ventricular ejection fraction, to arrhythmias in the long-term ECG, and to infarction localization as well. The patients were significantly older though (67 years versus 61 years), and they frequently had an additional arterial hypertension. Eye-catching was also the higher proportion of diabetics in the group with pathological test results (30% versus 19%).

Follow-up

With the exception of two patients, all patients could be observed for an overall follow-up of 2 years. In the course of this follow-up 21 patients died, 16 of cardiac causes (4 of those from sudden cardiac death), 5 died of unknown origin.

In the patient group with a pathological deep breath test, the mortality was 26%; in the group with a normal deep breath test, it was only 11% (p = 0.04). Also in the patient group with a pathological Valsalva maneuver, the cardiac 2-year mortality was higher than in the group with normal findings (31% versus 13%) (p = 0.03).

Evaluation of the Results

The results which have been gained from this still ongoing study are very promising. They show that patients with reduced vagal activity have an increased risk of cardiac events. This result correlates to the findings of the studies on BRS.

If cardiovascular reflex tests are used in measuring similar things as the tests on the BRS, namely, the dynamic activity of the ANS, then one might actually prefer the cardiovascular reflex tests. They are carried out more easily and are less stressful for the patient. This conclusion would, however, be wrong. The study carried out by ourselves is too small in number and as a result, the univariate analysis with regard to clinical differences between the collective with pathological stress test and that with normal results must be evaluated with the greatest reserve. The trends lead to the assumption that in a numerical increase of the patient population, several other variables will become significant. Only a multivariate analysis can then test the possible independent value of the test procedure in the frame of a risk stratification. Also, the tests should not be overestimated in their clinical relevance. They are carried out easily, a result is calculated easily as well. The interpretation, however, still presents difficulties.[17,20] It should therefore be asked, to control the clinical value of the test procedures in an even larger study on risk stratification. The planning of such a study has been started.

Conclusion

Cardiovascular reflex tests are useful tools for measuring autonomic nervous dysfunction. The tests are easy to perform, standardized and put little stress on the patient and the operator.

Some preliminary results concerning the predictive value of the tests in patients following myocardial infarction are promising. However, their independent prognostic value in the frame of risk stratification in postmyocardial infarction patients and other cardiac diseases has to be established.

References

1. Lown B, Verrier RL. Neutral activity and ventricular fibrillation. N Engl J Med 1976; 294:1165-1170.
2. Lown B. Sudden cardiac death: the major challenge confronting contemporary cardiology. Am J Cardiol 1979; 43:313-328.
3. Schwartz PJ, La Rovere MT, Vanoli E. Autonomic nervous system and sudden cardiac death: experimental basis and clinical observations for post-myocardial infarction risk stratification. Circulation 1992; 85(suppl 1):4.

4. Schwartz PJ, Stone HL. The role of the autonomic nervous system in sudden cardiac death. Ann N Y Acad Sci 1982; 382:162-180.

5. Kleiger GE, Miller JP, Bigger JT Jr, et al. Heart rate variability: a variable predicting mortality following acute myocardial infarction. Am J Cardiol 1987; 59:256-262.

6. Bigger JT, Keiger RE, Fleiss JL, et al. Components of heart rate variability measured during healing of acute myocardial infarction. Am J Cardiol 1988; 61:61-215.

7. Malik M, Farrell T, Cripps T, et al. Heart rate variability in relation to prognosis after myocardial infarction: selection of optimal processing techniques. Eur Heart J 1989; 10:1060-1074.

8. Scharpey-Schafer EP. Effects of Valsalva's manoeuvre in normal and failing circulation. Br Med J 1955; 1:693-695.

9. Korner PI, Tonkin AM, Uther JB. Reflex and mechanical circulatory effects of graded Valsalva maneuvre in normal man. J Appl Physiol 1976; 40:434-440.

10. Hamilton WF, Woodbury RA, Harper HT. Physiologic relations between intrathoracic, intraspinal, and arterial pressure. JAMA 1936; 107:853-856.

11. Booth RW, et al. Hemodynamic changes associated with the Valsalva maneuvre in normal men and women. J Lab Clin 1962; 59:275-285.

12. Brooker JZ, Alderman EL, Harrison DC. Alterations in left ventricular volumes induced by Valsalva maneuvre. Br Heart J 1974; 36:713.

13. Delius W, et al. Maneuvres affecting sympathetic outflow in human muscle nerves. Acta Physiol Scand 1972; 84:82.

14. Robertson D, et al. Comparative assessment of stimuli that release neutronal and adrenomedullary catecholamines in man. Circulation 1979; 59:637.

15. Eckberg D. Parasympathetic cardiovascular control in human disease: a critical review of methods and results. Am J Physiol 1980; 239:H581-H593.

16. Spodick DH, Meyer MB, Quarry Pigott VM. Effect of β-adrenergic blockade in beat-to-beat response to Valsalva manoeuvre. Br Heart J 1974; 36:1082-1986.

17. Benarroch EE, Opfer-Gehrking TL, Low PA. Use of photoplethysmographic technique to analyze the Valsalva maneuvre in normal man. Muscle Nerve 1991; 14:1165-1172.

18. Ewing DJ. Cardiac autonomic neuropathy. In: Jarrett RJ (ed). Diabetes and Heart Disease. Amsterdam: Elsevier, 1984; 99-132.

19. Watkins PJ, Mackay JD. Cardiac denervation in diabetic neuropatrhy. Ann Intern Med 1980; 92:304-307.

20. Pfeifer MA, et al. Quantitative evaluation of cardiac parasympathetic activity in normal and diabetic man. Diabetes 1982; 31:339-346.

21. Ewing DJ, et al. Immediate heart rate response to standing: simple test of autonomic neuropathy in diabetes. Br Med J 1978; 1:145-147.

22. Ewing DJ, et al. Autonomic mechanisms in the initial heart rate response to standing. J Appl Physiol 1980; 49:809-814.

23. Kirchheim HR. Systemic arterial baroreceptor reflexes. Physiol Rev 1976; 56:100-177.

24. Malliani A, Recordati G, Schwartz PJ. Nervous activity of afferent cardiac sympathetic fibers with atrial and ventricular endings. J Physiol 1973; 229:457-469.

25. Thoren PN. Activation of left ventricular receptors with non-medullated vagal afferent fibers during occlusion of a coronary artery in the cat. Am J Cardiol 1976; 37:1046-1051.

26. Eckberg DL, et al. A simplified neck suction device for activation of carotid baroreceptors. J Lab Clin Med 1975; 85:167-173.

27. Heidorn GH, McNamara AP. Effect of carotid sinus stimulation on the electrocardiograms of clinically normal individuals. Circulation 1956; 14:1104-1113.

28. Schwartz PJ, Zaza A, Pala M, et al. Baroreflex sensitivity and its evolution during the first year after myocardial infarction. JACC 1988; 12(3):629-636.

29. Bennett T, et al. Assessment of vagal control of the heart in diabetes. Br Heart J 1977; 39:25-28.

30. Dyrberg T, et al. Prevalence of diabetic autonomic neuropathy measured by simple bedside tests. Diabetologia 1981; 20:190-194.

31. MacKay JD. Respiratory sinus arrhythmia in diabetic neuropathy. Diabetologia 1983; 24:253-256.

32. Barber MJ, Mueller TM, Davies BG, et al. Interruption of sympathetic and vagal-mediated afferent responses by transmural myocardial infarction. Circulation 1985; 72:623-631.

33. Corr PB, Gillis RA. Role of the vagus nerves in the cardiovascular changes induced by coronary occlusion. Circulation 1974; 49:86-97.

34. Locatelli A, et al. Mental arithmetic stress as a test for evaluation of diabetic sympathetic autonomic neuropathy. Diabetic Med 1989; 6:490-495.

35. La Rovere MT, Specchia G, Mortara A, et al. Baroreflex sensitivity, clinical correlates, and cardiovascular mortality among patients with a first myocardial infarction: a prospective study. Circulation 1988; 78:816-824.

36. Bigger JT, La Rovere MT, Steinman RC, et al. Comparison of baroreflex sensitivity and

heart period variability after myocardial infarction. J Am Coll Cardiol 1989; 14: 1511-1518.

37. Hohnloser SH, Klingenheber T, van de Loo A, et al. Reflex versus tonic vagal activity as a prognostic parameter in patients with sustained ventricular tachycardia or ventricular fibrillation. Circulation 1994; 89(3): 1068-1073.

38. Farell TG, Odemuyiwa O, Bashir J, et al. Prognostic value of baroreflex sensitivity testing after acute myocardial infarction. Br Heart J 1992; 67:129-137.

39. Cardone C, et al. Autonomic mechanisms in the heart rate response to coughing. Clin Sci 1987; 72:55-60.

40. Heath MA, Downey JA. The cold face test (diving reflex) in clinical autonomic assessment: methodological considerations and repeatability of responses. Clin Sci 1990; 78:139-147.

Chapter 22

Effects of Pharmacological Interventions on Heart Rate Variability: Animal Experiments and Clinical Observations

Lü Fei

Since autonomic activity plays an important role in both electrical and mechanical activities of the heart, pharmacological modulation of autonomic activity has been of great interest. In 1962, Black and Stephenson[1] pointed out in their initial study on a β-blocker ICI 38174 that "we are hoping that this compound will be sufficiently active to examine some pharmacological and clinical problems. For example, will conditions such as atrial and ventricular tachycardia, be helped by reducing the cardiac sympathomimetic responses to anxiety, emotion and exercise? Again, will myocardial adrenergic blockade reduce the myocardial demand for oxygen, and, if so, will this be helpful to patients with angina? These are some of the problems we are currently investigating with compound 38174." However, little was known about drug effects on autonomic activity, since there was no established method available for the assessment of autonomic function during normal daily activities until the recent emergence of heart rate variability (HRV) analysis. The influence of autonomic agents on HRV has greatly improved our understanding of the physiological basis underlying HRV and in turn, analysis of HRV can be used to assess the autonomic effects of various drugs. This chapter reviews the literatures (published before January 1994) addressing the effects of drugs on HRV in animals and in humans.

Physiological Basis of Heart Rate Variability

HRV is usually analyzed in the time and frequency domains. Most time-domain parameters reflect the overall autonomic modulation of heart rate (HR) but provide no information regarding sympathetic and parasympathetic activity individually (except pNN50, which has been reported to reflect mostly parasympathetic activity).[2] In contrast, spectral analysis of HRV can par-

From: Malik M., Camm AJ (eds.): *Heart Rate Variability*. Armonk, NY. Futura Publishing Company, Inc., © 1995.

tially separate parasympathetic from sympathetic effects on the heart. It is generally accepted that overall HRV is mainly mediated by vagal activity, although the contribution of sympathetic activity to the low-frequency (LF) component of HRV under certain conditions remains controversial.[3] The high-frequency (HF) component (0.15 to 0.40 Hz) of spectral HRV is almost exclusively mediated by vagal activity and the LF component (0.04 to 0.15 Hz) gives a measure of sympathetic activity with some influence from vagal activity. The sympatho-vagal balance may be assessed by examining either the low-to-high ratio or the normalized LF and HF components.[4] An increased low-to-high ratio suggests increased sympathetic and/or decreased parasympathetic activity. It has been shown that direct electrical stimulation of the vagus nerve causes a decrease in the LF component, an increase in the HF component and a decrease in the low-to-high ratio.[5] In addition to numerous drugs, however, HRV is affected by many influencing factors including age,[6,7] mean HR,[8,9] posture,[10,11] physical exercise,[12-15] emotional stress,[16,17] cardiac function,[18-21] myocardial ischemia/infarction,[22-26] and autonomic neuropathy.[27] Ventricular arrhythmias may also have a significant influence on HRV.[28,29]

Reproducibility of Heart Rate Variability

Reproducibility of HRV measures is a prerequisite for the evaluation of drug effects on HRV. Several investigators have demonstrated that HRV is essentially stable over a short period in normal subjects,[30-33] and in patients with decreased cardiac function[34] or ventricular arrhythmias,[35] despite significant interindividual HRV variations. This is also true in patients on drug therapy.[36] An example of the correlation between two separate recordings is shown in Figures 1 and 2. It has been shown that there is no significant effect of placebo on HRV in normal subjects[34] and in patients with and without cardiac failure.[37-39] These observations suggest that analysis of HRV can be used for the assessment of the effect of pharmacological intervention on cardiac autonomic activity.

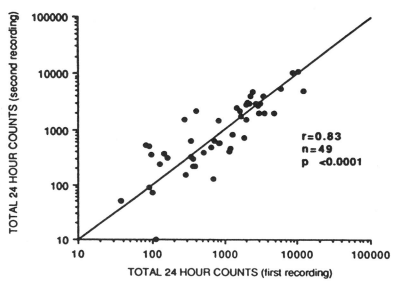

Figure 1. Correlation of HRV (pNN50) between two separate recordings (median: 192 days) in 49 patients with ventricular arrhythmias. Reproduced with permission from Zuanetti et al.[36]

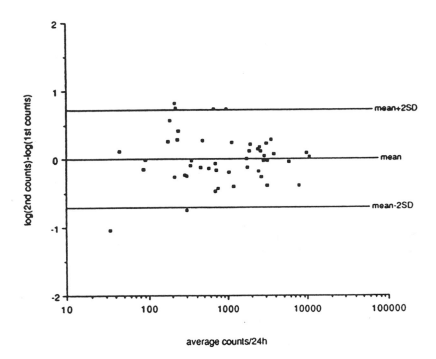

Figure 2. Bland and Altman plot for the reproducibility of HRV between two separate recordings based on the same data as in Figure 1. Reproduced with permission from Zuanetti et al.[36]

Effects of Autonomic Agents on Heart Rate Variability in Normal Subjects

Initially the physiological basis of HRV was mainly studied using autonomic blocking and stimulating agents. For example, Akselrod et al[40] observed that in the power spectrum of HRV obtained from a 5-minute recording in adult conscious dogs, three distinct components can be distinguished: an HF peak at approximately 0.4 Hz; a mid-frequency peak at approximately 0.15 Hz; and an LF peak at approximately 0.05 Hz. The HF and mid-frequency peaks were abolished, and the power of the LF peak was reduced by selective parasympathetic blockade, while combined beta-sympathetic and parasympathetic blockade abolished all frequency components of HRV.

The effect of *atropine* on HRV has been comprehensively studied. Several studies have demonstrated that atropine decreases HRV in animals[41-43] and in humans.[33,39,44,45]

Hayano et al[44] demonstrated a typical S-shaped dose-response curve for atropine-induced changes in HR. Since vagal modulation of HR contributes to both the LF and HF components of HRV, not surprisingly, atropine reduces overall HRV including the LF and HF components. It has been shown that central anticholinergic agents also decrease HRV,[46] suggesting that central cholinergic receptors may also be involved in the modulation of HR. Ali Melkkila et al[47] reported that high-dose atropine decreases HRV, while low-dose atropine may increase HRV. *Glycopyrrolate*,[47] and *hyoscine butylbromide*[48,49] also reduce HRV.

Vagal activity is also modulated by vagomimetic agents, such as scopolamine. In contrast to the peripheral vagolytic action of high-dose scopolamine, low-dose scopolamine exerts a vagomimetic effect. Low-dose transdermal scopolamine has been shown to increase HRV in normal subjects.[50,51]

β-adrenergic stimulation by *isoproterenol* increases the LF component of HRV in normal subjects.[45,52,53] However, β-blockade has variable effects on HRV. It may increase,[48,54] decrease,[41,55,56] or not affect[44] HRV. Basal autonomic tone may account for the different responses of HRV to β-blockade. This variable effect of β-blockade on HRV is consistent with observations of the uncertain significance of the contribution of sympathetic activity to HRV.[3] Bittiner and Smith[49] reported that increased HRV accompanies β-blockade only in the absence of intrinsic sympathetic activity when bradycardia ensues. Therefore, increase in HRV may reflect augmented vagal tone induced by β-blockade.[49] Although β-blockade has significant influence on HRV, the effects of α-blockade on HRV remain to be defined.[57,58] It has recently been shown that propranolol suppresses the increase in all frequency components of HRV during tilt in patients with vasovagal syncope.[59] It is interesting to note that HRV is usually decreased in certain clinical settings associated with increased sympathetic activity. This depressed HRV associated with increased sympathetic activity may be partially explained by subsequent sympatho-vagal interaction.

Effects of Antiarrhythmic Drugs on Heart Rate Variability

Since the autonomic nervous system (ANS) plays an important role in the pathogenesis of ventricular tachyarrhythmias, the effects of antiarrhythmic drugs on HRV is of special clinical interest. Schwartz[60] recently pointed out that ANS function may influence the efficacy of antiarrhythmic drugs under some circumstances. Currently available data suggest that most antiarrhythmic agents decrease HRV. This may be due to their vagolytic or β-blocking properties.[36] In a study of 15 patients with ventricular arrhythmias, for example, Lombardi et al[61] showed that propafenone significantly decreases the LF component (52±6 versus 28±4 nu, p<0.05) but increases the HF component of HRV (39±6 versus 55±5 nu,

p<0.05), resulting in a significant decrease in the low-to-high ratio (2.0±0.4 versus 0.6±0.1, p<0.05) (Figure 3). Zuanetti et al[36] also reported a significant decrease in HRV (pNN50) in patients with ventricular arrhythmias treated with flecainide or propafenone. This decrease in HRV was reversible with discontinuation of treatment and was not related to arrhythmia suppression, since 24-hour HRV was similar during treatment irrespective of the presence or absence of frequent arrhythmias. This study, using pNN50 as a measure of HRV, does not preclude a possible relationship between the effects of antiarrhythmic drugs on arrhythmias and those on spectral HRV. A significant relationship between increase in pNN50 and suppression of ventricular ectopic beats has recently been demonstrated.[62] In the study of Zuanetti,[36] amiodarone was found to have no significant influence on pNN50 in patients with ventricular arrhythmias. We have also noted that low-dose amiodarone (200 mg daily) does not significantly influence spectral HRV in patients with hypertrophic cardiomyopathy although it significantly reduces HR and prolongs QT and QTc intervals. Hohnloser et al[63] have reported that sotalol produces a significant increase in the HF component of HRV, but causes no change in the LF component. Several studies have demonstrated that drug effects on HRV are independent of their effects on HR.[49,61,63] There is evidence that chronic adrenergic blockade leads to a reduction in sympathetic efferent activity and a change in myocardial electrophysiological properties, whereas acute blockade may not have the same effects.[64,65] However, both acute and chronic administration of propranolol has been shown to significantly alter HRV.[40,44,62,66,67] Although the effects of antiarrhythmic drugs on autonomic activity are of important clinical significance, our knowledge in this field is limited. For example, reports on the effects of propranolol on HRV in patients with ventricular arrhythmias are scarce, and conclusive data are still

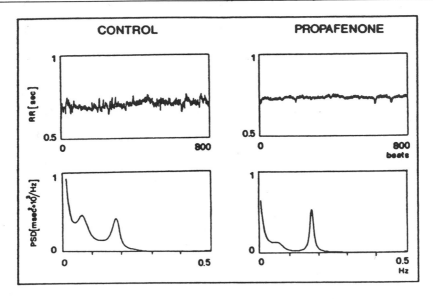

Figure 3. Effects of propafenone on spectral HRV in patients with ventricular arrhythmias. The top diagram is tachograms and the bottom shows autospectra. Note the decreased LF component and an increased HF component of HRV after propafenone. PSD = power spectrum density. Reproduced with permission from Lombardi et al.[61]

lacking. The effects of antiarrhythmic drugs on HRV are summarized in Table 1.

It has been reported that nonpharmacological methods, such as exercise training, reduce the risk of death in patients following myocardial infarction.[71] Exercise training has been shown to increase vagal activity in normal subjects,[72,73] in patients with congestive heart failure,[74] and in patients following myocardial infarction.[75] Cowen et al[76] have also reported that biofeedback or self-management training increases vagal tone in sudden cardiac death survivors. However, data on the relationship between antiarrhythmic drug-induced alterations of HRV and their antiarrhythmic and proarrhythmic actions are scarce, although this relationship is obviously important for our understanding of the mechanisms underlying the electrophysiological effects of antiarrhythmic drugs.

The Effects on Heart Rate Variability in Hypertensive Subjects

It is well known that blood pressure is under the influence of the ANS and en-hanced sympathetic activity may play an important role in the pathogenesis of hypertension.[77] However, little is known about vagal activity in hypertensive patients. Guzzetti et al[78] reported that compared with normotensive controls, hypertensive patients demonstrated an increased LF component and a decreased HF component of HRV suggesting that there is an increased sympathetic and/or decreased vagal drive to the heart in these patients. Abnormality of HRV in hypertensive patients has recently been confirmed by Chakko et al[79] and by Langewitz et al.[80] The circadian rhythm of HR and HRV is also altered in hypertensive patients.[79] Using spectral analysis of HRV, Murakawa et al[81] demonstrated that parasympathetic activity plays an important role in the modulation of the circadian variability of HR in healthy subjects and in patients with coronary artery disease or diabetic mellitus. Impaired vagal activity may also contribute to the altered circadian rhythm of HR and HRV in hypertensive patients. β-blockade (*atenolol*) has been shown to partially normalize the abnormal spectrum of HRV in hypertensive patients.[78]

Table 1
Effects of Antiarrhythmic Drugs on HRV

Drug		Effect on HRV
Class I		
Ia	Procainamide	Decreases CV and spectral HRV but does not affect SD and pNN50 in patients with VT.[68]
Ib	Mexiletin	Decreases RR variance but does not affect normalized LF and HF components in patients with ventricular arrhythmias.[69]
Ic	Propafenone	Decreases all absolute values of time-domain[36,61,62,69] and spectral HRV[61,62,69] in absolute value but increases HF component in normalized units[61,69] in patients with ventricular arrhythmias.
	Flecainide	Decreases RR variance[69] and pNN50[36] but does not affect normalized LF and HF components[69] in patients with ventricular arrhythmias.
Class II*		
Metoprolol		Increases SD and pNN50[37] but decreases SD in the supine position and LF component during tilt[70] in patients following MI.
Propranolol		Increases SD, pNN50 and HF component in patients with ventricular arrhythmias.[62]
Class III		
Amiodarone		Does not affect pNN50 in patients with ventricular arrhythmias.[36]
Sotalol		Increases SD, rMSSD, pNN50 and HF component but does not affect TF and LF components.[63]
Class IV		
Diltiazem		Decreases SD in the supine position and increases LF component during tilt in patients after MI.[70]
Nifedipine		No consistent changes in HRV in patients after MI.[70]

*See also under the section of "effects of autonomic agents on HRV in normal subjects." HF = high frequency component; LF = low frequency component; MI = myocardial infarction; VT = ventricular tachycardia; SD = standard deviation; CV = coefficient of variance of all normal RR intervals.

Several studies have demonstrated that *clonidine*[82-86] reduces HRV, but *angiotensin converting enzyme inhibitors* either increase or do not affect HRV.[87-90] Janssen et al[87] studied the effects of five antihypertensive drugs on HR in spontaneously hypertensive rats. They demonstrated that HRV, defined as the standard deviation of HR calculated by averaging 60-minute values of HR over 24-hour periods (not the conventional HRV parameter SD), was lower in spontaneously hypertensive rats than in Wistar-Kyoto normotensive control rats (26±3 versus 31±3, $p < 0.05$). HRV was significantly decreased by *metoprolol* (18±3, $p < 0.05$) and was increased by *prazosin* (33±3, $p < 0.05$) but was not changed significantly by *captopril* (25±3, NS), *clonidine* (24±4, NS) or *hydralazine* (24±2, NS). They suggested that the circadian rhythm of HRV is under sympathetic control in spontaneously hypertensive rats and is not influenced by nonsympatholytic vasodilators. Considering the findings of Murakawa et al,[81] both sympathetic and parasympathetic activity may significantly contribute to the impairment of the circadian rhythm of HRV in hypertensive patients. However, the effects of these drugs on HRV remain to be fully defined due to the insensitive methods used for computation of animal HRV in this study. The effects of antihypertensive drugs on HRV are summarized in Table 2.

The Effects of Drugs on Heart Rate Variability following Myocardial Infarction

Myocardial infarction is known to cause autonomic disturbance. Inferior myo-

Table 2
Effects of Antihypertensive Drugs on HRV

Drug	Effect on HRV
Atenolol	Decreases LF component and increases HF component in uncomplicated essential hypertension.[78]
Captopril	Does not affect SD in rats.[87,88]
Cilazapril	Does not affect LF component of HRV in mild hypertensive patients.[90]
Clonidine	Decreases SD and spectral HRV in animals[82,83] and in humans[84,85] but does not significantly affect CV in patients subjected to surgery.[86]
Delapril	Does not affect HRV in essential hypertension.[91]
Guanethidine	Does not affect SD or CV in rats.[92]
Hydralazine	Does not affect SD in rats[87] but chronic administration may increase heart rate variance in conscious Wistar rats.[93]
Metoprolol	Decreases SD in rats.[87]
Nadolol	Decreases CV in essential hypertension.[94,95]
Prazosin	Increases SD in rats.[87]
Ramipril	Increases HRV in normal subjects.[89]
Trandolapril	Does not affect SD in hypertensive men.[96]

The abbreviations are the same as in Table 1.

cardial infarction may cause vagal predominance leading to bradycardia with or without hypotension. In contrast, enhanced sympathetic activity is indicated by tachycardia with transient hypotension and occurs especially in patients with anterior myocardial infarction. These changes in autonomic activity may be due either to autonomic reflexes elicited by direct effects on the chemoreceptors and mechanoreceptors in the infarcted area, or to adrenaline secretion from the adrenal medulla. Correction of autonomic disturbance may cause a significant reduction in mortality following myocardial infarction.[97]

Although the predictive value of HRV has been well studied in patients following acute myocardial infarction, few studies have been done to address the effect of drugs on HRV in this clinical setting. As in normal subjects, β-blockers can either decrease (*propranolol*)[98] or increase (*metoprolol*)[37] HRV in patients following acute myocardial infarction. Bekheit et al[70] reported that *metoprolol* reduces the LF component of HRV during tilt in patients following myocardial infarction. Since propranolol is a nonselective β-blocker, and metoprolol is a β$_1$-blocker, whether the differential effects of β$_1$- and β$_2$-blockade on HRV contribute to the inconsistent results of β-blockade observed remains unknown.

There is evidence from animal experiments that β-adrenergic blockade causes a significant increase in HR and a decrease in the HF component (0.24 to 1.04 Hz), and in the SD of HRV in animals with myocardial infarction.[99] These changes tend to be greater in animals susceptible to ventricular fibrillation than in resistant animals, although there are no significant differences in HR and HRV between susceptible and resistant animals in the drug free state. If this observation can be verified in humans, the response of HRV to autonomic blockade may be useful in the risk stratification of patients following acute myocardial infarction. However, this observation needs to be fully defined in both animals and humans.

Scopolamine increases HRV in patients following acute myocardial infarction,[100,101] as in normal subjects.[50,51] In a randomized, placebo-controlled study of 61 patients (mean age: 58±10 years, LVEF 44.7±15.5%) 6 days (median) following acute myocardial infarction, Vybiral et al[100] demonstrated that time-domain HRV increases 26% to 35% in patients given low-dose scopolamine (n = 30) compared with patients given placebo (n = 31). These authors suggest that this effect of scopolamine on autonomic tone may provide an alternative approach to autonomic modulation for the prevention of sudden cardiac death, particularly in patients in whom β-blockers are contraindicative.

Bekheit et al[70] have reported that *diltiazem* reduces the LF component of HRV, but *nifedipine* does not have consistent effects on HRV in patients following myocardial infarction. It appears that *thrombolytic therapy* does not affect HRV, but HRV has been shown to correlate with the patency of the infarct-related artery.[102] However, it has been reported that recombinant tissue-type plasminogen activator (*rt-PA*) may increase HRV.[25] There is evidence that exercise training increases HRV[75] and reduces mortality in patients following myocardial infarction.[71] Whether drug-induced autonomic alteration in HRV is also associated with a change in prognosis following acute myocardial infarction has yet to be determined. HRV has been shown to vary with time following acute myocardial infarction.[103] This spontaneous decrease in HRV should be taken into account when studying the effect of drugs on HRV following acute myocardial infarction.

The Effects of Drugs on Heart Rate Variability in Patients with Congestive Heart Failure

There is substantial evidence of autonomic imbalance in patients with congestive heart failure.[104] This autonomic dysfunction may contribute to the pathophysiology of congestive heart failure. Modification of autonomic activity may alter prognosis in these patients. HRV is significantly decreased in congestive heart failure. Angiotensin converting enzyme inhibition may not significantly affect HRV in subjects without cardiac dysfunction. However, *angiotensin converting enzyme inhibitors* consistently improve the depressed HRV in patients with congestive heart failure (Figure 4).[38,105,106] Augmentation of parasympathetic tone by angiotensin converting enzyme inhibitors may contribute to their beneficial effect in the treatment of patients with congestive heart failure.[107]

It has been noted that angiotensin II produces a decrease in vagal tone and an increase in sympathetic activity, and blockade of the renin-angiotensin system is involved in the modulation of HRV (LF component).[40] The mechanism underlying the effect of angiotensin converting enzyme inhibition on autonomic tone may involve the removal of central suppression of vagal tone by angiotensin II.[38] In patients with heart failure, there is an abnormal autonomic response to changes in arterial and/or intracardiac pressure[108] and baroreflex sensitivity (BRS) is also significantly altered.[109] There is evidence that angiotensin II inhibits the baroreceptor reflex both in animals and in humans[110,111] and that angiotensin converting enzyme inhibitor therapy improves BRS in patients with congestive heart failure. This improvement in BRS may contribute to the augmentation of HRV in these patients. Benedict et al[112] have recently reported that decreased left ventricular ejection fraction plays an important role in the activation of neurohormones in patients with heart failure. Since HRV is significantly related to left ventricular function, drug-induced alteration of autonomic tone may be, at least partly, secondary to the improvement of pathophysiology of this disease caused by drug therapy (including cardiac function and peripheral hemodynamic changes).

Due to the failure of encainide and flecainide to reduce mortality after myocardial infarction[113] and the uncertain role of low-dose amiodarone in the prevention of sudden cardiac death and/or reduction of overall mortality in patients with decreased left

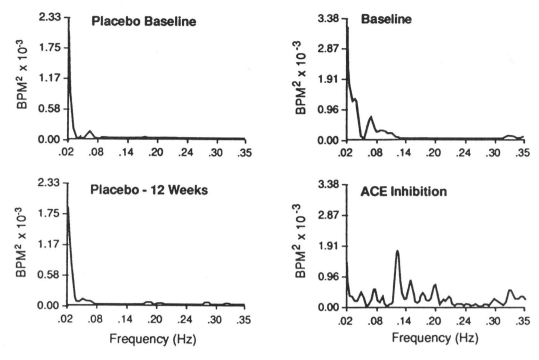

Figure 4. Effect of the angiotensin converting enzyme (ACE) inhibitor zofenopril on spectral HRV in patients with congestive heart failure. There is no significant change in HRV before and after placebo (left), while there is a marked augmentation of HRV after zofenopril (right). BPM^2 = beats/min^2. Reproduced with permission from Binkley et al.[38]

ventricular function,[114-117] attention has been shifted to other treatment strategies. β-adrenergic blockers may serve as one of such strategies for the prevention of sudden cardiac death in patients with left ventricular dysfunction since trials have shown that β-blockers lead to a consistent reduction in mortality in patients following myocardial infarction with and without ventricular arrhythmias and depressed left ventricular function.[118,119] Correction of autonomic dysfunction may explain contribution to improved survival in patients with congestive heart failure. Angiotensin converting enzyme inhibition also reduces the incidence of sudden cardiac death in patients with congestive heart failure.[120] Whether an improvement in autonomic balance is involved in the mechanism underlying the reduction of mortality in these patients is not yet clear. *Digoxin* may also affect HRV in patients with congestive heart failure.[8]

Effects of Anesthetics on Heart Rate Variability

A central nervous system mechanism may be involved in the negative influence of sedatives, analgesics and anesthetics on HRV. Adinoff et al[121] reported that *diazepam* decreases HRV in a dose-dependent manner. Several studies[122-124] have demonstrated that HRV is decreased by anesthesia. Mental activity may also significantly influence HRV in normal subjects and in patients following myocardial infarction.[17] Elimination of emotional influences might, therefore, contribute to the changes in HRV observed during anesthesia.

Effects of Drugs on Fetal Heart Rate Variability

Fetal HRV, as seen in a fetal HR tracing, has been regarded as a clinical indicator of fetal neurocardiovascular integration.[125] Alterations of fetal and neonatal HRV have been found in several conditions including hypoxia, fetal compromise and sudden infant death syndrome.[126] Maternal medication may cause significant changes in fetal HRV. Several drugs have been reported to decrease fetal HRV, for example, *meperidine*[127,128] and *scopolamine*.[129] The effects of *meperidine* on fetal HRV have been reviewed by Petrie.[130] *Glucose*[131] and *ephedrine*[132] increase fetal HRV, while *atropine*,[133,134] *glycopyrrolate*,[133,134] *propofol*,[135] and *antiepiletic therapy*[136,137] do not significantly influence fetal HRV. Although *general anesthesia* in pregnancy causes a profound depression in fetal HRV,[138] *epidural anesthesia* may not lead to significant changes.[139] However, this observation has been questioned by Viscomi et al.[140] *Magnesium sulphate* may decrease[141] or may not significantly influence[142] fetal HRV.

The methodology used for computation of fetal HRV and its underlying pathophysiological basis and clinical significance, which may be quite different from those in adult cardiology, are beyond the scope of this chapter. The reader is therefore directed to the individual references above for details.

Effects of Alcohol, Smoking and Caffeine on Heart Rate Variability

The effect of acute *alcohol* ingestion on short-term HR fluctuations was reported by Gonzalez-Gonzalez et al.[143] They demonstrated that acute ingestion of a low dose of alcohol (0.3 g/kg) in 18 normal volunteers did not alter mean HR, but spectral HRV was significantly changed: the LF oscillation (0.02 to 0.06 Hz) increased, while middle (0.08 to 0.15 Hz) and HF (0.20 to 0.35 Hz) oscillations decreased. Acute alcohol intoxication (0.7 g/kg) also reduces HRV.[144] Murata et al[145] reported that moderate drinking habits might not strongly influence HRV.

Hayano et al[146] have demonstrated that cigarette *smoking* causes a transient and significant decrease in the HF component and an increase in the LF component of HRV. Reduction in the HF component of HRV caused by acute cigarette smoking was recently confirmed by Niedermaier et al.[147] Long-term heavy smoke was also shown to cause a decrease in the HF component of HRV.[146] *Caffeine* has been shown to increase HRV in women.[148]

Effects of Other Agents on Heart Rate Variability

Several agents are effective in provoking panic attacks in the laboratory setting. Gorman et al[149] demonstrated that HRV does not change during *lactate*-induced panic attacks. *Yohimbine* significantly increases HRV in both normal subjects and patients with panic disorder.[150] *Imipramine* also decreases HRV in panic and depressed patients.[151] HRV is significantly decreased during *vincristine* treatment of acute lymphoblastic leukemia.[152] Hrushesky et al[153] reported a decreased HRV in doxorubicin-induced cardiomyopathy. *Aldose reductase inhibitor* therapy improves symptoms of autonomic neuropathy but does not cause significant changes in HRV.[154,155] The evidence that HRV decreases after treatment in patients with thyrotoxicosis[156] suggests that *thyroid hormones* may increase HRV. Lethal doses of cocaine have been shown to cause a marked decrease in HRV prior to sudden death in conscious ferrets.[157]

Conclusions

Many drugs have a significant influence on HRV, either directly or indirectly (eg, through drug-induced hemodynamic changes).[69,158] The majority of these findings may be explained by their parasympathetic and/or sympathetic blocking or stimulating effects. However, the results of different studies do not always agree. This discrepancy may be due to a different basal state of cardiac autonomic tone under various study conditions. In addition, other factors influencing drug effects, such as underlying heart disease and left ventricular dysfunction, may also contribute to inconsistent drug effects on HRV. Nonetheless, analysis of HRV has provided a useful tool for the assessment of pharmacological modulation of cardiac autonomic function, although drug effects on HRV have not been extensively studied in clinical practice. Our knowledge in this field, however, will undoubtedly expand in the next few years. Drugs which influence HRV, other than ordinary muscarinic and adrenergic agonists and antagonists, should be included in the category of autonomic pharmacology (such as antiarrhythmic drugs). Assessment of drug effects on HRV will further improve our understanding of their pharmacological mechanisms and may serve as a guide in treatment strategies.

References

1. Black JW, Stephenson JS. Pharmacology of a new adrenergic beta-receptor blocking compound (Nethalide). Lancet 1962; 2:311-314.
2. Ewing DJ, Neilson JM, Travis P. New method for assessing cardiac parasympathetic activity using 24-hour electrocardiograms. Br Heart J 1984; 52:396-402.
3. Pagani M, Lombardi F, Malliani A. Heart rate variability: disagreement on the markers of sympathetic and parasympathetic activities. J Am Coll Cardiol 1993; 22:951. Letter.
4. Malliani A, Lombardi F, Pagani M. Power spectrum analysis of heart rate variability: a tool to explore neural regulatory mechanisms. Br Heart J 1994; 71:1-2. Editorial.
5. Kamath M, Fallen E, Upton A, et al. Neurocardiac responses to vagal electrostimulation in man. PACE 1992; 15:519. Abstract.
6. Kleiger RE, Miller JP, Bigger JT Jr, et al. Decreased heart rate variability and its association with increased mortality after acute myocardial infarction. Am J Cardiol 1987; 59:256-262.
7. O'Brien IA, O'Hare P, Corrall RJ. Heart rate variability in healthy subjects: effect of age and the derivation of normal ranges for test of autonomic function. Br Heart J 1986; 55:348-354.
8. Rich MW, Saini JS, Kleiger RE, et al. Correlation of heart rate variability with clinical and angiographic variables and late mortality after coronary angiography. Am J Cardiol 1988; 62:714-717.
9. Fleiss JL, Bigger JT Jr, Rolnitzky LM. The correlation between heart period variability and mean period length. Stat Med 1992; 11:125-129.
10. Pomeranz B, Macaulay RJ, Caudill MA, et al. Assessment of autonomic function in humans by heart rate spectral analysis. Am J Physiol 1985; 248:H151-153.
11. Vybiral T, Bryg RJ, Maddens ME, et al. Effect of passive tilt on sympathetic and parasympathetic components of heart rate variability in normal subjects. Am J Cardiol 1990; 63:1117-1120.
12. Arai Y, Saul JP, Albrecht P, et al. Modulation of cardiac autonomic activity during and immediately after exercise. Am J Physiol 1989; 256:H132-141.
13. Yamamoto Y, Hughson RL, Peterson JC. Autonomic control of heart rate during exercise studied by heart rate variability spectral analysis. J Appl Physiol 1991; 71:1136-1142.
14. Kamath MV, Fallen EL, McKelvie R. Effects of steady state exercise on the power spectrum of heart rate variability. Med Sci Sports Exerc 1991; 23:428-434.
15. Bernardi L, Salvucci F, Suardi R, et al. Evidence for an intrinsic mechanism regulating heart rate variability in the transplanted and the intact heart during submaximal dynamic exercise? Cardiovasc Res 1990; 24:969-981.
16. Langewitz W, Ruddel H. Spectral analysis of heart rate variability under mental stress. J Hypertens 1989; 7:S32-33.
17. Pagani M, Mazzuero G, Ferrari A, et al. Sympathovagal interaction during mental stress. A study using spectral analysis of heart rate variability in healthy control subjects and patients with a prior myocardial infarction. Circulation 1991; 83(II):43-51.
18. Saul JP, Arai Y, Berger RD, et al. Assessment of autonomic regulation in chronic congestive heart failure by heart rate spectral analysis. Am J Cardiol 1988; 61:1292-1299.
19. Casolo G, Balli E, Taddei T, et al. Decreased spontaneous heart rate variability in congestive heart failure. Am J Cardiol 1989; 64:1162-1167.
20. Nolan J, Flapan AD, Capewell S, et al. Decreased cardiac parasympathetic activity in chronic heart failure and its relation to left ventricular function. Br Heart J 1992; 67:482-485.
21. Fei L, Keeling PJ, Gill JS, et al. Heart rate variability and its relation to ventricular arrhythmias in congestive heart failure. Br Heart J 1994; 71:322-328.

22. Airaksinen KE, Ikäheimo MJ, Linnaluoto M, et al. Impaired vagal heart rate control in coronary artery disease. Br Heart J 1987; 58:592-597.

23. Hull SS, Evans AR, Vanoli E, et al. Heart rate variability before and after myocardial infarction in conscious dogs at high and low risk of sudden death. J Am Coll Cardiol 1990; 16:978-985.

24. Luria MH, Sapoznikov D, Gilon D, et al. Early heart rate variability alterations after acute myocardial infarction. Am Heart J 1993; 125:676-681.

25. Casolo GC, Stroder P, Signorini C, et al. Heart rate variability during the acute phase of myocardial infarction. Circulation 1992; 85:2073-2079.

26. Bigger JT Jr, Fleiss JL, Rolnitzky LM, et al. Time course of recovery of heart period variability after myocardial infarction. J Am Coll Cardiol 1991; 18:1643-1649.

27. Bernardi L, Ricordi L, Lazzari P, et al. Impaired circadian modulation of sympatho-vagal activity in diabetes. A possible explanation for altered temporal onset of cardiovascular disease. Circulation 1992; 86:1443-1452.

28. Vybiral T, Bryg RJ, Maddens MA. Impact of arrhythmias on heart rate variability. Strategies to deal with imperfect clinical data. In: Murray A, Ripley KL (eds). Computers in Cardiology. Los Alamitos: IEEE Computer Society Press, 1990; 251-254.

29. Woo MA, Stevenson WG, Moser DK. Effects of ventricular ectopy on sinus R-R intervals in patients with advanced heart failure. Heart Lung 1992; 21:515-522.

30. Huikuri HV, Kessler KM, Terracall E, et al. Reproducibility and circadian rhythm of heart rate variability in healthy subjects. Am J Cardiol 1990; 65:391-393.

31. van Hoogenhuyze D, Weinstein N, Martin GJ, et al. Reproducibility and relation to mean heart rate of heart rate variability in normal subjects and in patients with congestive heart failure secondary to coronary artery disease. Am J Cardiol 1991; 68:1668-1676.

32. Molgaard H, Sorensen KE, Bjerregaard P. Circadian variation and influence of risk factors on heart rate variability in healthy subjects. Am J Cardiol 1991; 68:777-784.

33. Tapp WN, Knox FS III, Natelson BH. The heart rate spectrum in simulated flight: reproducibility and effects of atropine. Aviat Space Environ Med 1990; 61:887-892.

34. Kleiger RE, Bigger JT Jr, Bosner MS, et al. Stability over time of variables measuring heart rate variability in normal subjects. Am J Cardiol 1991; 68:626-630.

35. Bigger JT Jr, Fleiss JL, Rolnitzky LM, et al. Stability over time of heart period variability in patients with previous myocardial infarction and ventricular arrhythmias. Am J Cardiol 1992; 69:718-723.

36. Zuanetti G, Latini R, Neilson JM, et al. Heart rate variability in patients with ventricular arrhythmias: effect of antiarrhythmic drugs. J Am Coll Cardiol 1991; 17:604-612.

37. Molgaard H, Mickley H, Pless P, et al. Effects of Metoprolol on heart rate variability in survivors of acute myocardial infarction. Am J Cardiol 1993; 71:1357-1359.

38. Binkley PF, Haas GJ, Starling RC, et al. Sustained augmentation of parasympathetic tone with angiotensin-converting enzyme inhibition in patients with congestive heart failure. J Am Coll Cardiol 1993; 21:655-661.

39. Parati G, Pomidossi G, Casadei R, et al. Role of heart rate variability in the production of blood pressure variability in man. J Hypertens 1987; 5:557-560.

40. Akselrod S, Gordon D, Ubel FA, et al. Power spectrum analysis of heart rate fluctuation: a quantitative probe of beat-to-beat cardiovascular control. Science 1981; 213(4504):220-222.

41. Ferrari AU, Daffonchio A, Albergati F, et al. Inverse relationship between heart rate and blood pressure variabilities in rats. Hypertension 1987; 10:533-537.

42. Jansen HT, Dellinger JA. Comparing the cardiac vagolytic effects of atropine and methylatropine in rhesus macaques. Pharmacol Biochem Behav 1989; 32:175-179.

43. Zwiener U, Richter A, Schumann NP, et al. Heart rate fluctuations in rabbits during different behavioural states. Biomed Biochim Acta 1990; 49:59-68.

44. Hayano J, Sakakibara Y, Yamada A, et al. Accuracy of assessment of cardiac vagal tone by heart rate variability in normal subjects. Am J Cardiol 1991; 67:199-204.

45. Binkley PF, Nunziata E, Haas GJ, et al. Parasympathetic withdrawal is an integral component of autonomic imbalance in congestive heart failure: demonstration in human subjects and verification in a paced canine model of ventricular failure. J Am Coll Cardiol 1991; 18:464-472.

46. Lacroix D, Logier R, Kacet S, et al. Effects of consecutive administration of central and peripheral anticholinergic agents on respiratory sinus arrhythmias in normal subjects. J Auton Nerv Syst 1992; 39:211-217.

47. Ali Melkkila T, Kaila T, Antila K, et al. Effects of glycopyrrolate and atropine on heart rate variability. Acta Anaesthesiol Scand 1991; 35:436-441.

48. Coker R, Koziell A, Oliver C, et al. Does the sympathetic nervous system influence sinus arrhythmia in man? Evidence from combined autonomic blockade. J Physiol 1984; 356:459-464.

49. Bittiner SB, Smith SE. Beta-adrenoceptor antagonists increase sinus arrhythmia, a vagotonic effect. Br J Clin Pharmacol 1986; 22: 691-695.

50. Vybiral T, Bryg RJ, Maddens ME, et al. Effects of transdermal scopolamine on heart rate variability in normal subjects. Am J Cardiol 1990; 65:604-608.

51. Dibner-Dunlap ME, Eckberg DL, Magid NM, et al. The long-term increase of baseline and reflexly augmented levels of human vagal-cardiac nervous activity induced by scopolamine. Circulation 1985; 71:797-804.

52. Davis PB, Simpson DM, Paget GL, et al. Beta-adrenergic responses in drug-free subjects with asthma. J Allergy Clin Immunol 1986; 77:871-879.

53. Rote WE II, Connor JD. Autonomic mechanisms in heart rate variability after isoproterenol-induced myocardial damage in rats. J Auton Nerv Syst 1992; 38:37-44.

54. Cook JR, Bigger JT Jr, Kleiger RE, et al. Effect of atenolol and diltiazem on heart period variability in normal persons. J Am Coll Cardiol 1991; 17:480-484.

55. Elghozi JL, Japundzic N, Grichois ML, et al. Nervous mechanisms of spontaneous oscillations of systolic blood pressure and heart rate. Arch Mal Coeur Vaiss 1990; 83: 1065-1068.

56. Coumel P, Hermida JS, Wennerblöm B, et al. Heart rate variability in left ventricular hypertrophy and heart failure, and the effects of beta-blockade. A non-spectral analysis of heart rate variability in the frequency domain and in the time domain. Eur Heart J 1991; 12:412-422.

57. Rimoldi O, Furlan R, Pagani MR, et al. Analysis of neural mechanisms accompanying different intensities of dynamic exercise. Chest 1992; 101:226S-230S.

58. Akselrod S, Gordon D, Madwed JB, et al. Hemoodynamic regulation: investigation by spectral analysis. Am J Physiol 1985; 249:H867-875.

59. Theodorakis GN, Kremastinos DT, Stefankis GS, et al. The effectiveness of β-blockade and its influence on heart rate variability in vasovagal patients. Eur Heart J 1993; 14:1499-1507.

60. Schwartz PJ. Antiarrhythmic drugs and the autonomic nervous system: an intriguing and potentially dangerous interaction. New Trends Arrhythmias 1994; IX(1):193-199.

61. Lombardi F, Torzillo D, Sandrone G, et al. Beta-blocking effect of propafenone based on spectral analysis of heart rate variability. Am J Cardiol 1992; 70:1028-1034.

62. Filipecki A, Trusz-Gluza M, Szydlo K, et al. Effect of propranolol and propafenone on heart rate variability in patients with ventricular arrhythmias. PACE 1993; 16:1157. Abstract.

63. Hohnloser SH, Klingenheben T, Zabel M, et al. Effect of sotalol on heart rate variability assessed by Holter monitoring in patients with ventricular arrhythmias. Am J Cardiol 1993; 72:67A-71A.

64. Wallin BG, Sundlöf G, Strömgren E, et al. Sympathetic outflow to muscles during treatment of hypertension with metoprolol. Hypertension 1984; 6:557-562.

65. Edvardsson N, Olsson SB. Effects of acute and chronic beta-receptor blockade on ventricular repolarisation in man. Br Heart J 1981; 45:628-636.

66. Pagani M, Lombardi F, Guzzetti S, et al. Power spectral analysis of heart rate and arterial pressure variabilities as a marker of sympatho-vagal interaction in man and conscious dog. Circ Res 1986; 59:178-193.

67. Syutkina EV. Effect of autonomic nervous system blockade and acute asphyxia on heart rate variability in the fetal rat. Gynecol Obstet Invest 1988; 25:249-257.

68. Bailey JR, Crossley GH, Simmons TW, et al. Effect of procainamide on time and frequency domain analysis of heart rate variability. Circulation 1993; 88:I-116. Abstract.

69. Lombardi F, Torzillo D, Sandrone G, et al. Autonomic effects of antiarrhythmic drugs and their importance. Eur Heart J 1992; 13(suppl F):38-43.

70. Bekheit S, Tangella M, el Sakr A, et al. Use of heart rate spectral analysis to study the effects of calcium channel blockers on sympathetic activity after myocardial infarction. Am Heart J 1990; 119:79-85.

71. O'Connor GT, Buring JE, Yusuf S, et al. An overview of randomized trials of rehabilitation with exercise after myocardial infarction. Circulation 1989; 80:234-244.

72. Costa O, Freitas J, Puig J, et al. Spectrum analysis of the variability of heart rate in athletes. Rev Port Cardiol 1991; 10:23-28.

73. Goldsmith RL, Bigger JT Jr, Steinman RC, et al. Comparison of 24-hour parasympathetic activity in endurance-trained and untrained young men. J Am Coll Cardiol 1992; 20:552-558.

74. Adamopoulos S, Piepoli M, McCance A, et al. Comparison of different methods for assessing sympathovagal balance in congestive heart failure secondary to coronary ar-

tery disease. Am J Cardiol 1992; 70: 1576-1582.

75. La Rovere MT, Mortara A, Sandrone G, et al. Autonomic nervous system adaptations to short-term exercise training. Chest 1992; 101:299S-303S.

76. Cowen MJ, Kogan H, Burr R, et al. Power spectral analysis of heart rate variability after biofeedback training. J Electrocardiol 1990; 23(suppl):85-94.

77. Folkow B. Physiological aspects of primary hypertension. Physiol Rev 1982; 62:347-504.

78. Guzzetti S, Piccaluga E, Casati R, et al. Sympathetic predominance in essential hypertension: a study employing spectral analysis of heart rate variability. J Hypertens 1988; 6:711-717.

79. Chakko S, Mulingtapang RF, Huikuri HV, et al. Alterations in heart rate variability and its circadian rhythm in hypertensive patients with left ventricular hypertrophy free of coronary artery disease. Am Heart J 1993; 126:1364-1372.

80. Langewitz W, Rüddel H, Schächinger H. Reduced parasympathetic cardiac control in patients with hypertension at rest and under mental stress. Am Heart J 1994; 127:122-128.

81. Murakawa Y, Ajiki K, Usui M, et al. Parasympathetic activity is a major modulator of the circadian variability of heart rate in healthy subjects and in patients with coronary artery disease or diabetic mellitus. Am Heart J 1993; 126:108-114.

82. Blanc J, Grichois ML, Elghozi JL. Effects of clonidine on blood pressure and heart rate responses to an emotional stress in the rat: a spectral study. Clin Exp Pharmacol Physiol 1991; 18:711-717.

83. Grichois ML, Japundzic N, Head GA, et al. Clonidine reduces blood pressure and heart rate oscillations in the conscious rat. J Cardiovasc Pharmacol 1990; 16:449-454.

84. Elghozi JL, Laude D, Janvier F. Clonidine reduces blood pressure and heart rate oscillations in hypertensive patients. J Cardiovasc Pharmacol 1991; 17:935-940.

85. Yeragani VK, Pohl R, Balon R, et al. Effects of clonidine on heart rate variability. Jpn Heart J 1992; 33:359-364.

86. Pluskwa F, Bonnet F, Saada M, et al. Effects of clonidine on variation of artery blood pressure and heart rate during carotid artery surgery. J Cardiothorac Vasc Anesth 1991; 5:431-436.

87. Janssen BJ, Tyssen CM, Struyker-Boudier HA. Modification of circadian blood pressure and heart rate variability by five different antihypertensive agents in spontaneous hypertensive rats. J Cardiovasc Pharmacol 1991; 17:494-503.

88. Longo VL, Farah VM, Gutierrez MA, et al. Attenuation of neurogenic hypertension by chronic converting enzyme inhibition. J Hypertens 1989; 7:S44-45.

89. Sugimoto K, Kumagai Y, Tateishi T, et al. Effects on autonomic function of a new angiotensin converting enzyme inhibitor, ramipril. J Cardiovasc Pharmacol 1989; 13:S40-44.

90. Pagani M, Pizzinelli P, Mariani P, et al. Effects of chronic cilazapril treatment on cardiovascular control: a spectral analysis approach. J Cardiovasc Pharmacol 1992; 19: S110-116.

91. Miyakawa T, Minamisawa K, Yamada Y, et al. A study of the effects of delapril, a new angiotensin converting enzyme inhibitor, on the diurnal variation of arterial pressure in patients with essential hypertension using indirect and direct arterial pressure monitoring methods. Am J Hypertens 1991; 4:29S-37S.

92. Julien C, Kandza P, Barres C, et al. Effects of sympathetectomy on blood pressure and its variability in conscious rats. Am J Physiol 1990; 259:H1337-1342.

93. Grichois ML, Blanc J, Deckert V, et al. Differential effects of enalapril and hydralazine on short-term variability of blood pressure and heart rate in rats. J Cardiovasc Pharmacol 1992; 19:863-869.

94. Mancia G, Ferrari A, Pomidossi G, et al. Twenty-four hour hemodynamic profile during treatment of essential hypertension by once-a-day nadolol. Hypertension 1983; 5:573-578.

95. Mancia G, Ferrari A, Pomidossi G, et al. Twenty-four hour blood pressure profile and blood pressure variability in untreated hypertension and during antihypertensive treatment by once-a-day nadolol. Am Heart J 1984; 108:1078-1083.

96. Dutrey-Dupagne C, Girard A, Ulmann A, et al. Effects of the converting enzyme inhibitor trandolapril on short-term variability of blood pressure in essential hypertension. Clin Auton Res 1991; 1:303-307.

97. Webb SW, Adgey AA, Pantridge JE. Autonomic disturbance at onset of acute myocardial infarction. Br Med J 1972; 3(818):89-92.

98. Snisarenko AA. Cardiac rhythm in cats during physiological sleep in experimental myocardial infarction and beta-adrenergic receptor blockade. Cor Vasa 1986; 28:306-314.

99. Billman GE, Hoskins RS. Time-series analysis of heart rate variability during submaximal exercise. Evidence for reduced cardiac

vagal tone in animals susceptible to ventricular fibrillation. Circulation 1989; 80:146-157.

100. Vybiral T, Glaeser DH, Morris G, et al. Effects of low dose transdermal scopolamine on heart rate variability in acute myocardial infarction. J Am Coll Cardiol 1993; 22:1320-1326.

101. de Ferrari GM, Mantica M, Vanoli E, et al. Scopolamine increases vagal tone and vagal reflexes in patients after myocardial infarction. J Am Coll Cardiol 1993; 22:1327-1334.

102. Dorado M, Gonzalez-Hermosillo JA, Garcia-Arenal F, et al. Influence of the permeability of the artery responsible for the infarction on the variability of heart rate and late potentials. Its importance in the risk stratification after myocardial infarction. Rev Esp Cardiol 1993; 46:71-83.

103. Camm AJ, Fei L. Risk stratification after myocardial infarction. PACE 1994; 17:401-416.

104. Floras JS. Clinical aspects of sympathetic activation and parasympathetic withdrawal in heart failure. J Am Coll Cardiol 1993; 22:72A-84A.

105. Flapan AD, Nolan J, Neilson JM, et al. Effect of captopril on parasympathetic activity in congestive cardiac failure secondary to coronary artery disease. Am J Cardiol 1992; 69:532-535.

106. Townend JN, West JN, Davies MK, et al. Effects of quinapril on blood pressure and heart rate in congestive heart failure. Am J Cardiol 1992; 69:1587-1590.

107. The Acute Infarction Ramipril Efficacy (AIRE) Study Investigators. Effect of ramipril on mortality and morbidity of survivors of acute myocardial infarction with clinical evidence of heart failure. Lancet 1993; 342:821-828.

108. Olivari MT, Levine TB, Cohn JN. Abnormal neurohumoral response to nitroprusside infusion in congestive heart failure. J Am Coll Cardiol 1983; 2:411-417.

109. Zucker IH, Wang W. Modulation of baroreflex and baroreceptor function in experimental heart failure. Basic Res Cardiol 1991; 86(suppl):133-148.

110. Lumbers ER, McCloskey DI, Potter EK. Inhibition by angiotensin II of baroreceptor evoked activity in cardiac vagal efferent nerves. J Physiol 1979; 294:69-80.

111. Mace PJ, Watson RD, Skan W, et al. Inhibition of the baroreceptor heart rate reflex by angiotensin II in normal man. Cardiovasc Res 1985; 19:525-527.

112. Benedict CR, Weiner DH, Johnstone DE, et al. Comparative neurohormonal responses in patients with preserved and impaired left ventricular ejection fraction: results of the Studies of Left Ventricular Dysfunction (SOLVD) Registry. J Am Coll Cardiol 1993; 22:146A-153A.

113. Cardiac Arrhythmia Suppression Trial (CAST) Investigators. Preliminary report: effects of encainide and flecainide on mortality in a randomized trial of arrhythmia suppression after myocardial infarction. N Engl J Med 1989; 321:406-412.

114. Cairns JA, Connolly SJ, Gent M, et al. Post-myocardial infarction mortality in patients with ventricular premature depolarizations. Canadian Amiodarone Myocardial Infarction Arrhythmia Trial Pilot Study. Circulation 1991; 84:550-557.

115. Nicklas JM, McKenna WJ, Stewart RA, et al. Prospective, double blind, placebo-controlled trial of low-dose amiodarone in patients with severe heart failure and asymptomatic frequent ventricular ectopy. Am Heart J 1991; 122:1016-1021.

116. Navarro-Lopez F, Cosin J, Marrugat J, et al. Comparison of the effects of amiodarone versus metoprolol on the frequency of ventricular arrhythmias and mortality after acute myocardial infarction. Am J Cardiol 1993; 72:1243-1248.

117. Nul DR, Doval H, Grancelli H, et al. Amiodarone reduces mortality in severe heart failure. Circulation 1993; I-603. Abstract.

118. Friedman LM, Byington RP, Capone RJ, et al. Effect of propranolol in patients with myocardial infarction and ventricular arrhythmia. J Am Coll Cardiol 1986; 7:1-8.

119. Lichstein E, Hager WD, Gregory JJ, et al. Relation between beta-adrenergic blocker use, various correlates of left ventricular function and the chance of developing congestive heart failure. J Am Coll Cardiol 1990; 16:1327-1332.

120. Cohn JN, Johnson G, Ziesche S, et al. A comparison of enalapril with hydralazine-isosorbide dinitrate in the treatment of chronic congestive heart failure. N Engl J Med 1991; 325:303-310.

121. Adinoff B, Mefford I, Waxman R, et al. Vagal tone decreases following intravenous diazepam. Psychiatry Res 1992; 41:89-97.

122. Galletly DC, Corfiatis T, Westenberg AM, et al. Heart rate periodicities during induction of propofol-nitrous oxide-isoflurane anaesthesia. Br J Anaesth 1992; 68:360-364.

123. Komatsu T, Kimura T, Sanchala V, et al. Effects of fentanyl-diazepam-pancuronium anesthesia on heart rate variability: a spectral analysis. J Cardiothorac Vasc Anesth 1992; 6:444-448.

124. Latson TW, McCarroll SM, Mirhej MA, et al. Effects of three anesthetic induction techniques on heart rate variability. J Clin Anesth 1992; 4:265-276.

125. Martin CB Jr. Physiology and clinical use of fetal heart rate variability. Clin Perinatol 1982; 9:339-352.

126. van Ravenswaaij-Arts CM, Kollée LA, Hopman JC, et al. Heart rate variability. Ann Intern Med 1993; 118:436-447.

127. Baxi LV, Peterie RH, James LS. Human fetal oxygenation (tcPo2), heart rate variability and uterine activity following maternal administration of meperidine. J Perinat Med 1988; 16:23-30.

128. Zimmer EZ, Divon MY, Vadasz A. Influence of meperidine on fetal movements and heart rate beat-to-beat variability in the active phase of labor. Am J Perinatol 1988; 5:197-200.

129. Ayromlooi J, Tobias M, Berg P. The effects of scopolamine and ancillary analgesics upon the fetal heart rate recording. J Reprod Med 1980; 25:323-326.

130. Petrie RH. Influence of meperidine on fetal movements and heart rate beat-to-beat variability in the acute phase of labor. Am J Perinatol 1988; 5:306. Editorial.

131. Ferrer-Barriendos J, Llaneza P, Hurtado E, et al. The glucose perfusion test: value in detecting fetal distress. J Gynecol Obstet Biol Reprod (Paris) 1989; 18:479-486.

132. Wright RG, Shnider SM, Levinson G, et al. The effect of maternal administration of ephedrine on fetal heart rate and variability. Obstet Gynecol 1981; 57:734-738.

133. Abboud T, Raya J, Sadri S, et al. Fetal and maternal cardiovascular effects of atropine and glycopyrrolate. Anesth Analg 1983; 62:426-430.

134. Murad SH, Couklin KA, Tabsh KM, et al. Atropine and glycopyrrolate: hemodynamic effects and placental transfer in the pregnant ewe. Anesth Analg 1981; 60:710-714.

135. Alon E, Ball RH, Gillie MH, et al. Effects of propofol and thiopental on maternal and fetal cardiovascular and acid-base variables in the pregnant ewe. Anesthesiology 1993; 78:562-576.

136. van Geijn HP, Swartjes JM, van Woerden EE, et al. Fetal behavioural states in epileptic pregnancies. Eur J Obstet Gynecol Reprod Biol 1986; 21:309-313.

137. Swartjes JM, van Geijn HP, Meinardi H, et al. Fetal heart rate patterns and chronic exposure to antiepiletic drugs. Epilepsia 1992; 33:721-728.

138. van Buul BJ, Nijhuis JG, Slappendel R, et al. General anesthesia for surgical repair of intracranial aneurysm in pregnancy: effects on fetal heart rate. Am J Perinatol 1993; 10:183-186.

139. Lavin JP, Samuels SV, Miodovnik M, et al. The effects of bupivacaine and chloroprocaine as local anesthetics for epidural anesthesia of fetal heart rate monitoring parameters. Am J Obstet Gynecol 1981; 141:717-722.

140. Viscomi CM, Hood DD, Melone PJ, et al. Fetal heart rate variability after epidural fentanyl during labor. Anesth Analg 1990; 71:679-683.

141. Lin CC, Pielet BW, Poon E, et al. Effect of magnesium sulfate on fetal heart rate variability in preeclamptic patients during labor. Am J Perinatol 1988; 5:208-213.

142. Canez MS, Reed KL, Shenker L. Effect of maternal magnesium sulfate treatment on fetal heart rate variability. Am J Perinatol 1987; 4:167-170.

143. Gonzalez-Gonzalez J, Mendez-Llorens A, Mendez-Novoa A, et al. Effect of acute alcohol ingestion on short-term heart rate fluctuations. J Stud Alcohol 1992; 53:86-90.

144. Weise F, Krell D, Brinkhoff N. Acute alcohol ingestion reduces heart rate variability. Drug Alcohol Depend 1986; 17:89-91.

145. Murata K, Landrigan PJ, Araki S. Effects of age, heart rate, gender, tobacco and alcohol ingestion on R-R interval variability in human ECG. J Auton Nerv Syst 1992; 37:199-206.

146. Hayano J, Yamada M, Sakakibara Y, et al. Short- and long-term effects of cigarette smoking on heart rate variability. Am J Cardiol 1990; 65:84-88.

147. Niedermaier ON, Smith ML, Beightol LA, et al. Influence of cigarette smoking on human autonomic function. Circulation 1993; 88:562-671.

148. Kolodiichuk EV, Arushanian EB. The effect of caffeine on the cardiac intervalogram indices depending on the ovarian cycle phase in women. Farmakol Toksikol 1991; 54:28-30.

149. Gorman JM, Davies M, Steinman R, et al. An objective maker of lactate-induced panic. Psychiatry Res 1987; 22:341-348.

150. Yeragani VK, Berger R, Pohl R, et al. Effects of yohimbine on heart rate variability in panic disorder patients and normal controls: a study of power spectral analysis of heart rate. J Cardiovasc Pharmacol 1992; 20:609-618.

151. Yeragani VK, Pohl R, Balon R, et al. Effect of imipramine treatment on heart rate variability measures. Neuropsychobiology 1992; 26:27-32.

152. Hirvonen HE, Salmi TT, Heinponen E, et al. Vincristine treatment of acute lymphoblastic leukemia induces transient autonomic cardioneuropathy. Cancer 1989; 64:801-805.

153. Hrushesky WJ, Fader DJ, Berestka JS, et al. Diminishment of respiratory sinus arrhythmia foreshadows doxorubicin-induced cardiomyopathy. Circulation 1991; 84:697-707.

154. Green A, Jaspan J, Kavin H, et al. Influence of long-term aldose reductase inhibitor therapy on autonomic dysfunction of urinary bladder, stomach and cardiovascular systems in diabetic patients. Diabetes Res Clin Pract 1987; 4:67-75.

155. Gill JS, Williams G, Ghatei MA, et al. Effect of the aldose reductase inhibitor, ponalrestat, on diabetic neuropathy. Diabetes Metab 1990; 16:296-302.

156. Northcote RJ, MacFarlane P, Kesson CM, et al. Continuous 24-hour electrocardiography in thyrotoxicosis before and after treatment. Am Heart J 1986; 112:339-344.

157. Stambler BS, Morgan JP, Mietus J, et al. Cocaine alters heart rate dynamics in conscious ferrets. Yale J Biol Med 1991; 64:143-153.

158. McCabe PM, Yongue BG, Ackles PK, et al. Changes in heart period, heart-period variability, and a spectral analysis estimate of respiratory sinus arrhythmia in response to pharmacological manipulations of the baroreceptor reflex in cats. Psychophysiology 1985; 22:195-203.

Chapter 23

Circadian Rhythms of Heart Rate Variability

Ernest L. Fallen, Markad V. Kamath

Introduction

Contained within most biophysical systems are physiological rhythms which oscillate at specific frequencies. The periodicities of these cyclic phenomena have a broad range within each 24-hour interval. For instance, the beat-to-beat variability of heart rate (HRV), when transposed to the frequency domain, reveals a power density spectrum whose peak amplitudes have periodicities ranging from less than 0.003 Hz[1,2] to 24-hour cycles[3,4] depending on how long a data set is used for analysis. It is now recognized that some of these oscillations, especially those lying between 0.02 Hz and 0.40 Hz, are modulated by autonomic regulatory signals from centers in the midbrain.[5-8] A circadian rhythm, strictly speaking, refers to a time event series with a principal frequency of one cycle in 24 to 26 hours. Therefore, the minimum recording time to confirm a rhythm as circadian ought to be no less than 48 hours. It turns out that most time- or frequency-domain analyses of HRV derive from RR interval sequences of either shorter data sets (2.2 to 5 minutes)

which may provide clues to autonomic balance,[9,10] or longer data sets (1 minute to 24 hours) which may contain useful prognostic information.[11,12] Much has been written on the circadian distribution of HRV as a manifestation of autonomic regulation in health and disease.

Why the Interest in Circadian Rhythms?

It is now accepted that the onset of acute cardiovascular events does not occur randomly, but rather in a characteristic diurnal pattern with a prominent peak in the morning hours between 6 am and 12 noon.[13] This striking preponderance of morning events has been demonstrated for acute myocardial infarction,[14,15] sudden cardiac death,[16] thrombotic stroke,[17] and transient myocardial ischemia,[18,19] to name a few (Figure 1).

Because of this unique circadian distribution of event onset, efforts have been made to ascribe a possible linkage with those physiological rhythms known to have

From: Malik M., Camm AJ (eds.): *Heart Rate Variability*. Armonk, NY. Futura Publishing Company, Inc., © 1995.

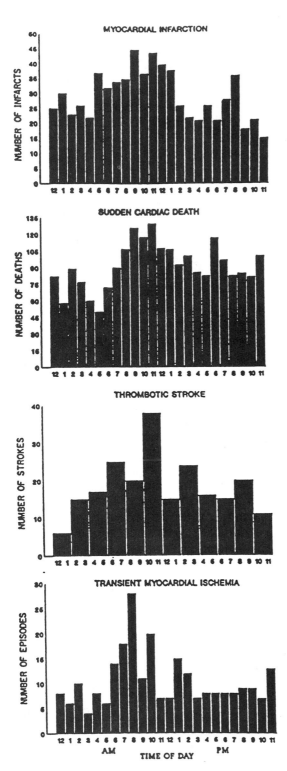

a similar diurnal variation. For example, it is well known that potential triggers of increased vascular tone have their peak activity in the morning hours indistinguishable from that of event onset. Examples include plasma catecholamines,[20] cortisol secretion,[21] platelet aggregability,[22] alpha adrenergic tone,[23] and fibrinogen activity.[24] All exhibit circadian patterns with the crest of activity occurring between 6 am and 12 noon. This coupled with the rapid rate of change of heart rate (HR) and blood pressure upon awakening[25] has prompted some investigators to attribute a causal link between the diurnal nature of the sleep-wake cycle and an abrupt imbalance in autonomic processes governing steady state cardiovascular regulation.[26,27] Support for these inferences come from several interesting observations. For instance, in one study, exercise performance in patients with stable angina was shown to be worse in the morning when forearm vascular resistance (and, presumably, coronary vascular resistance) was significantly higher than at night.[28] In the BHAT trial, the group assigned beta-blocker therapy had significantly fewer episodes of sudden cardiac death occurring in the morning hours compared to the remainder of the day.[29]

Although early morning arousal or the sleep-wake cycle presents a logical explanation for the circadian onset of vascular events, there remains several inconsistencies. First, the sleep-wake cycle, as a trigger, fails to explain the early evening peak seen in most circadian rhythms of event onset.[30,31] Note the late peak in Figure 1. Second, certain physiological processes such as cortisol secretion and platelet aggregability have similar circadian patterns but are independent of daily activity. Third, there appears

Figure 1. Bar graphs of time of day of onset of myocardial infarction, sudden cardiac death, stroke and transient myocardial ischemia. The number of events is shown on the y-axis and the hour of the day on the x-axis. From Muller JT et al. Circulation 1989; 79:734. With permission.

to be marked differences in diurnal patterns of event onset among certain patient subgroups.[32] Included are those with non-Q myocardial infarction, smoking, diabetes mellitus, prior congestive heart failure and beta-blocker use. Finally, therapeutic attempts to modify the cyclic variation of event onset, although at times altering the circadian rhythm, have so far not led to conclusive results.[33,34] In summary, the extent to which the circadian pattern of event onset reflects either the natural rhythmic oscillations of physiological triggers independent of the sleep/wake cycle or external factors coincident with arousal remains to be resolved. The circadian rhythms cited so far refer to isolated clinical or physiological events within a 24-hour period.

It turns out that many of these physiological processes contain inherent rhythmicities, the study of which may shed further light on the mechanism by which clinical event onset occurs. Consequently, attention has recently been directed towards study of the variability of time event parameters among which the most extensively analyzed is HRV.

Circadian Patterns of Heart Rate Variability: Measurement Issues

There exists a wide array of methodological approaches to estimating HRV. A comprehensive assessment and comparison of these measures are detailed in Chapters 3, 4 and 5. To determine the circadian distribution of beat-to-beat HR fluctuations, at least four general methodologies have been employed. They are:

1. chronobiologic techniques[4,35];
2. long-term time-domain measurements which are, in turn, broadly classified as: descriptive statistics applied to variable cycle lengths such as the standard deviation of all normal sinus conducted RR intervals over 24 hours (SDNN)[36,37] or; measurements of the differences between successive RR intervals expressed, as the percentage of RR interval differences which exceed 50 milliseconds (pNN50) or the root mean square of the standard deviation of successive RR interval differences (rMSSD) or the baseline width of the RR interval histogram[38-40];
3. frequency domain or power spectral indices usually applied to short data lengths of 2.2 to 5 minute sequences[41,42] and;
4. nonlinear techniques such as the plot of log spectral power versus log frequency or the 1/f statistic.[43]

As previously mentioned, a true definition of a circadian HRV cycle requires at least 48 to 50 hours of continuous electrocardiogram (ECG) monitoring to capture cycles with a 24-hour periodicity. Here, the essential circadian nature of an event is perhaps best estimated from standard chronobiologic methods. For example, HRV is commonly expressed as the standard deviation of normal cardiac cycle lengths during successive 5-minute intervals averaged hourly and displayed throughout a 24-hour cycle.[44] Applying chronobiologic methods, one can provide a statistical summary of the point and interval estimates of the rhythm adjusted mean, the peak amplitude of the 24-hour cycle, and the lag or acrophase which defines the time interval from any reference time to the peak amplitude of the oscillant.[4] Such cosine analyses have been determined and appear to validate a circadian rhythm for HRV accounting for more than 80% of the total variance (Figure 2).

However, there are rhythms within rhythms. As an analogy consider a pendulum oscillating at a specific frequency. Its principal harmonic can be inscribed as a simple sine wave with a specific amplitude and frequency. However, the oscillatory pattern of several pendulums in series reveals superimposed sine waves each with separate, but distinct, periodicities and amplitudes. The same can be surmised with

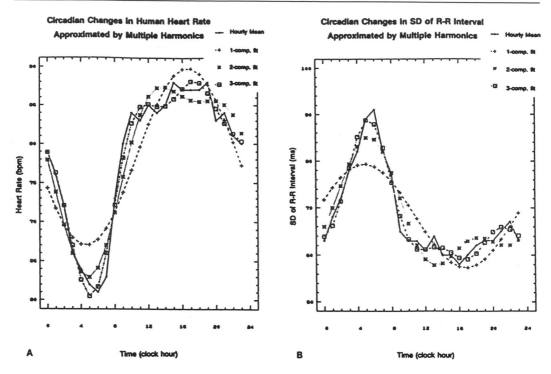

Figure 2. Circadian rhythm of (A) heart rate and in (B) standard deviation of RR intervals approximated by a 24-hour cosine cure alone or with 1 (12 hour) or 2 (12 and 8 hour) harmonic components. From Cornelissen et al. Am J Cardiol 1990; 66:864. With permission.

HRV. Examination of the variability of all RR intervals over 24 hours defines a cyclic pattern approximating a true circadian rhythm (Figure 2). The standard deviation of all normal RR intervals over 24 hours has been shown to be a powerful prognostic indicator of mortality following acute myocardial infarction.[11] If, on the other hand, the circadian pattern of HRV is derived from the standard deviation of RR intervals over 5-minute segments and averaged hourly over 24 hours, a similar reduction in variability is highly correlated with mortality in post-MI patients.[45,46] As with the pendulum analogy, the influence of the 24-hour circadian waveform on the variability of RR intervals of shorter data sets results in some attenuation.[47] When HR changes rather abruptly just prior to or on awakening, these ultradian rhythms (shorter periodicities in the 24-hour spectrum) are amplified in the sequences of shorter cycle lengths.[25] The broad based statistical measurements of cycle lengths reflect diurnal rhythms which are influenced by shorter cycle length changes and HR trends. Alternatively, time-domain measurements of RR interval differences such as the p-NN50 or root mean square of successive differences (r-MSSD) are said to be independent of diurnal or secular trends and exhibit a strong correlation with parasympathetic tone.[48,49]

Similar correlations are seen when the 24-hour period is analyzed in the frequency domain,[50,51] although studies of diurnal variation using power spectrum are comparatively sparse.

Using the Fast Fourier Transform (FFT), Rottman et al[50] compared the HR power spectrum computed over 24 hours with the spectrum derived from successive nonoverlapping 5-minute segments. The instantaneous heart period was rendered free of noise and ectopic beats by a process of linear interpolation. They demonstrated a remarkably tight concordance (r values >0.97) between the natural logarithm of either the low-frequency (LF) or high-frequency (HF) power from 5-minute segments and the corresponding power from the 24-hour total FFT.

It is generally acknowledged that our understanding of autonomic modulation of HRV is best derived from heart period power spectra obtained from short data sets especially under controlled conditions. Controversy exists over the physiological interpretation of individual spectral components when different lengths of data sets are used.[52,53] For instance, when the LF power is characterized in terms of the 24-hour spectrum, it appears to behave similar to those time-domain indices which reflect changes in parasympathetic tone.[49] Conversely, the spectral composition of an RR interval time series computed over 2.2 to 5 minutes exposes at least two distinct bands representing different autonomic regulatory processes. In a carefully conducted series of experiments designed to perturb cardiac autonomic tone during short-term controlled conditions (tilt, mild exercise, mental stress, pharmacological blockade and cardiac sympathetic denervation), Malliani and his associates have shown that the LF power consistently increased in response to sympathetic activation.[54-57] However, from a circadian perspective successive short-term power spectra viewed over 24 hours shows a clear reduction in the LF power during the night in healthy subjects, whereas the total amplitude of this spectral band is attenuated in those with cardiovascular disease where, presumably, there should be heightened sympathetic tone.[49] As with the pendulum analogy, the apparent differences in interpretation could be ascribed to the influence of the wide variance seen with long-term (nighttime) data sets on shorter term series. Whether measured by time- or frequency-domain methods, there is no controversy in asserting that vagal efferent regulation of sinus node activity is represented by the HF component of the power spectrum coincident with respiratory sinus arrhythmia. It is unlikely that the LF band, under steady state resting supine conditions, contains exclusively,

sympathetic information.[58] On the other hand, there can be no question that in response to maneuvers which predictably augment sympathetic tone, the LF and HF power show a reciprocal relationship with a dominant increase in the LF amplitude.

It turns out that short- and long-term data sets each have unique advantages which make them complementary in any assessment of diurnal variation of HRV. From power spectral analysis of short data lengths over 24 hours the advantages are:

1. the ability to determine the state of sympatho-vagal balance at specified intervals during the day[9];
2. the ability to control for movement artifacts, noise, respiratory variation and ectopic beats by examining subjects under controlled experimental conditions at specified times during the 24 hours of recording[59] (NB these are, paradoxically, its disadvantages if the power spectrum is computed from unrestricted ambulatory Holter ECG recordings); and
3. the ability to capture important transients such as the rapid changes in HR seen prior to or upon awakening in order to gain some insight into the underlying autonomic physiology of these events.

In a complementary fashion, the unique advantages of long-term time- and frequency-domain measures include:

1. the ability to uncover other frequencies; especially spectra in the very low-frequency (VLF) ranges which appear to have important prognostic significance for post-MI patients,[49] even though their physiological mechanism has yet to be explained;
2. a measure of total spectral power in those conditions where the signal-to-noise ratio is borderline, eg, congestive heart failure,[60] autonomic

neuropathy,[61] postcardiac transplantation,[62] etc.; and

3. less dependency on artifact-free and arrhythmia-free records, although careful editing and annotation are still essential.

Both approaches offer useful, albeit overlapping, information and are therefore complementary as analytic approaches to the study of circadian rhythms of HRV. Regardless of which system is employed, it is well to remember that HRV is, in the final analysis, an output signal from an exceedingly complex biophysical system.

Various computational techniques, some based on nonlinear models, are currently being explored to more faithfully represent the physiological mechanism underlying the day-to-day changes in HRV.[63-65] A detailed analysis of these experimental methods is beyond the scope of this review. Finally, it should be pointed out that the majority of methods discussed so far actually measures heart period variability as opposed to HRV. We use the term HRV in conformity with conventional usage.

Circadian Variation of Heart Rate Variability in Healthy Subjects

Using chronobiologic methods, Malps and Purdie[66] fitted a series of harmonic sine curves (24, 12, and 6 hours) to the standard deviations of successive RR interval differences of 30-minute duration in 11 healthy control subjects. They showed a significant circadian variation of HRV with a dominant 24-hour harmonic term. Of interest, the amplitudes at the 12- and 6-hour harmonics were comparatively negligible. The modeled curves revealed a maximum variation during sleep when the time to peak amplitude was 0356 hours. Although there is a temptation to ascribe this pattern to vagal influences, a similar pattern was seen in both diabetics and alcoholics with vagal neuropathy. The authors postulate that the origin of this circadian variation is likely

due to sympathetic withdrawal coinciding with the trough level of circulating catecholamines at round 0400 hours. However, in another study, when shorter segments of the HR record were subjected to frequency analysis, there appeared to be a decrease in HRV during sleep.[67] The latter, strictly speaking, was not a true circadian analysis but nonetheless focused on relevant autonomic changes over shorter time periods.

Sapoznikov et al[68] reported circadian patterns of HRV using both time domain and power spectral data from 50 subjects (age: 37 ± 16 years) without heart disease. The power spectrum was performed using a 16th order autoregressive model on 5 minute epochs and compared with the standard deviation of epochal mean RR intervals. They found that the HR and total RR interval variability was reduced at night despite an increase in the HF amplitude. In 77 healthy controls, Ewing et al[69] determined the HRV measured as the number of beat-to-beat differences greater than 50 milliseconds over 24 hours, an expression of cardiac parasympathetic activity. They found a significant inverse correlation between age and the difference in mean hourly counts between wakefulness and sleep. There was much higher variability at night, especially in the younger subjects. Of interest was the loss of diurnal variation in both HR and HRV during a period of sleep deprivation in eight subjects.

Using the HR autospectrum, Furlan et al[25] examined the 24-hour variation in autonomic modulation of sinus node activity in 28 healthy subjects. They found significantly reduced sympathetic modulation (LF power) between 11 pm and 5 am directly opposite the enhanced power contained in the HF (vagal) band. The rate of HR change in the early morning hours coincided with a rise in the LF power and a decrease in the HF power corresponding to the time of most frequent onset of major cardiovascular events. This reciprocal relationship, an expression of sympatho-vagal balance, was most noticeable at night. By contrast, Hayano et al[70] also employing an autoregressive model, showed a higher HF (vagal) component in the morning compared to late afternoon among eight healthy control subjects. The LF component did not change substantially throughout the day. The duration of their recording was from 0700 to 2300 and consequently did not include a sleep epoch.

Stability of Heart Rate Variability Measurements

Huikuri et al[71] estimated the reproducibility of HRV from repeated 24-hour ECG recordings in 22 healthy young adults. The mean and standard deviation of cardiac cycle lengths during successive 5-minute epochs were analyzed. A negative correlation was reported between the 24-hour means of HRV and the mean HR over 24 hours. HRV increased during sleep with its peak occurring within 3 hours of awakening. The mean intraindividual coefficient of variation for the 24-hour HRV was an acceptable 7±6% for repeated studies, whereas considerable intraindividual variation was seen for hour-to-hour HRV (coeff. of var: 23±10%). The wide temporal variability in HRV of shorter data sets presumably reflects the extent of fluctuation of vagal tone throughout the day. There was considerably less variation in repeated 24-hour measures of HR itself (a mixture of both sympathetic and vagal tone). Kleiger et al[38] documented the stability of time-domain measures with repeated monitoring of 14 healthy subjects. Using the intraclass correlation coefficient as a measure of individual variability, they found that the group means and standard deviations for a number of variables (SDNN, pNN50, r-MSSD) were virtually identical for repeated measures. The intraclass correlation coefficient for the differences measurements exceeded 0.9 making them suitable for both follow-up monitoring and for study of interventions (Table 1).

Influence of Modifying Factors

The influence of selected risk factors on circadian variation of HRV has been reported by Molgaard et al.[72] As an index of vagal tone they used the percentage of successive RR intervals that varied >6%. Among 140 healthy subjects, 95% of the beat-to-beat variability during a 24-hour period varied less than 6%. The percentage of successive RR intervals that varied >6% was significantly higher in subjects who were more physically trained. Age, on the other hand, correlated with a decrease in the percent of interval differences >6%; a reflection of decreasing cardiac vagal tone with increasing age. Likewise, smokers had lower variability scores especially during the day. Gender differences were also seen with a higher variability at night for men.

In summary, a diurnal variation of HRV with more pronounced interbeat variabilities at night is a normal and reproducible feature of heathy individuals. Whether one uses time-domain or frequency-domain analysis, there is a distinct day/night difference with maximum variance in the early morning hours just prior to awakening. The rise in HRV at night is mostly attributable to increased vagal tone, whereas changes in variability during the day are due to more complex interactions between sympathetic and vagal modulation of sinus node activity. Younger healthy subjects exhibit wider fluctuations of interbeat intervals especially at night, while advancing age appears to attenuate the vagal influence and, hence, the extent of 24-hour HRV.

Circadian Variation of Heart Rate Variability in Clinical Disorders

Myocardial Ischemia

In patients with stable coronary artery disease, the occurrence of ischemic episodes during the day follows a typical bimodal distribution with a prominent peak between 6 am and 11 am, and a second smaller amplitude peak between 6 pm and 9 pm.[73,74] From ambulatory ECG monitoring of patients with exercise-induced ischemia, Benhorin et

Table 1
Correlations for 14 Placebo and Baseline Records

	r-MSSD	pNN50	SDNN	NDDiff	RR	RR.N	RR.D	SDNNIDX
pNN50	0.96							
24-Hour standard deviation of NN intervals (ms) (CLV)	0.78	0.71						
Night/day difference	0.52	0.38	0.78					
Average NN interval for 24 hours (ms)	0.84	0.89	0.80	0.40				
Average nighttime NN interval (ms)	0.87	0.84	0.92	0.72	0.92			
Average daytime NN interval (ms)	0.76	0.88	0.66	0.19	0.97	0.82		
Mean of standard deviation of 5-minute NN intervals over 24 hours (SDNN index)	0.97	0.94	0.85	0.53	0.89	0.91	0.85	
Total power	0.94	0.92	0.87	0.57	0.86	0.90	0.85	1.0
Low-frequency power	0.91	0.81	0.85	0.71	0.72	0.86	0.63	0.92
High-frequency power	0.98	0.92	0.68	0.45	0.74	0.77	0.71	0.90

	Total Power	Low Frequency Power
Low-frequency power	0.93	
High-frequency power	0.88	0.89

Abbreviations: NNDDiff = Night/day differences; NN = normal cycle interval; pNN50 = percent of difference between adjacent normal cycle intervals >50 ms computed over the entire 24-hour ECG recording: r-MSSD = root mean square successive difference.
From Kleiger RE, Bigger JT, Bosner MS, et al. Stability over time of variables measuring heart rate variability in normal subjects. Am J Cardiol 68:526, 1991. With permission.

al[75] determined the circadian variation of both ischemic episodes and ischemic thresholds; the latter defined as the HR at which 1 mm ST segment depression was first observed. Both phenomena exhibited distinct circadian distributions. Whereas there was a typical bimodal pattern for ischemic episodes, only a single maximum peak for thresholds occurred with a slight morning lag between 10 am and 1 pm (Figure 3). These authors postulate that the absence of a secondary peak for ischemic threshold at night implies a different triggering mechanism for each peak; namely, a demand (increased sympathetic tone with arousal/activity) outstripping supply in the morning as opposed to a primary supply mechanism at night where changes in coronary vascular tone may occur in the absence of any change in demand.

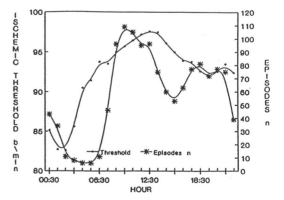

Figure 3. Plot of diurnal distribution of ischemic episodes and threshold of ischemia in 41 patients who had 1,371 ischemic episodes. From Benhorin J et al. Circulation 1993; 87:809. With permission.

Andrews et al[76] also demonstrated that over 80% of daily ischemic episodes during ambulatory ECG monitoring were preceded by an increase in HR and the peak activity occurred between 6 am and 9 pm. Although highly suggestive of a causal link between the time of increased oxygen demand and the onset of silent ischemia, HR is only one variable among many in the complex supply-demand equation associated with ischemia. A potentially fruitful approach to the study of silent ischemia would be the determination of a circadian pattern of short-term power spectral indices in these patients to shed some light on the role of autonomic regulation especially during the late afternoon/evening peak where there may be primary changes in vasomotor tone.

Congestive Heart Failure

In congestive heart failure, HRV is reduced (Figure 4) and the pattern of diurnal fluctuations of HRV is significantly flattened.[77-79] Using mean hourly HR standard deviations, there was marked depression of HRV throughout the day in 20 CHF patients studied by Casolo et al.[60] There was also virtual disappearance of the normal 24-hour HRV and a tenfold decrease in absolute power of spectral components. This resembles the pattern seen with diabetic autonomic neuropathy[80] and postcardiac transplantation[81]; two partially denervated states. The reduction in HRV affects all spectral components including the LF or sympathetic component where one would expect heightened sympathetic activity. However, this is not entirely surprising when one considers that patients with advanced CHF exhibit marked changes in neurohormonal activation.[82] Hence, an increase in circulating catecholamines and angiotensin II coupled with a depression of baroreceptor sensitivity, may account for the suppression of normal autonomic regulatory activity.

This phenomenon of decreased spectral power is also seen with standard time-domain indices in patients with CHF. It should be pointed out that the absence of a circadian pattern in CHF is not an all or none phenomenon, but varies depending on the degree of LV dysfunction.[83] In fact, there may be several distinct spectral patterns during the course of CHF based on the relationship between integrity of baroreceptor function and neurohormonal activation. For instance, preservation of nocturnal HF power has been reported in CHF patients, while augmented LF power has also been seen.[84]

Myocardial Infarction

The clinical potential of HRV measurements came to the fore when it was shown that diminished variance of the RR interval over 24 hours was a powerful and independent predictor of mortality following acute myocardial infarction.[11,12] Much attention has since focused on the circadian pattern of HRV measured either in the time or frequency domains postinfarction (Figure 5). It turns out that both short-term spectral indices as well as long-term time-domain indices offer equal prognostic power in predicting post-MI outcome despite the differing mechanistic interpretations ascribed to the two methodologies.[36,85] Hence, whether the 24 heart period is measured as

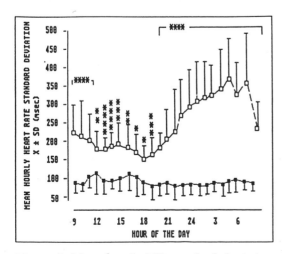

Figure 4. Mean hourly HR standard deviation in control subjects (white squares) and CHF patients (dark squares). Values are means ± SD (ms). *=p<0.05; **=p<0.01; ***=p<0.005; ****= p<0.001. From Casolo G et al. Am J Cardiol 1989; 64:1164. With permission.

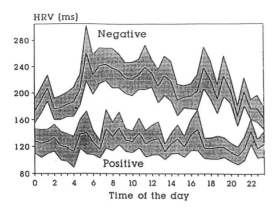

Figure 5. Mean short-term HRV from separate 40-min intervals in Positive group (20 post-MI patients who suffered death or sustained VT) and Negative group (20 post-MI patients who remained free of complications). HRV measured as baseline width (ms) of the RR interval frequency distrubution. From Malik M et al. Am J Cardiol 1990; 66:1050 with permission.

total SD, pNN50, r-MSSD, base width of the RR interval histogram, total spectral power or individual spectra ranging from as low as 0.003 Hz to the HF peak (0.15 to 0.5 Hz), these fractionated time series appear equally strong as predictors of outcome following an infarct, and therefore, can be used interchangeably.

Of equal importance is the observation that these indices, even with a background of a previous MI with or without ventricular arrhythmias, are stable and reproducible over time allowing for study of therapeutic interventions.[38] Bigger et al[49] presents evidence that the ultra LF power, as well as being prognostically important, is probably biologically generated despite the fact that the physiological explanation for this component remains unresolved. Moreover, in high-risk post-MI patients, the power contained in all spectral bands are depressed, including the LF component wherein lies sympathetic modulation. This may not be too surprising considering the attenuation of power in all spectral bands among high-risk patients with depressed LV function in CHF as previously noted. And so, when it comes to selecting an HRV time series for prognostic information, it appears that the

circadian distribution of any heart period measurement is useful. On the other hand, if one wishes to identify specific alterations in the balance between sympathetic and vagal modulation, any of the frequency-domain analyses is preferred. Bigger et al[40] found a high correlation between the various measures of 24-hour time- and frequency-domain parameters reflecting parasympathetic activity. However, there was a poor correlation between indices of pNN50 and r-MSSd with measures of baroreceptor sensitivity.[36] One is an approximate reflection of tonic vagal activity during a 24-hour period, while the other is an index of a complex interaction involving vagal stress performed at one time during the day.

Since any of the longer data sets for HRV appear equally effective as post-MI prognosticators, and since many of the measures described so far can be tedious due to the need for operator intervention in assuring records free of noise and artifacts, other simpler but effective methodologies have been proposed. Using, as an index, the width of the frequency distribution of RR intervals over 24 hours, Malik et al[12] explored different portions of the 24-hour ECG record to identify the time sequence most predictive of malignant arrhythmias in the post-MI period. They selected 20 patients who developed sudden cardiac death or sustained VT and matched them to a case control group of 20 post-MI patients who remained free of complications. There was a typical diurnal variation in the control group with a significant increase in RR variability at night and a decrease during the day. The time sequence with the highest predictive value for the high-risk group started at 6 am and lasted up to 8 hours. Note was made of another evening peak at 8 pm.

The issue of short versus long data sets was also addressed in this and related studies by the same authors.[12,86,87] It was clear that analysis of shorter data sets failed to provide reliable prognostic information when compared to long-term analysis using time-domain indices. Therefore, it is safe to conclude that measurement of HRV in post-MI patients should not be restricted to short ECG strips. They also observed that HRV, when measured as short-term 20-minute intervals, varied substantially with low values frequently seen in very low-risk patients. They offer a word of caution that time-domain data processing methods are still prone to some errors and provide only rough estimates of HRV. Likewise, long-term frequency-domain measures are equally coarse unless performed under stringent conditions of stationariness. In this regard, circadian rhythms of long cycle length with strong vagal influence may overwhelm the power contained in lower frequency components when viewed over prolonged periods. This dispute regarding the physiological nature of different frequency components between short and long segments could be better resolved when the short-term spectral analysis is performed under controlled conditions with attention to respiratory frequency, posture and stationariness. Even under these conditions, the signal-to-noise ratio is precariously low, especially in patients with LV dysfunction. Therefore, it is suggested that standardized interventions known to predictably alter sympatho-vagal balance (eg, tilt) be incorporated as part of the assessment. Hence, the decision for selecting between short-term frequency or long-term time-domain methods rests with the fundamental question being asked. Simply put, is the objective to ascertain prognosis or pathophysiology?

Several studies have examined the circadian variation in power spectral indices shortly following an acute myocardial infarction. Lombardi et al[85] compared the spectral indices of HRV throughout a 24-hour period between 20 post-MI patients and 20 matched controls. In the post-MI patients, they demonstrated enhanced sympathetic activity (elevated LF power) throughout the 24 hours with an attenuated increase in the vagal HF component at night. The RR interval variance was decreased in the post-MI population despite the fact that these were uncomplicated infarcts. It was also noted that both LF and HF components were reduced in absolute units. Using similar autoregressive techniques, Kamath and Fallen[88] reported a diurnal variation in 24 patients within 4 days of an acute MI. They found that under steady state wakeful conditions, HF power was more pronounced during the late evening (11 to 12 pm) compared to early morning (7 to 8 am) hours. There was also a shift towards relative sympathetic dominance during the early morning and mid-afternoon (3 to 4 pm) hours.

In summary, a predisposition to malignant ventricular tachyarrhythmias and sudden cardiac death following an acute MI can be foretold by monitoring the diurnal variation of HRV. A depressed 24-hour HR variance is strongly prognostic of mortality. There appears to be heightened sympathetic tone, especially in the morning hours, and a blunted vagal tone at night in the early postinfarction phase. The spectral composition of all components is generally depressed in these patients.

Sudden Cardiac Death

HRV is a powerful prognosticator of overall mortality. Algra et al[89] examined RR interval variability from 24-hour ECG records in 245 sudden death patients from a cohort of 6693 patients followed over a 2-year period. They found that those with low parasympathetic activity defined as low short-term RR interval variability had a substantially increased risk for sudden death independent of other risk factors. Decreased HRV has also been demonstrated in the same ambulatory ECG as the occurrence of ventricular fibrillation.[3] And yet, working back from the time of onset of ventricular fibrillation, Vybiral et al[90] demonstrated no change in the pattern of HRV prior to the onset of ventricular fibrillation.

Other Disease Entities

The same relationship between indices of depressed autonomic function and mortality can be seen for several noncardiac diseases such as diabetes[91] and alcoholic neuropathy.[92] Using 24-hour spectral analysis of HRV in 54 diabetic subjects, Bernardi et al[93] showed a marked reduction in the HF oscillations during the night and early morning hours. The day/night rhythm was reduced or absent in diabetics regardless of whether they had autonomic neuropathy or not. Using the number of beat-to-beat differences greater than 50 milliseconds during 24-hour ECG monitoring, Ewing et al[69] found that about half of 343 diabetic patients showed significantly reduced mean hourly counts. The percentage of abnormal counts increased with increasing autonomic abnormality in these patients. As expected, the circadian pattern of HRV post-heart transplantation is significantly attenuated.[62] However, there appears to be partial functional reinnervation as early as 7 months posttransplant reflected in a reappearance of a circadian variation in both BP and HRV.[94]

Effect of Interventions

Although there are numerous studies on the pharmacological effects of various agents on HRV, there are comparatively few studies specifically directed to circadian effects of drugs. Parmley et al[95] showed that long acting nifedipine attenuated the circadian pattern and frequency of episodes of myocardial ischemia in 207 patients with angina. Andrews et al[76] showed, in 50 patients with stable coronary disease, that ischemic episodes were related to HR increases in a circadian pattern with a daytime peak at 6 am to 10 pm. As predicted, propranolol reduced rate-related episodes during the day, but actually was associated with an increased proportion of non-HR related episodes compared with placebo. Nifedipine exerted the opposite effect, suggesting that spontaneous ischemia unassociated with HR change and occurring later in the day may be related to sudden changes in vasomotor tone.

Atenolol has been shown to increase time-domain measures of RR interval differences (pNN50 and r-MSSD) with little or no effect on total 24-hour SD in normal subjects.[96] It is reasonable to conclude from this and other studies[97] that beta-blockers have a direct effect on increasing vagal tone presumably through a central mechanism. Conversely, several type 1C antiarrhythmic agents (encainide and propaphenone) decrease the number of successive RR intervals exceeding 50 milliseconds (an expression of vagal tone) in a group of patients with ventricular arrhythmias.[98] While ACE inhibitors do not appear to alter HRV significantly,[99] digoxin increases the variance of all time-domain indices due, most likely, to its central vagal effect.[99]

Using power spectral analysis, Lambert et al[100] showed that the 24-hour periodicity of day/night ischemic episodes was attenuated with beta-blockade. However, some residual ischemia remained that was characterized by a shift in peak spectral activity to a period of 5 to 7 hours rather than 24 hours. In the Physicians Health Study where 342 nonfatal MIs occurred over a 5-year period, aspirin was associated with a 60% reduction in risk during the morning hours compared with a 34% risk reduction for the rest of the day.[101] Overall, there was a 44% risk reduction. The authors postulate that the circadian effect of aspirin is due to the increase in platelet aggregability during morning hours and upon rising. Goldsmith et al[102] compared the 24-hour beat-to-beat heart period variability between endurance trained and untrained young men. They found that the geometric mean of HF power was significantly more pronounced in the trained group during both day and night sequences. These authors interpret the findings to indicate that parasympathetic activity is substantially greater in trained than untrained men, a finding substantiated by others.[103]

The above observations raise the tantalizing suggestion that interventions which shift sympatho-vagal balance towards sustained and heightened vagal tone may be protective against sudden cardiac death. There are now a variety of interventions known to augment and possibly sustain increased vagal tone. These include exercise training, beta-blockade, low-dose atropine[104] including its derivatives such as transdermal scopolamine,[105] and vagoafferent electrostimulation.[106] Caution, however, is urged because any apparent association between a so-called favorable shift in autonomic activity and a decreased event rate does not necessarily imply a cause and effect relationship. Like ventricular arrhythmias, a depressed HRV may be nothing more than a marker rather than a direct precipitant of a catastrophic event. Furthermore, as mentioned several times in this review, the association between the predictive power of any HRV index and its physiological correlates remains unresolved. Circadian variation of HRV, therefore, is a useful means to characterize abnormalities of neurocardiac function but further refinement of these methods are required to more fully understand the basis of many interacting physiological processes.

References

1. Bigger JT, Fleiss JL, Steinman RC, et al. Frequency domain measures of heart rate period variability and mortality after myocardial infarction. Circulation 1992; 85:164-171.

2. Goldberger A, Findley LJ, Blackburn MR, et al. Nonlinear dynamics in heart failure: implications of long-wavelength cardiopulmonary oscillations. Am Heart J 1984; 107:612.

3. Myers GA, Martin GJ, Magid NM, et al. Power spectral analysis of heart rate variability in sudden cardiac death: comparison to other methods. IEEE Trans Biomed Eng 1986; 33:1149-1156.

4. Cornelissen G, Bakken E, Delmore P, et al. From various kinds of heart rate variability to chronocardiology. Am J Cardiol 1990; 66:863-868.

5. Sayers BM. Analysis of heart rate variability. Ergonomics 1973; 16:17.

6. Kitney RI. An analysis of nonlinear behaviour of human thermal vasomotor control system. J Theor Biol 1975; 52:231-248.

7. Akselrod S, Gordon D, Ubel FA, et al. Power spectrum analysis of heart rate fluctuation: a quantitative probe of beat-to-beat cardiovascular control. Science 1981; 213:220.

8. Malliani A, Pagani M, Lombardi F, et al. Cardiovascular neural regulation explored in the frequency domain. Circulation 1991; 84:482-492.

9. Pagani M, Lombardi F, Guzetti S, et al. Power spectral analysis of heart rate and arterial pressure variabilities as a marker of sympatho-vagal interaction in man and conscious dog. Circ Res 1986; 59:178-193.

10. Appel ML, Saul JP, Berger RD, et al. Closed loop identification of cardiovascular regulatory mechanisms. Comp Cardiol 1989; 16:3-8.

11. Kleiger RE, Miller JP, Bigger JT, et al. Decreased heart rate variability and its association with increased mortality after acute myocardial infarction. Am J Cardiol 1987; 59:256-262.

12. Malik M, Farrell T, Camm AJ. Circadian rhythm of heart rate variability after acute myocardial infarction and its influence on the prognostic value of heart rate variability. Am J Cardiol 1990; 66:1049.

13. Muller JE, Tofler GH, Stone PH. Circadian variation and triggers of onset of acute cardiovascular disease. Circulation 1989; 79:733-743.

14. Muller JE, Stone PH, Turi ZG, et al. Circadian variation in the frequency of onset of acute myocardial infarction. N Engl J Med 1985; 313:1315-1322.

15. Thompson DR, Blandford RL, Sutton TW, et al. Time of onset of chest pain in acute myocardial infarction. Int J Cardiol 1985; 7:139-146.

16. Muller JE, Ludmer PL, Willich SN, et al. Circadian variation in the frequency of sudden cardiac death. Circulation 1987; 75:131-138.

17. Tsementzis SA, Gill JS, Hitchcock ER, et al. Diurnal variation of and activity during the onset of stroke. Neurosurgery 1985; 42:459-904.

18. Rocco MB, Barry J, Campbell S, et al. Circadian variation of transient myocardial ischemia in patients with coronary artery disease. Circulation 1987; 75:395-400.

19. Nademanee K, Intarachot V, Josephson MA, et al. Circadian variation in occurrence of transient overt and silent myocardial ischemia in chronic stable angina and comparison with Prinzmetal angina in men. Am J Cardiol 1987; 60:494-498.

20. Linsell CR, Lightman SL, Mullen PE, et al. Circadian rhythms of epinephrine and nor-

epinephrine in man. J Clin Endocrinol Metab 1985; 60:1210-1215.

21. Weitzman ED, Fukushima D, Nogeire C, et al. Twenty-four hour pattern of the episodic secretion of cortisol in normal subjects. J Clin Endocrinol Metab 1971; 33:14-22.

22. Tofler GH, Brezinski DA, Schafer AI, et al. Concurrent morning increase in platelet aggregability and the risk of myocardial infarction and sudden cardiac death. N Engl J Med 1987; 316:1514-1518.

23. Panza JA, Epstein SE, Quyyumi AA. Circadian variation in vascular tone and its relation to α-sympathetic vasoconstrictor activity. N Engl J Med 1991; 325:986-990.

24. Andreotti F, Davies GJ, Hacket DR, et al. Major circadian fluctuations in fibrinolytic factors and possible relevance to time of onset of myocardial infarction, sudden cardiac death and stroke. Am J Cardiol 1988; 62:635-637.

25. Furlan R, Guzzetti S, Crivellaro W, et al. Continuous 24-hour assessment of the neural regulation of systemic arterial pressure and RR variabilities in ambulant subjects. Circulation 1990; 81:537-547.

26. Willich SN, Maclure M, Mittleman M, et al. Sudden cardiac death. Support for a role of triggering in causation. Circulation 1993; 87:1442-1450.

27. DeWood MA, Spores J, Notske R, et al. Prevalence of total coronary occlusion during the early hours of transmural myocardial infarction. N Engl J Med 1980; 303:897-902.

28. Kaneko M, Zechman FW, Smith RE. Circadian variation in human peripheral blood flow levels and exercise responses. J Appl Physiol 1968; 25:109-114.

29. Peters RW, Muller JE, Goldstein S, et al. Propranolol and the morning increase in the frequency of sudden cardiac death (BHAT Study). Am J Cardiol 1989; 63:1518-1520.

30. Kiowski W, Osswald S. Circadian variation of ischemic cardiac events. J Cardiovasc Pharmacol 1993; 21:S45-S48.

31. Mulcahy D, Cunningham D, Crean P, et al. Circadian variation of the total ischemic burden and its alteration with anti-anginal agents. Lancet 1988; 2:755-759.

32. Hjalmarson A, Gilpin EA, Nicod P, et al. Differing circadian patterns of symptom onset in subgroups of patients with acute myocardial infarction. Circulation 1989; 80:267-275.

33. Pitt B. The role of β-adrenergic blocking agents in preventing sudden cardiac death. Circulation 1992; 85(suppl I):I107-I111.

34. Peters RW, Mitchell LB, Pawitan Y, et al. Circadian pattern of sudden arrhythmic death in patients receiving encainide or flecainide in the Cardiac Arrhythmia Suppression Trial (CAST). Circulation 1990; 82(suppl III): III-138. Abstract.

35. Halberg F, Drayer JIM, Cornelissen G, et al. Cardiovascular reference data base for recognizing circadian mesor- and amplitude-hypertension in apparently healthy men. Chronobiologia 1984; 11:275-298.

36. Bigger JT, LaRovere MT, Steinman RC, et al. Comparison of baroreflex sensitivity and heart period variability after myocardial infarction. J Am Coll Cardiol 1989; 14:1511.

37. Farrel TG, Bashir Y, Cripps T, et al. Risk stratification for arrhythmic events in post-infarction patients based on heart rate variability, ambulatory electrocardiographic variables and the signal-averaged electrocardiogram. J Am Coll Cardiol 1991; 18:687.

38. Kleiger RE, Bigger JT, Bosner MS, et al. Stability over time of variables measuring heart rate variability in normal subjects. Am J Cardiol 1991; 68:626.

39. Ewing DJ, Neilson JMM, Travis P. New method for assessing cardiac parasympathetic activity using 24 hour electrocardiograms. Br Heart J 1984; 52:416.

40. Malik M, Cripps T, Farrell T, et al. Prognostic value of heart rate variability after myocardial infarction: a comparison of different data-processing methods. Med Biol Eng Comput 1989; 29:603.

41. Akselrod S, Gordon D, Madwed JB, et al. Hemodynamic regulation: investigation by spectral analysis. Am J Physiol 1985; 249:H867.

42. Fallen El, Kamath MV, Ghista DN. Power spectrum of heart rate variability: a noninvasive test of integrated neurocardiac functions. Clin Invest Med 1988; 11:331-340.

43. Kobayashi M, Musha T. 1/f fluctuations of heart beat period. IEEE Trans Biomed Eng 1982; 29:456.

44. Heslegrave RJ, Ogilvie JC, Furedy JJ. Measuring baseline-treatment differences in heart rate variability: variance versus successive difference mean square and beats per minute versus interbeat intervals. Psychophysiology 1979; 16:11.

45. Kleiger RE, Miller JP, Krone RJ, et al. The independence of cycle length variability and exercise testing on predicting mortality of patients surviving acute myocardial infarction. Am J Cardiol 1990; 65:408.

46. Malik M, Farrell T, Cripps TR, et al. Heart rate variability in relation to prognosis after myocardial infarction: selection of optimal processing techniques. Eur Heart J 1989; 10:1060.

47. Malik M, Farrell TG, Camm AJ. Evaluation of receiver-operator characteristics. Optimal time of day for the assessment of heart rate variability after acute myocardial infarction. Int J Biomed Comput 1991; 29:175.

48. Von Neumann J, Kent RH, Bellinson HR, et al. The mean square successive difference. Ann Math Stat 1941; 12:153.

49. Bigger JT, Albrecht P, Steinman RC, et al. Comparison of time- and frequency domain-based measures of cardiac parasympathetic activity in Holter recordings after myocardial infarction. Am J Cardiol 1989; 64:536-538.

50. Rottman JN, Steinman R, Albrecht P, et al. Efficient estimation of the heart period power spectrum suitable for physiologic or pharmacologic studies. Am J Cardiol 1990; 66:1522-1524.

51. Saul JP, Albrecht P, Brger RD et al. Analysis of long term heart rate variability. Comput Cardiol 1988; 419-422.

52. Pagani M, Lombardi F, Malliani A. Heart rate variability: disagreement on the markers of sympathetic and parasympthetic activities. JACC 1993; 22:951-954. Letter.

53. Goldsmith RL, Bloomfield D, Rottman J, et al. Heart rate variability: disagreement on the markers of sympathetic and parasympathetic activities. JACC 1993; 22:952-953. Letter.

54. Pagani M, Lombardi F, Guzzetti F, et al. Power spectral analysis of heart rate and arterial pressure variabilities as a marker of sympathovagal interaction in man and conscious dog. Circ Res 1986; 59:178.

55. Pagani M, Malfatto G, Pierini S, et al. Spectral analysis of heart rate variability in the assessment of autonomic diabetic neuropathy. J Auton Nerv Syst 1988; 23:143.

56. Pagani M, Furlan R, Pizzinelli P, et al. Spectral analysis of R-R and arterial pressure variabilities to assess sympatho-vagal interaction during mental stress in humans. J Hypertens 1989; 7(suppl 6):S14-S15.

57. Pagani M, Somers V, Furlan R, et al. Changes in autonomic regulation induced by physical training in mild hypertension. Hypertension 1988; 12:600-610.

58. Pomeranz B, Macauley RJB, Shannon DC, et al. Assessment of autonomic function in humans by heart rate spectral analysis. Am J Physiol 1985; 248:H151-153.

59. Bianchi A, Bontempi B, Cerutti S, et al. Spectral analysis of heart rate variability signal and respiration in diabetic subjects. Med Biol Eng Comput 1990; 28:205-211.

60. Casolo G, Balli E, Fazi A, et al. Twenty-four hour spectral analysis of heart rate variability in congestive heart failure secondary to coronary artery disease. Am J Cardiol 1991; 67:1154-1158.

61. Lishner M, Akselrod S, Mor Avi V, et al. Spectral analysis of heart rate fluctuations. A non-invasive, sensitive method for early diagnosis of autonomic neuropathy in diabetes mellitus. J Auton Nerv Syst 1987; 19:119-125.

62. Sands KEF, Appel ML, Lilly LS, et al. Power spectrum analysis of heart rate variability in human cardiac transplant recipients. Circulation 1989; 79:76.

63. Saul JP, Berger RD, Albrecht P, et al. Transfer function analysis of circulation: unique insights into cardiovascular regulation. Am J Physiol 1991; 261:H1231.

64. Kaplan DT, Furman MI, Pincus SM, et al. Aging and complexity of cardiovascular dynamics. Biophys J 1991; 59:945.

65. Lefebvre JH, Goodings DA, Kamath MV, et al. Predictability of normal heart rhythms and deterministic chaos. CHAOS, 1993; 3:267-276.

66. Malpas SC, Purdie GL. Circadian variation of heart rate variability. Cardiovasc Res 1990; 24:210-213.

67. Ichimaru Y, Clark KP, Ringler J, et al. Effect of sleep stage on the relationship between respiration and heart rate variability. Comput Cardiol 1990; 17:657.

68. Sapoznikov D, Luria MH, Mahler Y, et al. Day vs night ECG and heart rate variability patterns in patients without obvious heart disease. J Electrocardiol 1992; 25:175-184.

69. Ewing DJ, Neilson JMM, Shapiro CM, et al. Twenty-four hour heart rate variability: effects of posture, sleep and time of day in healthy controls and comparison with bedside tests of autonomic function in diabetic patients. Br Heart J 1991; 65:239-244.

70. Hayano J, Sakakibara Y, Yamada M, et al. Diurnal variations in vagal and sympathetic cardiac control. Am J Physiol 1990; 258(Heart Circ Physiol 27):H642-H646.

71. Huikuri HV, Kessler KM, Terracall E, et al. Reproducibility and circadian rhythm of heart rate variability in healthy subjects. Am J Cardiol 1990; 65:391-393.

72. Molgaard H, Sorensen KE, Bjerregaard P. Circadian variation and influence of risk factors on heart rate variability in healthy subjects. Am J Cardiol 1991; 68:777-784.

73. Cecchi AG, Dovellini EV, Marchi F, et al. Silent myocardial ischemia during ambulatory electrocardiographic monitoring in patients with effort angina. J Am Coll Cardiol 1983; 1:934-939.

74. Fox K, Mulcahy D, Keegan J, et al. Circadian patterns of myocardial ischemia. Am Heart J 1989; 118:1084-1086.

75. Benhorin J, Banai S, Moriel M, et al. Circadian variations in ischemic threshold and their relation to the occurrence of ischemic episodes. Circulation 1993; 87:808-814.

76. Andrews TC, Fenton T, Toyosaki N, et al. Subsets of ambulatory myocardial ischemia based on heart rate activity. Circulation 1993; 88:92-100.

77. Casolo G, Balli E, Taddei T, et al. Decreased spontaneous heart rate variability in congestive heart failure. Am J Cardiol 1989; 64:1162.

78. Binkley PF, Nunziata E, Haas Gj, et al. Parasympathetic withdrawal is an integral component of autonomic imbalance in congestive heart failure: demonstration in human subjects and verification in a paced canine model of ventricular failure. J Am Coll Cardiol 1991; 18:464-472.

79. Eckberg DL, Drabinsky M, Braunwald E. Defective parasympathetic control in patients with heart disease. N Engl J Med 1971; 285:877-883.

80. Thomaseth K, Cobelli C, Bellavere F, et al. Heart rate spectral analysis for assessing autonomic regulation in diabetic patients. J Auton Nerv Syst 1990; 30:S169-S172.

81. Fallen EL, Kamath MV, Ghista DN, et al. Spectral analysis of heart rate variability following human heart transplantation: evidence for functional reinnervation. J Auton Nerv Syst 1988; 23:199-206.

82. Packer M, Lee WH, Kessler PD, et al. Role of neurohormonal mechanisms in determining survival in patients with severe chronic heart failure. Circulation 1987; 75(suppl IV):IV80-IV87.

83. Saul JP, Arai Y, Berger RD, et al. Assessment of autonomic regulation in chronic congestive heart failure by heart rate spectral analysis. Am J Cardiol 1988; 61:1292-1299.

84. van de Borne P, Abramowicz M, Degre S, et al. Effects of chronic congestive heart failure on 24-hour pressure and heart rate patterns: a hemodynamic approach. Am Heart J 1992; 123:998-1004.

85. Lombardi F, Sandrone G, Mortara A, et al. Circadian variation of spectral indices of heart rate variability after myocardial infarction. Am Heart J 1992; 123:1521-1529.

86. Cripps TR, Malik, M, Farrell TG, et al. Prognostic value of reduced heart rate variability after myocardial infarction: clinical evaluation of a new analysis method. Br Heart J 1991; 65:14-19.

87. Malik M, Camm AJ. Heart rate variability: from facts to fancies. JACC 1993; 22:566-568.

88. Kamath MV, Fallen EL. Diurnal variations of neurocardiac rhythms in acute myocardial infarction. Am J Cardiol 1991; 68:155-160.

89. Algra A, Tijssen JGP, Roelandt JRTC, et al. Heart rate variability from 24-hour electrocardiography and the 2-year risk for sudden death. Circulation 1993; 88:180-185.

90. Vybiral T, Glaeser DH, Goldberger AL, et al. Conventional heart rate variability analysis of ambulatory electrocardiographic recordings fails to predict imminent ventricular fibrillation. JACC 1993; 22:557-565.

91. Ewing DJ, Campbell IW, Clarke BF. Assessment of cardiovascular effects in diabetic autonomic neuropathy and prognostic implications. Ann Intern Med 1980; 92(part 2):308-311.

92. Johnson RH, Robinson BJ. Mortality in alcoholics with autonomic neuropathy. J Neurol Neurosurg Psychiatry 1988; 51:476.

93. Bernardi L, Ricordi L, Lazzari P, et al. Impaired circadian modulation of sympathovagal activity in diabetes. A possible explanation for altered temporal onset of cardiovascular disease. Circulation 1992; 86:1443-1452.

94. van de Borne P, Leeman M, Primo G, et al. Reappearance of a normal circadian rhythm of blood pressure after cardiac transplantation. Am J Cardiol 1992; 69:794-801.

95. Parmley WW, Nesto RW, Singh BN, et al. Attenuation of the circadian patterns of myocardial ischemia with nifedipine GITS in patients with chronic stable angina. JACC 1992; 19:1380-1389.

96. Cook JR, Bigger JT, Kleiger RE, et al. Effect of atenolol and diltiazem on heart rate variability in normal persons. J Am Coll Cardiol 1991; 17:480.

97. Coker R, Koziell A, Oliver C, et al. Does the sympathetic nervous system influence sinus arrhythmia in man? Evidence from combined autonomic blockade. J Physiol 1984; 356:459-464.

98. Zuanetti G, Latini R, Nielson JMM, et al. Heart rate variability in patients with ventricular arrhythmias: effect of antiarrhythmic drugs. J Am Coll Cardiol 1991; 17:604.

99. Bosner MS, Kaufman ES, Stein PK, et al. The effect of enalapril and digoxin on heart rate variability in normal subjects. Circulation 1991; 84(suppl II):II-616.

100. Lambert CR, Coy K, Imperi G, et al. Influence of beta-adrenergic blockade defined by time series analysis on circadian variation of heart rate and ambulatory myocardial ischemia. Am J Cardiol 1989; 64:835-839.

101. Ridker PM, Manson JE, Buring JE, et al. Circadian variation of acute myocardial infarction and the effect of low-dose aspirin

in a randomized trial of physicians. Circulation 1990; 82:897-902.

102. Goldsmith RL, Bigger JT Jr, Steinman RC, et al. Comparison of 24-hour parasympathetic activity in endurance-trained and untrained young men. JACC 1992; 20:552-558.

103. Dixon EM, Kamath MV, McCartney N, et al. Neural regulation of heart rate variability in endurance athletes and sedentary controls. Cardiovasc Res 1992; 26:713-719.

104. Weise F, Baltrusch K, Heydenreich F. Effect of low-dose atropine on heart rate fluctuations during ortho-static load: a spectral analysis. J Auton Nerv Syst 1989; 26:223.

105. Vybiral T, Bryg RJ, Maddens ME, et al. Effects of transdermal scopolamine on heart rate variability in normal subjects. Am J Cardiol 1990; 65:604.

106. Kamath MV, Upton ARM, Talalla A, et al. Neurocardiac responses to vagoafferent electrostimulation in humans. PACE 1992; 15:235.

Chapter 24

Relationships Between Heart Rate, Respiration and Blood Pressure Variabilities

Peter Sleight, Barbara Casadei

Introduction

The origins of respiratory sinus arrhythmia have intrigued physicians and physiologists for many years (for recent comprehensive reviews see Eckberg,[1] and Eckberg and Sleight).[2] The most generally accepted explanation is that this waxing and waning of the pulse rate is caused by a central nervous medullary "oscillator" which becomes entrained to the respiratory rate as a result of afferent input from bronchopulmonary receptors.

There is ample evidence for such an oscillating circuit in the medulla oblongata of animals.[3,4] There is also evidence that the cells involved in autonomic control do receive inputs from respiratory afferents which alter their resting membrane potential.[5]

Since the range of heart rate (HR) change can be increased by deeper breathing,[6,7] the central mechanism cannot be a simple entrainment of an oscillator; but it would not be difficult to envisage modifica-tion of the amplitude of the oscillation by the influence of such respiratory afferents on cardiovascular motor neurones. This central nervous network continues to oscillate in the absence of respiratory movements.[8]

However, as in the study by Shykoff, many of the studies on respiratory sinus arrhythmia have been carried out on anesthetized preparations. There is evidence that baroreflex mechanisms (ie, not solely central), may be more important in conscious animals, and conscious humans.[7,9]

Blood Pressure Changes Linked to Respiration

There is some confusion in the literature about the precise changes in blood pressure (BP) which occur during breathing. The general view is that systemic BP falls during inspiration, particularly systolic BP.[6,7]

However, Eckberg et al[10] found that during inspiration, diastolic BP surprisingly

From: Malik M., Camm AJ (eds.): *Heart Rate Variability*. Armonk, NY. Futura Publishing Company, Inc., © 1995.

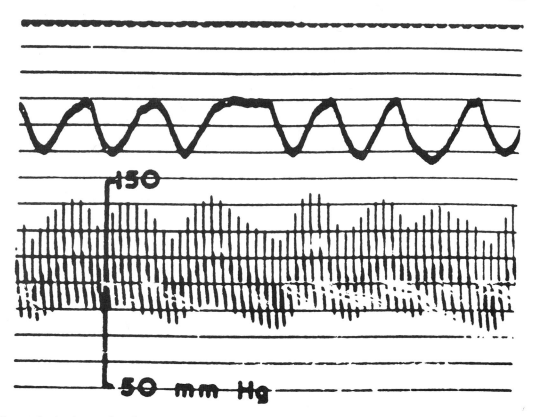

Figure 1. An interpolated expiratory pause demonstrates that the fall of pressure accompanying inspiration does not depend on it, but on the preceding expiration. Recordings from above down: Time 1 sec, respiratory record (inspiration downwards), brachial intra arterial pressure. Note the fall in arterial pressure, during the pause in respiration, at the time of what would have been the next inspiration. From Dornhorst et al[12] with permission.

rose during inspiration, at a time when HR increased (ie, vagal tone reduced) and sympathetic output to muscle nerves (MNSA) decreased. In other words, there was an unusual response in that a rise in BP would be expected to cause a reflex fall in HR (not seen), and reduction in sympathetic discharge (seen).

On the other hand, several other studies (see Laude et al[7]) have documented clear decreases in systolic BP on inspiration, which would then be quite compatible (on a reflex basis) with the normally observed inspiratory tachycardia and increase in MSNA. It is now possible to reconcile these seemingly opposed results.

DeBoer et al[11] have pointed out that changes in diastolic BP with respiration are generally small, since the inspiratory tachy-

cardia tends to reduce any inspiratory fall in diastolic pressure (since there is less time for diastolic pressure run off). During expiration, the longer pulse interval buffers any change in diastolic pressure caused by the increase in stroke volume, so diastolic pressure may correlate poorly with reflex changes. Dornhorst et al[12] carried out an elegant series of experiments in which they not only examined changes in both breathing rate and depth, but also separated the mechanical effects of respiration from a central neural mechanism by introducing a respiratory pause. They showed (Figure 1) that when such a pause is introduced, the inspiratory fall in BP is unchanged—demonstrating that it was the result of the previous inspiration, before the pause. It is hard to better their original explanation for the changes in stroke volume caused by inspiration, and the way in which increases in respiratory frequency alter the relationships.

Mechanism of Stroke Volume Modulation

It is generally agreed that respiratory modulation of stroke volume is produced as follows: inspiration lowers intrathoracic pressure and enhances filling of the right heart from the extrathoracic veins. Right ventricular stroke volume thus increases, and hence the effective (distending) pressure of the lesser circulation rises. The rise in effective pressure in the pulmonary veins leads to increased filling of the left heart and so to increased left ventricular stroke volume.

The dynamic implications of this mechanism have not, so far as we are aware, been recognized. It can be seen that the resistance and the hydraulic capacitances of the lesser circulation interpose a "lag" mechanism between inspiration and right ventricular output increase on the one hand, and the rise of effective pulmonary venous pressure and left ventricular filling on the other. It follows that, for a given depth of respiration, stroke volume modulation will decrease with increasing respiratory rate. Moreover, while there is a primary phase relationship between inspiration and increased stroke volume, with increasing rates, the phase of the stroke volume change will lag increasingly behind the corresponding respiratory phase. It thus comes about that at moderately rapid rates stroke volume (and BP) is falling throughout most of inspiration, the fall being due not to the accompanying inspiration, but to the preceding expiration. The true causal connections may be displayed by interrupting breathing for a few seconds at different points in the cycle.

They also noted that the right ventricular stroke volume was more responsive to changes in filling pressure when this was lower, in the upright, compared with the supine position. They further commented that during inspiration the lowered intrathoracic pressure distends pulmonary veins and left atrium more than the less compliant left ventricle, whose filling gradient is thus reduced, so that the resultant immediate decrease in stroke volume coincides with the fall in left sided stroke volume which follows the modulation of right ventricular stroke volume (by the previous breath).

Constancy of Diastolic Blood Pressure During Breathing

The relative constancy of diastolic BP during respiration (see Eckberg above) is well illustrated by Figure 2, from Laude's more exhaustive and statistical analysis of these complex interrelations.[7] She and her colleagues confirmed Dornhorst's views.[12] Figure 3 shows the relationship between breathing rate and tidal volume, and the HR and SBP changes (lower panel). HR changes are greatest with larger tidal volumes and slower breathing rates (9/minute). The phase relation between inspiration and BP are shown in Figure 4. With slower breathing (9 and 12 per minute), inspiration is related to a fall in SBP and a later fall in HR which is probably baroflex related (see below). With faster breathing (18 and 24 per minute) the HR increase now lags somewhat. Both oscillations are reduced by tachypnoea, since smaller faster breaths have less influence on venous return.

These authors conclude that these findings lend considerable support to the De Boer model[11] which attributes the HR changes to baroreflex responses to BP changes caused by mechanically induced cycling of left ventricular stroke volume, caused mainly by inspiratory increases in venous return. Comparisons between spontaneous free breathing and controlled breathing at the same rate and depth suggest no important differences in autonomic control between these two conditions, although one might speculate that the effort of following the command to breathe might decrease baroreflex gain (see below).[43]

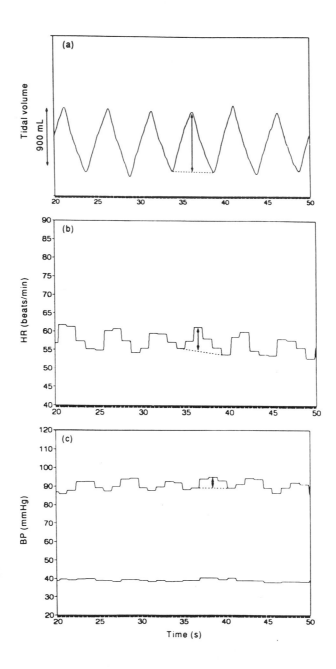

Figure 2. Computer displays of tidal volume (VT), inspiration upwards (a), HR (b), SBP and DBP (c) in a respresentative subject. Thirty seconds of data are shown during voluntary control of VT and breathing frequency (BF). Note the nearly constant value of DBP. The amplitude of changes in VT, HR and SBP are calculated as the perpendicular distance between each respective peak and a straight line drawn between successive nadirs of each signal, and show the usual inspiratory tachycardia and expiratory rise in SBP. From Laude et al[7] with permission.

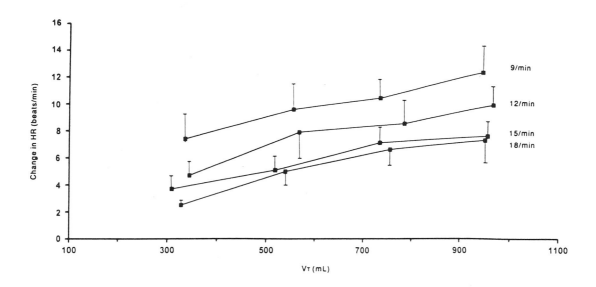

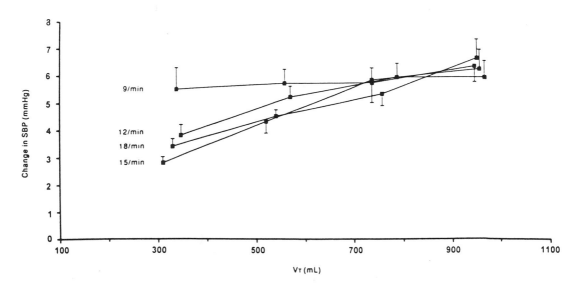

Figure 3. Effects of VT and BF on HR (upper panal). The average change in HR and SBP during respiratory cycle is shown on the vertical axes, and average VT is shown on the horizontal axis. Mean data and s.e.m. ($n = 8$) are shown for each of four VT at each of the four different BF. From Laude et al[7] with permission.

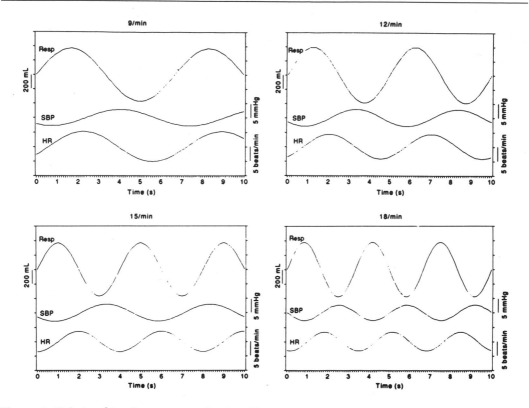

Figure 4. Relationships between respiration (Resp), inspiration upwards, SBP and HR at four different BF with a fixed VT of 700 mL. Mean data of the eight subjects were used. Note the inspiritory fall in BP and rise in HR. From Laude et al[7] with permission.

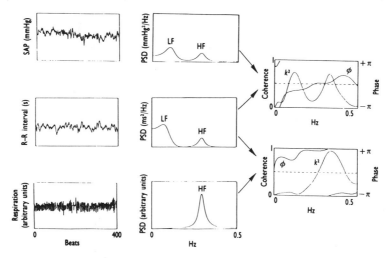

Figure 5. Example of time series (left panels) and autospectra (middle panels) of RR interval (center), systolic arterial pressure (SAP) (top) and respiration (bottom) in a control subject at rest. The right panels illustrate the results of the cross-spectral analysis between RR and SAP variabilities (top) and between RR variability and respiration (bottom). Note the high value (>0.5) of the coherence (K^2) function in correspondence of the LF and HF components, in the case of RR interval and SAP variabilities cross-spectra (top panel). On the contrary, spectral analysis of RR interval variability and respiration (botton panel) indicates a high level (>5.0) of coherence only in correspondence of the HF components. From Lucini et al[15] with permission.

Importance of Respiratory Coherence Measures in Power Spectral Analyses of Cardiovascular Variation

As we have seen, respiration induced changes in circulatory variables are of great importance. This underlies the need to measure respiration, particularly when carrying out studies using power spectral methodology. Unless this is done, occasional slow breaths can cause oscillations which fall in the low-frequency (LF) (0.1 Hz) part of the power spectrum. Respiration can be conveniently recorded using changes in chest impedance changes between the electrodes on the chest also used to record the ECG.[13]

In order to avoid this, it is necessary to examine for coherence with the respiratory signal (see Figure 5).[14] This presentation allows one to identify correctly the peaks related to respiration. If the PSA data are presented as a pie chart representing the vagal and "sympathetic" balance, the size of the circle gives a visual impression of total power. In Figure 6, we can see this type of display for changes with posture; the upright position not only increases the relative contribution of the sympathetic (LF) component, but decreases the overall variability (smaller circle).[16]

Non-neural Mechanisms for Respiratory Sinus Arrhythmia

In addition to the neurally mediated changes, it is now well established that inspiratory increases in HR are also seen in the denervated hearts of human

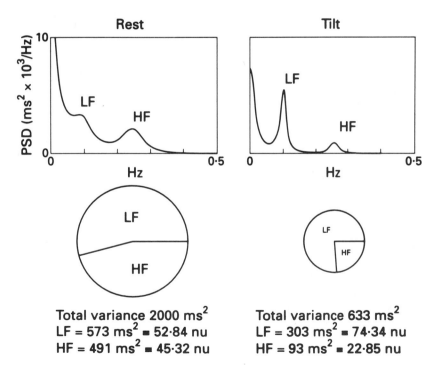

Figure 6. Example of spectral analysis of RR interval variability in a healthy subject examined at rest and during a passive tilt. At rest, there are two major components (LF and HF) of similar power, whereas during tilting the LF component predominates. In this case, the total variance during tilting is markedly reduced, so both LF and HF powers are diminished when expressed in absolute units. The use of normalized units (nu) clearly indicates the altered relation between the two spectral components induced by tilting. The pie charts show this relative distribution together with the absolute power of the two components (represented by the area). From Malliani et al[16] with permission.

transplant patients.[13] The respiratory HR increases are considerably smaller than in normal increases, and are thought to be related to direct effects of increased stretch of the sinus node caused by inspiratory increases in venous return.[17]

Is There a Peripheral Component Which Drives Respiratory Sinus Arrhythmia?

The central oscillator hypothesis has held sway for many decades. More recently (in a series of impressive theses) Karemaker, DeBoer, Ten Voorde and colleagues[11,18-20] have used mathematical modeling techniques and found that the oscillations in HR and BP could be explained by baroreflex responses to the fluctuations in BP produced by respiration, but not by a central oscillator model.[20]

As we have seen above, the relation between systemic BP and respiration is complex; for the first two or three beats following inspiration, blood, as well as air, is sucked into the thorax, and then into the right atrium and ventricle. This increases right ventricular stroke volume and leads to the familiar inspiratory delay in the sound of pulmonary closure valve heard with the stethescope[21]; this is also accompanied by earlier aortic closure on inspiration due to the inspiratory fall in LV stroke volume[22] (see Dornhorst quotation above). The surge of right ventricular pressure and flow is slightly damped as it passes through the pulmonary circulation, but still causes a respiratory related oscillation in systemic BP. At normal rates of breathing, this systemic pressure rise coincides with expiration and is responsible for the reflex bradycardia seen during expiration. Similarly, falls in systemic BP (and hence reflex tachycardia) are seen during inspiration (see Figure 1).

DeBoer/Karemaker Model of Respiratory Sinus Arrhythmia

The Dutch group have thus constructed a model which closely mimicked actual variations in RR interval seen during various respiratory maneuvers. The model (Figure 7) depends on:

1. respiratory fluctuations in right, then left ventricular stroke volume;
2. rapid baroreflex responses in HR (vagal); and
3. slower baroreflex responses in vascular tone (sympathetic).

As well as explaining the more obvious peaks in the power of HR and BP seen at the respiratory frequency (generally at about 0.25 Hz, 15 breaths per minute—high-frequency (HF) peak in power spectrum), they showed that baroreflex driven changes could also explain variations in the LF area (about 0.1 Hz) of the power spectrum. These LF variations were the result of the inability of the reflex sympathetic neural outflow to follow beat-to-beat changes in BP sensed by the arterial and other baroreceptors. This is particularly pronounced when baroreflex vagal responses are responding on a faster, beat-to-beat, basis. This "inefficient" feedback loop generated a resonance in the BP and RR interval spectrum in their model at about 0.1 Hz, ie, the LF peak seen in analyses of actual BP recordings of steady state conditions in man.

Newer Data on the Derivation of Peaks in the Power Spectrum of Heart Rate and Blood Pressure Variability

Power spectral analysis methods are increasingly used to shed light on the behavior of the autonomic nervous system (ANS).[14-16,23-25] Interest has increased considerably since it has been shown that low HF and high LF may help in identifying cardiac

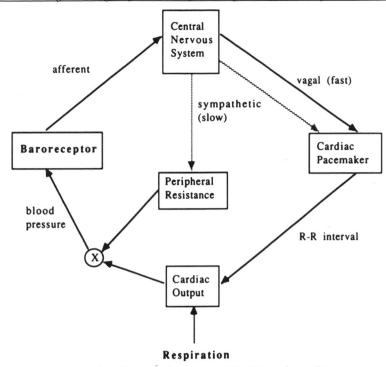

Figure 7. Schematic diagram of cardiovascular system. BP affects, through baroreceptors and central nervous system, both interval length and peripheral resistance (baroreflex). *Dashed line* indicates slow sympathetic control. Cardiac output is determined by HR (or RR interval). Peripheral resistance and cardiac output determine new BP value. These simulations suggest that respiration first affects BP possibly through mechanical effects. From DeBoer et al[11] with permission.

patients with a poor prognosis, eg, associated with heart failure, arrhythmia, or after a myocardial infarction.[26] There is general agreement that the HF or respiratory peak (0.25 Hz, HF) is determined by reflex vagal activity largely determined by increases in inspiratory venous return (see above). There is a good deal of evidence that the LF peak is in some way related to the sympathetic outflow[16]; however in some conditions (eg, exercise and heart failure) measures of muscle sympathetic nerve activity, or plasma catecholamines show clear evidence of increased sympathetic tone, yet PSA methods show reduced LF power. We should remember that PSA measures the amount of variability seen at 0.1 Hz (LF) or 0.25 Hz (HF); this does not necessarily always equate with the mean level of discharge.

Low Frequency Power: A Baroreflex Phenomenon?

One of the puzzling aspects of the LF peak is that it is strikingly reduced by atropine, a vagal blocking agent. This would be difficult to explain if the LF peak were just a simple marker of sympathetic discharge. DeBoer and colleagues (see above) suggested that the LF peak was caused by the rather slow baroreflex response to beat-to-beat changes in arterial pressure. Unlike the vagus which responds within one beat of a pressure change,[27] the sympathetic does not respond for 2 to 3 seconds.[28] This delayed response is an inefficient servo control, and leads to oscillations in pressure (and hence RR interval) at a period of about 0.1 Hz. This oscillation can be modeled by the baroreflex reacting only through the sympathetic; but is accentuated by interaction between the sympathetic response with the rapid vagal response.[11] This could explain why vagal motor blockade by atropine reduces the LF as well as the expected reduction in the HF peak.

Experimental Data in Favor of the DeBoer Model

We have used neck suction with a modified Eckberg collar[29] transiently to perturb the circulation, in order to test the DeBoer hypothesis.[30]

We used a 600 millisecond-40 mm Hg negitive pressure stimulus to the carotid baroreceptors, delivered in the early part of a 20-second period of apnea, starting at end expiration. This was delivered in random order with an "anticipation" control (held expiration, no stimulus) and an alerting control (loud noise, no neck stimulus). The "pure" baroreflex stimulus (ie, neck suction minus alerting control) resulted in an immediate bradycardia and hypotension which in turn resulted in a further baroreflex response of tachycardia and rise in pressure, and so on to produce a damped oscillation in RR interval (Figure 8). The period of this oscillation in response to the very brief initial neck suction was closely and significantly related to the spontaneous LF peak seen during quiet respiration at rest in each of the 11 subjects tested, thus supporting the DeBoer model (Figure 9). The DeBoer/Karemaker mathematical model (which suggests that the arterial baroreflex can account for the RSA) has recently been expanded further by the Karemaker group,[11,18-20] and seems to fit very well with observed perturbations such as the Valsalva maneuver, and also with the testing we have described above.

More recently, with colleagues in the Fondazione Clinica del Lavoro, Pavia, we have applied the DeBoer model to patients with heart failure who had differing baroreflex sensitivity (BRS), and to normals, examining both the spontaneous variations in the power spectrum, and also using the technique of neck stimulation at a frequency close to, but different from the controlled breathing frequency.[50] We found that the LF peak was present in the spontaneous power spectrum, ie, without neck stimulation) only if the baroreflex was relatively intact. In the heart failure patients with poor HR responses to baroreflex stimulation, we could generate RR-LF by neck suction, but this needed a powerful stimulus. It was not possible to generate LF in the BP spectrum unless the baroreflex was relatively intact. This infers that it is too simplistic to use PSA as a simple measure of autonomic control without consideration of the gain of the baroreflex arc. Of course there is often (but not always) a correlation between gain of the reflex control of HR (the Oxford phenylephrine or related tests) and autonomic balance.

Methods of Assessment of Baroreflex Sensitivity

For recent reviews in detail, the reader should consult Eckberg & Sleight,[2] Veerman,[19] and/or Faes.[20] It is not possible to review all methods of assessing BRS here. Early methods, such as the tachycardic response to standing are only semiquantitative, and have been replaced with more precise measures such as HR (or rather, pulse interval) change in response to rising or falling pressure produced by drugs[31] or to graded neck suction.[29]

It is now relatively simple to use minimally or noninvasive tests of baroreflex suction, such as the computerized generation of "mini baroreflex sensitivity slopes" developed by Mancia's group using analyses of sequences of 3 to 7 beats of a continuous Finapres arterial pressure record, where the pulse-interval and BPs are changing spontaneously, but are inversely related, as might be expected if they were reflexly induced.[32]

Another surrogate measure which correlates well with the Oxford phenylephrine method[27] is the use of the HR (or pulse-interval) response to a deep breath.[33] Caretta and his colleagues used two other noninvasive methods instead of recording arterial

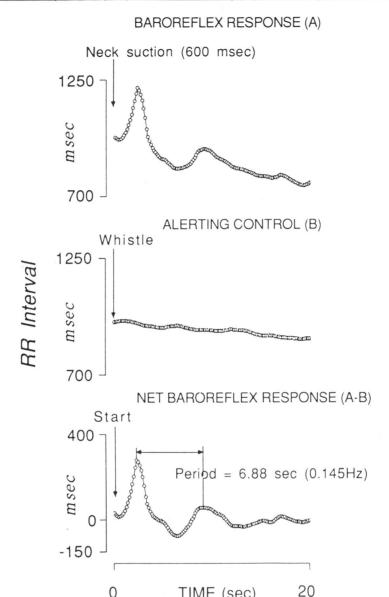

Figure 8. Sequence of RR intervals during the 20 seconds of voluntary apnea, after neck suction, after an alert timulus (whistle), and effect of subtraction of the two signals. Neck suction and alert signals are averaged on 10 interventions. Each circle represent a time interpolation of 150 msec. The frequency of the baroreceptor transient-induced oscillation was 0.145 Hz. In this subject the spontaneous LF was 0.12 Hz. From Bernardi et al[30] with permission.

pressure. Reflex changes in carotid peak velocity measured by echo-doppler[34] gave an extremely good (negative) correlation between beat-to-beat doppler flow and beat-to-beat RR interval change (falls in peak velocity clearly correlated with rises in arterial pressure, so peak velocity is a useful alterna-tive to arterial pressure measurement); this method correlated well with the Oxford phenylephrine technique.[2] Similarly, they found significant positive correlations between ultrasonically derived radial artery diameter changes and pulse-interval.[35] Similar plots can be obtained by spectral analysis

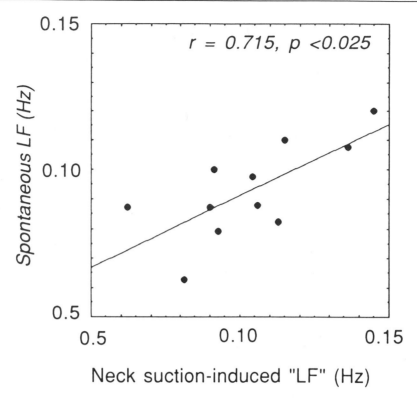

Figure 9. Relationship between the frequency of the damped oscillation obtained on the RR interval after neck suction (and subtraction of the alerting response), LF, and the frequency of the spontaneous LF oscillation recorded in supine position for each subject, during controlled breathing at 15/min, evaluated by autoregressive power spectral analysis (PSA). From Bernardi et al[30] with permission.

techniques by dividing the power of the HRV by that of the BP variability to yield the so-called alpha index (Figure 10),[15] which also correlates well with the phenylephrine slopes. This can be done for both LF and HF power separately. In the original description of the phenylephrine technique,[27] we found that beats falling in inspiration yielded a flatter slope (ie, reduced BRS), compared with those falling in expiration. Thus, part of the mechanisms of inspiratory tachycardia could be the result of central "gating" of afferent impulses from baroreceptors or central resetting of baroreflex gain.

Can We Suppress or Augment Respiratory Sinus Arrhythmia by Baroreflex Maneuvers

We next used the neck suction technique to further test more directly the De-

Boer model (that respiratory sinus arrhythmia was mainly determined by arterial baroreceptors rather than by a central oscillator). We asked three questions:

1. During apnea, can RSA be simulated solely by cyclical neck suction at the frequency of respiration?
2. To what extent can RSA be suppressed by appropriately timed neck suction, cycled at the previous respiratory frequency, which was designed to counteract the respiratory related changes in carotid arterial pressure? and
3. Is it possible to distinguish between respiratory related changes in pulse-interval (which might be generated by a medullary oscillator) and/or pulse rate modulation by a pure baroreceptor stimulus?

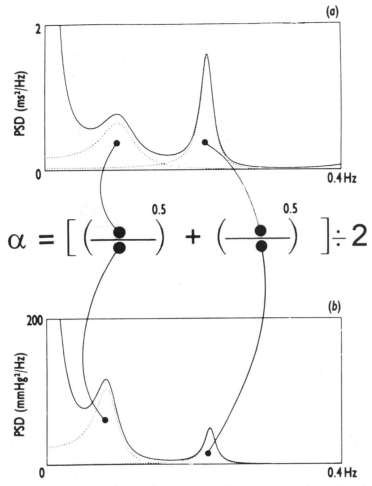

Figure 10. Schematic example of the method employed to compute the index alpha (baroreflex gain) from the simultaneous RR interval (a) and systolic arterial pressure (b) autospectra. From Lucini et al[15] with permission.

The answer to all of these questions was yes.[36]

During apnea, some oscillations in both BP and pulse interval do occur, but they are generally small in amplitude and slower than the normal respiratory sinus arrhythmia. We found that it was always possible to reproduce the full HR changes of the previous sinus arrhythmia during apnea by cycled neck suction at the respiratory frequency.

During controlled breathing, (15 per minute) in 13 subjects using appropriately phased (trial and error) neck suction, we were able to suppress the HF component of RSA by about 40%; there was also a signifi-

cant, though smaller reduction in LF, as might be expected from the DeBoer model (see above). This was achieved by rather small neck pressure swings of only about 5 to 10 mm Hg (at the respiratory frequency)—quite physiologically plausible.

Finally, we attempted to separate the respiratory effects on RSA from the baroreflex effects by breathing at 15 breaths per minute, while applying neck suction at a different frequency (12 per minute). By increasing the amplitude of the neck suction stimulus, it was possible to change the dominant peak in the RSA LF spectrum from the time of respiration to that of the neck suction stimulus.[36]

We believe that these data underline the importance of the baroreflex in the generation of the HF (but also the LF) rhythms in the power spectra associated with respiration. These data from conscious man are supported by studies from Jänigs group,[9] who studied the control of thoracic sympathetic preganglionic motor neurones with cardiac rhythmicity.

Very Low and Ultra Low Frequency Peaks in the Power Spectra of Circulatory Variables

So far we have dealt solely with the more conventional measures of autonomic control, namely the LF (10 seconds, 0.1 Hz) rhythm, which as we have seen is strongly dependent both on the arterial baroreflex and reflex variations in vagal tone, and the respiratory frequency HF rhythm. These rhythms are best seen during controlled breathing (which avoids contamination of the LF by occasional slow breathing). They are also best seen during the steady state—so-called "stationarity." These conditions, therefore, generally preclude recordings of longer than a few minutes. For this reason, very little attention has been paid to the information contained in the frequency range below 0.1 Hz. These very or ultra LF zones (VLF and ULF) contain most of the power in PSA analyses of long (ie, 24-hour) ECG recordings, but the origins of these lower frequency variations are poorly researched or understood. It has been suggested that these rhythms may be related to thermo-regulation or perhaps to hormonal fluctuations.

Interest in this LF zone has recently increased since Bigger and his colleagues[37] examined the prognostic significance of HRV in 24-hour Holter ECG recordings in patients who had recovered from a recent myocardial infarction. These showed, somewhat surprisingly, that low VLF was the best predictor of morbidity and mortality, rather than the more understandable reduction in vagal, or increase in sympathetic tone seen in the HF and LF bands.

However, Bernardi and colleagues have shown that these LF variabilities can be powerfully influenced by activity.[38] In a study of normal subjects, they showed that 3 hours of normal random activity strongly increased VLF compared with 3 hours resting, awake. Not surprisingly, the biggest increase was seen when the subjects carried out alternate 15-minute periods of rest/activity.

Tiberi and Casadei, in Oxford (personal communication, 1994) have recently studied HRV in 24-hour recordings in a group of 12 young people of (spontaneously) varying fitness. They found that ULF variability had the best correlation with fitness, as judged by maximal oxygen uptake (and lower HR). Surprisingly, there was no correlation with HF power.

Effects of Training on Autonomic Control

Exercise has many beneficial effects, which do not concern us here. One area of physical fitness which does concern us is that there are now many studies which show that training (long known to cause a physiological bradycardia both at rest and on submaximal exercise) can increase baroreflex gain (particularly for vagal control),[39] increase indices of vagal tone[39] and decrease sympathetic tone and the sympathetic component of the arterial baroreflex.[40]

These are the long-term effects, which are reversed by detraining.[41] Many of the deleterious effects of heart disease can be attributed to the rise in sympathetic tone, which follows from spontaneous or enforced inactivity.

On the other hand, during exercise, baroreflex gain is reduced.[42] This is immediate and is almost certainly due to inhibition of the baroreflex arc by downward neuronal inputs from higher centers such as the motor cortex. Similar suppression of the baroreflex occurs with arousal, and even more so with mental arithmetic.[43,44] These changes in gain are rapid, and coincide with reciprocal changes in BP and HR.

The increase in baroreflex gain with physical training could be protective, particularly for arrhythmia and sudden death (see Chapter 31).

Augmentation of Baroreflex Control by Low-Dose Atropine

It has long been known that low doses of muscarinic receptor blocking agents such as atropine or scopolamine can (paradoxically) increase vagal tone. The mechanism is unclear, but may act via the central nervous system.

We have used this in a double blind trial of the effects of a seasickness patch (scopoderm-Ciba) in patients with ischemic heart disease or heart failure.[46] We found a significant bradycardia, both at rest and on exercise, and on 24-hour Holter recording. This was associated with increased baroreflex gain, and increased heart rate variability. These short-term (1 to 2 days) experiments need to be tested under long-term conditions.

Pharmacological "Exercise" Training

Adamopoulos et al[47] in our laboratory, have found that daily and careful sequential dose increases of infusions of dobutamine (which increased HR and cardiac output) had exactly similar effects on autonomic function over several weeks, as did exercise training, with similar increases in baroreflex gain and HRV.

Effects of Long-Term Vagal Stimulation in Man

Vagal nerve electro stimulation with an implanted vagal pacemaker has been used to treat intractable epilepsy. Fallen and his colleagues[48] have studied a patient with this implanted device to examine the effects of prolonged (hours) vagal stimulation on power spectral analyses. Using a continuous stimulus of 1.25v, 300 μsec, at a rate of 20 Hz they found an increase in HF power and a decrease in LF/HF ration with the stimulator on, and a reproducible and dramatic 60% increase in LF power and a decrease in HF power when it was switched off.

This experiment shows directly, that increased vagal stimulation can change these autospectra, but raises many questions. Surprisingly, there was no bradycardia when the stimulator was on (but they were stimulating only the left vagus). Was the stimulator causing these effects by afferent or efferent vagal stimulition?

Conclusion

Respiratory sinus arrhythmia is thus a complex process, involving interactions between the mechanical effects of inspiratory increases in venous return which lead to delayed baroreflex responses, because of the time taken for this inspiratory bolus of blood to traverse the pulmonary circulation. In turn, these reflex responses generate complex resonances, largely as a result of the mismatch in response times between the baroreceptor beat-to-beat afferent information, and the inefficiently slow response of the sympathetic efferent system, which causes a resonance at 0.1 Hz. This resonance is powerfully enhanced when there is an efficient reflex response in HR by the vagus. Reflex vagal stimulation also rapidly (within 1 beat) reduces left ventricular stroke volume,[49] adding to the timing mismatch in sympathetic and vagal responses.

RSA is now an important marker of autonomic disturbance in disease, and we now have a much better understanding of the way in which RSA is generated. It is easy to understand how a reduction in vagal, and an increase in sympathetic tone might be adverse factors, particularly for arrhythmia or sudden death. It is less easy to say anything about the generation of VLF variability. This does seem an important marker of prognosis. It is increased by activity. Obviously, this in itself may be a confounding factor. Future studies will need to take this into account, and also exclude any periods of slow respiratory rates in any future clinical correlations between VLF and prognosis.

References

1. Eckberg DL. Respiratory sinus arrhythmia and other cardiovascular neural periodicities. In: Dempsey JA, Pack A (eds). Regulation of Breathing. New York, NY: Marcel-Dekker, 1993.
2. Eckberg DL, Sleight P. Human Arterial Baroreceptors. New York, NY: Oxford University Press, 1992.
3. Richter DW, Ballantyne D, Remmers JE. How is the respiratory rhythm generated? A model. News in Physiological Sciences 1986; 1:109-112.
4. Richter DW, Spyer KM. Cardio-respiratory control. In: Loewy AD, Spyer KM (eds). Central Regulation of Autonomic Functions. New York, NY: Oxford University Press, 1990; 189-207.
5. Langhorst P, Schultz G, Lambertz M, et al. Processing of the information from baroreceptors by neurons in the dorso-medial part of the nucleus of the solitarii tract. In: Sleight P (ed). Arterial Baroreceptors and Hypertension. New York, NY: Oxford University Press, 1980; 268-275.
6. Hirsch JA, Bishop B. Respiratory sinus arrhythmia in humans: how breathing pattern modulates heart rate. Am J Physiol 1981; 241(Heart Circ Physiol 10):H620-H629.
7. Laude D, Goldman M, Escourrou P, et al. Effect of breathing pattern on blood pressure and heart rate oscillations in humans. Clin Exp Pharmacol Physiol 1993; 20:619-626.
8. Shykoff BE, Nagvi SS, Menon AS, et al. Respiratory sinus arrhythmia in dogs. J Clin Invest 1991; 87:1621-1627.
9. Boczek-Funcke A, Dembowsky K, Häbler H-J, et al. Respirtory-related activity patterns in preganglionic neurones projecting into the cat cervical sympathetic trunk. J Physiol 1992; 457:277-296.
10. Eckberg DL, Nerhed C, Wallin BG. Respiratory modulation of muscle sympathetic and vagal cardiac outflow in man. J Physiol 1985; 365:181-196.
11. DeBoer RW, Karemaker JM, Strackee J. Hemodynamic fluctuations and baroreflex sensitivity in humans: a beat-to-beat model. Am J Physiol 1987; 253(Heart Circ Physiol 22):680-689.
12. Dornhorst AC, Howard P, Leathart GL. Respiratory variations in blood pressure. Circulation 1952; 6:553-558.
13. Bernardi L, Salvucci F, Suardi R, et al. Evidence for an intrinsic mechanism regulating heart rate variability in the transplanted and the intact heart during submaximal dynamic exercise. Cardiovasc Res 1990; 24:969-981.
14. Baselli G, Cerruti S, Civardi S, et al. Spectral and cross-spectral analysis of heart rate and arterial blood pressure variability signals. Comput Biomed Res 1986; 19:520-634.
15. Lucini D, Pagani M, Mela GS, et al. Sympathetic restraint of baroreflex control of heart period in normotensive and hypertensive subjects. Clin Sci 1994; 86:547-556.
16. Malliani A, Lombardi F, Pagani M. Power spectrum analysis of heart rate variability: a tool to explore neural regulatory mechanisms. Br Heart J 1994; 71:1-2.
17. Blinks JR. Positive chronotropic effect of increasing right atrial pressure in the isolated mammalian heart. Am J Physiol 1956; 186:299-303.
18. ten Voorde BJ. Modeling the Baroreflex, a Systems Analysis Approach. Amsterdam: University of Amsterdam, 1992. MD Thesis.
19. Veerman DP. Clinical Studies on Blood Pressure Variibility. Amsterdam: University of Amsterdam, 1994. MD Thesis.
20. Faes Th. JC. Assessment of Cardiovascular Autonomic Function. An Inquiry into Measurement. Amsterdam: University of Amsterdam, 1992. MD Thesis.
21. Leatham A. Splitting of the first and second heart sounds. Lancet 1954; ii:607-613.
22. Shafter HA. Splitting of the second heart sound. Am J Cardiol 1960; 6:1013-1022.
23. Penáz J. Frequency response of the cardiac chronotropic action of the vagus in the rabbit. Arch Int Physiol Biochim 1962; 70:636-650.
24. Penáz J. Photoelectric measurement of blood pressure, volume and flow in the finger. In: Digest of the 10th International Conference on Medical and Biologic Engineering; 1973; Dresden.
25. Penáz J, Honzikova N, Fiser B. Spectral analysis of resting variability of some circulatory parameters in man. Physaiologia Bohemoslovaca 1978; 27:349-357.
26. Malik M, Camm AJ. Heart rate variability and clinical cardiology. Br Heart J 1994; 71: 3-6.

27. Smyth HS, Sleight P, Pickering GW. Reflex regulation of arterial pressure during sleep in man. A quantitative method of assessing baroreflex sensitivity. Circ Res; 24:109-121.

28. Pickering TG, Davies J. Estimation of the conduction time of the baroreceptor-cardiac reflex in man. Cardiovasc Res 1973; 7:213-219.

29. Eckberg DL, Cavanaugh MS, Mark AL, et al. A simplified neck suction device for activition of carotid baroreceptors. J Appl Physiol 1975; 85:167-173.

30. Bernardi L, Leuzzi S, Radaelli A, et al. Low frequency spontaneous fluctuations of RR interval and blood pressure in conscious humans: a baroreceptor or central phenomenon? Clin Sci 1994 87:649-654.

31. Pickering TG, Gribbin B, Sleight P. Comparison of the reflex heart rate response to rising and falling arterial pressure in man. Cardiovasc Res 1972; 6:277-283.

32. Parati G, Di Rienzo M, Bertinieri G, et al. Evaluation of the baroreceptor-heart rate reflex by 24-hour intra-arterial blood pressure monitoring in humans. Hypertension 1988; 12:214-219.

33. Bennett T, Farquar IK, Hosking DJ, et al. Assessment of methods for estimating autonomic nervous control of the heart in patients with diabetes mellitus. Diabetes 1978; 27:1167-1174.

34. Caretta R, Bardelli M, Bulli G, et al. An ultrasonographic method to measure the sensitivity of the baroreflex in clinical practice: application to pharmacological studies. J Hypertens 1991; 9(suppl 3):S33-S36.

35. Caretta R, Bardelli M, Fabris B, et al. Ultrasonographic assessment of baroreceptor reflex sensitivity. A new method based on the measurement of pulsatile arterial diameter changes. High Blood Press 1992; 1:51-56.

36. Sleight P, Leuzzi S, Piepoli M, et al. Evidence that respiratory sinus arrhythmia (RSA) in humans originates from arterial baroreceptors. In: Proceedings: 32 Congress IUPS Glasglow; 1993.

37. Kleiger RE, Miller JP, Bigger JT Jr, et al. Decreased heart rate variability and its association with increased mortality after acute myocardial infarction. Am J Cardiol 1987; 59:256-262.

38. Bernardi L, Valle F, Coco M, et al. Physical activity is a major determinant of heart rate variability and of its "very low" frequency components in the Holter ECG. 1995. Submitted for publication.

39. Somers VK, Conway J, Johnston J, et al. Effects of endurance training on baroreflex sensitivity and blood pressure in borderline hypertension. The Lancet 1991; 337:1363-1368.

40. Kingwell BA, Dart AM, Jennings GL, et al. Exercise training reduces the sympathetic component of the blood pressure-heart rate baroreflex in man. Clin Sci 1992; 82:357-362.

41. Coats AJS, Adamopoulos S, Radaelli A, et al. Controlled trial of physical training in chronic heart failure: exercise performance, hemodynamics, ventilation and autonomic function. Circulation 1992; 85:2119-2131.

42. Pickering TG, Gribbin B, Strange Petersen E, et al. Comparison of the effects of exercise and posture on the baroreflex in man. Cardiovasc Res 1971; 5:582-586.

43. Conway J, Boon N, Jones JV, et al. Involvement of the baroreceptor reflexes in the changes in blood pressure with sleep and mental arousal. Hypertension 1983; 5(5):746-748.

44. Conway J, Boon N, Davies C, et al. Neural and humoral mechanisms involved in blood pressure variability. J Hypertens 1984; 2:203-208.

45. Conway J, Boon N, Floras J, et al. Impaired control of heart rate leads to increased blood pressure variability. J Hypertens 1984; 3:S395-396.

46. Casadei B, Pipilis A, Sessa F, et el. Low doses of scopolamine increase cardiac vagal tone in the acute phase of myocardial infarction. Circulation 1993; 88:353-357.

47. Adamopoulos S, Piepoli M, Qiang F, et al. Upregulating-Adrenoceptors and enhancing chronotropic responsiveness with pulsed inotrope therapy in chronic heart failure: short- and long-term effects. Circulation 1993; 88:I-257.

48. Kamath MV, Upton ARM, Tallala A, et al. Effect of vagal nerve electrostimulation on the power spectrum of heart rate variability in man. PACE 1992; 15:235-243.

49. Casadei B, Meyer TE, Coats AJS, et al. Baroreflex control of stroke volume: an effect mediated by tha vagus. J Physiol 1992; 448:539-550.

50. Sleight P, La Rovere MT, Mortura A, et al. Physiology and pathophysiology of heart rate and blood pressure variability in humans: is power spectral analysis largely an index of baroreflex gain? Clin. Sci 1995; 88:103-109.

Part IV

Clinical Implications and Use of Heart Rate Variability

Chapter 25

Heart Rate Variability and Risk Stratification After Myocardial Infarction

Matthew S. Bosner, Robert E. Kleiger

The majority of patients who survive acute myocardial infarction (MI) do well, however some develop recurrent angina, re-infarction, ventricular arrhythmias, or sudden death. Thus, a major goal of risk stratification is to identify the population at risk for subsequent morbidity and mortality. To date, age, sex, infarct location (interior and anterior), the extent and location of the index infarction, presence of electrocardiographic Q waves, acute congestive heart failure (CHF) or recurrent ischemia, and concomitant medical conditions such as diabetes and renal insufficiency, are among the variables investigated and defined as clinically significant risk stratifying factors in the post-MI period. Additional laboratory-defined parameters investigated include coronary anatomy, exercise capacity, left ventricular systolic function, ischemia on radionuclide scintigraphy, electrical instability suggested by the presence of ventricular arrhythmias on electrocardiographic monitoring, and late potentials on the signal-averaged electrocardiogram. Although extensive, this set is not complete; those most easily obtained provide only limited prognostic information; pursuing more meaningful data is often difficult, expensive, and associated with increased morbidity.[1] Assessment of heart rate variability (HRV) based on ambulatory electrocardiographic monitoring is an inexpensive, and noninvasive technique that is becoming widely available on commercial Holter scanning equipment. This method is an excellent noninvasive assessment of cardiac autonomic tone.[2-7] The absence of variability is a highly significant risk factor for adverse outcomes following acute MI, including all cause mortality,[8] arrhythmic,[9] and sudden death.[10-12] The initial studies of HRV in the post-MI setting were motivated by the wealth of experimental and clinical evidence linking abnormalities of the autonomic nervous system (ANS) to the development of ventricular tachyarrhythmias a primary precipitating factor for sudden death during myocardial ischemia.[13,14]

From: Malik M., Camm AJ (eds.): *Heart Rate Variability*. Armonk, NY. Futura Publishing Company, Inc., © 1995.

The normal heartbeat is not characterized by clockwork regularity.[2,3,5,15] Changes in heart rate (HR) occur secondary to physical or mental stress, exercise, respiration, metabolic changes, and various other influences. Both the basic HR and its modulation are primarily due to alterations in autonomic tone, parasympathetic or vagal tone slowing the HR, and sympathetic stimulation increasing HR. In healthy individuals, small changes in the interval between successive sinus beats (the normal RR, or "NN" interval) are common and called sinus arrhythmia. The cardiac cycle will alter at a high-frequency (HF) secondary to respiration (respiratory variation) throughout the day and night and, in addition, more sudden HR changes occur secondary to acute alterations in autonomic tone. In addition, very slow circadian changes occur mediated by neural and hormonal influences.[3,16] It is clear that changes in the cardiac cycle may be measured by a number of techniques and that these measurements provide information about autonomic tone.[2-4,6,17]

We will briefly review how HRV is measured, since this is extensively covered in recent reviews[5] and in this text. HRV is a misnomer, since the "heart period," cycle length or RR interval, is most often used in calculating various indices of variability. The two measurements are reciprocal; instantaneous HR is generally measured in beats per minute, and the RR interval or cycle length in milliseconds. In practical terms the conclusions drawn from either are to be essentially interchangeable.

Before HRV can be calculated, electrocardiographic recordings are scanned and QRS complexes identified and labeled (beat annotation). HRV can be assessed from short-term (5- to 15-minute) and, more commonly, long-term (24-hour) electrocardiographic recordings. This is performed using standard Holter processing equipment in the (most common) case of 24-hour recordings. It is important that the beat annotation be as accurate as possible, because most measures of variability are based on the timing changes between two normal (sinus) QRS complexes. Most HRV measurements attempt to exclude analysis of non-normal intervals; those between successive ectopic beats or between normal and ectopic beats, and those inaccurately measured because of artifact. Changes in tape speed can also alter timing intervals; this can be minimized by recording an external timing signal, and appropriate calibration and validation.

A variety of approaches are utilized to minimize erroneous calculations and the need for extensive human editing. These include eliminating from analysis intervals that vary by more than 20% from preceding intervals, and then calculating indices of HRV from all cycles, including those with ectopic beats. This method makes the assumption that such intervals represent a distinct minority of the total number of intervals and will only marginally affect the final calculation. This assumption appears to be valid only when there are <10 ectopic beats per hour. Another approach, taken by Malik and Camm, is to construct a frequency plot or histogram of the measured intervals.[11,18-20] This is termed the HRV index. The most frequently occurring interval (modal frequency) is determined and, using a variety of calculations, a baseline RR interval that depends on the distribution of frequencies and excludes the outliers calculated. Such a system may obviate or significantly reduce the need for human editing. Direct comparisons between these different approaches are currently being completed.

A cycle stream of intervals is collected, and variables related to HRV computed. These variables can be divided into two broad classes: time domain and frequency domain. Roughly, time-domain variables are computed directly from the NN intervals; frequency-domain variables result from mathematical techniques that analyze the sequence of NN intervals and describe the periodicity of patterns in this sequence. The technical details of the computation of frequency-domain measures is outside of the scope of this discussion, but will be found in accompanying chapters. Bigger has defined the frequency spectra into four frequency bands: HF power (between 0.15 to 0.40 Hz), low-frequency (LF) power (0.04 to 0.15 Hz), very low-frequency (VLF) power (0.0033 to 0.04 Hz) and ultra low-frequency (ULF) power (1.15×10^{-5} to 0.0033 Hz).[9,21] Generally, the variables include HF power centered near the respiratory frequency, and has been shown under experimental conditions to primarily reflect vagal tone; LF power, reflecting both sympathetic and parasympathetic tone, and even lower frequency components of uncertain physiological basis. Total power (or total variability) measured by frequency- and time-domain analyses is identical.

Time-domain measurements themselves can be broadly divided into two classes: those variables computed directly from the NN intervals; and those in which intervals are considered in the context of their surrounding intervals. Examples of the former are mean HR or mean cycle length for the entire recording period, standard deviations of the HR (SDNN) or cycle length (CLV), means of the HR over shorter recording segments (eg, five minutes), means of the standard deviation of normal cycle intervals or the difference in mean daytime intervals and mean nighttime intervals (after having defined some period of the recording as day or night interval). All of these variables tend to be broad-based measures of HRV; their magnitude depends on short-term changes in HR secondary to respiration, diurnal influences, and secular trends in HR (those independent of short-term trends).

The second class of variables analyzes the differences in adjacent cycles. These measurements include the standard deviation of the difference between adjacent normal cycles (the root mean square successive differences, where each difference is squared and summed, and the square root of the mean obtained rMSSD), and the proportion of the differences between adjacent cycles that exceed an arbitrary limit, such as 50 milliseconds (pNN50) or 6.25% (pNN6.25) of the preceding cycle interval.

These variables are virtually independent of diurnal or other secular trends in HR and reflect almost wholly alterations in autonomic tone that are predominantly vagally mediated.

Not surprisingly, time- and frequency-domain measure of HRV are related. For every time-domain measure, there is a frequency-domain measure that strongly correlates with it (>0.85).[22] HF correlates with r-MSSD and pNN50, LF and VLF correlate with SDNNIDX and ULF correlates well with SDNN and SDANN. Total power is identical to the square of SDNN, since both are measures of the variance in the HR signal. Thus, certain time-domain measures which are generally easier to calculate may act as surrogates for frequency measures and thus broaden the utilization of these measures in both the clinical and research communities.[22]

Clinical Studies

HRV analysis has been utilized in noncardiac disorders that likely influences the cardiovascular system including but not limited to: aging,[4,7,23–25] fetal HR monitoring,[26,27] thyroid disease,[28] diabetes,[23,29] and various neuropathic states.[30] However, the most extensive investigations have been done in the analysis of cardiac physiology, pharmacology, and disease states, including sudden death,[12,13,31–33] post-MI,[1,8–11,18–20,34–37] CHF,[38] and hypertension.[24,39]

There is a wealth of experimental evidence linking abnormalities of the ANS to ventricular arrhythmias during myocardial ischemia or CHF. Norepinephrine is reflexively released from sympathetic nerve terminals to maintain blood pressure (BP) in response to decreased cardiac output; however, catecholamines also stimulate ventricular arrhythmias, by a variety of mechanisms.[14,32] Ventricular arrhythmias are accepted as significant risk factors for sudden death in patients with ischemic or nonischemic ventricular dysfunction.[1,13] Factors that increase sympathetic nervous system activity increase the likelihood of ventricular arrhythmias, whereas those that decrease sympathetic nervous system activity decrease the likelihood of ventricular arrhythmias. Conversely, an increase in parasympathetic nervous system (vagal) activity tends to prevent ventricular arrhythmias, whereas a decrease in its activity tends to promote them.

Schwartz et al have shown in the dog that experimentally induced MI causes a decrease in the baroreceptor reflex slope, measured as the increase in RR interval as a function of an increase in BP on phenylephrine infusion.[12,32] Exercise training of dogs after MI increased the baroreceptor reflex slope and decreased susceptibility to ventricular fibrillation [VF]. LaRovere et al showed baroreceptor reflex slope was reduced in some of the 78 patients with recent MI.[40] They found that baroreceptor reflex slope was inversely correlated with age and, surprisingly, not related to left ventricular ejection fraction (LVEF) or exercise capacity. The baroreceptor reflex slope was significantly lower for the six patients who died during follow-up than in the 72 survivors. The authors concluded that, as in the dog model, many post-MI patients developed reduced parasympathetic activity, tipping the autonomic balance in favor of the sympathetic nervous system. Thus, it appears that sympathetic predominance in the year after MI may be related to a higher death rate.

Lombardi et al compared sympathovagal interactions in 70 patients studied 2 weeks after MI with those in 26 age-matched controls by analyzing spectral components of HR.[6] They found that after infarction, patients had smaller HF peaks (representing primarily vagal activity) and larger LF peaks (representing primarily sympathetic activity) compared to the control group. This finding was interpreted as a shift in autonomic balance toward sympathetic predominance at 2 weeks postinfarction. Thirty patients were studied at 6 months and 1 year after MI. These studies suggested that autonomic balance returned

to normal by 6 months; ie, the LF/HF ratio was lower. However, since paired observations were not reported, it is possible that the patients who were studied late had more normal autonomic balance to begin with. The increase in the amplitude of the LF peak during passive tilt testing to 90° was markedly blunted at 2 weeks after MI in 24 subjects. The interpretation of this finding is uncertain. The increased sympathetic tone at rest may have down-regulated myocardial beta receptors. This interesting finding needs further investigation.

The first large study which documented the importance of HRV measures in as a significant risk stratifier in the postinfarction period was published by Kleiger et al who used cycle length variability (CLV; the standard deviation of normal RR intervals within one 24-hour period) as a measure of HRV in 808 patients who had a 24-hour electrocardiographic recording 11+/−3 days after MI. The CLV is a broad-based measure reflecting to ultra LF variability as well as LF and HF variability. It was related to mortality during an average follow-up of 31 months. Patients with a CLV <50 milliseconds represented 16% of the sample and had a relative mortality risk 5.3 times as high as those with a CLV >100 milliseconds (upper 25% of the sample). Figure 1 demonstrates the Kaplan Meier survival curves for the population over 4 years of follow-up. The differences in mortality among the three groups continued to increase over time. This study also investigated the correlation between CLV and other predictors of risk. It was most strongly correlated with average RR interval (r = 0.52), LVEF (r = 0.25), and age (r = 0.19). Correlations with ventricular premature depolarization (VPD) frequency (r = 0.07) and the occurrence of VPD runs (r = 0.02) were very weak. Cox proportional hazards models were fitted using the best Multicenter Postinfarction Project (MPIP) predictors of mortality (ie, rales on presentation to the hospital, LVEF <30%, VPD frequency >10 per hour, New York Heart Association functional Class III or IV), and then CLV was added

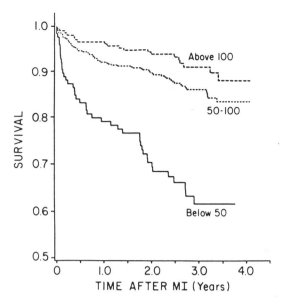

Figure 1. Cumulative survival over total follow-up period as a function of heart rate variability. Survival curves were calculated by the method of Kaplan Meier. Significant by log-rank <50ms from both other groups (p<0.0001). MI = myocardial infarction.[8]

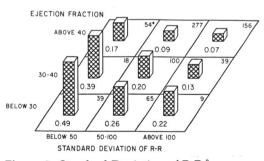

Figure 2. Standard Deviation of R-R.[8]

to the model. Even when simultaneous adjustments were made for these risk predictors and for heart period, CLV was significantly and independently associated with mortality. Figure 2 demonstrates the independence of CLV at any level of ejection fraction. Even in the group with an ejection fraction below 30%, low CLV more than doubles the risk. The authors suggested that the increased sympathetic tone, decreased parasympathetic tone, or both resulted in the observed reduction CLV.[8]

Subsequently, Bigger et al found that a variety of other indices of heart period

variability were reduced in patients with low CLV.[34] A time-domain measure of parasympathetic nervous system activity, pNN50, was markedly reduced in patients with low CLV (<50 milliseconds) compared to those with high CLV (>100 milliseconds), indicating that patients with low heart period variability after MI have reduced vagal (parasympathetic) activity.

Malik, Camm, Farrell and coworkers in London have extended the findings on HRV in the postinfarction population.[11,18–20,35,36] They correlated HRV based on baroreceptor sensitivity (BRS), and their unique HRV baseline width index with mortality, arrhythmic death, ventricular tachycardia and sudden death with other risk variables including ejection fraction, abnormal late potentials, ventricular tachycardia induced by programmed extra stimuli, and high grade ventricular arrhythmias on Holter monitoring. On their initial report on 68 patients postinfarction they noted that depressed BRS and decreased HRV, measured both by their index and by CLV, were predictors of spontaneous ventricular tachycardia and that induced by programmed stimulation. In this study, depressed BRS was a better predictor for events than electrocardiographic derived measures of HRV.[36]

In subsequent clinical studies from the same group, findings were reported in 487 postinfarction patients.[11] Holter derived indices of HRV were used rather than BRS. The decision to do this was due to the greater practicality of assessing HRV from Holter rather than from BRS measurements which require arterial cannulation and phenylephrine infusion and data which suggested that decreased HRV determined by 24-hour electrocardiographic analysis was at least equivalent in predictive strength to decreased BRS. Odemuyiwa et al[19,20] on 417 and 477 patients respectively, compared the sensitivity and specificity of their HRV index and ejection fraction in predicting all cause mortality, arrhythmic events and sudden death. HRV index was obtained from Holter monitors obtained 7 days postinfarction, and left ventricular

Table 1

Ranked Univariate Relation of Variables to Cardiac Mortality in 416 Patients

	Log-Rank Analysis	Cox Proportional Hazards Regression Coefficient	Proportional Hazards Chi-Square	Relative Risk (95% CI)
Heart rate variability <20 ms	0.0000	1.90	36.6	6.67 (3.6–12.3)
Ventricular ectopic beats >10/h	0.0001	1.10	13.57	2.99 (1.7–5.4)
Repetitive ventricular forms	0.0014	0.93	9.54	2.53 (1.4–4.6)
Mean RR interval <750 ms	0.0000	1.25	17.52	3.49 (2.0–6.2)
Late positive potentials	0.0075	0.79	16.8	2.21 (1.2–4.0)
Killip class ≥2	0.0000	1.73	34.52	5.64 (3.2–10.0)
Exercise test	0.002	0.98	8.98	2.66 (1.4–5.0)
Age >65 yr	0.0000	1.14	14.81	3.13 (1.75–5.6)
Left ventricular ejection fraction <40%	0.0000	1.30	19.58	3.67 (2.1–6.5)

The initial relation between variables and arrhythmic events is expressed as the Kaplan-Meier product estimate of the survival function (log-rank) multivariate analysis: the relative risk is calculated from the Cox analysis. Abbreviation as in Table 2.[45]

ejection fraction calculated from either angiograms or radionuclide studies. Receiver operator curves were created comparing sensitivity and specificity for events at given sensitivities for each of the endpoints. At a sensitivity of 75% a decreased HRV index of <30 units had greater specificity for sudden death and arrhythmic events than decreased ejection fraction, and a marginally better specificity for prediction of total death. The combination of decreased HRV index and low ejection fraction increased both the sensitivity and specificity for all three endpoints (arrhythmic events, sudden cardiac death and total death).

Farrell et al[11,36] described 416 survivors of acute MI and univariate predictors of arrhythmic events included impaired HRV, abnormal late potentials, frequency and repetitiveness of ventricular ectopic beats, decreased left ventricular ejection fraction and advanced Killip class. On multivariate analysis the combination of impaired HRV and abnormal late potentials was the best independent combination for predicting arrhythmic events (Table 1).[45] For cardiac mortality, the strongest univariate predictor of mortality was HRV <20 milliseconds followed by Killip class and repetitive ventricular forms (Figure 3).[45] Thus, diminished

HRV, implying disordered autonomic function, predicted both death and arrhythmic events with greater sensitivity and specificity than conventional predictors such as left ventricular ejection fraction. Decreased HRV index and other abnormal risk variables indentify subgroups with particularly high risk of adverse events.

The data from these postinfarction studies clearly demonstrates that decreased indices of HRV such as CLV,[8] or the HRV index,[11,19] or baroreceptor sensitivity[36,40] are associated with increased mortality and increased arrhythmic death following infarction. Using combinations of these indices and other variables predictive of mortality or arrhythmias such as low ejection fraction, decreased exercise tolerance, high PVC frequency on Holter or abnormal late potentials identify subgroups of patients with very high risk for mortality and malignant arrhythmias.

Although most of the large studies of HRV after MI as a risk variable have assessed time-domain variables, BRS or geometric measures, several investigators have studied frequency-domain measures. Bigger et al,[9] utilizing the MPIP population, studied 715 patients postinfarction. In univariate analysis, all of the frequency bands, as well as total power, were highly correlated with each other and inversely related to mortality. In multivariate analysis only total power, ULF, and VLF power were independently associated with mortality and the strongest relationship was noted between ULF and mortality.[9] The addition of VLF or LF power measurement improved the predictive ability of HRV measurement. A fascinating finding in this report was the stronger association of VLF with only arrhythmic death, than all cardiac death or total mortality. This was the only variable exhibiting this property and needs confirmation in further studies. This group further extended their studies by calculating spectral density of VLF, LF, and HF power from short 2- to 15-minute periods both during day and night and correlating these short-term measurements with total power and ULF calculated from the 24-hour tape. There were very high correlation greater than or equal to 0.75 between the estimates of power obtained from short segments of recording time and those obtained from the total 24 hours. Moreover, like the long-term frequency measures, there was a highly significant inverse relationship to mortality and spectral density. The predictive value of the short-term measurements was somewhat weaker than those of the long-term. As demonstrated now in multiple studies, HRV remained an independent predictor of

mortality even after controlling for standard risk variables such as Killip class, rales, ventricular ectopy etc.

Bigger et al have also studied patients late after MI. In 331 patients from the CAPS study, 24-hour ambulatory tapes obtained 1 year after the index infarction were analyzed. Subsequent mortality risk was strongly correlated with low HRV measures, particularly depressed VLF power. Similar to the results of the MPIP study, low HRV remained a predictor of mortality even when controlling for other adverse risk factors as CHF, low ejection fraction, and ventricular ectopy. The relative risk of all cause mortality using the optimal cutoff point and optimal variable VLF power was 5.6.[21]

There have been few studies in which repeat measures of HRV have been performed over time. The issue of stability of these measures is vital if HRV is to be a valid tool for clinical studies. This is analogous to the problem of interpreting changes in ectopic frequency or number of ischemic episodes on recording which show marked change variation from recording to recording.[41] Kleiger et al examined 14 normal patients with repeat monitoring, one recording at baseline, and one on placebo medication.[22] The intervals between recordings ranged from 3 to 65 days. Various time-domain measures were determined, including CLV, r-MSSD, pNN50, mean

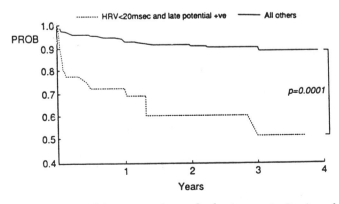

Figure 3. Kaplan-Meier survivorship curves for arrhythmic events (top) and cardiac mortality (bottom) in patients with depressed heart rate variability (HRV) <20 ms and positive (+ve) late potentials (LP) and ventricular ectopic beats. The p values refer to differences in event rates between subgroups (log-rank analysis). PROB = probability.

standard deviation of normal RR intervals calculated for each 5-minute interval, mean RR interval, and mean difference between night and day RR interval. The authors calculated the mean and standard deviations for these measures and also the intraclass correlation coefficient, a measure of individual variability. They showed that the group means and standard deviations for the variables were virtually identical for the baseline and placebo recordings. Moreover, for some of the time-domain variables such as pNN50 and r-MSSD, the intraclass correlations exceeded .9, demonstrating not only group stability but individual stability in measurement. They concluded that the stability of these variables over time, the lack of placebo effect, and the limited individual variability in their measurement made them suitable variables for the study of interventions on autonomic tone. This has been verified in a population with CHF (PE Stein Ph.D, unpublished observations).

The multiple studies described herein demonstrate a strong and independent relationship between low HRV measures and mortality following acute MI pose interesting and important clinical questions. The physiological mechanisms responsible for decreased HRV have not been completely defined, yet it seems likely that whatever mechanisms are responsible for a low HRV, potentially are related to those which pre-dispose to poor survival in the postinfarction period. Although most HRV variables predict total cardiac mortality and primary arrhythmic death equally, the finding of Bigger et al[9] that low VLF predicted arrhythmic death preferentially may lead to a better understanding of the physiological causes of increased mortality and arrhythmic death. Although there is no direct proof that altering autonomic tone will affect survival in specific patient populations, animal and clinical research to date suggest that interventions that increase (or do not alter) HRV may be desirable. An additional hypothesis that is now being actively investigated is that alterations in cardiac autonomic note as reflected by HRV secondary to pharmacological or other interventions such as revascularization may reflect physiological changes that may either increase or decrease risk of mortality in ischemic disease, particularly those secondary to arrhythmic events. A subsequent chapter by Dr. Peter Schwartz will cover in detail the effects on HRV of such diverse drugs as beta-blockers, scopolamine and I-C antiarrhythmic agents, drugs commonly used in these patients which have been shown to alter HRV postischemic events both in experimental models and in clinical experience. Cardiac autonomic balance as reflected by HRV may potentially be modified and the subsequent risk of mortality altered in the postinfarction period.

References

1. Krone RJ. The role of risk assessment in the early management of a myocardial infarction. Ann Intern Med 1992; 116:223–237.
2. Appel ML, Berger RD, Saul JP, et al. Beat to beat variability in cardiovascular variables: noise or music? J Am Coll Cardiol 1989; 14:1139–1148.
3. Eckberg DW. Parasympathetic cardiovascular control in human disease: a critical review of methods and results. Am J Physiol 1980; 241:H581–593.
4. Gautschy B, Weidmann P, Gnümadinger MP. Autonomic function tests as related to age and gender in normal man. Klin Wochenscrift 1986; 64:499–505.
5. Kleiger RE, Bosner MS, Rottman J. Time domain measures of heart rate variability in the assessment of cardiac autonomic tone. J Ambul Monitor 1993; 6:1–18.
6. Lombardi F, Sandrone G, Pernproner S, et al. Heart rate variability as an index of sympathovagal interaction in patients after myocardial infarction. Am J Cardiol 1987; 59:256–263.
7. Pfeifer MA, Weinberg CR, Cook D, et al. Differential changes of autonomic nervous system function with age in man. Am J Med 1983; 75:249–258.
8. Kleiger RE, Miller JP, Bigger JT, et al. Decreased heart rate variability and its association with increased mortality after acute myo-

cardial infarction. Am J Cardiol 1987; 59:256–262.

9. Bigger JT, Fleiss J, Steinman RC, et al. Frequency domain measures of heart period variability and mortality after myocardial infarction. Circulation 1992; 85:164–171.

10. Ewing DJ. Heart rate variability: an important new risk factor in patients following myocardial infarction. Clin Cardiol 1991; 14:683–685.

11. Farrell TG, Bashir Y, Cripps T, et al. Risk stratification for arrhythmic events in postinfarction patients based on heart rate variability, ambulatory electrocardiographic variables and the signal-averaged electrocardiogram. J Am Coll Cardiol 1991; 18:687–697.

12. Hull SS, Evans AR, Vanoli E, et al. Low sodium diet increases risk for sudden death in conscious dogs after myocardial infarction. J Am Coll Cardiol 1990; 16:978–985.

13. Martin GJ, Magid NM, Myers G, et al. Heart rate variability and sudden death secondary to coronary artery disease during ambulatory electrocardiographic monitoring. Am J Cardiol 1987; 60:86–89.

14. Sharma AD, Corr PB. Adrenergic factors in arrhythmogenesis in the ischemic and reperfused myocardium. Eur Heart J 1983; 4(suppl D):79–90.

15. Denton TA, Diamond GA, Helfant RH, et al. Fascinating rhythm: a primer on chaos theory and its application to cardiology. Am Heart J 1990; 120:1419–1440.

16. Molgaard H, Sorensen KE, Bjerregaard P. Circadian variation and influence of risk factors on heart rate variability in healthy subjects. Am J Cardiol 1991; 68:777–784.

17. O'Brien IA, O'Hare P, Corrall RJM. Heart rate variability in healthy subjects: effect of age and the derivation of normal ranges for tests of autonomic function. Br Heart J 1986; 55:348–354.

18. Malik M, Cripps T, Farrell T, et al. Prognostic value of heart rate variability after myocardial infarction: a comparison of different data-processing methods. Med Biol Eng Comput 1989; 29:603.

19. Odemuyiwa O, Malik M, Farrell T, et al. Multifactorial prediction of arrhythmic events after acute myocardial infarction. Combination of heart rate variability and left ventricular ejection fraction with other variables. PACE 1991; 14:1986–1991.

20. Odemuyiwa O, Malik M, Farrell T, et al. Comparison of the predictive characteristics of heart rate variability index and left ventricular ejection fraction for all-cause mortality, arrhythmic events and sudden death

after acute myocardial infarction. Am J Cardiol 1991; 68:434–439.

21. Bigger JT, Fleiss JL, Rolnitzky LM, et al. Frequency domain measures of heart period variability to assess risk late after myocardial infarction. J Am Coll Cardiol 1993; 21:729–736.

22. Kleiger RE, Bigger JT, Bosner MS, et al. Stability over time of variables measuring heart rate variability in normal subjects. Am J Cardiol 1991; 68:626–630.

23. Cripps TR, Kraegen EW, Zelenka GS, et al. Cardiac beat to beat variation: age related changes in the normal population and abnormalities in diabetics. Aust N Z J Med 1981; 11:614–629.

24. Gribbin B, Pickering TG, Sleight P, et al. The effect of age and high blood pressure on baroreflex sensitivity in man. Circ Res 1971; 29:424.

25. Waddington JL, MacCulloch MJ, Sambrooks JE. Resting heart rate variability in man declines with age. Experientia 1979; 35:1197–1198.

26. Modanlou HD, Freeman RK, Braly P. A simple method of fetal and neonatal heart rate beat-to-beat variability quantification. Am J Obstet Gynecol 1977; 129:861–868.

27. Valimaki IA, Nieminen T, Antila KJ, et al. Heart rate variability and SIDS. Examination of heart rate patterns using an expert system generator. Ann NY Acad Sci 1988; 533:228–237.

28. Northcote RJ, MacFarlane P, Kesson CM, et al. Continuous 24-hour electrocardiography in thyrotoxicosis before and after treatment. Am Heart J 1986; 112:339–344.

29. Masaoka S, Lev-Ran A, Hill LR, et al. Heart rate variability in diabetes; relationship to age and duration of the disease. Diabetes Care 1985; 8:64–68.

30. Niklasson U, Olofsson BO, Bjerle P. Autonomic neuropathy in familial amyloidotic polyneuropathy. A clinical study based on heart rate variability. Acta Neurol Scand 1989; 79:182–187.

31. Myers GA, Martin GJ, Magid NM, et al. Power spectral analysis of heart rate variability in sudden cardiac death: comparison to other methods. IEEE Trans Biomed Eng 1986; 33:1149–1156.

32. Schwartz PJ. Manipulation of the autonomic nervous system in the prevention of cardiac sudden death. In: Brugada PW, Wellens HJJ (eds). Cardiac Arrhythmias: Where Do We Go From Here? Mount Kisco, NY: Futura Publishing Co., 1987; 741–765.

33. Singer DH, Martin GJ, Magid N, et al. Low heart rate variability and sudden cardiac death. J Electrocardiol 1988; 21:S46–55.

34. Bigger JT, Kleiger RE, Fleiss JL, et al. Components of heart rate variability measured during healing of acute myocardial infarction. Am J Cardiol 1988; 61:208–215.

35. Cripps TR, Malik M, Farrell TS, et al. Prognostic value of reduced heart rate variability after myocardial infarction: clinical evaluation of a new analysis method. Br Heart J 1991; 65:14–19.

36. Farrell TG, Paul V, Cripps TR, et al. Baroreflex sensitivity and electrophysiological correlates in postinfarction patients. Circulation 1991; 83:945–950.

37. Pipilis A, Flather M, Ormerod O, et al. Heart rate variability in acute myocardial infarction and its association with infarct site and clinical course. Am J Cardiol 1991; 67:1137–1139.

38. Casolo G, Balli E, Fazi A, et al. Twenty-four hour spectral analysis of heart rate variability in congestive heart failure secondary to coronary artery disease. Am J Cardiol 1991; 67:1154–1158.

39. Somers VK, Conway J, Johnston J, et al. Effects of endurance training on baroreflex sensitivity and blood pressure in borderline hypertension. Lancet 1991; 337:1363–1368.

40. LaRovere MT, Specchia G, Mazzolenaetc C, et al. Baroreflex sensitivity in post myocardial infarction patients. Circulation 1986; 74(suppl):II–514. Abstract.

41. Morganroth J, Michelson EL, Horowitz LN, et al. Limitations of routine long-term electrocardiographic monitoring to assess ventricular ectopic frequency. Circulation 1978; 58:408–412.

42. Bigger JT, Fleiss JL, Kleiger R, et al. The relationships among ventricular arrhythmias, left ventricular dysfunction and mortality in the two years after myocardial infarction. Circulation 1984; 69:250–258.

43. Kleiger RE, Miller JP, Krone RJ, et al. The independence of cycle length variability and exercise testing on predicting mortality of patients surviving acute myocardial infarction. Am J Cardiol 1990; 408–411.

44. Lown B, Verrier RL. Neural activity and ventricular fibrillation. N Engl J Med 1976; 294:1165–1170.

45. Farrell TG, Bashir Y, Cripps T, et al. Risk stratification for arrhythmic events in postinfarction patients based on heart rate variability, ambulatory electrocardiographic variables and the signal-averaged electrocardiogram. J Am Coll Cardiol 1991; 18:687–697.

Chapter 26

Short-Term and Long-Term Assessment of Heart Rate Variability for Postinfarction Risk Stratification

Lü Fei, Marek Malik

Analysis of heart rate variability (HRV) provides a noninvasive method for the assessment of autonomic influence on the heart. HRV is depressed in various clinical settings.[1,2] Depressed HRV is a powerful risk predictor in patients following acute myocardial infarction, independent of other established risk factors.[3-6] Assessment of HRV for postinfarction risk stratification is extensively reviewed in Chapters 25, 27, 28, and 29. The predictive value of HRV has almost exclusively been derived from data analyzed from 24-hour Holter electrocardiograms (ECGs). Unfortunately, the technical difficulties limit the assessment of HRV from ambulatory 24-hour Holter recordings. Short-term recordings are obviously more practical in the clinical application of HRV assessment. However, data on short-term analysis of HRV for postinfarction risk stratification is scarce and inconclusive.[7,8] Bigger et al[8] reported that spectral HRV from short-term recordings (2 to 15 minutes) randomly selected from 24-hour Holter ECGs, strongly predicts postinfarction mortality. However, the predictive power of short-term HRV (positive predictive accuracy up to 31%)[8] seems to be lower than that of HRV calculated from 24-hour recordings (positive predictive accuracy up to 41%).[9] The cost-effectiveness of short- and long-term assessments of HRV for postinfarction risk stratification remains to be fully defined. We have therefore studied the predictive value of short- and long-term HRV based on data from the St. George's Post-Infarction Survey Program.

Methods

Patients

Seven hundred consecutive patients with documented acute myocardial infarction admitted to St. George's Hospital were enrolled in this study. The definition

From: Malik M., Camm AJ (eds.): *Heart Rate Variability*. Armonk, NY. Futura Publishing Company, Inc., © 1995.

Table 1
The Clinical Characteristics of Patients Following Acute Myocardial Infarction

Age (years)	57 ± 9
Sex (male/female) (n)	555/145
Anterior MI (n)	355
Prior MI (n)	107
LVEF (%)	48 ± 15
VPCs (hourly)	21 ± 114
Thrombolysis (n)	391
β-blockers (n)	277

LVEF: left ventricular ejection fraction; MI: myocardial infarction; n: number of patients; VPCs: ventricular premature complexes.

of infarction, enrollment criteria, data acquisition techniques and follow-up have previously been published.[5] All patients underwent a risk stratification research protocol before hospital discharge between days 5 and 8 following acute myocardial infarction. This included symptom-limited treadmill exercise test (Bruce protocol), signal-average ECG, and 24-hour Holter monitoring. Left ventricular ejection fraction was assessed by either cardiac catheterization (exercise test positive) or radionuclide-gated blood pool scanning (exercise test negative). The clinical characteristics of the 700 patients are summarized in Table 1. All patients were followed up for at least 1 year. All cause cardiac mortality during the first year following acute myocardial infarction was used as the endpoint in this study.

Analysis of Heart Rate Variability

Short-term HRV was computed as the standard deviation of all sinus RR intervals from a short (5 to 20 minutes) clean and stable period ECG recording (SDNN). This short period was selected according to the following: sinus rhythm with no ectopic beats or artifacts (clean); and none of the RR intervals during the entire period differed from the first RR interval by more than 20% (stationarity). The first segment of ECG fulfilling these criteria from the beginning of the 24-hour Holter ECG recordings was used for the short-term HRV analysis. This method of selection of ECG recording periods for analysis of HRV was used in an attempt to simulate practical standardized ECG recording conditions, such as the supine position at rest.

Long-term HRV was computed as the HRV index from 24-hour Holter recordings using a previously described method.[5,10] The method used for the geometrical calculation of the HRV index is discussed in detail in Chapter 4.

Statistical Analysis

All data are expressed as mean ± standard deviation. Student's t-test, analysis of variance and multivariant linear correlation were used where appropriate. A two-tailed p value <0.05 was considered statistically significant.

Results

Analysis of Short-Term Heart Rate Variability

Of the 700 patients, a 5-minute stationary period suitable for short-term analysis could be identified in 663 patients. Suitable stationary recordings of 10, 15 and 20 minute duration could be identified in 641, 610 and 575 patients respectively. There was no significant difference in SDNN between these different durations. Five or more non-overlapping suitable 5-minute segments were found in 646 patients. Suitable 5-minute period of ECGs could not be identifed in 37 patients due to either ectopy or artifacts. These 37 patients were excluded from further analysis of short-term HRV in this study. The SDNNs calculated from different duration of recordings (5 to 20 minutes) were significantly related to each other (correlation coefficient r ranged from 0.71 to 0.85, all p <0.001). Figure 1 shows a plot of the relationship between 5- and 20-minute SDNNs. Correlation between 5-minute stationary SDNN and 24-hour HRV index was also significant, but was relatively poor (r = 0.51, p <0.001) (Figure 2).

Stationary 5 min SDNN [ms]

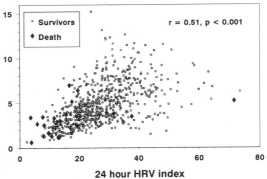

Figure 2. The correlation between the standard deviation of all normal RR intervals over 5-minute stationary periods (SDNN) and HRV index over 24 hours.

Predictive Power of Short- and Long-Term Heart Rate Variability

During 1-year follow-up, 45 patients died from cardiac causes. The HRV index was significantly lower in patients who died than in survivors (18±12 versus 28±10 units, p<0.001). Short-term HRV was also significantly lower in patients who died (Table 2). Since there was no significant difference in SDNN between the different short duration of recordings, we used the 5-minute SDNN for further analyses. Figure 3 shows the survival curves for short- and long-term HRV for all cause cardiac mortality during the year following acute myocardial infarction. Figure 4 shows the positive predictive accuracy curve of HRV. The long-term HRV index was clearly superior to 5-minute SDNN for the prediction of 1-year cardiac mortality, although the 5-minute SDNN was also significantly associated with increased cardiac mortality in these patients.

Analysis of Long-Term Heart Rate Variability After Preselection by Short-Term Assessment

In order to seek more cost-effective methods of HRV analysis for postinfarction

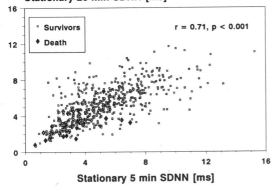

Figure 1. The correlation between the standard deviations of all normal RR intervals (SDNN) over 5- and 20-minute stationary periods in ambulatory Holter ECG recordings.

Table 2
Short-Term Heart Rate Variability in Patients Following Acute Myocardial Infarction

Time Period	Survivors	Death	p Value
5 min	5.07 ± 2.44	3.16 ± 1.42	0.0001
10 min	5.16 ± 2.30	3.37 ± 1.53	0.0001
15 min	5.16 ± 2.15	3.09 ± 1.34	0.0001
20 min	5.20 ± 2.07	3.24 ± 1.42	0.0001

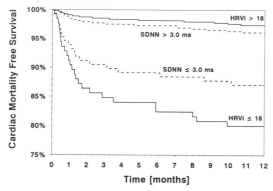

Figure 3. The Kaplan-Meier survival curves for all cause cardiac mortality during the year following acute myocardial infarction (both p<0.001). HRVi: HRV index over 24-hour periods; SDNN: the standard deviation of all normal RR intervals over 5-minute stationary periods.

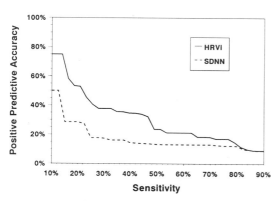

Figure 4. The positive predictive accuracy curves of HRV for all cause cardiac mortality during the year following acute myocardial infarction. HRVi: HRV index over 24-hour periods; SDNN: the standard deviation of all normal RR intervals over 5-minute stationary periods.

risk stratification, we studied all cause cardiac mortality in 10% and 15% of the total population who had the lowest values of HRV based on different strategies of HRV assessment. This approach models the planning of a hypothetical clinical trial in which the number of patients to be included is a fixed proportion of the total screened population. The aim of such a strategy would be to include a patient population with the highest likelihood of mortality.

First, we analyzed 5-minute SDNN and 24-hour HRV index in relation to 1-year total cardiac mortality in all patients. The 1-

year cardiac mortality in the 10% of patients who had the lowest values of 5-minute SDNN and 24-hour HRV index was 17% and 27%, respectively. Short-term (5-minute) analysis of HRV (SDNN) is simpler and less expensive than the analysis of long-term (24-hour) HRV. We therefore used depressed short-term SDNN to select out a population of patients from the total population for 24-hour analysis of HRV index, with the aim of achieving the highest 1-year cardiac mortality in the 10% of patients who had the lowest HRV index. The effect of selecting from 20% to 50% (in steps of 5%) of the total population with the lowest 5-minute SDNN for 24-hour analysis was assessed (ie, HRV index was only assessed in 20% to 50% of all patients who had the lowest 5-minute SDNN). In the 10% of patients who had the lowest HRV index after preselection by the lowest SDNN in this way, all cause cardiac mortality was higher than that identified by 5-minute SDNN alone (Figure 5). Analysis of 24-hour HRV index in ≥35% of patients who had the lowest 5-minute SDNN values was able to yield 1-year cardiac mortality as high as analysis of HRV

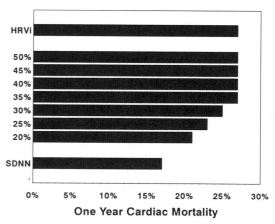

Figure 5. The 1-year cardiac mortality in 10% of the total patient population with the lowest HRV values, taken from groups of patients preselected as the given proportion of the total population with the lowest SDNN values. Percentage (%): the percentage of all patients in which HRV is assessed (see text for details). HRVi: HRV index over 24-hour periods; SDNN: the standard deviation of all normal RR intervals over 5-minute stationary periods.

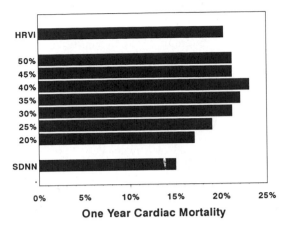

Figure 6. The 1-year cardiac mortality in 15% of patients who had the lowest HRV values (as in Figure 5). Percentage (%): the percentage of all patients in which HRV is assessed (see text for details). HRVi: HRV index over 24-hour periods; SDNN: the standard deviation of all normal RR intervals over 5-minute stationary periods.

index in all the patients (27%). Similarly, we studied the mortality in 15% of total patient population who had the lowest HRV values and the results are presented in Figure 6. This approach may provide a cost-effective method of risk stratification, with the more expensive and more cumbersome long-term (24-hour) HRV analysis performed only in patients with depressed short-term HRV values.

Discussion

Heart Rate Variability Assessment for Postinfarction Risk Stratification

Use of HRV analysis for the assessment of autonomic nervous system function has greatly improved our understanding of the pathophysiology of a variety of diseases, particularly those related to ventricular arrhythmias and heart failure.[1] Both the short- and long-term predictive value of HRV in patients following myocardial infarction are now well established. The predictive value of HRV has been shown to be independent of other postinfarction risk factors, such as left ventricular ejection fraction, ventricular ectopic activity and late potentials. For prediction of all-cause mortality, the value of HRV is similar to that of left ventricular ejection fraction, while HRV is superior to left ventricular ejection fraction in predicting arrhythmic events.[11] The positive predictive accuracy of HRV over a clinically important range of sensitivity (25% to 75%) for cardiac mortality and arrhythmic events was around 20% to 30%. Combination with other risk factors significantly improves the positive predictive accuracy of HRV.[12]

Short- and Long-Term Heart Rate Variability Assessment

The value of depressed HRV for postinfarction risk stratification is well established. However, the clinical application of HRV assessment is limited by a lack of standardized methodology for HRV measurement. Analysis of HRV over long-term recordings, especially those of poor quality, is time-consuming and may be misleading due to technical difficulties in dealing with noise in the computation of HRV. Often, it is necessary to assess HRV from these poor quality recordings. We have previously examined the relationship between short- and long-term HRV during different physical maneuvers in patients at risk of sudden cardiac death.[13] We found a significant correlation in all the frequency components of spectral HRV between short- and long-term recordings. Unfortunately, these correlations were not strong enough for short-term HRV to replace 24-hour assessment. The relatively poor measuring agreement between short- and long-term HRV was also observed in this study (Figure 2). Our data suggest that depressed short-term HRV is significantly associated with 1-year mortality in patients following acute myocardial infarction, despite its poor correlation with 24-hour values. The predictive power of 5-minute SDNN alone, however, was significantly lower than that of the 24-hour HRV index. This is consistent with the findings in the studies of Bigger et al.[8,9]

Clinical Implications

We conclude that depressed short-term HRV is associated with increased cardiac mortality in patients following acute myocardial infarction. But the predictive power of short-term analysis is lower than that of long-term HRV. Our observations suggest that assessment of HRV over 5-minute stationary periods can be used for screening patients at risk of cardiac death. The suspected patients as detected by depressed 5-minute SDNN may undergo 24-hour Holter monitoring and other risk stratification assessments. This may provide a cost-effective method of HRV assessment for postinfarction risk stratification. Specific cut-off points have not been addressed in this study. They depend on the proportion of population to be finally stratified. In other words, they depend on the nature of treatment or clinical investigation to which the stratified patients are subjected.

References

1. Malliani A, Pagani M, Lombardi F, et al. Cardiovascular neural regulation explored in the frequency domain. Circulation 1991; 84:482-492.
2. Kjellgren O, Gomes JA. Heart rate variability and baroreflex sensitivity in myocardial infarction. Am Heart J 1993; 125:204-215.
3. Kleiger RE, Miller JP, Bigger JT Jr, et al. Decreased heart rate variability and its association with increased mortality after acute myocardial infarction. Am J Cardiol 1987; 59:256-262.
4. Cripps TR, Camm AJ. Prediction of arrhythmic events in patients following myocardial infarction. Clin Cardiol 1989; 12:661-665.
5. Farrell TG, Bashir Y, Cripps T, et al. Risk stratification for arrhythmic events in postinfarction patients based on heart rate variability, ambulatory electrocardiographic variables and the signal-averaged electrocardiogram. J Am Coll Cardiol 1991; 18:687-697.
6. Pedretti R, Etro MD, Laporta A, et al. Prediction of late arrhythmic events after acute myocardial infarction from combined use of noninvasive prognostic variables and inducibility of sustained monomorphic ventricular tachycardia. Am J Cardiol 1993; 71:1131-1141.
7. Malik M, Camm AJ. Significance of long term components of heart rate variability for the further prognosis after acute myocardial infarction. Cardiovasc Res 1990; 24:793-803.
8. Bigger JT, Fleiss JL, Rolnitzky LM, et al. The ability of several short-term measures of RR variability to predict mortality after myocardial infarction. Circulation 1993; 88:927-934.
9. Bigger JT Jr, Fleiss JL, Rolnitzky LM, et al. Frequency domain measures of heart period variability to assess risk late after myocardial infarction. J Am Coll Cardiol 1993; 21:729-736.
10. Cripps TR, Malik M, Farrell TG, et al. Prognostic value of reduced heart rate variability after myocardial infarction: clinical evaluation of a new analysis method. Br Heart J 1991; 65:14-19.
11. Odemuyiwa O, Malik M, Farrell TG, et al. Comparison of the predictive characteristics of heart rate variability index and left ventricular ejection fraction for all-cause mortality, arrhythmic events and sudden cardiac death after acute myocardial infarction. Am J Cardiol 1991; 68:434-439.
12. Camm AJ, Lü Fei. Risk stratification after myocardial infarction. PACE 1994; 17:401-416.
13. Lü Fei, Sttaters DJ, Anderson MH, et al. Relationship of short- and long-term measurements of heart rate variability in patients at risk of sudden cardiac death. PACE 1994; 17:2194-2200.

Chapter 27

Heart Rate Variability and Risk Stratification Post-myocardial Infarction Physiological Correlates

Emilio Vanoli, Philip B. Adamson, Donatella Cerati,
Stephen S. Hull Jr

Introduction

The comprehension of the pathophysiological mechanisms linking occurrence of a myocardial infarction and the consequent alteration in heart rate variability (HRV) represents the necessary path to properly use this variable in risk stratification in post-myocardial infarction patients. As described elsewhere in this book, HRV reflects the influences of both limbs of the autonomic nervous system (ANS) on the heart. Caution has been suggested in extrapolating information obtained from markers of the autonomic control of heart rate (HR) to the neural influences on the ventricle.[1] However, the experimental observation of an existing link between cardiac reflexes elicited by acute myocardial ischemia and the physiological reflex and tonic control of HR[2] indicated the possibility that the analysis of functional aspects of the ANS could contribute to identify individuals at higher risk for lethal event, specifically at the time of an acute ischemic episode, after a myocardial infarction.[3] This observation was obtained in an experimental preparation in conscious dogs with a healed myocardial infarction in which two subgroups of animals at high and low risk for lethal arrhythmias can be unambiguously identified.[4]

One of the primary anatomical and functional links between autonomic mechanisms of HR control and cardiac reflexes of ventricular origin is represented by the nucleus tractus solitarius (NTS).[5] The NTS receives afferent inputs from the pulmonary, atrial, ventricular and baroreceptors. Furthermore, this important nucleus also receives information from all areas controlled by the ANS.[5] Thus, via the NTS, afferent information from areas other than the cardiopulmonary may influence cardiovascular reflexes.

From: Malik M., Camm AJ (eds.): *Heart Rate Variability.* Armonk, NY. Futura Publishing Company, Inc., © 1995.

In the present chapter the following issues will be discussed:

1. the analysis of the information that generated the hypothesis of a link between autonomic markers and risk for lethal events after myocardial infarction;
2. the neural mechanisms by which an ischemic damage, acute and/or chronic, of the heart can influence the autonomic control of HR; and
3. the consequences of the ischemia-dependent autonomic derangements on cardiac electrical stability.

Analysis of Autonomic Markers in Conscious Dogs Before and After Myocardial Infarction

Experimental and clinical evidence have established the concept that dominance of sympathetic or vagal reflexes during acute myocardial ischemia markedly increases or decreases, respectively, the risk for developing lethal arrhythmias and sudden death.[4,6-9] A very important step in the comprehension and in the recognition that ANS activity is a major determinant in the prognosis of coronary artery disease patients is represented by the experimental evidence that the likelihood of having predominant sympathetic or vagal reflexes during acute myocardial ischemia could be predicted by the analysis of the autonomic control of HR prior to the occurrence of the ischemic event.[2,10] This hypothesis was initially developed by using baroreflex sensitivity,[2,10] that is marker of reflex vagal activity. However, the increasing use of HRV,[11] marker of tonic autonomic control of HR,[12] provided new insights on the autonomic mechanisms involved in the genesis of lethal events after myocardial infarction.

The experimental model that generated this information has been already described in several circumstances.[2-4,9,10] It combines three elements highly relevant to the genesis of malignant arrhythmias in man[8]: a healed myocardial infarction, acute myocardial ischemia, and physiologically elevated sympathetic activity. In brief, 30 days after an anterior wall myocardial infarction, chronically instrumented dogs perform a submaximal exercise stress test (Figure 1). When HR reaches approximately 210 to 220 bpm, a 2-minute occlusion of the circumflex coronary artery is performed by means of a pneumatic occluder previously positioned around the vessel. After 1 minute, exercise stops while the occlusion continues for another minute. The outcome of the test is highly reproducible over time in the same animal, and allows to the clear separation of two groups: animals that develop ventricular fibrillation and are defined "susceptible" to sudden death. They represent 40% to 50% of the total population; and dogs that survive and are defined "resistant." "Resistant" dogs very often have marked heart rate reduction despite the ongoing exercise, while susceptible dogs had an opposite response (a significant increase in HR). The reflex HR increase during ischemia could be attributed to the combination of the baroreflex response to the decline in arterial blood pressure (BP) and of the excitatory cardiocardiac sympathetic reflex.[13] However, in the susceptible dogs the reflex tachycardia does not depend upon a greater hemodynamic impairment, since mean BP and dP/dt just before the occurrence of ventricular fibrillation are not different from that of resistant dogs at the same moment.[14] The unexpected HR reduction induced by

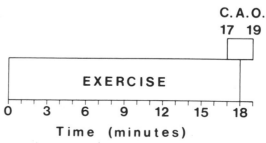

Figure 1. Diagram illustrating the protocol of the exercise and ischemia test (see text for detail). From Schwartz et al.[4]

myocardial ischemia in the resistant dogs is dependent on a vagal reflex, as it could be prevented by atropine.[15] Given the preferential distribution of vagal sensory endings in the inferior ventricular wall,[16] the manifestation of a vagal reflex following occlusion of the circumflex coronary artery would have been expected at rest but its overriding nature during exercise and in the presence of a prior myocardial infarction indicates a very powerful reflex.

Baroreflex sensitivity (BRS) in the experimental preparation was assessed by the method described by Sleight's group.[17] Briefly, BRS is expressed by the slope of the regression line correlating consecutive RR intervals with the increasing values of systolic BP due to the bolus injection of phenylephrine. The changes at the sinus node level after injection of phenylephrine reflect primarily vagal reflex activity but are significantly influenced by the concomitant level of sympathetic activity.[18,19] In the 86 resistant dogs, BRS was 17.7 ± 6.0 ms/mm Hg compared to 9.1 ± 6.5 ms/mm Hg in the 106 susceptible dogs (p<0.001).[10] This indicated that the capability of reflexly increasing vagal activity was significantly lower in those dogs that were at higher risk for developing ventricular fibrillation. An important observation of this study, relevant to the use of autonomic markers for post-MI risk stratification and that can be obtained only in an experimental setting, originated from measuring BRS before and after myocardial infarction. This analysis documented that the reductions in BRS caused by myocardial infarction were not significantly different between resistant and susceptible dogs. Indeed, the difference in BRS between the two groups was, to some degree, already present before the myocardial infarction. In 68 dogs studied prior to the myocardial infarction, those that would have died either during the recovery phase after the anterior myocardial infarction or during the exercise and ischemia test already had a lower (p <0.001) BRS (16.2 ± 5.9 mm Hg) compared to the dogs that would have survived (22.2 ± 6.2 mm Hg). Thus, the depressed BRS

observed after MI in dogs at high risk for ventricular fibrillation was consequent to the effects of the ischemic injury but also to a preexisting lesser capability of activating vagal reflexes.

As a step further in the study of the autonomic mechanisms in our conscious animal model for sudden cardiac death,[4] we examined the prognostic value of HRV, measured in a 30-minute period, taking again the advantage of the possibility of performing the study both before and after the myocardial infarction.[20] The study was performed in 25 dogs identified during the exercise and ischemia test as "susceptible" and in 25 identified as "resistant" to sudden death. Two were the main findings of the study. Thirty days after myocardial infarction, HRV, measured by the standard deviation of RR intervals (Std) from 30-minute ECG recording, was significantly lower in susceptible groups. However, the difference in Std was largely independent of the difference in HR as indicated by the fact that the coefficient of variance, which corrects the standard deviation for HR, provided similar results. The resistant dogs had a significantly (p <0.05) higher coefficient of variance (+48%, 0.277 ± 0.012) than susceptible dogs (0.187 ± 0.012) (Figure 2). Overall, this would simply confirm, in a more controlled environment of the experimental laboratory, the observation obtained in patients. A novel observation was obtained, as for BRS by studying, by internal control analysis, HRV before and after myocardial infarction in dogs susceptible and resistant to ventricular fibrillation. It was found that before myocardial infarction, susceptible and resistant dogs had almost an identical HRV (226 ± 30 versus 233 ± 30 milliseconds) and that the myocardial infarction produced a significant reduction in the susceptible (-53%, to 106 ± 9 milliseconds) but not in the resistant dogs (-10%, to 209 ± 13 milliseconds). Even in this case, the significance of the change was independent of HR increase after MI, as indicated by the analysis of the coefficient of variance (Figure 3). Thus, as for a reduced BRS, a depressed

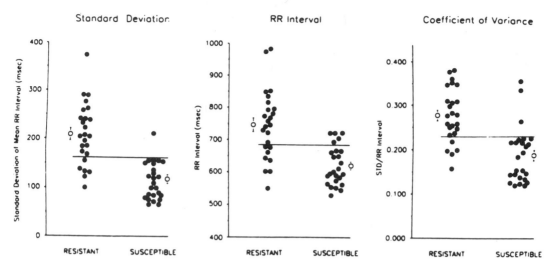

Figure 2. Scattergrams of the standard deviation of the mean, RR interval, and coefficient of variance in 25 resistant and in 25 susceptible animals. Group mean values (±SEM) are displayed adjacent to scatter data; discriminator placed at the midpoint of group mean values (P<0.05). From Hull et al.[20]

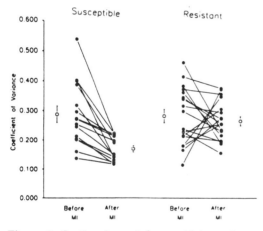

Figure 3. Scatterplots of the coefficient of variance in 15 susceptible dogs and in 18 resistant dogs before and 1 month after myocardial infarction. From Hull et al.[20]

HRV effectively distinguishes between individuals at high and low risk after myocardial infarction. On the other hand, at variance from BRS, HRV before myocardial infarction is not different among dogs destined to be resistant or susceptible to sudden death. The prognostic value of HRV after MI seems to be entirely due to the fact that myocardial infarction influences HRV of susceptible dogs only, or, that only if MI decreases HRV the dog becomes susceptible

to lethal arrhythmias. Of interest is the fact that the greater autonomic imbalance in susceptible dogs is not due to a greater myocardial infarction. In this study, as well as in others,[21,22] the infarct size, measured by tetrazolium blue, was similar in susceptible and resistant dogs. Specifically, in the study where HRV was measured, infarct size was 13.9 ± 0.8% of the left ventricular mass in susceptible dogs and 12.6 ± 1.8% in the resistant dogs (NS).

Patterns of Recovery of Heart Rate Variability After Myocardial Infarction

Important insights on the pathophysiological mechanisms of HRV depression after MI can be obtained by the analysis of the time-course of this measure after MI. Recent clinical observations had indicated that the depression of HRV after MI is transient and that a trend toward a recovery of the autonomic control of HR can be observed within 2 to 6 months after MI (see Chapter 28).[23,24] Such a recovery parallels the progressive reduction in risk for lethal events. On the other hand, recent clinical evidence indicates that a depressed HRV identifies high-risk patients even 1 year after MI.[25] This observation is potentially in conflict with the concept of a recovery of HRV and raises the question that such a recovery may not involve all post-MI patients. The clinical studies conducted so far involved a relatively limited number of patients with a low mortality rate within the first year after MI. Consequently, these studies could not explore the relation between pattern of recovery of HRV after MI and risk for lethal events.

We recently extended the information in our experimental preparation for sudden death by studying HRV in 22 dogs before and every 3 days after myocardial infarction. HRV was periodically measured after MI beginning from the first day in which sinus rhythm was evident. The information from these 22 dogs, prepared with the anterior MI, was compared with data from 8 sham operated dogs.[26] Of the 22 post-MI dogs, 10 had ventricular fibrillation during the exercise and ischemia test performed 30 days later, while 12 were resistant. Prior to MI, HRV was not different among the three groups, as previously described.[20] However, after beta-blockade with atenolol (1 mg/kg), the group of dogs destined to be resistant to lethal arrhythmias during a new ischemic episode occurring after MI showed a significant increase in HRV, measured as Std of RR intervals, by 27%. At variance, this did not happen in the susceptible group where the increase in HRV was only 4.8%.

The recovery pattern of HRV after MI in the 22 dogs as a whole showed a picture reproducing the information that already emerged from the clinical studies (Figure 4). However, the analysis based on the outcome from the exercise and ischemia test (VF or not VF) revealed that the two groups of dogs differed significantly in their HRV time course (Figure 5). At 5 days after MI, HRV was similarly depressed in susceptible and resistant dogs. This would indicate that the acute effects of MI on HRV is similar in all dogs and that the capability to recover

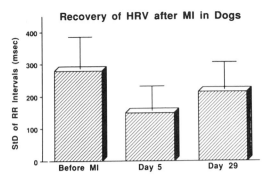

Figure 4. The bar graph shows mean HRV, expressed by Std of RR intervals from 30 minutes of ECG recording, in the same 22 dogs in control conditions, at 5 and 29 days after MI. The analysis on the group as a whole shows that, by the 29th day after MI, HRV has returned close to control.

from this acute situation is the key factor to also recover from a condition of high risk for lethal arrhythmias. As matter of fact, within 10 days after MI, resistant dogs had HRV measures that were not different from those observed prior to MI. On the contrary, susceptible dogs showed only a minimal trend toward a recovery. At the ninth day after MI, Std of RR intervals was 133 ± 22 milliseconds in susceptible dogs and 240 ± 23 milliseconds in the resistant dogs ($p<0.03$). Susceptible dogs continued to have a depressed HRV and, in association with it, had ventricular fibrillation during the exercise and ischemia test 30 days after MI. Sham prepared dogs had only a minimal reduction in HRV 2 to 3 days after the surgical intervention and recovered their normal autonomic balance within a few days. This rules out the possibility that the surgical trauma may contribute to a significant degree to the observation obtained in post-MI dogs. Thus, the depression in HRV after MI has a markedly different temporal recovery between high- and low-risk dogs. The lack of recovery of autonomic control of HR in susceptible dogs is likely an important contributing mechanism to their high-risk status.

Overall, the data presented indicated three important concepts that have significant clinical implications:

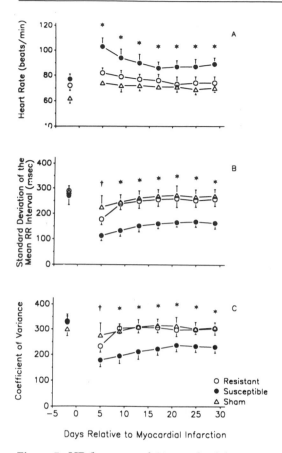

Figure 5. HR (bpm, panel A), standard deviation of RR intervals (milliseconds, panel B), and coefficient of variance from 10 dogs susceptible (closed circles), 12 dogs resistant (open circles) to ventricular fibrillation and 8 sham prepared dogs (open triangles). Measures were made 3 days before and periodically after an anterior wall myocardial infarction or surgery (sham). * indicates significant differences ($p<0.01$) when susceptible dogs are compared to both resistant and sham dogs. † indicates significant difference ($p<0.05$) when susceptible and resistant dogs are compared with the sham group. Values are mean ±SEM. From Adamson et al.[26]

1. the high risk for lethal events, as it can be identified by the analysis of HRV, is due to the negative effect of MI on HRV;

2. at the time when the healing process of the MI is completed in a dog, ie, 10 to 15 days after coronary artery ligation, autonomic control of HR recovers in resistant dogs that are then able to survive a new episode of

acute myocardial ischemia. In high risk individuals, the healing process is not accompanied by such a recovery, the autonomic imbalance is permanent and the dogs remain at high risk for lethal arrhythmias even at distance from the occurrence of the first MI; and

3. the great individual diversity in the functional aspects of the ANS contains elements likely to contribute to the depression in HRV observed after MI.

Neural Mechanisms After Myocardial Infarction

The mechanisms involved in the observed reduction in HRV after MI, and by which HRV reflects the neural response to acute myocardial ischemia, are not yet fully described. No clinical or experimental evidence exists describing neural activity at a distance from an MI and thus, the neural mechanisms involved in the chronic alteration in HRV and in the consequent high risk for lethal arrhythmias can be only extrapolated from data obtained in anesthetized preparation in which neural activity is recorded during acute myocardial ischemia.

Acute myocardial ischemia activates ventricular endings connected to both sympathetic[27,28] and vagal[29-31] afferent fibers. Several factors may contribute to the rapid activation of autonomic reflexes. Mechanoreceptors may be excited in the ischemic region and the border zone by dyskinesia[28]; chemoreceptors may be excited by bradykinin,[32,33] acidosis[34] hyperkaliemia,[35] serotonin,[36] prostaglandins.[37] In case of a significant depression of myocardial contractile function by ischemia, reflexes from the atrial, pulmonary and systemic baroreceptors may also be elicited. The activation of vagal afferent fibers, mainly C fibers,[29-31] results in bradycardia and hypotension because of both an increase of vagal efferent activity and a decrease of sympathetic efferent activity directed to the heart and blood vessels. Experimental studies performed in anesthetized animals suggest that a prevailing depressor response is more likely to originate from large compared to small ischemic areas[38] and from inferoposterior ischemic areas.[16] These studies are in agreement with the traditional concept of greater parasympathetic activation caused in patients by inferior, as compared to anterior wall myocardial ischemia or infarction.[6]

Myocardial ischemia induces an excitatory cardiocardiac sympathetic reflex,[13] and this increase in sympathetic efferent discharge following coronary artery occlusion closely parallels the increase in the vulnerability to ventricular fibrillation.[39] The degree of such a response is significantly greater when the ischemia is transmural.[40] This is probably because of the preferential distribution of the sympathetic fibers in the epicardium,[41] at least in dogs. The deleterious role of the cardiocardiac sympathetic reflex is supported by the evidence that the section of the dorsal roots—a maneuver that interrupts sympathetic afferent fibers—significantly decreases the severity of ventricu-

lar arrhythmias following coronary artery occlusion.[42]

If the information emerging from data obtained during acute myocardial ischemia are transposed in the setting of a chronic damage, it is possible that the changes in the geometry of a beating heart secondary to the presence of a necrotic and noncontracting segment may increase, beyond normal, the firing of sympathetic afferent fibers by mechanical distortion of their sensory endings.

The depressed vagal and increased sympathetic activity after MI may be explained by the fact that excitation of sympathetic afferents depresses the physiological activity of vagal fibers directed to the sinus node.[43] Figure 6 shows the demonstration of this phenomenon obtained by directly recording the activity of single neural fiber from the cardiac branch of right vagus. Relevant to the present discussion is the fact that the electrical stimulation of afferent sympathetic fibers markedly decreases the activity of efferent vagal fibers activated by the BP rise. In a more recent series of experiments, vagal efferent activity was recorded prior to and after removal of the left stellate gan-

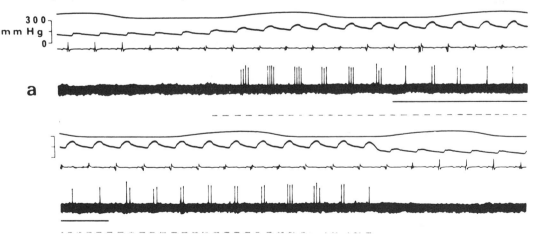

Figure 6. Effects of BP increase, by aortic occlusion, and of sympathetic afferent activation, by electrical stimulation of the cut central end of the left inferior cardiac nerve, on the discharge of a single efferent vagal fiber in an intact, anesthetized cat. The broken line indicates stenosis of the aorta, and the solid line indicates sympathetic stimulation. The two strips are continuous recordings. The tracings in each section from top to bottom are: respiration, systemic arterial BP, electrocardiogram, and neural activity. This vagal fiber begins to fire only in response to BP elevation (baroreceptor reflex) and the concurrent afferent sympathetic stimulation is able to interfere with this response. Modified from Schwartz et al.[43]

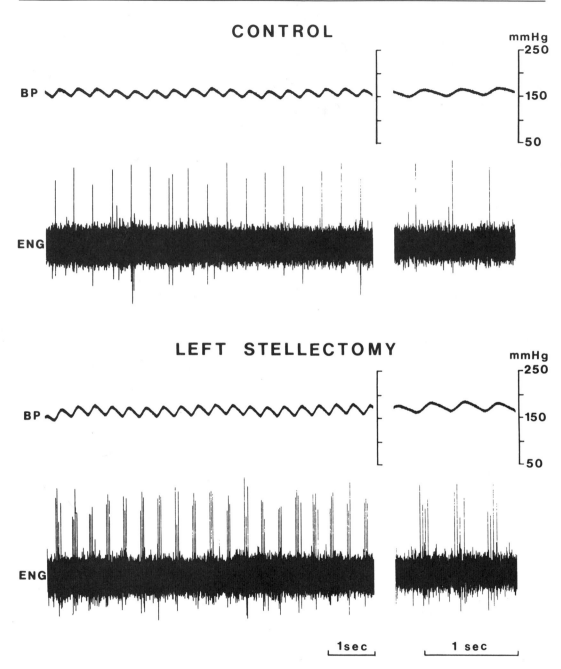

Figure 7. Tracings showing activity of a single cardiac vagal efferent fiber, at the same (BP) levels induced by phenylephrine before (top panel) and after (bottom panel) left stellectomy. The fiber shows a pulse-synchronous activity. In each panel, the upper tracing shows the BP, and the lower tracing shows the electroneurogram. From Cerati et al.[44]

glion.[44] After left stellectomy tonic vagal activity was higher (Figure 7) and also the reflex increase following the rise in BP was significantly potentiated. In 16 anesthetized cats removal of the left stellate ganglion in-

creased resting level of vagal activity from 1.2 ± 0.2 impulses per second to 2.1 ± 0.3 impulses per second, (+75%, p<0.01). In the same cats, vagal activity during similar BP rises induced by phenylephrine was also higher after left stellectomy (4.7 ± 0.7 versus 2.2 ± 0.4 imp/sec, p<0.001), with an increment of 134 ± 24 versus 86 ± 18%, (p<0.05) above the resting level. This information has an equivalent in the evidence that section of the dorsal roots significantly augmented the bradycardic reflex response during BP rise.[19] Overall, these studies support the concept that sympathetic activation exerts a restraining effect on vagal reflexes of cardiac origin.

The study by Cerati and Schwartz[44] also provided important insights on the relation between reflex control of HR and vagal reflex activity during acute myocardial ischemia. This was obtained in 17 anesthetized cats by correlating the cardiac vagal activity recorded during phenylephrine-induced BP rise and during a 60-minute occlusion of the left anterior descending coronary artery. The main finding was that the cats that had a reflex increase in cardiac vagal activity during acute myocardial ischemia (+48% versus control, p<0.01)) survived while the cats that did not have this reflex vagal activation (-18% versus control) developed ventricular fibrillation within a few minutes after the beginning of the coronary artery occlusion. The cats destined to survive the coronary artery occlusion also showed a greater reflex vagal activation during BP rise induced by phenylephrine (+246% versus +80%, p<0.01) than the cats that developed ventricular fibrillation during acute myocardial ischemia. This study, performed in anesthetized open chest preparations, described vagal activation during acute myocardial ischemia and indicated a tight correlation between vagal activity, directly measured and not extrapolated from "markers," during acute myocardial ischemia and during reflex responses to BP rise.

Central Mechanisms

The experimental evidence presented above describes a correlation between autonomic control of HR and cardiac reflex activation during acute myocardial ischemia.

The understanding of the central pathways involved in the control of the autonomic function contributes to explain this relation.

The NTS is the major visceral sensory relay cell group in the brain and, as such, it receives inputs from all the major visceral organs.[45] The afferent information projects into the NTS in two ways. The first is based on an organ-specific projection pattern in individual NTS subnuclei (Figure 8). The second involves overlapping informations projecting into a common region, the commisural NTS (Figure 9). However, most, if

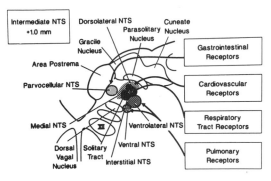

Figure 8. Drawing showing the viscerotopic pattern of innervation of the NTS. This drawing illustrates the NTS of the cat in the transverse plane and the number given indicates the distance from the obex. The nomenclature used follows that presented by Loewy and Burton (1978). From Loewy.[45]

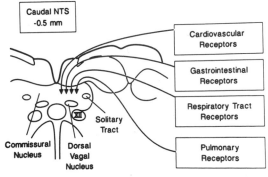

Figure 9. Drawing illustrating a common site of projection for various visceral afferent in the NTS in the cat. It is not yet certain whether this common area of projection receives overlapping projections or whether the fibers carrying different visceral modalities converge on specific commissuralmedial NTS neurons. The number indicates the position relative to the obex. From Loewy.[45]

not all, visceral afferent fibers make connections with other NTS subnuclei besides their main "organ-specific" receptive one.[46] Specifically relevant to the subject of the present chapter is the evidence that afferences from cardiovascular, respiratory and gastrointestinal systems project in an overlapping, and possibly convergent fashion, to neurons in the commisural NTS. The information from the NTS is sent to the brain stem neurons that project either directly to the vagal neurons or the sympathetic preganglionic neurons or, indirectly, via the interneurons that regulate them.[45]

Thus, the NTS is the central site of integration of visceral reflexes where the anatomical and functional pathway exists that can explain the interaction between baroreceptive reflexes and reflexes originating from receptors than can be activated by acute myocardial ischemia. On the other hand, the evidence that afferent information from other viscera projects in the NTS and overlap with projections from the cardiovascular system, indicates the possibility of multiple influences originating from all organs controlled by the ANS on autonomic control of HR, ie, on HRV. Relevant to this issue is the multiple experimental evidence that stimulation of afferents with endings in the stomach,[47] gallbladder,[48] and pancreas[49] increases HR, BP and contractility. This experimental evidence has clinical counterparts. Cohan and colleagues demonstrated that patients with Syndrome X have decreased coronary blood flow and increased incidence of anginal attacks after acidification of the distal esophagus.[50] Gastroesophageal reflux is a rather frequent event during sleep. We recently documented that the ratio between the power in the low-frequency (LF) and the high-frequency (HF) band of the spectral analysis of HRV significantly increases in normal subjects during REM sleep, (Figure 10) and is even higher after myocardial infarction.[51] Preliminary data from an ongoing study indicate that the surge in power in the LF band during REM sleep is exaggerated in the presence of esophageal acidification.[52]

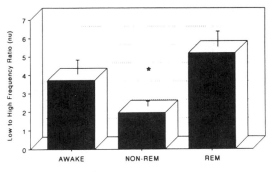

Heart Rate Variability During Sleep

Figure 10. Bar graph illustrating the ratio between the power comprised in the LF and HF band of spectral analysis of HR in three different conditions: awake, non-REM and REM sleep.

The notion of an important interplay among information from the different organs innervated by the ANS cannot be forgotten in the interpretation of the analysis of HRV, as it often occurs when this is based only on pathologies involving the cardiovascular system.

Autonomic Balance and Risk for Lethal Arrhythmias

The evidence that the two limbs of the ANS have opposite effects on arrhythmogenesis represents the principal background for the use of HRV in risk stratification in post-MI patients. A large number of experimental and clinical evidence has established, for many years, the arrhythmogenic effects of sympathetic hyperactivity.[53] This information has its counterpart in the widespread and successful use of antiadrenergic interventions in high-risk patients.[54,55]

At variance from the sympathetic nervous system, the influences of the vagus on arrhythmogenesis has been clarified only recently by a series of experiments. The potential influences of the vagus on the ventricle were already proposed in the early 1900s. In 1909, Thomas Lewis, among several conclusions drawn from his experiments on arrhythmogenesis following coronary artery occlusion, indicated that: "in the dog the ventricle is certainly under control of the vagus, in some instances at least."[56] However, until the 1970s it was generally accepted that vagal hyperactivity was either uninfluential or actually detrimental on the likelihood of ventricular arrhythmias, mainly because of the supposed absent or insufficient innervation of the ventricles[57,58] or because of the negative effects of bradycardia. Experimental studies have shown that, in the normal heart, bradycardia was associated with an increase in temporal dispersion of refractory periods and decreased the ventricular fibrillation threshold (VFT).[59] These experimental findings appeared to have a clinical correlate in the observations, made in the first coronary care units, that in patients with acute myocardial infarction, marked bradycardia was often associated with the occurrence of ventricular arrhythmias.[6]

In the 1970s, one group of investigators readdressed, in a series of publications, the issue of vagal activity. Kent et al[60] indicated that, during ischemia, vagal stimulation markedly increased, rather than decreased, the VFT. Goldstein et al found that vagal stimulation did not change the incidence of ventricular arrhythmias during anterior myocardial ischemia in closed-chest dogs[61]; Myers et al[62] found that vagal stimulation, initiated before the onset of anterior myocardial ischemia, delayed the time of onset of ventricular fibrillation and reduced its incidence, both when the HR was allowed to decrease and also when it was kept constant by right ventricular pacing.

Later, Kolman et al[63] found that, in anesthetized dogs, vagal stimulation prevented the decrease in VFT induced by simultaneous left stellate ganglion stimulation. Similar conclusions were drawn by Furey and Levy,[64] utilizing the repetitive extrasystole threshold, which is strongly related to VFT.[65] Since vagal stimulation also counteracted the effect of isoproterenol infusion, it was possible to show that a significant part of the vagosympathetic antagonism was occurring postjunctionally, by primarily acting on cyclic AMP.[66]

Morphine significantly increased the repetitive extrasystole threshold in anesthetized dogs.[67] This effect was due to the vagotonic action of the opiate, since it was completely blocked by atropine or vagotomy. In the same animal preparation, the IV infusion of the muscarinic agonist methacholine induced a marked increase in the repetitive extrasystole threshold,[68] which appeared to be greater than the one caused by cervical vagosympathetic trunk stimulation, although the two interventions were not directly compared. Interestingly, after the administration of propranolol, the addition of methacholine did not allow any further increase in the repetitive extrasystole threshold.

Vagal Reflexes and Stimulation in the Conscious Experimental Preparation

Three sets of data obtained in the experimental preparation for sudden death described above will be presented here.

As a first step, we investigated whether vagal reflexes were involved in the capability of resistant animals to survive the 2-minute occlusion of the circumflex coronary artery.[15] In this study a group of resistant dogs, ie, that had survived the first test in control conditions, performed a second exercise and ischemia test, after atropine administration. In these conditions 23 of 45 dogs (51%) showed an arrhythmia worsening, and 11 of 45 (24%) developed ventricular fibrillation.

Based on this evidence, it was then rationale, as a second step, to test whether vagal stimulation was able to prevent ventricular fibrillation in dogs at high risk for lethal events. To address this issue we used a chronically implantable electrode for direct electrical stimulation of the vagus nerve in the conscious state.[69] Susceptible dogs underwent either a further exercise and ischemia test with no additional intervention (control group) or a trial in which electrical stimulation of the right vagus was started few seconds after the beginning of the occlusion. The intensity of the stimulation was adjusted to produce an HR reduction of 30 to 40 bpm. Ventricular fibrillation occurred in 23/25 (92%) control animals but only in 3 of 30 (10%) vagally stimulated dogs.[70] The relative role of the reduction in HR was assessed by experiments with atrial pacing. In nine dogs HR was maintained at the same level attained during the control exercise and ischemia test and five of the nine dogs (55%) survived the test. This indicates that approximately half of the antifibrillatory effect is independent of the HR reduction caused by vagal stimulation. Thus, electrically produced vagal hyperactivity at the onset of an ischemic episode is capable of drastically reducing the incidence of lethal arrhythmia in this animal model.

As a third step, we evaluated the capability of a pharmacological parasympathomimetic intervention to prevent the occurrence of life-threatening arrhythmias. This study was preceded by another study where the antiarrhythmic potential of the muscarinic agonist oxotremorine[71] was tested in an acute feline animal model in which malignant arrhythmia are elicited by the combination of acute myocardial ischemia and sympathetic hyperactivity. A useful feature of this model is that it has been utilized[72] for analysis of the efficacy of several antiarrhythmic interventions,[73] so that comparisons between different drugs are possible and meaningful. Oxotremorine produced a significant HR decrease and a striking antiarrhythmic effect with the complete abolition of VF and clear-cut reduction in ventricular arrhythmias. The severity of the arrhythmias, and specifically, the incidence of ventricular fibrillation was still significantly lower even when HR was controlled by atrial pacing. Overall, the antiarrhythmic efficacy of oxotremorine was comparable to that observed with propranolol.

The study in anesthetized cats generated the background for the subsequent evaluation of two muscarinic agonists, that were compared with propranolol, in conscious dogs.[74] Eleven susceptible dogs underwent exercise and ischemia tests with the following treatments: saline, propranolol, methacholine and oxotremorine. Saline never prevented VF, whereas propranolol was effective in 90% of the dogs (p<0.001), methacholine in 40% (p = 0.035), and oxotremorine in 62.5% (p = 0.005). Propranolol and oxotremorine significantly reduced HR, compared to saline, but methacholine did not. Propranolol significantly reduced left ventricular dP/dt max, particularly during myocardial ischemia, when dP/dt max values with propranolol were approximately half compared to those observed with the other treatments (p<0.005). Therefore, compared to β-blockade, methacholine and oxotremorine provide a less marked, but still valid protection and caused a significantly smaller impairment of contractility.

Overall, these data clearly documented, in absence of the confounding effects of anesthesia, the antifibrillatory effect of vagal activation. They represent a strong experimental rationale for the use of tools able to detect alterations in the autonomic control of HR resulting in augmented sympathetic activity and reduced vagal activity. This will contribute to the early identification of subjects at higher risk of developing lethal arrhythmias in the event of an episode of acute myocardial ischemia.

Conclusions

The predictive value of HRV reflects the relation existing between autonomic control of HR and reflex responses to acute myocardial ischemia. The lower the HRV, the greater the probability that acute myocardial ischemia results in a dominance of sympathetic reflexes and, consequently, in a greater risk for the occurrence of lethal arrhythmias. Enhanced afferent sympathetic activity from the heart is a likely mechanism contributing to a depressed HRV after MI. A normal HRV after MI reflects a preserved physiological cardiac vagal activity that is protective against ventricular fibrillation.

Overall, the experimental data presented in this chapter suggest the concept that the predictive value of a depressed HRV primarily reflects the capability of this marker to identify post-MI subjects at higher risk of sudden cardiac death because of the arrhythmogenic interaction between acute myocardial ischemia and high reflex sympathetic activity.

References

1. Zipes DP, Miyazaki T. The autonomic nervous system and the heart: basis for understanding interactions and effects on arrhythmia development. In: Zipes DP, Jalife J (eds). Cardiac Electrophysiology: From Cell to Bedside. Philadelphia, Pa: WB Saunders Co., 1990; 312-330.

2. Billman GE, Schwartz PJ, Stone HL. Baroreceptor reflex control of heart rate: a predictor of sudden death. Circulation 1982; 66:874-880.

3. Schwartz PJ, Stone HL. The analysis and modulation of autonomic reflexes in the prediction and prevention of sudden death. In: Zipes DP, Jalife J (eds). Cardiac Arrhythmias: Mechanisms and Management. New York, NY: Grune and Stratton, 1985; 165-176.

4. Schwartz PJ, Billman GE, Stone HL. Autonomic mechanisms in ventricular fibrillation induced by myocardial ischemia during exercise in dogs with a healed myocardial infarction. An experimental preparation for sudden cardiac death. Circulation 1984; 69:790-800.

5. Spyer KM. The central nervous organization of reflex circulatory control. In: Loewy AD, Spyer KM (eds). Central Regulation of Autonomic Function. New York, NY: Oxford University Press, 1990; 168-188.

6. Webb SW, Adgey AAJ, Pantridge JF. Autonomic disturbance at onset of acute myocardial infarction. Br Med J 1972; 3:89-92.

7. Corr PB, Yamada KA, Witkowski FX. Mechanisms controlling cardiac autonomic function and their relation to arrhythmogenesis. In: Fozzard HA, Haber E, Jennings RB, et al (eds). The Heart and the Cardiovascular System. New York, NY: Raven Press, 1986; 1343-1404.

8. Meyerburg RJ, Kessler KM, Interian A Jr, et al. Clinical and experimental pathophysiology of sudden cardiac death. In: Zipes PD, Jalife J (eds). Cardiac Electrophysiology: From Cell to Bedside. Philadelphia, Pa: WB Saunders, 1990; 666-677.

9. Schwartz PJ, La Rovere MT, Vanoli E. Autonomic nervous system and sudden cardiac death: experimental basis and clinical observations for post-myocardial infarction risk stratification. Circulation 1992; 85(suppl I):I77-I91.

10. Schwartz PJ, Vanoli E, Stramba-Badiale M, et al. Autonomic mechanisms and sudden death. New insight from the analysis of baroreceptor reflexes in conscious dogs with and without a myocardial infarction. Circulation 1988; 78:969-979.

11. Malik M, Camm AJ. Heart rate variability: from facts to fancies. Am J Cardiol 1993; 22:566-568.

12. Eckberg DL. Human sinus arrhythmia as an index of vagal cardiac outflow. J Appl Physiol 1983; 54:961-966.

13. Malliani A, Schwartz PJ, Zanchetti A. A sympathetic reflex elicited by experimental coronary occlusion. Am J Physiol 1969; 217:703-709.

14. De Ferrari GM, Grossoni M, Salvati P, et al. Reflex response to acute myocardial ischemia in conscious dogs susceptible to ventricular fibrillation. Eur Heart J 1993; 14(suppl):41. Abstract.

15. De Ferrari GM, Vanoli E, Stramba-Badiale M, et al. Vagal reflexes and survival during acute myocardial ischemia in conscious dogs with healed myocardial infarction. Am J Physiol 1991; 261:H63-H69.

16. Thames MD, Klopfenstein HS, Abboud FM, et al. Preferential distribution of inhibitory cardiac receptors with vagal afferents to the inferoposterior wall of the left ventricle activated during coronary occlusion in the dog. Circ Res 1978; 43:512-519.

17. Smyth HS, Sleight P, Pickering GW. Reflex regulation of arterial pressure during sleep in man. Circ Res 1969; 24:109-121.

18. Goldstein DS. Arterial baroreflex sensitivity, plasma catecholamines, and pressor responsiveness in essential hypertension. Circulation 1983; 68:234-240.

19. Gnecchi Ruscone T, Lombardi F, Malfatto G, et al. Attenuation of baroreceptive mechanisms by cardiovascular sympathetic afferent fibers. Am J Physiol 1987; 253:H787-H791.

20. Hull SS, Evans AR, Vanoli E, et al. Heart rate variability before and after myocardial infarction in conscious dogs at high and low risk of sudden death. J Am Coll Cardiol 1990; 16:978-985.

21. Billman GE, Schwartz PJ, Gagnol JP, et al. The cardiac response to submaximal exercise

in dogs susceptible to sudden cardiac death. J Appl Physiol 1985; 59:890-897.

22. Schwartz PJ. An experimental approach to the problem of postinfarction angina and sudden cardiac death. Eur Heart J 1987; 7(suppl C):7-17.

23. Lombardi F, Sandrone G, Pernpruner S, et al. Heart rate variability as an index of sympathovagal interaction after acute myocardial infarction. Am J Cardiol 1987; 60:1239-1245.

24. Bigger JT Jr, Fleiss JL, Rolnitzky LM, et al. Time course of recovery of heart period variability after myocardial infarction. J Am Coll Cardiol 1991; 18:1643-1649.

25. Bigger JT, Fleiss JL, Rolnitzky LM, et al. Frequency domain measures of heart period variability and death in chronic heart disease (1 year after infarction). Circulation 1992; 86(suppl I):I-660.

26. Adamson PB, Huang MH, Vanoli E, et al. Unexpected interaction betweeen beta-adrenergic blockade and heart rate variability before and after myocardial infarction: a longitudinal study in dogs at high and low risk for sudden death. Circulation 1994; 90:976-982.

27. Malliani A, Recordati G, Schwartz PJ. Nervous activity of afferent cardiac sympathetic fibres with atrial and ventricular endings. J Physiol 1973; 229:457-469.

28. Uchida Y, Murao S. Excitation of afferent cardiac sympathetic nerve fibers during coronary occlusion. Am J Physiol 1973; 226:1094-1099.

29. Thoren PN. Activation of left ventricular receptors with non-medullated vagal afferent fibers during occlusion of a coronary artery in the cat. Am J Cardiol 1976: 37:1046-1051.

30. Recordati G, Schwartz PJ, Pagani M, et al. Activation of cardiac vagal receptors during myocardial ischemia. Experientia 1971; 27:1423-1424.

31. Thoren PN. Vagal reflexes elicited by left ventricular C-fibers during myocardial ischemia in cats. In: Schwartz PJ, Brown AM, Malliani A, et al (eds). Neural Mechanisms in Cardiac Arrhythmias. New York, NY: Raven Press, 1978; 179-190.

32. Lombardi F, Della Bella P, Casati R, et al. Effects of intracoronary administration of bradykinin on the impulse activity of afferent sympathetic fibers. Circ Res 1981; 48:69-75.

33. Reimann KA, Weaver LC. Contrasting reflexes evoked by chemical activation of cardiac afferent nerves. Am J Physiol 1980; 239:H316-H325.

34. Ueda H, Uchida Y, Kamisaka K. Distribution and responses of the cardiac sympathetic receptors to mechanically induced circulatory changes. Jpn Heart J 1969; 10:70-81.

35. Uchida Y, Murao S. Potassium-induced excitation of afferent cardiac sympathetic nerve fibers. Am J Physiol 1973; 226:603-607.

36. James TN, Isobe JH, Urthaler F. Analysis of components in a hypertensive cardiogenic chemoreflex. Circulation 1975; 52:179-192.

37. Staszewska-Barczak J, Ferreira S, Vane RJ. An excitatory nocioceptive cardiac reflex elicited by bradykinin and potentiated by prostaglandins and myocardial ischemia. Cardiovasc Res 1976; 10:314-323.

38. Lombardi F, Casalone C, Della Bella P, et al. Global versus regional myocardial ischemia: differences in cardiovascular and sympathetic responses in cats. Cardiovasc Res 1984; 18:14-23.

39. Lombardi F, Verrier RL, Lown B. Relationship between sympathetic neural activity, coronary dynamics, and vulnerability to ventricular fibrillation during myocardial ischemia and reperfusion. Am Heart J 1983; 105:958-965.

40. Minisi AJ, Thames MD. Activation of cardiac sympathetic afferents during coronary artery occlusion. Evidence for reflex activation of sympathetic nervous system during transmural myocardial ischemia in the dog. Circulation 1991; 84:357-367.

41. Barber MJ, Mueller TM, Davies BG, et al. Interruption of sympathetic and vagal-mediated afferent responses by transmural myocardial infarction. Circulation 1985; 72:623-631.

42. Schwartz PJ, Foreman RD, Stone HL, et al. Effect of dorsal root section on the arrhythmias associated with coronary occlusion. Am J Physiol 1976; 231:923-928.

43. Schwartz PJ, Pagani M, Lombardi F, et al. A cardiocardiac sympathovagal reflex in the cat. Circ Res 1973; 32:215-220.

44. Cerati D, Schwartz PJ. Single cardiac vagal fiber activity, acute myocardial ischemia, and risk for sudden death. Circ Res 1991; 69:1389-1401.

45. Loewy AD. Central autonomic pathways. In: Loewy AD, Spyer KM (eds): Central Regulation of Autonomic Function. New York, NY: Oxford University Press, 1990; 88-103.

46. Jordan D, Spyer KM. Brainstem integration of cardiovascular and pulmonary afferent activity. Prog Brain Res 1986; 67:295-314.

47. Longhurst JC, Ashton JH, Iwamoto GA. Cardiovascular reflexes resulting from capsaicin stimulated gastric receptors in anesthetized dogs. Circ Res 1980; 46:780-788.

48. Ordway GA, Langhurst JC. Cardiovascular reflexes arising from the gallbladder of the cat, effects of capsaicin, bradykinin and distension. Circ Res 1983; 52:26-35.

49. Ordway GA, Langhurst JC, Mitchell JH. Stimulation of pancreatic afferents reflexly activates the cardiovascular system in cats. Am J Physiol 1983; 245:R820-R826.

50. Chohan A, Petch MC, Schofield PM. Effect of aesophageal acid instillation on coronary blood flow. Lancet 1993; 341:1309-1310.

51. Vanoli E, Adamson PB, Lin B, et al. Heart rate variability during specific sleep stages: a comparison of healthy subjects with patients after myocardial infarction. Circulation 1995. In press.

52. Orr WC, Lin B, Adamson PB, et al. Effect of esophageal acidification on the autonomic regulation of cardiac activity. Gastroenterology 1993; 104:A562.

53. Schwartz PJ, Priori SG. Sympathetic nervous system and cardiac arrhythmias. In: Zipes DP, Jalife J (eds). Cardiac Electrophysiology: From Cell to Bedside. Philadelphia, Pa: WB Saunders Co, 1990; 330-343.

54. Yusuf S, Teo KK. Approaches to prevention of sudden death: need for fundamental re-evaluation. J Cardiovasc Electrophysiol 1991; 2(suppl):S233-S239.

55. Schwartz PJ, Motolese M, Pollavini G, et al. Prevention of sudden cardiac death after a first myocardial infarction by pharmacological or surgical antiadrenergic interventions. J Cardiovasc Electrophysiol 1992; 3:2-16.

56. Lewis T. The experimental production of paroxysmal tachycardia and the effects of ligation of the coronary arteries. Heart 1909; 1:98-137.

57. Wiggers CJ. Physiology in Health and Disease, 5th ed. Philadelphia, Pa: Lea & Febiger, 1949; 530.

58. Rosen MR, Hoffman BF. The vagus and the ventricle. Circ Res 1978; 42:1. Editorial.

59. Han J, Millet D, Chizzonitti B, et al. Temporal dispersion of recovery of excitability in atrium and ventricle as a function of heart rate. Am Heart J 1966; 71:481-487.

60. Kent KM, Smith ER, Redwood DR, et al. Electrical stability of acutely ischemic myocardium: influences of heart rate and vagal stimulation. Circulation 1973; 47:291-298.

61. Goldstein RE, Karsh RB, Smith ER, et al. Influence of atropine and of vagally mediated bradycardia on the recurrence of ventricular arrhythmias following acute coronary occlusion in closed chest dogs. Circulation 1973; 47:1180-1190.

62. Myers RW, Pearlman AS, Hyman RM, et al. Beneficial effects of vagal stimulation and bradycardia during experimental acute myocardial ischemia. Circulation 1974; 49:943-947.

63. Kolman BS, Verrier RL, Lown B. The effect of vagus nerve stimulation upon vulnerability of the canine ventricle: role of the sympathetic parasympathetic interactions. Circulation 1976; 52:578-585.

64. Furey SA III, Levy MN. Interactions among heart rate, autonomic activity, and arterial pressure upon the multiple repetitive extrasystole threshold in the dog. Am Heart J 1983; 106:1112-1120.

65. Matta RJ, Verrier RL, Lown B. Repetitive extrasystole as an index of vulnerability to ventricular fibrillation. Am J Physiol 1976; 230:1469-1473.

66. Brown AM. Regulation of heartbeat by G protein-coupled ion channels. Am J Physiol 1990; 259:H1621-H1628.

67. DeSilva RA, Verrier RL, Lown B. The effects of psychological stress and vagal stimulation with morphine on vulnerability to ventricular fibrillation (VF). Am Heart J 1978; 95:197-203.

68. Rabinowitz SH, Verrier RL, Lown B. Muscarinic effects of vagosympathetic trunk stimulation on the repetitive extrasystole (RE) threshold. Circulation 1976; 53:622-627.

69. Stramba-Badiale M, Vanoli E, De Ferrari GM, et al. Sympathetic-parasympathetic interaction and accentuated antagonism in conscious dogs. Am J Physiol 1991; 260:H335.

70. Vanoli E, De Ferrari GM, Stramba-Badiale M, et al. Vagal stimulation and prevention of sudden death in conscious dogs with a healed myocardial infarction. Circ Res 1991; 68:1471-1481.

71. De Ferrari GM, Vanoli E, Curcuruto P, et al. Prevention of life-threatening arrhythmias by pharmacologic stimulation of the muscarinic receptors with oxotremorine. Am Heart J 1992; 124:883-890.

72. Schwartz PJ, Vanoli E. Cardiac arrhythmias elicited by interaction between acute myocardial ischemia and sympathetic hyperactivity: a new experimental model for the study of antiarrhythmic drugs. J Cardiovasc Pharmacol 1981; 3:1251-1259.

73. Schwartz PJ, Vanoli E, Zaza A, et al. The effect of antiarrhythmic drugs on life-threatening arrhythmias induced by the interaction between acute myocardial ischemia and sympathetic hyperactivity. Am Heart J 1985; 109:937-948.

74. De Ferrari GM, Salvati P, Grossoni M, et al. Pharmacologic modulation of the autonomic nervous system in the prevention of sudden cardiac death. A study with propranolol, methacholine and oxotremorine in conscious dogs with a healed myocardial infarction. J Am Coll Cardiol 1993; 21:283-290.

Chapter 28

Heart Rate Variability and Risk Stratification After Acute Myocardial Infarction: Change in Heart Rate Variability After Acute Myocardial Infarction

Olusola Odemuyiwa

Acute myocardial infarction is associated with rises in plasma and urinary concentrations of catecholamines,[1] and with an impairment of parasympathetic reflexes[2,3] which gradually resolve with time. This chapter will address the change in heart rate variability (HRV) after acute myocardial infarction.

Rothschild et al[3] compared RR variation and RR intervals during beta-blockade in seven patients studied between 6 weeks and 6 months after infarction, and in 10 other patients 6 months or more after myocardial infarction: RR interval variation was significantly lower in the former group. Serial evaluation of HRV was not undertaken but the study drew attention to the possibility that HRV could change with time after infarction. Lombardi et al[4] extended these observations by comparing baseline HRV at 2 weeks in 70 patients with measurements

in 33 and 29 patients at 6 and 12 months, respectively. They concentrated on total RR variance and the low-frequency (LF) and high-frequency (HF) normalized power in 7 to 8 minutes of RR intervals. Their findings could be summarized as follows:

1. at 2 weeks after myocardial infarction, there was no difference in total RR variance between patients and controls; but compared with controls, there was a decrease in HF power and a rise in LF power. In other words, there was sympathetic predominance early after infarction. These differences persisted for about 6 months;

2. between 6 and 12 months, there was a gradual reversal of these differences; and

From: Malik M., Camm AJ (eds.): *Heart Rate Variability.* Armonk, NY. Futura Publishing Company, Inc., © 1995.

3. at 12 months there was no difference in total RR variance or the LF or HF power between patients and controls (Figure 1).

Bigger and colleagues[5] undertook serial measurement of HRV in 68 patients from the placebo arm of the Cardiac Arrhythmia Pilot Study[6] at a mean of 25 days and at 3, 6 and 12 months after acute myocardial infarction. Ultra-low frequency, very low frequency (VLF), LF and HF components and total power of the heart period power spectrum were derived from 24-hour Holter recordings:

1. at baseline, these indices of HRV were depressed by between 50% and 67% compared with age- and gender-matched controls;
2. there was a marked increase in the measures of HRV between the baseline and the 3-month recording, but little change between 3 and 12 months. In short, HRV had more or less recovered completely after 3 months; and
3. however, the results differed from those reported by Lombardi et al[4] in showing that even after 12 months, HRV was still markedly depressed

when compared with controls (Figure 2).

Differences between the studies account, at least in part, for their conflicting conclusions, particularly with respect to HRV at 12 months. Lombardi et al[4] studied at 12 months, only a small number of the patients who had had a baseline assessment of HRV. Moreover, Lombardi et al[4] derived HRV using short, 7- to 8-minute recordings, whereas Bigger et al[5] used 24-hour recordings, the results of which are more reproducible. Finally, where Bigger et al used fast Fourier analysis for deriving HRV, Lombardi et al[4] used an autoregressive method. These two techniques are discussed in more detail in Chapter 5. A more recent prospective study by Casolo et al[7] derived HRV in the time domain from 24-hour recordings in 54 patients at baseline, within 12 hours of the onset of chest pain, in 22 patients 30 days after discharge from the coronary care unit, and in 48 patients at 60 days. Near-normal HRV was observed at 60 days and intermediate values at 30 days. At 60 days, only 2 patients showed a low HRV: one had experienced repeated bouts of pulmonary edema after infarction and the other patient developed congestive heart failure. These results agree with those

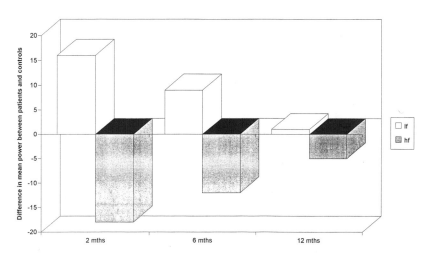

Figure 1. LF and HF power in controls and in survivors of myocardial infarction. Derived from Lombardi et al.[4]

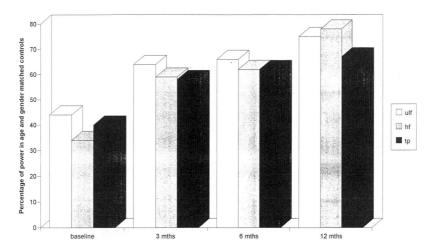

Figure 2. Recovery of different components of HRV after myocardial infarction. LF, HF, and Tp (total power). Derived from Bigger et al.[5]

reported by Mcalpine and colleagues[8] who found that the decline in plasma catecholamines in the week after infarction was attenuated in those with extensive infarction or heart failure. Luria et al[9] reported a more marked reduction in HRV after anterior than after inferior infarction, but did not examine whether the site of infarction influenced the subsequent course of HRV. Mazzuero et al[10] examined the changes in HRV in a selected group of patients at 4 to 6 weeks and again at 6 months in 38 patients after anterior infarction who were deemed suitable for long-term exercise training. Not surprisingly, HRV at baseline was almost within the normal range in this highly selected group of patients. An increase in the time-domain indices between baseline and the second assessment at 6 months was also reported. One unexpected finding, however, was the rise in the mean LF/HF ratio between assessments, indicating a shift towards sympathetic predominance. Whether this resulted from the highly selected patient population, the site of infarction or reflected the deficiencies of spectral analysis of HRV, is unclear. It appears that most indices of HRV are depressed for the first 2 to 3 months after acute myocardial infarction, the time-domain indices eventually rising to near normal values unless complicated by clinical features of heart failure while

the spectral indices of HRV show different patterns of recovery and may remain depressed for up to 6 or 12 months.

How far do these changes in HRV reflect real changes in cardiovascular function? By pretreating the patients with propranolol, Rothschild and colleagues[3] have shown that autonomic dysfunction after myocardial infarction was limited to cardiac parasympathetic function. Moreover, other tests of autonomic function including the Valsalva ratio and pupillary light responses were unaffected after myocardial infarction. Other workers have shown that the assessment of HRV is reproducible[11,12] and that its serial evaluation should therefore be able to distinguish changes due to cardiac disease from those due to random variation. Kleiger et al[11] recorded baseline and placebo 24-hour ambulatory electrocardiograms 3 and 65 days apart in 14 normal subjects aged 20 to 55 years. They found that the mean and standard deviations of these measures were virtually identical between placebo and baseline measurements and that both the time- and frequency-domain measures of HRV could be used interchangeably. Pagani et al[12] also showed that HRV in individual subjects remained constant on testing over a period of a year. Assessment of HRV is also reproducible in postinfarction patients with ventricular arrhythmias.[13]

Proposed causes of the changes in neuroendocrine activity seen after acute myocardial infarction come from studies in animals. These include activation or interruption of cardiac autonomic reflexes by direct ischemia or by mechanical distortion or disruption of cardiac afferent nerve receptors, as well as activation or interruption of reflexes because nerves which themselves may not be ischemic may be lying in an ischemic milieu.[14] The severity, duration and causes of the changes in autonomic function and in HRV in particular may vary with the extent and site of myocardial damage and whether infarction is transmural or nontransmural.[14] Diuretic therapy,[15] anxiety and anger[16] may also contribute to these changes. The gradual improvement in autonomic indices has been attributed to a reversal of ischemia, the washing out of ischemic metabolites, receptor necrosis and the adaptation of receptors to continuing mechanical and chemical stimuli.[17,18] What are the clinical implications of these findings? The most marked depression in HRV occurs when mortality after myocardial infarction is relatively high. If a reduction in parasympathetic tone or relative increase in sympathetic activity explain both the depressed HRV early after infarction and an increased susceptibility to ventricular arrhythmias,[19] then the predictive value of low HRV measured early after infarction for sudden arrhythmic deaths should decline with time. This will occur either because some patients with these markers will die suddenly soon after infarction and because the tendency is for the abnormalities to improve spontaneously with time in the other patients. A recent study appears to confirm this hypothesis by showing that low HRV was an independent predictor of sudden death only during the first 6 months after infarction.[20] The findings also agree with the suggestion by Rothschild and colleagues[3] that patients with low HRV soon after infarction may not remain at risk indefinitely and that an assessment at 6 months may help to reevaluate the risk. This may be particularly apposite in predicting sudden death in patients with other features of impaired left ventricular function.

Further studies of the relation between the evolution of various measures of cardiac function and prognosis in postinfarction patients may help to establish the best time to repeat these measurements. The findings also imply that prospective studies into the prevention of sudden death after myocardial infarction should be based on a recent assessment of HRV. Whether therapy directed at increasing the rate of recovery of HRV after myocardial infarction will improve prognosis is unknown.[21,22]

References

1. Forssman O, Hansson G, Jensen CC. The adrenal function in coronary thrombosis. Acta Med Scand 1952; 142:441-449.
2. Ryan C, Hollenberg M, Harvey DB, et al. Impaired parasympathetic responses in patients after myocardial infarction. Am J Cardiol 1976; 37:1013-1018.
3. Rothschild M, Rothschild A, Pfeifer M. Temporary decrease in cardiac parasympathetic tone after acute myocardial infarction. Am J Cardiol 1988; 62:637-639.
4. Lombardi F, Sandrone G, Pernpruner S, et al. Heart rate variability as an index of sympatho-vagal interaction in patients after myocardial infarction. Am J Cardiol 1987; 60 1239-1245.
5. Bigger TJ, Fleiss JL, Rolnitzky LM, et al. Time course of recovery of heart period variability after myocardial infarction. J Am Coll Cardiol 1991; 18:1643-1649.
6. The Cardiac Arrhythmia Study (CAPS) Investigators. Recruitment and baseline description of patients in the Cardiac Arrhythmia Pilot Study. Am J Cardiol 1988; 61:704-709.
7. Casolo GC, Stroder P, Signorini C, et al. Heart rate variability during the acute phase of myocardial infarction. Circulation 1992; 85:2073-2079.
8. Mcalpine HM, Morton JJ, Leckie B, et al. Neuroendocrine activation after acute myocardial infarction. Br Heart J 1988; 60:117-124.
9. Luria MH, Sapoznikov D, Gilon D, et al. Early heart rate variability alterations after acute myocardial infarction. Am Heart J 1993; 125:676-681.
10. Mazzuero G, Lanfranchi P, Colombo R, et al. Long-term adaptability of 24-hour heart

rate variability after myocardial infarction. Chest 1992; 101:304S-308S.

11. Kleiger RE, Bigger JT, Bosner MS, et al. Stability overtime of variables measuring heart rate variability in normal subjects. Am J Cardiol 1991; 68:626-630.

12. Pagani M, Lombardi F, Guzzetti S, et al. Power spectral analysis of heart rate and arterial pressure variabilities as a marker of sympatho-vagal interaction in man and conscious dog. Circ Res 1986; 59:178-193.

13. Bigger JT, Fleiss JL, Rolnitzky LM, et al. Stability over time of heart period variability in patients with previous myocardial infarction and ventricular arrhythmias. Am J Cardiol 1992; 69:718-723.

14. Zipes DP. Influence of myocardial ischaemia and infarction on autonomic innervation of heart. Circulation 1990; 82:1095-1105.

15. Hull SS Jr, Adamson PB, Vanoli E, et al. Dietary sodiumalters heart rate response to acute myocardial ischaemia inconscious dogs after myocardial infarction. Eur Heart J 1991; 12:217.

16. Buchanan LM, Cowan M, Burr R, et al. Measurement of recovery from myocardial infarction using heart rate variability and psychological outcomes. Nurs Res 1993; 42(2):74-78.

17. Barber MJ, Mueller TM, Henry DD, et al. Transmural myocardial infarction in the dog produces sympathectomy in noninfarcted myocardium. Circulation 1983; 67:787-796.

18. Bishop VS, Malliani A, Thoren PN. Cardiac-mechanoceptors. In: Handbook of Physiology. The Cardiovascular System, Volume 3, Part 2. Bethesda, MD: American Physiological Society, 1983; 497-555.

19. Gillis RA. Role of the nervous system in the arrhythmias produced by coronary occlusion in the cat. Am Heart J 1971; 81:677-684.

20. Odemuyiwa O, Poloniecki J, Malik M, et al. Temporal influences on the prediction of postinfarction mortality using heart rate variability. A comparison with the left ventricular ejection fraction. Br Heart J 1994; 71:521-527.

21. La Rovere MT, Mortara A, Sandrone G, et al. Autonomic nervous system adaptations to short-term exercise training. Chest 1992; 101(suppl 5):299S-303S.

22. Casadei B, Pipilis A, Sessa F, et al. Low doses of scopolamine increase cardiac vagal tone in the acute phase of myocardial infarction. Circulation 1993; 88:353-357.

Chapter 29

Risk Stratification Following Myocardial Infarction: Heart Rate Variability and Other Risk Factors

A. John Camm, Lü Fei

Introduction

Patients after acute myocardial infarction (MI) are at increased risk of sudden cardiac death (SCD), largely due to ventricular tachyarrhythmias.[1] Until recently, the risk assessment of patients following MI has been based on the evaluation of residual ischemia, persistent left ventricular dysfunction and recurrent ventricular arrhythmias. The stratification procedure identifies postinfarction patients at increased risk of major medical events, such as reinfarction, arrhythmic events (sustained ventricular tachycardia/fibrillation), and death (SCD, cardiovascular death and all cause mortality). Current research work in this field is mainly focused on the identification of patients at risk of SCD, including life-threatening arrhythmic events. Since this catastrophic arrhythmia seems to be due to an electrical accident rather than to terminal, irreversible myocardial damage, survival

could be improved by a successful intervention. Several powerful techniques are now available for the stratification of patients following acute MI into subgroups at high and low risk of postinfarction morbidity and mortality. Accumulating knowledge of postinfarction risk stratification has begun to provide a rational foundation for individualizing diagnostic and therapeutic strategies.

The aim of post-MI risk stratification is two-fold: to identify patients at very low risk of subsequent events after MI, and to identify patients at high risk of specific postinfarction events such as reinfarction, heart failure, SCD, or arrhythmic events. In the former case, a test with extremely high negative predictive accuracy is essential. In any event, since most serious outcomes following MI are rare (say <10%), any useful test must have a negative predictive accuracy much greater than 90%. When attempting to predict an adverse outcome, the statistical

From: Malik M., Camm AJ (eds.): *Heart Rate Variability*. Armonk, NY. Futura Publishing Company, Inc., © 1995.

characteristics of an ideal test designed to identify the patient at risk must take into account possible therapeutic strategies which might result from the identification of a patient at risk. For example, if an expensive or potentially complicated therapy (such as an implantable cardioverter defibrillator) is envisaged, the patients to be treated must be selected using a test with a very high positive predictive accuracy so that as few patients as possible are unnecessarily exposed to the treatment. Obviously, the sensitivity of the test should be as high as possible, without allowing the positive predictive accuracy to fall below the critical level of about 50%. On the other hand, if the proposed treatment is cheap and relatively safe (such as β-blockers), a test with a high sensitivity is essential. In this instance the positive predictive accuracy need not be high, since it does not matter much if some patients receive unnecessary therapy.

Recently, assessment of heart rate variability (HRV) has provided a new powerful noninvasive technique for postinfarction risk stratification. The predictive value of HRV is independent of other established risk factors for postinfarction risk stratification, such as left ventricular ejection fraction (LVEF), ventricular ectopy and late potentials. However, the positive predictive accuracy of all of these risk factors is relatively low, and their combination is often necessary. For example, combination with other techniques significantly improves the positive predictive accuracy of HRV with only a modest reduction of sensitivity. The currently used stratification techniques, including assessment of ventricular arrhythmias, ventricular function, late potentials, exercise test, electrophysiological testing and other relevant clinical variables, as well as HRV and the relationship of HRV to other risk factors, will be reviewed in this chapter. Assessment of baroreflex sensitivity (BRS) for postinfarction risk stratification is also discussed in the context of other risk predictors.

Since many statistical terms are used in this chapter, their definition as applied to postinfarction risk stratification are summarized in Table 1. An example of such calculations is shown in Table 2. 'Receiver Operating Characteristic' (ROC) curve (ie, a plot of *sensitivity* versus *specificity*) provides a useful graphical approach for making the choice of the 'best' cut-point of a measurement (Figure 1). This curve is particularly useful when comparing two or more competing methods. For single test it does not add anything to a table, but it is preferable when there are many possible cut-off values.

Another important issue in postinfarction risk stratification is the specification of the endpoint of observations. Different risk factors are likely to predict specific risks differently. For example, ventricular premature complexes (VPCs) may be associated with development of arrhythmic events, while LVEF may be more likely to be associated with death secondary to circulatory failure. In principle, the Hinkle-Thaler classification of deaths[2] has been used to distinguish the endpoints in clinical trials (Table 3). Death is assigned as arrhythmic death, circulatory failure death or not classifiable (noncardiac death). Arrhythmic death is defined as abrupt loss of consciousness and disappearance of pulse without prior collapse of the circulation. Circulatory failure is defined as collapse of circulation before disappearance of the pulse. The Hinkle-Thaler approach was further refined in the Cardiac Arrhythmia Suppression Trial (CAST),[3] where death was judged to be due to arrhythmia if it was characterized in any of the following ways:

1. witnessed and instantaneous, without new or accelerating symptoms;
2. witnessed and preceded or accompanied by symptoms attributable to myocardial ischemia in the absence of shock or Class IV congestive heart failure as categorized by the New York Heart Association;

Table 1
The Commonly Used Definitions for Postinfarction Risk Stratification

Sensitivity = number of true positives detected/total number of positives in the group tested
Specificity = number of true normals detected/total number of normals in the group tested
Accuracy = number of true test results (true positives + true negatives)/total number of tests performed
  True positive = abnormal test results in individual who has or will have the event
  False positive = abnormal test result in one who does not and will not have the event
  True negative = normal test result in one who does not and will not have the event
  False negative = normal test result in one who has or will have the event
Positive predictive value = true positives/the apparent (true + false) positives
Negative predictive value = true negatives/the apparent (true + false) negatives
Relative risk = the incidences in the group with risk factor(s)/the incidence in the group without risk factor(s)

Table 2
An Example for Calculation of Sensitivity, Specificity and Predictive Value

		Outcome		
		+	−	*total*
test result	+	a	b	a + b
	−	c	d	c + d
total		a + c	b + d	n = a + b + c + d

sensitivity = a/(a + c); specificity = d/(b + d); positive predictive value = a/(a + b); and negative predictive value = d/(c + d).

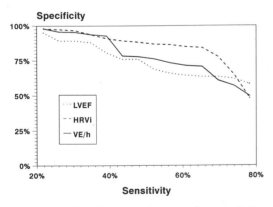

Figure 1. Receiver operator characteristics (ROC) curves for stratifying 1-year arrhythmic events (sustained ventricular tachycardia and sudden cardiac death) based on the data from the St. George's Post-Infarction Survey Program. HRVi: heart rate variability index; LVEF: left ventricular ejection fraction; VE/h: ventricular ectopic beats per hour.

3. witnessed and preceded by symptoms attributable to cardiac arrhythmia, eg, syncope or near syncope; or

4. unwitnessed but without evidence of another cause. In the Postinfarction Survey Program at St. George's Hospital, London, we use all cause cardiac mortality and arrhythmic events (sustained ventricular arrhythmias and arrhythmic death) as major endpoints.

Signal-Averaged Electrocardiography

Late potentials, detected using the signal-averaged electrocardiogram (ECG), suggest the presence of slow and inhomogeneous ventricular conduction. Late potentials have been shown to predict both spontaneous[4-7] and inducible ventricular tachycardia[6,8-11] and SCD.[4-7,12] At the time of discharge from hospital following acute MI, the incidence of late potentials and/or other abnormalities of the signal-averaged ECG

Table 3
Hinkle-Thaler Classification of Deaths After Myocardial Infarction

1. Arrhythmic deaths
   i. not preceded by heart failure
   ii. preceded by heart failure, not disabling
   iii. preceded by heart failure, disabling
2. Circulatory failure deaths
   i. peripheral circulatory failure
   ii. myocardial failure
3. Death not classifiable (noncardiac)

ranges from 30% to 50%. A higher prevalence of late potentials has been found in association with inducible ventricular tachycardia than with ventricular fibrillation in both animals and humans. In a prospective study of 306 patients after MI, Denniss et al[6] demonstrated that 19% of patients with late potentials have arrhythmic events compared with 4% of patients without late potentials during a 12-month follow-up period. Abolition of late potentials during follow-up in patients who had an abnormal signal-averaged ECG at the time of hospital discharge does not necessarily imply an improved prognosis.[13]

Using multiple regression analysis, Ohnishi et al[14] have demonstrated that among variables analyzed from the signal-averaged ECG, echocardiography, cardiac catheterization and Holter monitoring, ventricular arrhythmias were most strongly associated with late potential duration. Although the signal-averaged ECG, Holter monitoring and radionuclide ventriculography are independently significant in predicting outcome, the combined use of these variables can improve predictive accuracy (with a sensitivity of 80% and specificity of 89%).[4,15] Application of the signal-averaged ECG alone in risk stratification, however, is limited by its low sensitivity and positive predictive accuracy,[4,5,7,8] inconsistent effects of antiarrhythmic drugs on late potentials,[16-18] and the unknown optimum time of recording after MI.[15] Recently, ambulatory (Holter) electrocardiography signal-averaging has provided a new method for recording late potentials.[19,20] In contrast

to the conventional methods of detecting late potentials from the surface ECGs recorded at rest, ambulatory monitoring records from patients during normal daily activity over a prolonged period may provide new and, importantly, dynamic information. However, the predictive value of such potentials has not yet been thoroughly evaluated.

Assessment of Ventricular Function

Traditionally, left ventricular function is considered to be the best predictor of cardiac mortality after MI. It has been shown that the presence of clinical signs of left ventricular failure is a strong predictor of poor prognosis following MI.[21-26] LVEF prior to hospital discharge independently predicts 1-year mortality following acute MI.[21,23,24,27-30] Many other prognostic indicators, for example, programmed electrical stimulation,[8,31] have been found to be at least partially determined by the extent of left ventricular dysfunction. Univariate analysis has shown a progressive increase in 1-year cardiac mortality following MI with decreasing LVEF below 40%. Bigger et al[32] reported that after adjusting for other variables, LVEF <30% was an independent predictor for subsequent cardiac death (3.5 times that of patients with higher LVEF). Among several variables including the signal-averaged ECG, Holter monitoring and radionuclide ventriculography, stepwise logistic regression analysis showed that LVEF was the most powerful predictor of mortality (β = 2.8, p <0.005).[4]

The prognostic importance of left ventricular function after MI is well established, but the predictive value of LVEF at rest is low. Assessment of the response of left ventricular function to exercise may be of additional predictive value. Several investigators have demonstrated that exercise testing with radionuclide ventriculography[33] or echocardiography[34] at the time of hospital discharge is a sensitive method for the prediction of mortality or ischemic events after MI. Hung et al[35] have reported that in patients who underwent evaluation 3 weeks after a clinically uncomplicated MI, exercise radionuclide ventriculography contributed independent prognostic information to that provided by symptom-limited treadmill testing.

Electrophysiological Testing

During the past 2 decades, programmed electrical stimulation has greatly improved our understanding of arrhythmology. Programmed electrical stimulation has an excellent sensitivity, specificity and reproducibility in patients with chronic coronary artery disease and sustained ventricular tachycardia. Electrophysiological study is used in order to characterize the inducibility and the morphology, rate and hemodynamic consequences of arrhythmias; and guide treatment strategies including the selection of antiarrhythmic drug therapy (serial electrophysiological testing) and the suitability for antiarrhythmic surgery or implantation of an implantable cardioverter defibrillator. This invasive technique has been used for risk stratification of patients after MI.

Approximately 10% to 25% of patients have inducible sustained ventricular tachycardia soon after MI,[36-40] but early thrombolytic therapy reduces the incidence of inducible ventricular tachycardia.[41,42] In patients with recurrent ventricular tachycardia occurring within 8 weeks of MI, sustained uniform ventricular tachycardia is inducible in approximately 85% of patients.[43] The presence of ventricular arrhythmias on the Holter monitoring and late potentials in the signal-averaged ECGs increases the likelihood of inducing sustained ventricular tachycardia, but exercise-induced ST depression does not. The likelihood of inducing sustained ventricular tachycardia by programmed electrical stimulation increases with infarct size.[44] Preliminary observations suggest that the inducibility of sustained ventricular arrhythmias may vary with time following acute MI, but conclusive data are still lacking.[5,45,46]

Several studies[38-40,47] have demonstrated a predictive value of programmed electrical stimulation after MI. However, the predictive accuracy is relatively low (20%-35%) for the development of sustained ventricular tachycardia and/or SCD.[6,38] The role of electrophysiological testing as a tool to predict patients who will have arrhythmic events or SCD is still controversial, due to the relatively small number of patients that have been studied.[36,48-50] Bourke et al[50] have recently reported the results of programmed electrical stimulation in a relatively large cohort of survivors of acute MI. Electrophysiological testing was performed in 1,209 patients (37% of 3,286 consecutive patients hospitalized for acute MI) without complications at the time of hospital discharge. Sustained monomorphic ventricular tachycardia was inducible in 75 patients (6.2%). The incidence of spontaneous ventricular tachycardia/fibrillation in the absence of new ischemic events is 19% in patients with inducible ventricular tachycardia and 2.9% in those without inducible ventricular tachycardia (p <0.0005). It is concluded that electrophysiological testing is the single best predictor of spontaneous ventricular tachycardia/fibrillation in patients following acute MI. The authors also suggest that decreased left ventricular function may serve as a crude preselector to screen for survivors of acute MI most likely to benefit from electrophysiological testing.

In contrast to inducible ventricular tachycardia, the predictive significance of ventricular fibrillation induced by programmed electrical stimulation is negligible.[6] It seems that absence of an inducible arrhythmia in response to an aggressive protocol (at least three extrastimuli at two drive cycle lengths) indicates extremely low risk. The role of programmed electrical stimulation guided therapy at the time of hospital discharge remains to be defined in patients following an acute MI, although it may improve outcome in patients with remote MI.[51] In a randomized pilot trial in 136 patients with inducible ventricular tachyarrhythmias 1 to 4 weeks following acute MI, Denniss et al[52] demonstrated that prophylactic therapy with Class I antiarrhythmic agents at a 'therapeutic' serum level did not alter the prognosis during 3-year follow-up. Whether the inducibility of ventricular arrhythmias can be predicted by other clinical variables is still disputed.[39,53] The timing of electrophysiological testing significantly influences the inducibility of sustained ventricular arrhythmias after MI.[54] The optimum time for performing electrophysiological testing is not yet clear.[55,56] Furthermore, the sensitivity and specificity differ when using different protocols of stimulation. These limitations make this invasive and relatively expensive technique less popular for risk stratification after acute MI.

Assessment of Ventricular Arrhythmias

Since malignant ventricular tachyarrhythmias are the major cause of death after hospital discharge in the first year following acute MI,[57] ventricular ectopic activity has been evaluated for postinfarction risk stratification. The frequency and complexity of ventricular ectopy fluctuate with time after MI. Most large studies in which ventricular arrhythmias were detected on Holter monitoring were made about 10 days after acute MI. The prevalence of VPCs is not high.

Only 15% to 20% of patients have ≥10 VPCs per hour. However, the frequency of ventricular arrhythmias may rise substantially from 2 weeks to 3 months after hospital discharge, and then remain approximately constant.[58,59] Recurrent ventricular tachycardia occurring ≥48 hours after acute MI usually signifies the presence of a pathophysiological substrate from which recurrent sustained ventricular tachycardia and/or SCD may evolve. It has been shown that frequent (≥10 beats per hour), repetitive VPCs (couplets and salvos) or sustained ventricular tachycardia following MI heralds a poor prognosis.[24,27,32,60,61] Not only the frequency of ventricular tachyarrhythmias, but also the presence of ventricular bradycardias have prognostic implications.[57,62,63] Recently Hodges et al[64] reported that an average of even one VPC per hour is associated with increased postinfarction mortality. These authors also found that nonsustained ventricular tachycardia predicts mortality independently of LVEF and the frequency of VPCs. An S-shaped curve describes the relationship between mortality rate and VPC frequency.[65]

Data in 680 patients of whom 379 received early thrombolytic therapy from St. George's Hospital demonstrated that VPC frequency is more highly predictive of prognosis in thrombolyzed than nonthrombolyzed patients following acute MI. The mean frequency of VPCs on predischarge Holter recordings after acute MI is significantly higher in patients suffering from all cause mortality, SCD and arrhythmic events in both thrombolyzed and nonthrombolyzed patients. At a sensitivity of 40% the positive predictive accuracy is greater in thrombolyzed patients (19.4% for cardiac death and 25.8% for arrhythmic events) than in nonthrombolyzed patients (16% for cardiac death and 16% for arrhythmic events). The optimal dichotomy frequency of VPCs is 25 and 10 per hour in thrombolyzed and nonthrombolyzed populations, respectively. Figures 2A and B show the Kaplan-Meier survival curves of VPCs dichotomized at 25 per hour in patients with

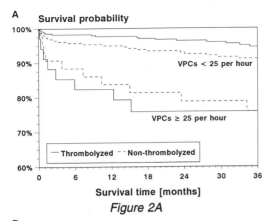

Figure 2A

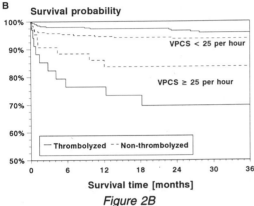

Figure 2B

Figures 2A-B. Cumulative Kaplan-Meier survival curves of ventricular ectopic frequency on 24-hour Holter monitoring in patients following myocardial infarction from the Post-Infarct Survey Program of St. George's Hospital Medical School. VPC: ventricular premature complexes. VPC is dichotomized at 25 per hour. A: for total cardiac mortality (p <0.001 for both thrombolyzed and nonthrombolyzed patients); B: for arrhythmic events (sudden cardiac death and sustained ventricular tachycardia) (p <0.001 for thrombolyzed patients and p <0.05 for nonthrombolyzed patients).

and without thrombolysis. It has been reported that the risk of ventricular fibrillation is reduced over the hospital course in thrombolyzed patients, although there is no significant change in the likelihood of developing ventricular fibrillation in the first few hours after thrombolysis.[66]

Despite some concordance between ventricular arrhythmias and left ventricular dysfunction,[67,68] both ventricular ectopic activity and ventricular tachycardia have been

regarded as independent risk factors after MI.[61,69,70] However, there is no evidence to suggest a cause-and-effect relationship between ventricular ectopic activity and cardiac death. Since ventricular arrhythmias may be provoked and aggravated by left ventricular dysfunction, the independent predictive significance of ventricular ectopic activity has been questioned.[30,67,71] This has been further supported by the low mortality of patients in the placebo limb of the Cardiac Arrhythmia Suppression Trial (CAST).[72]

Exercise Testing

Exercise testing prior to hospital discharge has been used extensively in postinfarction risk stratification. Exercise testing can identify residual ischemia, assess exercise tolerance, and may provoke exercise-induced ventricular arrhythmias.[73] An abnormal ST segment response during an early symptom limited exercise test (or angina in-hospital) is a strong predictor of mortality within 1 year, but not thereafter.[74] Late mortality correlates better with markers of poor left ventricular function. Theroux et al[75] reported that 1 mm of ST segment depression during a low-level treadmill exercise test was highly predictive of the 1-year mortality rate and was significantly associated with the occurrence of SCD during this period. More marked ST depression (>0.2 mV) carried no extra prognostic significance in this study.

Krone et al[76] noted that an increased 1-year mortality after MI was found in patients who had one or more of the following independent predictors during exercise testing:

1. failure to achieve an increased systolic blood pressure of ≥110 mmHg (18% versus 3%, p <0.001);
2. inability to complete the 9-minute exercise test (8% versus 3%, p <0.01); and

3. presence of ventricular couplets (13% versus 4%, p <0.05) or any VPCs during or after the test (7% versus 4%, <0.05).

Angina during or after the exercise test predicts cardiac mortality in the first year (9% versus 4%, p <0.05) independent of ST segment changes. Myocardial ischemia is manifested not only by traditional indices such as exercise-induced ST segment depression and angina pectoris and by reversible thallium perfusion defects, but also by a low peak treadmill word load and by a decrease in LVEF during exercise.[35] Pharmacological stress imaging using dipyridamole, adenosine, or dobutamine, combined with ^{201}Tl scintigraphy, radionuclide ventriculography, or two-dimensional echocardiography, can be used in patients unable to exercise.[77] Recently the application of exercise testing for risk stratification after thrombolytic therapy has been questioned.[78] However, it now seems that the negative response to exercise may identify a group of patients at low risk after MI treated by thrombolysis (negative predictive accuracy was 89%). The addition of cardiac imaging techniques has augmented the predictive capacity of exercise testing. The value of planar thallium[-201] imaging in postinfarction risk stratification has been reviewed recently by Gibson and Watson.[79]

Residual ischemia may also be assessed by ambulatory electrocardiographic monitoring. Langer et al[80] have recently reported that approximately one third of survivors of acute MI have ST segment depression on Holter monitoring, regardless of the use of thrombolytic therapy. Patients who had ST segment depression on Holter monitoring had an unfavorable prognosis. Although silent and symptomatic dipyridamole-induced ischemia after MI may have comparable clinical and prognostic significance,[81,82] Gill et al[83] have recently reported that silent ischemia on Holter monitoring early after MI provides better prognostic information than exercise testing. It has been shown that the predictive value of ischemia detected from either Holter monitoring or exercise testing is low. However, a combination of the two techniques significantly increases prognostic significance.[84]

The echocardiogram has been shown to be of considerable value in postinfarction risk stratification for acquisition of prognostic information in addition to that derived from left ventricular ejection fraction.[85,86] Several investigators have demonstrated that assessment of wall motion abnormalities by two-dimensional echocardiography,[87-89] particularly during or shortly after exercise,[90-92] is valuable in postinfarction risk stratification. It has been reported that echocardiographic imaging before and immediately after treadmill exercise can be accomplished in 85% to 95% of patients.[34] New or worsening wall motion abnormalities identify 63% to 80% of patients who will suffer cardiac events and correctly predict 78% to 95% of those who will not. Multivessel coronary disease may be detected using exercise echocardiography (with a sensitivity of 80% and a specificity of 90%).[34]

Coronary Angiography

Although left ventricular dysfunction is the major determinant of mortality after MI, multivessel coronary disease independently increases the risk of death.[21,93] Prognosis in the first year after MI is directly related to the extent of coronary obstruction, as well as to the degree of left ventricular dysfunction.[21,94] Both can be assessed by contrast angiography. Coronary and left heart angiography by evaluating coronary anatomy and jeopardized myocardium defines patients at risk for complications or premature death who may benefit from revascularization. The importance of early cardiac catheterization and angiography has recently been emphasized by Kulick and Rahimtoola.[95] Patients with clinical evidence of Killip Class III or IV heart failure, hypotension, ongoing myocardial ischemia, malignant arrhythmias, or evidence of mechanical complications are at high risk and should undergo early cardiac catheterization.[96] The possible indications for early coronary angiography after MI include[65,95]:

1. angina with ST depression;
2. non-Q wave infarction (especially anterior);
3. inferior infarction with a positive exercise test; and
4. anterior infarction and an LVEF <30%.

Other Clinical Variables

Clinical variables are readily available from the patient's history and have been shown to provide useful predictive information.[97-99] It has been demonstrated that *ST segment depression* on the admission ECG in patients with acute MI is an independent predictor of mortality in the year following infarction.[100] Patients with resting ECG ST segment depression may have more extensive coronary artery disease.[101] Persistent ST depression is a strong predictor of increased long-term mortality.[102] Approximately one third of patients had *early postinfarction angina*.[24] Early postinfarction angina suggests ongoing ischemia and is associated with an increased risk of further coronary events.[103,104] In general, angina with ECG changes portends a poorer prognosis than angina without these changes. *Recurrent infarction* in the first year has been shown to be a stronger predictor for long-term total mortality (relative risk = 4.76) than angina or ST segment depression during exercise testing.[105] Since myocardial dysfunction is primarily associated with the extent of myocardial damage, examination of *infarct size* may be of importance in postinfarction risk stratification. Determination of the myocardial band fraction of serum creatine phosphokinase (CPK-MB) activity has been used for quantitative assessment of the extent of MI.[106-108] Other techniques, such as myocardial scintigrams with ^{99m}Tc pyrophosphate,

can also be used for assessment of the extent of myocardium involved in the infarct.[109-114]

A prolonged QTc interval has been demonstrated to be associated to increased risk of SCD in patients following acute MI. For example, Schwartz and Wolf[115] demonstrated that QTc was prolonged in patients following MI and a prolonged QTc carried 2.16 times greater risk for SCD. In a larger population of patients with MI, Ahnve et al[116] demonstrated that the QT interval was longer in nonsurvivors. Patients with QT <400 milliseconds had very low mortality (3 of 171 patients, <2%) and 10 of 30 patients with a QTc >400 milliseconds died (33%). Recently there is interest in assessment of QT dynamics and QT dispersion for risk stratification. By examination of the QT/RR relationship, Viñolas et al[117] have demonstrated that postinfarction patients with life-threatening sustained ventricular arrhythmias demonstrated different QT dynamics compared with those without arrhythmias and with normal subjects.

It is thought that QT dispersion may be served as a measure of inhomogeneity of ventricular repolarization. Therefore, it may be of importance in postinfarction risk stratification. It has been shown that QT dispersion increases reversibly during ischemia in patients with chronic coronary artery disease.[118,119] The increase in dispersion contrasts with the decrease seen during exercise in normal subjects.[119,120] QT dispersion measured from recordings made within days of MI is higher in patients who later develop ventricular arrhythmias compared with those who do not. Potratz et al[121] reported that increased QTc dispersion may be useful for postinfarction risk stratification. These authors demonstrated that QTc dispersion ≥85 milliseconds determined on the third day after acute MI is significantly associated with the high prevalence of SCD and arrhythmic events during follow-up (sensitivity = 62%, specificity = 90%, positive predictive value = 42%, and negative predictive value = 89%). However, the predictive value of QT dispersion was not confirmed in the studies of Dritsas et al[122] and

Zareba et al.[123] Two groups[124,125] have demonstrated that QT dispersion on admission may predict primary ventricular fibrillation, and successful thrombolytic therapy may reduce QT dispersion.[125]

Other clinical variables which have been suggested to be associated with a worse prognosis include anterior MI,[126,127] decreased blood pressure,[128] longer QRS duration,[129] hypokalemia,[130] elevated atrial natriuretic peptide,[131,132] and elevated cholesterol concentrations.[133] However, the predictive value of these variables remains to be fully defined.

Assessment of Heart Rate Variability

Recently there has been increased interest in the analysis of HRV for risk stratification. HRV decreases after MI and depressed HRV is associated with a susceptibility to ventricular arrhythmias in animal experimental models.[134] HRV is decreased in patients early after MI (from a few hours to 2 to 3 weeks after acute MI)[135-137] and begins to increase back towards normal levels within a few weeks following MI.[137,138] HRV is maximally recovered by 6 to 12 months after MI,[139] but never attains normal values. HRV recovery occurs within approximately the same time taken for the mortality rate to stabilize.[137]

Heart Rate Variability for Postinfarction Risk Stratification

The predictive value of HRV in patients following MI was first suggested in a brief report by Wolf et al[140] in 1978. However, the predictive significance of HRV was not well recognized until 1987, when Kleiger et al[141] reported that decreased HRV was associated with increased mortality in 808 survivors of acute MI. The authors found that the relative risk of mortality was 5.3 times higher in the group with depressed HRV (standard deviation of normal RR intervals over 24-hour recordings <50 milliseconds)

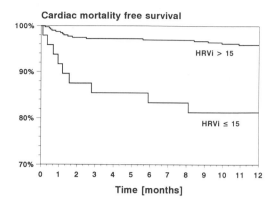

Figure 3. Cumulative Kaplan-Meier survival curves of HRV index (HRVi) for cardiac mortality in patients following myocardial infarction based on the data of the Post-Infarct Survey Program of St. George's Hospital Medical School.

than in the group with preserved HRV. The findings of Kleiger et al were later confirmed and expanded by Farrell et al[142] and Bigger et al.[143,144] Both the short-term (in-hospital) and long-term predictive value of HRV in patients following acute MI has now been well established (Figure 3). There is evidence that there is sometimes an alteration in heart rate (HR) and/or HRV preceding the onset of ventricular tachycardia episodes in patients with and without coronary artery disease. Whether there is a change of HRV immediately before the onset of ventricular fibrillation remains uncertain.[145,146]

Relationship of Heart Rate Variability to Other Risk Factors

HRV may be significantly related to other risk factors, such as age, LVEF, and the angiographic severity of coronary artery disease. As in normal subjects, HRV declines with age in patients who have sustained MI. It has been shown that the relationship between HRV and age is lost in patients with congestive heart failure, which is probably due to the overwhelming influence of severe cardiac dysfunction and/or to differences in the physiological basis underlying HRV in patients with congestive heart failure.[147] Several investigators have demonstrated that HRV is most strongly associated with LVEF in patients following acute MI, as well as in patients with congestive heart failure. However, it seems that there is no significant association between HRV and left ventricular function in normal subjects and in patients without reduced cardiac function.

Patients with anterior MI may have lower HRV than those with inferior MI,[135] but this observation has been questioned by some other investigators. Little is known about the relationship between HRV and the infarct size. A significant relationship between HRV and peak creatine kinase (CPK)- MB has been demonstrated in the early stage of acute MI.[136] HRV tends to be lower in patients with late potentials than in patients with a normal signal-averaged ECG.[148] Whether the difference in HRV in terms of late potentials is related to the patency of the infarct-related artery is not clear. Decreased HRV may correlate with the angiographic severity of coronary artery disease,[149] but this has recently been disputed by Nolan et al.[150] The relationship between HRV and the angiographic severity of coronary artery disease in patients following acute MI remains to be defined. All frequency components of HRV are related to mean HR in normal subjects and in patients with and without cardiac dysfunction. In addition to the autonomic modulation of both HR and HRV, a mathematical relationship between HR and HRV may also be contributory.

Despite the relationship between HRV and the above mentioned clinical variables, the predictive value of depressed HRV is independent of other established prognostic predictors, including other Holter features, signal-averaged ECG and LVEF.[141,151,152] In a study of 416 consecutive survivors of acute MI, the value of HRV, ambulatory ECG and the signal-averaged ECG was assessed before hospital discharge.[142] Impaired HRV, late potentials, frequent and repetitive VPCs, decreased LVEF and Killip class were identified as significant univariate pre-dictors of arrhythmic events. Stepwise Cox regression analysis showed that impaired HRV (followed by late potentials and repetitive ventricular ectopy) was the most powerful independent predictor of arrhythmic events. For prediction of all cause mortality, the value of HRV is similar to that of LVEF, while HRV is superior to LVEF in predicting arrhythmic events (SCD and ventricular tachycardia) (Figures 4A and B).[153]

Singer et al[154] have reported that HRV in inducible SCD survivors was found to be significantly lower than 'asymptomatic VPC' noninducible patients. This observation suggests the potential utility of HRV as a possible noninvasive clinical variable to screen patients for invasive electrophysiological assessment. In contrast, Raymenants et al[155] failed to demonstrate a significant difference of HRV between patients with inducible and noninducible sustained monomorphic ventricular tachycardia, although there was a lower HRV in patients with a history of malignant ventricular tachyarrhythmias compared to those without. However, the data on the relationship between HRV and inducibility during programmed electrical stimulation in patients following acute MI are scarce. Recently Huikuri et al[156] reported that in patients following acute MI the low-frequency (LF) component (particularly the very low-frequency (VLF) component) of HRV is significantly reduced in high-risk (with a history of sustained ventricular tachycardia or cardiac arrest) patients with inducible ventricular tachycardia compared with low-risk (no arrhythmic events) noninducible patients. This suggests that reduced HRV is not only a marker of increased mortality following acute MI, but it may also be involved in the pathogenesis of ventricular arrhythmias in these patients.

Combination of Heart Rate Variability With Other Predictors

The predictive value of HRV alone is modest (predictive accuracy up to 40%).

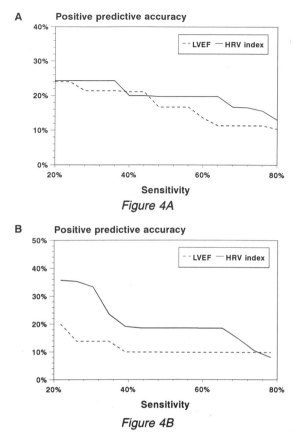

Figures 4A-B. The positive predictive accuracy curves of left ventricular ejection fraction (LVEF) and heart rate variability (HRV) index in patients following myocardial infarction based on the data of the St. George's Post-Infarction Survey Programme. A: for total cardiac mortality. B: for arrhythmic events (sudden cardiac death and sustained ventricular tachycardia).

HRV combined with other risk factors yields a better positive predictive accuracy. Bigger et al[143] have demonstrated that combining HRV with other risk factors (LVEF and VPC) yields a positive predictive accuracy of around 50% (LVEF or VPC alone is 26% and 24%, respectively). Unfortunately, the 95% confidence intervals around the point estimates for positive predictive accuracy are wide. The data on the higher positive predictive accuracy are derived from lower than conventional frequency components (VLF and ultra low-frequency power). The physiological basis underlying these lower frequency components is unclear. Data from our Postinfarction Survey Program at St. George's hospital showed that at 50% sensitivity, LVEF or VPCs has 10% to 20% positive predictive accuracy for ar-

rhythmic events within 1 year after MI. The combination of HRV with other risk factors significantly improves positive predictive accuracy (Figures 5A and B). More recently Bigger et al[157] have reported that short-term (2 to 15 minutes) HRV also provides prognostic information (predictive accuracy 24% to 31%). All the short-term measures of HRV are added to previously established risk factors. The positive predictive accuracy of other established risk predictors (LVEF, New York Heart Association functional Class III and IV, and rales in the coronary care unit greater than bibasilar) is 26% to 33%.[157] Combination of these established risk predictors with the short-term HRV measures, the positive predictive accuracy is significantly improved between 23% and 47%. It is worth noting that the predictive

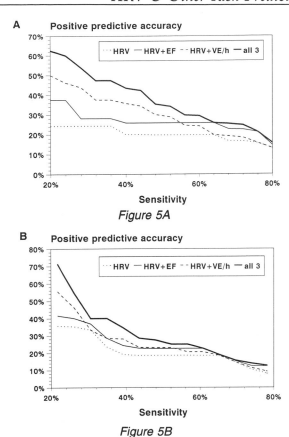

Figures 5A-B. The positive predictive accuracy curves of heart rate variability (HRV) index (HRVi), alone and in combination with left ventricular ejection fraction (EF) and ventricular premature complexes (VPCs), in patients following myocardial infarction based on the data from the St. George's Post-Infarction Survey Programme. A: for total cardiac mortality. B: for arrhythmic events (sudden cardiac death and sustained ventricular tachycardia).

accuracy of HRV measured from the short-term recordings, singly or in combination with other established risk factors, is lower than that derived from 24-hour recordings.

Pedretti et al[152] reported a combined use of invasive and noninvasive methods for postinfarction risk stratification in 303 patients of whom 19 died over a 15-month follow-up. Left ventricular dysfunction, late potentials and prolonged filtered QRS duration, frequent (>6 beats/hour) and complex (paired or ≥2 runs) VPCs, mean HR and HRV were all univariate predictors of late arrhythmic events. Multivariate analysis showed that only low LVEF, prolonged QRS duration, reduced HRV and the presence of ≥2 runs of nonsustained ventricular tachycardia remained as independent risk predictors. The authors also demonstrated that noninvasive risk factors may be used for selecting a sufficiently high-risk group of patients for invasive electrophysiological evaluation. A positive electrophysiological study is found to be the strongest independent predictor with an 81% sensitivity for arrhythmic events in patients preselected by noninvasive testing. Unfortunately, HRV is not included in the preselection criteria in this study. Nonetheless, assessment of HRV, singly or in combination with other established risk factors, provides a new powerful method for stratifying patients following MI into low- and high-risk groups. The identified high-risk patients may then undergo further invasive evaluation and/or aggressive management.

Table 4
Clinical Application of Holter Monitoring in Postinfarction Risk Stratification

1. Assessment of cardiac arrhythmias (including bradycardias)
2. Assessment of HRV
3. Assessment of ST segment alterations
4. Assessment of QT intervals and its relationship to RR intervals
5. Assessment of late potentials

Ahmed et al[158] have demonstrated that in SCD survivors the survival curves for inducibility by programmed electrical stimulation and depressed HRV are comparable for up to 8 years follow-up. Combination of the electrophysiological and autonomic assessments correctly identified all patients who died.

It has been shown that exercise elicited a greater reduction in the high-frequency component of HRV in animals susceptible to ventricular fibrillation.[159] This may be of clinical importance since exercise-induced autonomic and metabolic changes may contribute to the pathogenesis of ventricular arrhythmias and SCD. However, this observation has not yet been verified in patients following acute MI. There are no data on the tilt- or exercise-induced changes in HRV for risk stratification in patients following acute MI. Further studies should be aimed at improving our understanding about effect of pharmacological (particularly autonomic agents) and nonpharmacological interventions (such as exercise) on HRV and their value for postinfarction risk stratification and treatment.

Ambulatory electrocardiographic (Holter) monitoring has gained widespread application in clinical practice since it was introduced in 1961.[160] Assessment of HRV has expanded its clinical significance. This noninvasive technique has played an important role in postinfarction risk stratification. The clinical application of Holter monitoring in postinfarction risk stratification is summarized in Table 4. Combined analysis of these variables from the ambulatory ECG may be cost-effective making this noninvasive technique important in postinfarction risk stratification.

Baroreflex Sensitivity and Heart Rate Variability

BRS is decreased in patients following MI, and a severely depressed BRS identifies a subgroup at higher risk of arrhythmic events.[161-163] Unlike HRV, BRS before and after an acute MI was shown in animal experiments to predict the susceptibility to development of ventricular fibrillation during an induced ischemic episode.[164] It has been reported that BRS testing can be safely performed 7 to 10 days after acute MI.[163] Farrell et al[162] have demonstrated that BRS (expressed as the slope of the regression line of increase in beat-to-beat RR interval against the increase in the preceding systolic arterial pressure induced by phenylephrine) is significantly reduced in patients in whom sustained monomorphic ventricular tachycardia was inducible by programmed electrical stimulation. The authors concluded that programmed electrical stimulation might be appropriately limited to patients with depressed BRS without loss of predictive accuracy. During 1-year follow-up in 122 patients following acute MI, Farrell et al[163] demonstrated that depressed BRS was a strong predictor of arrhythmic events (relative risk: 23.1).

The baroreceptor reflex plays an important role in the modulation of HR. Bigger et al[165] have reported that there is a weak ($\tau = 0.57 - 0.63$) but significant correlation between BRS and HRV. However, no significant relationship between BRS and HRV was found in the study by Farrell et al.[162] These observations suggest that HRV and BRS may reflect different aspects of autonomic activity ('tonic' and 'phasic,' respectively). A close relationship between BRS and cardiac vagal tone (defined by the change in RR interval after complete cholinergic blockade by atropine) has been demonstrated.[166] Nonetheless, impaired autonomic activity, measured by either decreased HRV or depressed BRS, is significantly associated with an increased incidence of arrhythmic events in patients following MI during 1-year follow-up.[163] Assessment of autonomic activity has provided a powerful new method for risk stratification after MI.

Although depressed LVEF (<40%) is a powerful predictor of postinfarction mortality, approximately two thirds of the 1-year mortality predicted by LVEF is non-sudden in nature. Thus depressed LVEF leads to predict death due to pump failure rather than arrhythmic death. On the other hand, depressed BRS accurately predicts arrhythmic events, predominantly sustained ventricular tachyarrhythmias, to a lesser extent SCD, and to only a small degree pump failure deaths. Usually left ventricular function is not impaired prior to MI, but a depressed BRS is present prior to MI according to experiments with a canine model which are able to distinguish between dogs vulnerable and resistant to SCD after MI. HRV is depressed because of at least two major perturbations: poor left ventricular function and its consequences, and depressed cardiovascular reflexes, particularly baroreceptor reflexes. It is not surprising, therefore, that depressed HRV predicts death due to pump failure, SCD and arrhythmic events (Figure 6).

In summary, the predictive value of HRV is independent of other parameters established for postinfarction risk stratification, such as LVEF, VPCs and late potentials. For prediction of all cause mortality, the value of HRV is similar to that of LVEF. While HRV is superior to LVEF in predicting arrhythmic events. Combination with other techniques improves the positive predictive accuracy of HRV over a clinically important range of sensitivity (25% to 75%) for cardiac mortality and arrhythmic events. For example, at 50% sensitivity, LVEF or

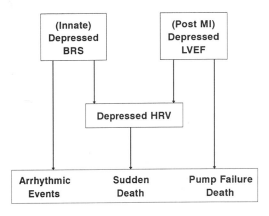

Figure 6. Contribution of unbalanced autonomic activity and depressed mechanical function of the heart to the development of arrhythmic events and cardiac death. BRS: baroreflex sensitivity; HRV: heart rate variability; MI: myocardial infarction; LVEF: left ventricular ejection fraction.

VPCs 10% to 20% positive predictive accuracy for arrhythmic events within 1 year after MI. HRV alone or combined with LVEF or VPCs provides 20% to 30% positive predictive accuracy. Current observations suggest that depressed HRV may not only be a marker of increased mortality, but may also be involved in the pathogenesis of ventricular arrhythmias and SCD. A more important observation in the field of HRV and BRS will evolve from a large ongoing multicenter trial, ATRAMI (Autonomic Tone and Reflexes in Acute Myocardial Infarction), involving multiple centers in Europe, Asia and North America and investigating the predictive value of HRV, BRS and their combination following MI.

Postinfarction Risk Stratification in Thrombolytic Era

Prognosis following acute MI has changed since the introduction of interventional and thrombolytic therapies.[167-169] Such interactions also complicate the interpretation of established methods of risk assessment.[167,170] For example, additional ST segment elevation early during thrombolytic therapy in patients with anterior infarction may suggest a more favorable clinical outcome.[171] McCallister et al[167] have reported that patients with a large MI (more than 40% of the left ventricle) can survive without heart failure. The Gruppo Italiano per lo Studio della Sopravvivenza nell' Infarto Miocardio (GISSI)-2 trial data base[170] shows that there is a 24% reduction in 6-month mortality in survivors of acute MI after thrombolysis. In GISSI-2, the 6-month mortality predictors identified by the Cox model include ineligibility for exercise (relative risk = 3.30), early left ventricular failure (relative risk = 2.41), echocardiographic evidence of recovery phase left ventricular dysfunction (relative risk = 2.41), advanced age (relative risk = 1.81), frequent and/or complex ventricular arrhythmias (relative risk = 1.70), late left ventricular failure (relative risk = 1.54), previous MI (relative risk = 1.47) and a history of treated hypertension (relative risk = 1.32). Early post-MI angina, a positive exercise test, female gender, a history of angina, a history of insulin-dependent diabetes, and anterior site of MI were not identified as risk factors. The lack of an independent adverse influence of early postinfarction angina on 6-month survival represents a major difference between this study and those in the prethrombolytic era. However, it has been reported that thrombolytic therapy may not significantly influence long-term prognosis.[172] Similarly, when data were analyzed for mortality at 5 weeks after trial entry, the second International Study of Infarct Survival (ISIS-2) investigators[168] observed that the 8,592 patients assigned to streptokinase treatment experienced 786 (9.1%) cardiovascular deaths compared with 1,016 such deaths (11.8%) in 8,595 patients assigned to receive placebo, a 23% reduction (p <0.00001). These observations suggest that the value of established predictors of prognosis is altered by thrombolytic therapy.[170,173] The postinfarction risk stratification techniques continue to evolve. Further studies should be aimed at improving our understanding of the underlying risk mechanisms following acute MI. This understanding is of fundamental importance since the purpose of postinfarction risk stratification is to decrease the subsequent mortality rate.

HRV has been shown to be correlated with the patency of the infarct related artery.[174] It has been reported that recombinant tissue-type plasminogen activator (rt-PA) may increase HRV.[136] Zabel et al[175] recently reported that thrombolysis-induced reperfusion of the infarct-related artery results in higher vagal tone (assessed by pNN50, the proportion of RR intervals 50 milliseconds greater than the preceding RR interval) during early thrombolytic therapy. This increase in vagal tone is unrelated to infarct location, but it is associated with a trend toward a lower incidence of ventricular fibrillation during the acute phase of acute MI. However, these observations remain to be further investigated since there were no proper controls in this study.

Future Perspective

Many retrospective studies have now conclusively demonstrated that HRV is a powerful predictor of postinfarction mortality, SCD and arrhythmic events. However, no study has prospectively assigned precise dichotomy limits and established the sensitivity, specificity and predictive accuracy of an abnormal HRV for the prediction of subsequent events. The forthcoming ATRAMI study (see above) will accomplish this objective. Presently it appears that depressed HRV is superior to depressed LVEF in its ability to predict postinfarction arrhythmic events and SCD. It is at least as good as LVEF in predicting all cause mortality. If this is confirmed by the results of the ATRAMI study, it will be appropriate to test antiarrhythmic therapy in mortality studies in which a high risk test population is selected because of the presence of depressed HRV (and/or BRS). In such a study, patients with very depressed left ventricular function (say LVEF ≤20%) could be excluded from the study on the basis that such patients die predominantly from pump failure or from severe bradyarrhythmias, neither of which would be expected to benefit from antiarrhythmic therapy such as Class III drugs or an implantable cardioverter defibrillator.

References

1. Marcus FI, Cobb LA, Edwards JE, et al. Mechanism of death and prevalence of myocardial ischemic symptoms in the terminal event after acute myocardial infarction. Am J Cardiol 1988; 61:8-15.
2. Hinkle LE Jr, Thaler HT. Clinical classification of cardiac death. Circulation 1982; 65:457-464.
3. Echt DS, Liebson PR, Mitchell LB, et al. Mortality and morbidity in patients receiving encainide, flecainide, or placebo. The Cardiac Arrhythmia Suppression Trial (CAST). N Engl J Med 1991; 324:781-788.
4. Kuchar DL, Thorburn CW, Sammel NL. Prediction of serious arrhythmic events after myocardial infarction: signal-averaged electrocardiogram, Holter monitoring and radionuclide ventriculography. J Am Coll Cardiol 1987; 9:531-538.
5. Gomes JA, Winters SL, Stewart D, et al. A new noninvasive index to predict sustained ventricular tachycardia and sudden death in the first year after myocardial infarction: based on signal-averaged electrocardiogram, radionuclide ejection fraction and Holter monitoring. J Am Coll Cardiol 1987; 10:349-357.
6. Denniss AR, Richards DA, Cody DV, et al. Prognostic significance of ventricular tachycardia and fibrillation induced at programmed stimulation and delayed potentials detected on the signal-averaged electrocardiograms of survivors of acute myocardial infarction. Circulation 1986; 74:731-745.
7. Steinberg JS, Regan A, Sciacca RR, et al. Predicting arrhythmic events after acute myocardial infarction using the signal-averaged electrocardiogram. Am J Cardiol 1992; 69:13-21.
8. Turitto G, Fontaine JM, Ursell S, et al. Risk stratification and management of patients with organic heart disease and nonsustained ventricular tachycardia: role of programmed stimulation, left ventricular ejection fraction, and signal-averaged electrocardiogram. Am J Med 1990; 88: 35N-41N.
9. Buxton AE, Simson MB, Falcone RA, et al. Results of signal-averaged electrocardiography and electrophysiologic study in patients with nonsustained ventricular tachycardia after healing of acute myocardial infarction. Am J Cardiol 1987; 60:80-85.
10. Turitto G, Fontaine JM, Ursell SN, et al. Value of the signal-averaged electrocardiogram as a predictor of the results of programmed stimulation in nonsustained ventricular tachycardia. Am J Cardiol 1988; 61:1272-1278.
11. Martinez-Rubio A, Shenasa M, Borggrefe M, et al. Electrophysiologic variables characterizing the induction of ventricular tachycardia versus ventricular fibrillation after myocardial infarction: relation between ventricular late potentials and coupling intervals for the induction of sustained ventricular tachyarrhythmias. J Am Coll Cardiol 1993; 21:1624-1631.
12. Kuchar DL, Thorburn CW, Sammel NL. Late potentials detected after myocardial infarction: natural history and prognostic significance. Circulation 1986; 74:1280-1289.
13. Kuchar DL, Thorburn CW, Sammel NL. Prognostic implications of loss of late potentials following acute myocardial infarction. PACE 1993; 16:2104-2111.
14. Ohnishi Y, Inoue T, Miwa S, et al. Determinants of late potentials in myocardial infarction. Jpn Circ J 1989; 53:1192-1198.
15. El-Sherif N, Ursell SN, Bekheit S, et al. Prognostic significance of the signal-averaged ECG depends on the time of recording in the postinfarction period. Am Heart J 1989; 118:256-264.
16. Denniss AR, Ross DL, Richards DA, et al. Effect of antiarrhythmic therapy on delayed potentials detected by the signal-averaged electrocardiogram in patients with ventricular tachycardia after acute myocardial infarction. Am J Cardiol 1986; 58:261-265.
17. Borbola J, Denes P. Oral amiodarone loading therapy. I. The effect on serial signal-averaged electrocardiographic recordings and the QTc in patients with ventricular tachyarrhythmias. Am Heart J 1988; 115:1202-1208.
18. Wechsler ME, Steinberg JS, Giardina EG. Time course of morcizine's effect on signal-averaged and 12-lead electrocardiograms: insights into mechanism of action. J Am Coll Cardiol 1991; 17:1626-1633.
19. Kelen G, Henkin R, Lannon M, et al. Correlation between the signal-averaged electrocardiogram from Holter tapes and from real-time recordings. Am J Cardiol 1989; 63:1321-1325.
20. Kennedy HL, Bavishi NS, Buckingham TA. Ambulatory (Holter) electrocardiography signal-averaging: a current perspective. Am Heart J 1992; 124:1339-1346.

21. Sanz G, Castaner A, Betriu A, et al. Determinants of prognosis in survivors of myocardial infarction: a prospective clinical angiographic study. N Engl J Med 1982; 306:1065-1070.

22. Norris RM, Caughey DE, Deeming LW, et al. Coronary prognostic index for predicting survival after recovery from acute myocardial infarction. Lancet 1970; 2(671):485-487.

23. Nicod P, Gilpin E, Dittrich H, et al. Influence on prognosis and morbidity of left ventricular ejection fraction with and without signs of left ventricular failure after acute myocardial infarction. Am J Cardiol 1988; 61:1165-1171.

24. The Multicenter Postinfarction Research Group. Risk stratification and survival after myocardial infarction. N Engl J Med 1983; 309:331-336.

25. Madsen EB, Gilpin E, Henning H. Evaluation of prognosis one year after myocardial infarction. J Am Coll Cardiol 1983; 1:985-993.

26. Arnold AE, Simoons ML, van de Werf F, et al. Recombinant tissue-type plasminogen activator and immediate angioplasty in acute myocardial infarction. One-year follow-up. Circulation 1992; 86:111-120.

27. Mukharji J, Rude RE, Poole WK, et al. Risk factors for sudden death after acute myocardial infarction: two-year follow-up. Am J Cardiol 1984; 54:31-36.

28. Schulze RA Jr, Strauss HW, Pitt B. Sudden death in the year following myocardial infarction. Relation to ventricular premature contractions in the late hospital phase and left ventricular ejection function. Am J Med 1977; 62:192-199.

29. Ahnve S, Gilpin E, Henning H, et al. Limitations and advantages of the ejection fraction for defining high risk after acute myocardial infarction. Am J Cardiol 1986; 58:872-878.

30. McClements BM, Adgey AA. Value of signal-averaged electrocardiography, radionuclide ventriculography, Holter monitoring and clinical variables for prediction of arrhythmic events in survivors of acute myocardial infarction in the thrombolytic era. J Am Coll Cardiol 1993; 21:1419-1427.

31. Hammill SC, Trusty JM, Wood DL, et al. Influence of ventricular function and presence or absence of coronary artery disease on results of electrophysiologic testing for asymptomatic nonsustained ventricular tachycardia. Am J Cardiol 1990; 65:722-728.

32. Bigger JT Jr, Fleiss JL, Kleiger R, et al. The relationships among ventricular arrhythmias, left ventricular dysfunction, and mortality in the 2 years after myocardial infarction. Circulation 1984; 69:250-258.

33. McGhie AI, Willerson JT, Corbett JR. Radionuclide assessment of ventricular function and risk stratification after myocardial infarction. Circulation 1991; 84:I167-176.

34. Crawford MH. Risk stratification after myocardial infarction with exercise and Doppler echocardiography. Circulation 1991; 84:I163-166.

35. Hung J, Goris ML, Nash E, et al. Comparative value of maximal treadmill testing, exercise thallium myocardial perfusion scintigraphy and exercise radionuclide ventriculography for distinguishing high- and low-risk patients after acute myocardial infarction. Am J Cardiol 1984; 53:1221-1227.

36. Roy D, Marchand E, Theroux P, et al. Programmed ventricular stimulation in survivors of an acute myocardial infarction. Circulation 1985; 72:487-494.

37. Hamer A, Vohra J, Hunt D, et al. Prediction of sudden death by electrophysiologic studies in high risk patients surviving acute myocardial infarction. Am J Cardiol 1982; 50:223-229.

38. Richards DA, Cody DV, Denniss AR, et al. Ventricular electrical instability: a predictor of death after myocardial infarction. Am J Cardiol 1983; 51:75-80.

39. Cripps T, Bennett ED, Camm AJ, et al. Inducibility of sustained monomorphic ventricular tachycardia as a prognostic indicator in survivors of recent myocardial infarction: a prospective evaluation in relation to other prognostic variables. J Am Coll Cardiol 1989; 14:289-296.

40. Iesaka Y, Nogami A, Aonuma K, et al. Prognostic significance of sustained monomorphic ventricular tachycardia induced by programmed ventricular stimulation using up to triple extrastimuli in survivors of acute myocardial infarction. Am J Cardiol 1990; 65:1057-1063.

41. Kersschot IE, Brugada P, Ramentol M, et al. Effects of early reperfusion in acute myocardial infarction on arrhythmias induced by programmed stimulation: a prospective, randomized study. J Am Coll Cardiol 1986; 7:1234-1242.

42. Bourke JP, Young AA, Richards DA, et al. Reduction in incidence of inducible ventricular tachycardia after myocardial infarction by treatment with streptokinase during infarct evolution. J Am Coll Cardiol 1990; 16:1703-1710.

43. Josephson ME. Clinical Cardiac Electrophysiology. Techniques and Interpretations. Philadelphia, Pa: Lea & Febiger, 1993; 616-629.

44. Gang ES, Bigger JT Jr, Livelli FD Jr. A model of chronic ischemic arrhythmias: the relation between electrically inducible ventricular tachycardia, ventricular fibrillation threshold and myocardial infarct size. Am J Cardiol 1982; 50:469-477.

45. Klein H, Trappe HJ, Hartwig CA, et al. Repeated programmed stimulation within the first year after myocardial infarction. Circulation 1985; 72:(III)359. Abstract.

46. Kuck KH, Costard A, Schlüter M, et al. Significance of timing programmed electrical stimulation after acute myocardial infarction. J Am Coll Cardiol 1986; 8:1279-1288.

47. Bhandari AK, Widerhorn J, Sager PT, et al. Prognostic significance of programmed ventricular stimulation in patients surviving complicated acute myocardial infarction: a prospective study. Am Heart J 1992; 124:87-96.

48. Marchlinski FE, Buxton AE, Waxman HL, et al. Identifying patients at risk of sudden death after myocardial infarction: value of the response to programmed stimulation, degree of ventricular ectopic activity and severity of left ventricular dysfunction. Am J Cardiol 1983; 52:1190-1196.

49. Dhingra RC. Electrophysiologic studies during acute myocardial infarction: do they prognosticate? J Am Coll Cardiol 1991; 18:789-791.

50. Bourke JP, Richards DA, Ross DL, et al. Routine programmed electrical stimulation in survivors of acute myocardial infarction for prediction of spontaneous ventricular tachyarrhythmias during follow-up: results, optimal stimulation protocol and cost-effective screening. J Am Coll Cardiol 1991; 18:780-788.

51. Rae AP, Greenspan AM, Spielman SR, et al. Antiarrhythmic drug efficacy for ventricular tachyarrhythmias associated with coronary artery disease as assessed by electrophysiologic studies. Am J Cardiol 1985; 55:1494-1499.

52. Denniss AR, Ross DL, Cody DV, et al. Randomized controlled trial of prophylactic antiarrhythmic therapy in patients with inducible ventricular tachyarrhythmias after recent myocardial infarction. Eur Heart J 1988; 9:746-757.

53. Santarelli P, Bellocci F, Loperfido F, et al. Ventricular arrhythmia induced by programmed ventricular stimulation after acute myocardial infarction. Am J Cardiol 1985; 55:391-394.

54. Costard A, Schluter M, Kunze KP, et al. Programmed electric stimulation following acute myocardial infarction. Significance of stimulation timing. Z Kardiol 1986; 75:589-597.

55. Bhandari AK, Au PK, Ross JS, et al. Decline in inducibility of sustained ventricular tachycardia from two to twenty weeks after acute myocardial infarction. Am J Cardiol 1987; 59:284-290.

56. Nogami A, Aonuma K, Takahashi A, et al. Usefulness of early versus late programmed ventricular stimulation in acute myocardial infarction. Am J Cardiol 1991; 68:13-20.

57. Rosenthal ME, Oseran DS, Gang E, et al. Sudden cardiac death following acute myocardial infarction. Am Heart J 1985; 109:865-876.

58. Kleiger RE, Miller JP, Thanavaro S, et al. Relationship between clinical features of acute myocardial infarction and ventricular runs two weeks to one year following infarction. Circulation 1981; 63:64-70.

59. Lichstein E, Morganroth J, Harrist R, et al. Effect of propranolol on ventricular arrhythmia. The beta-blocker heart attack trial experience. Circulation 1983; 67:I5-10.

60. Bigger JT Jr, Weld FM. Analysis of prognostic significance of ventricular arrhythmias after myocardial infarction. Shortcomings of Lown grading system. Br Heart J 1981; 45:717-724.

61. Bigger JT Jr, Fleiss JL, Rolnitzky LM. Prevalence, characteristics and significance of ventricular tachycardia detected by 24-hour continuous electrocardiographic recordings in the late hospital phase of acute myocardial infarction. Am J Cardiol 1986; 58:1151-1160.

62. Hindman MC, Wagner GS, JaRo M, et al. The clinical significance of bundle branch block complicating acute myocardial infarction. I. Clinical characteristics, hospital mortality, and one-year follow-up. Circulation 1978; 58:679-688.

63. Yano K, Grove JS, Reed DM, et al. Determinants of the prognosis after first myocardial infarction in a migrant Japanese population. The Honolulu Heart Program. Circulation 1993; 88:2582-2595.

64. Hodges M, Denes P, Morris M, et al. Ventricular arrhythmias and mortality after myocardial infarction: a follow-up study of 14,534 patients in the CAST Holter registry. J Am Coll Cardiol 1994; 23:296A.

65. Moss AJ, Bigger JT Jr, Odoroff CL. Postinfarct risk stratification. Prog Cardiovasc Dis 1987; 29:389-412.

66. Solomon SD, Ridker PM, Antman EM. Ventricular arrhythmias in trials of thrombolytic therapy for acute myocardial infarction. A meta-analysis. Circulation 1993; 88:2575-2581.

67. Schulze RA Jr, Rouleau J, Rigo P, et al. Ventricular arrhythmias in the late hospital phase of acute myocardial infarction. Relation to left ventricular function detected by gated cardiac blood pool scanning. Circulation 1975; 52:1006-1011.

68. Braat SH, de Zwaan C, Brugada P, et al. Value of left ventricular ejection fraction in extensive anterior infarction to predict development of ventricular tachycardia. Am J Cardiol 1983; 52:686-689.

69. Kostis JB, Byington R, Friedman LM, et al. Prognostic significance of ventricular ectopic activity in survivors of acute myocardial infarction. J Am Coll Cardiol 1987; 10:231-242.

70. Hallstrom AP, Bigger JT Jr, Roden D, et al. Prognostic significance of ventricular premature depolarizations measured 1 year after myocardial infarction in patients with early postinfarction asymptomatic ventricular arrhythmia. J Am Coll Cardiol 1992; 20:259-264.

71. Bluzhas J, Lukshiene D, Shlapikiene B, et al. Relation between ventricular arrhythmia and sudden cardiac death in patients with acute myocardial infarction: the predictors of ventricular fibrillation. J Am Coll Cardiol 1986; 8:69A-72A.

72. The Cardiac Arrhythmia Suppression Trial (CAST) Investigators. Preliminary report: effect of encainide and flecainide on mortality in a randomized trial of arrhythmia suppression after myocardial infarction. N Engl J Med 1989; 321:406-412.

73. Sami M, Kraemer H, DeBusk RF. The prognostic significance of serial exercise testing after myocardial infarction. Circulation 1979; 60:1238-1246.

74. Waters DD, Bosch X, Bouchard A, et al. Comparison of clinical variables and variables derived from a limited predischarge exercise test as predictors of early and late mortality after myocardial infarction. J Am Coll Cardiol 1985; 5:1-8.

75. Theroux P, Waters DD, Halphen C, et al. Prognostic value of exercise testing soon after myocardial infarction. N Engl J Med 1979; 301:341-345.

76. Krone RJ, Gillespie JA, Weld FM, et al. Low-level exercise testing after myocardial infarction: usefulness in enhancing clinical risk stratification. Circulation 1985; 71:80-89.

77. Bach DS, Armstrong WF. Dobutamine stress echocardiography. Am J Cardiol 1992; 69:90H-96H.

78. Stevenson R, Umachandran V, Ranjadayalan K, et al. Reassessment of treadmill stress testing for risk stratification in patients with acute myocardial infarction treated by thrombolysis. Br Heart J 1993; 70:415-420.

79. Gibson RS, Watson DD. Value of planar[201] Tl imaging in risk stratification of patients recovering from acute myocardial infarction. Circulation 1991; 84:I148-162.

80. Langer A, Minkowitz J, Dorian P, et al. Pathophysiology and prognostic significance of Holter-detected ST segment depression after myocardial infarction. J Am Coll Cardiol 1992; 20:1313-1317.

81. Bolognese L, Rossi L, Sarasso G, et al. Silent versus symptomatic dipyridamole-induced ischemia after myocardial infarction: clinical and prognostic significance. J Am Coll Cardiol 1992; 19:953-959.

82. Shimonagata T, Nishimura T, Uehara T, et al. Prognostic significance of scintigraphic silent myocardial ischemia detected by stress thallium scan in patients with recent myocardial infarction. Kaku Igaku 1991; 28:455-460.

83. Gill JB, Cairns JA, Roberts R, et al. Silent ischemia in survivors of acute myocardial infarction (SISAMI Study). Superior prognostic value of Holter monitoring early post myocardial infarction. Circulation 1993; 88:I-258. Abstract.

84. Jereczek M, Andersen D, Schröder J, et al. Prognostic value of ischemia during Holter monitoring and exercise after acute myocardial infarction. Am J Cardiol 1993; 72:8-13.

85. Kinney EL, Wright RJ. Echocardiographic score versus wall index for risk stratification after acute myocardial infarction. Angiology 1990; 41:112-117.

86. Launbjerg J, Berning J, Fruergaard P, et al. Sensitivity and specificity of echocardiographic identification of patients eligible for safe early discharge after acute myocardial infarction. Am Heart J 1992; 124:846-853.87. Gibson RS, Bishop HL, Stamm RB, et al. Value of early two-dimensional echocardiography in patients with acute myocardial infarction. Am J Cardiol 1982; 49:1110-1119.

88. Nishimura RA, Tajik AJ, Shub C, et al. Role of two-dimensional echocardiography in the prediction of in-hospital complications after acute myocardial infarction. J Am Coll Cardiol 1984; 4:1080-1087.

89. Shen WF, Cui LQ, Wang MH, et al. Spontaneous alterations in left ventricular regional wall motion after acute myocardial infarction. Chin Med J (Engl) 1990; 103:1015-1018.

90. Jaarsma W, Visser CA, Kupper AJ, et al. Usefulness of two-dimensional exercise echocardiography shortly after myocardial infarction. Am J Cardiol 1986; 57:86-90.

91. Ryan T, Armstrong WF, O'Donnell JA, et al. Risk stratification after acute myocardial infarction by means of exercise two-dimensional echocardiography. Am Heart J 1987; 114:1305-1316.

92. Applegate RJ, Dell'Italia LJ, Crawford MH. Usefulness of two-dimensional echocardiography during low-level exercise testing early after uncomplicated acute myocardial infarction. Am J Cardiol 1987; 60:10-14.

93. Muller DW, Topol EJ, Ellis SG, et al. Multivessel coronary artery disease: a key predictor of short-term prognosis after reperfusion therapy for acute myocardial infarction. Thrombolysis and Angioplasty in Myocardial Infarction (TAMl) Study Group. Am Heart J 1991; 121:1042-1049.

94. Taylor GJ, Humphries JO, Mellits ED, et al. Predictors of clinical course, coronary anatomy and left ventricular function after recovery from acute myocardial infarction. Circulation 1980; 62:960-969.

95. Kulick DL, Rahimtoola SH. Risk stratification in survivors of acute myocardial infarction: routine cardiac catheterization and angiography is a reasonable approach in most patients. Am Heart J 1991; 121:641-656.

96. Johnson TS, Wenger NK. Risk stratification after myocardial infarction. Curr Opin Cardiol 1993; 8:621-628.

97. Brugada P, Talajic M, Smeets J, et al. The value of the clinical history to assess prognosis of patients with ventricular tachycardia or ventricular fibrillation after myocardial infarction. Eur Heart J 1989; 10:747-752.

98. Steurer G, Brugada J, De Bacquer D, et al. Value of clinical variables for risk stratification in patients with sustained ventricular tachycardia and history of myocardial infarction. Am J Cardiol 1993; 72:349-351.

99. Pfisterer M, Salamin P, Schwendener R, et al. Clinical risk assessment after first myocardial infarction: is additional noninvasive testing necessary? Chest 1992; 102:1499-1506.

100. Krone RJ, Greenberg H, Dwyer EM, et al. Long-term prognostic significance of ST segment depression during acute myocardial infarction. J Am Coll Cardiol 1993; 22:361-367.

101. Miranda CP, Lehmann KG, Froelicher VF. Correlation between resting ST segment depression, exercise testing, coronary angiography, and long term prognosis. Am Heart J 1991; 122:1617-1628.

102. Gheorghiade M, Shivkumar K, Schultz L, et al. Prognostic significance of electrocardiographic persistent ST depression in patients with their first myocardial infarction in the placebo arm of the Beta-Blocker Heart Attack Trial. Am Heart J 1993; 126:271-278.

103. Dwyer EM Jr, McMaster P, Greenberg H. Nonfatal cardiac events and recurrent infarction in the year after acute myocardial infarction. J Am Coll Cardiol 1984; 4:695-702.

104. Bosch X, Theroux P, Pelletier GB, et al. Clinical and angiographic features and prognostic significance of early postinfarction angina with and without electrocardiographic signs of transient ischemia. Am J Med 1991; 91:493-501.

105. Kornowski R, Goldbout U, Zion M, et al. Predictors and long-term prognostic significance of recurrent infarction in the year after a first myocardial infarction. Am J Cardiol 1993; 72:883-888.

106. Roberts R, Henry PD, Sobel BE. An improved basis for enzymatic estimation of infarct size. Circulation 1975; 52:743-754.

107. Geltman EM, Ehsani AA, Campbell MK, et al. The influence of location and extent of myocardial infarction on long-term ventricular dysrhythmia and mortality. Circulation 1979; 60:805-814.

108. Hands ME, Lloyd BL, Robinson JS, et al. Prognostic significance of electrocardiographic site of infarction after correction for enzymatic size of infraction. Circulation 1986; 73:885-891.

109. Holman BL, Chisholm RJ, Braunwald E. The prognostic implications of acute myocardial infarct scintigraphy with ^{99m}Tc pyrophosphate. Circulation 1978; 57:320-326.

110. Schelbert HR, Henze E, Keen R, et al. C^{-11} palmitate for the noninvasive evaluation of regional myocardial fatty acid metabolism with positron-computed tomography. IV. In vivo evaluation of acute demand-induced ischemia in dogs. Am Heart J 1983; 106:736-750.

111. Gibbons RJ. Perfusion imaging with ^{99m}Tc-sestamibi for the assessment of myocardial area at risk and the efficacy of acute treatment in myocardial infarction. Circulation 1991; 84:I37-42.

112. Schelbert HR. Positron emission tomography for the assessment of myocardial viability. Circulation 1991; 84:I122-131.

113. Okada RD, Glover DK, Leppo JA. Dipyridamole ^{201}Tl scintigraphy in the evaluation of prognosis after myocardial infarction. Circulation 1991; 84:I132-139.

114. Cerqueira MD, Maynard C, Ritchie JL. Radionuclide assessment of infarct size and left ventricular function in clinical trials of thrombolysis. Circulation 1991; 84:I100-108.

115. Schwartz PJ, Wolf S. QT interval prolongation as predictor of sudden death in patients

with myocardial infarction. Circulation 1978; 57:1074-1077.

116. Ahnve S, Gilpin E, Madsen EB, et al. Prognostic importance of QTc interval at discharge after acute myocardial infarction: a multicenter study of 865 patients. Am Heart J 1984; 108:395-400.

117. Viñolas X, Homs E, Martí V, et al. QT/RR relationship in postmyocardial infarction patients with and without life-threatening ventricular arrhythmias. J Am Coll Cardiol 1993; 21:94A. Abstract.

118. Lee HS, Cross SJ, Rawles J, et al. QTc dispersion in patients with coronary artery disease—effect of exercise, dobutamine and dipyridamole myocardial stress. Eur Heart J 1993; 14:210. Abstract.

119. Perkiomaki, Koistinen J, Linnaluoto M, et al. Dispersion of QT-interval at rest and during exercise in healthy subjects and patients with coronary artery disease. Eur Heart J 1993; 14:254. Abstract.

120. Fu Z, Timothy K, Fox J, et al. Beta-blockers markedly affect QT dispersion during exercise in long QT syndrome patients. J Am Coll Cardiol 1993; 21:93A. Abstract.

121. Potratz J, Djonlagic H, Brandes A, et al. Prognostic significance of the QT-dispersion in patients with acute myocardial infarction. Circulation 1993; 88:I-307. Abstract.

122. Dritsas A, Sbarouni P, Nihoyannopoulos P, et al. Relation of QTc interval and QTc dispersion to ventricular arrhythmia in patients with previous myocardial infarction. Eur Heart J 1992; 13:344. Abstract.

123. Zareba W, Moss AJ, le Cessie S. Dispersion of ventricular repolarization and sudden cardiac death in ischemic heart disease. J Am Coll Cardiol 1994; 23:148A. Abstract.

124. Yunus A, Gillis A, Duff H, et al. Precordial QTc interval dispersion as a predictor of ventricular fibrillation in acute myocardial infarction. PACE 1994; 17:752.

125. van de Loo A, Klingenheben T, Zabel M, et al. Changes in QT dispersion after acute myocardial infarction: relation to success of thrombolysis and to the occurrence of ventricular fibrillation. PACE 1994; 17:752.

126. Stone PH, Raabe DS, Jaffe AS, et al. Prognostic significance of location and type of myocardial infarction: independent adverse outcome associated with anterior location. J Am Coll Cardiol 1988; 11:453-463.

127. Benhorin J, Moss AJ, Oakes D, et al. The prognostic significance of first myocardial infarction type (Q wave versus non-Q wave) and Q wave location. J Am Coll Cardiol 1990; 15:1201-1207.

128. The Coronary Drug Project Research Group. Blood pressure in survivors of myocardial infarction. J Am Coll Cardiol 1984; 4:1135-1147.

129. Zareba W, Moss AJ, le Cessie S. QRS duration as independent electrocardiographic predictor of cardiac death after myocardial infarction. Circulation 1993; 88:I-258. Abstract.

130. Nordrehaug JE. Malignant arrhythmia in relation to serum potassium in acute myocardial infarction. Am J Cardiol 1985; 56:20D-23D.

131. Omland T, Aarsland T, Aakvaag A, et al. Prognostic value of plasma atrial natriuretic factor, norepinephrine and epinephrine in acute myocardial infarction. Am J Cardiol 1993; 72:255-259.

132. Omland T, Bonarjee VV, Nilsen DW, et al. Prognostic significance of N-terminal proatrial natriuretic (1-98) in acute myocardial infarction: comparison with atrial natriuretic factor (99-126) and clinical evaluation. Br Heart J 1993; 70:409-414.

133. Wong ND, Wilson PW, Kannel WB. Serum cholesterol as a prognostic factor after myocardial infarction: the Framingham Study. Ann Intern Med 1991; 115:687-693.

134. Hull SS, Evans AR, Vanoli E, et al. Heart rate variability before and after myocardial infarction in conscious dogs at high and low risk of sudden death. J Am Coll Cardiol 1990; 16:978-985.

135. Luria MH, Sapoznikov D, Gilon D, et al. Early heart rate variability alterations after acute myocardial infarction. Am Heart J 1993; 125:676-681.

136. Casolo GC, Stroder P, Signorini C, et al. Heart rate variability during the acute phase of myocardial infarction. Circulation 1992; 85:2073-2079.

137. Bigger JT Jr, Fleiss JL, Rolnitzky LM, et al. Time course of recovery of heart period variability after myocardial infarction. J Am Coll Cardiol 1991; 18:1643-1649.

138. Flapan AD, Wright RA, Nolan J, et al. Differing patterns of cardiac parasympathetic activity and their evolution in selected patients with a first myocardial infarction. J Am Coll Cardiol 1993; 21:926-931.

139. Lombardi F, Sandrone G, Pernpruner S, et al. Heart rate variability as an index of sympathovagal interaction after acute myocardial infarction. Am J Cardiol 1987; 60:1239-25.

140. Wolf MM, Varigos GA, Hunt D, et al. Sinus arrhythmia in acute myocardial infarction. Med J Aust 1978; 2:52-53.

141. Kleiger RE, Miller JP, Bigger JT Jr, et al. Decreased heart rate variability and its asso-

ciation with increased mortality after acute rnyocardial infarction. Am J Cardiol 1987; 59:256-262.

142. Farrell TG, Bashir Y, Cripps T, et al. Risk stratification for arrhythmic events in post-infarction patients based on heart rate variability, ambulatory electrocardiographic variables and the signal-averaged electro-cardiogram. J Am Coll Cardiol 1991; 18:687-697.

143. Bigger JT Jr, Fleiss JL, Steinman RC, et al. Frequency domain measures of heart period variability and mortality after myocardial infarction. Circulation 1992; 85:164-171.

144. Bigger JT Jr, Fleiss JL, Rolnitzky LM, et al. Frequency domain measures of heart period variability to assess risk late after myocardial infarction. J Am Coll Cardiol 1993; 21:729-736.

145. Singer DH, Martin GJ, Mahid N, et al. Low heart rate variability and sudden cardiac death. J Electrocardiol 1988; 21:S46-55.

146. Malliani A, Lombardi F, Pagani M, et al. Power spectral analysis of cardiovascular variability in patients at risk of sudden cardiac death. J Cardiovasc Electrophysiol 1994; 5:274-286.

147. Fei L, Keeling PJ, Gill JS, et al. Heart rate variability and its relation to ventricular arrhythmias in patients with congestive heart failure. Br Heart J 1994; 71:322-328.

148. Hermosillo AG, Dorado M, Casanova JM, et al. Influence of infarct-related artery patency on the indexes of parasympathetic activity and prevalence of late potentials in survivors of acute myocardial infarction. J Am Coll Cardiol 1993; 22:695-706.

149. Hayano J, Sakakibara Y, Yamada M, et al. Decreased magnitude of heart rate spectral components in coronary artery disease. Its relation to angiographic severity. Circulation 1990; 81:1217-1224.

150. Nolan J, Flapan AD, Reid J, et al. Cardiac parasympathetic activity in severe uncomplicated coronary artery disease. Br Heart J 1994; 71:515-520.

151. Cripps TR, Malik M, Farrell TG, et al. Prognostic value of reduced heart rate variability after myocardial infarction: clinical evaluation of a new analysis method. Br Heart J 1991; 65:14-19.

152. Pedretti R, Etro MD, Laporta A, et al. Prediction of late arrhythmic events after acute myocardial infarction from combined use of noninvasive prognostic variables and inducibility of sustained monomorphic ventricular tachycardia. Am J Cardiol 1993; 71:1131-1141.

153. Odemuyiwa O, Malik M, Farrell T, et al. Comparison of the predictive characteristics of heart rate variability index and left ventricular ejection fraction for all-cause mortality, arrhythmic events and sudden death after acute myocardial infarction. Am J Cardiol 1991; 68:434-439.

154. Singer DH, Martin GJ, Magid N, et al. Low heart rate variability and sudden cardiac death. J Electrocardiol 1988; S46-S55.

155. Raymenants E, Duran A, Miller K, et al. Relationship between heart rate variability and programmed ventricular stimulation in sudden death survivors and patients with ventricular arrhythmias. J Am Coll Cardiol 1992; 19:124A.

156. Huikuri H, Koistinen MJ, Yli-Mäyry S, et al. Impaired very low frequency oscillation of heart rate in patients with life threatening arrhythmias. J Am Coll Cardiol 1994; 23:38A.

157. Bigger JT Jr, Fleiss JL, Rolnitzky LM, et al. The ability of several short-term measures of RR variability to predict mortality after myocardial infarction. Circulation 1993; 88:927-934.

158. Ahmed M, Fintel D, Zhang F, et al. Survival post-sudden cardiac death: predictive value of heart rate variability vs inducibility. J Am Coll Cardiol 1992; 19:167A.

159. Billman GE, Hoskins RS. Time-series analysis of heart rate variability during submaximal exercise. Evidence for reduced cardiac vagal tone in animals susceptible to ventricular fibrillation. Circulation 1989; 80:146-157.

160. Holter NJ. New method for heart studies. Science 1961; 134:1214-1220.

161. La Rovere MT, Specchia G, Mortara A, et al. Baroreflex sensitivity, clinical correlates, and cardiovascular mortality among patients with a first myocardial infarction: a prospective study. Circulation 1988; 78:816-824.

162. Farrell TG, Paul V, Cripps TR, et al. Baroreflex sensitivity and electrophysiological correlates in patients after acute myocardial infarction. Circulation 1991; 83:945-952.

163. Farrell TG, Odemuyiwa O, Bashir Y, et al. Prognostic value of baroreflex sensitivity testing after acute myocardial infarction. Br Heart J 1992; 67:129-137.

164. Schwartz PJ, Vanoli E, Stamba-Badiale M, et al. Autonomic mechanisms and sudden death. New insights from analysis of baroreceptor reflexes in conscious dogs with and without a myocardial infarction. Circulation 1988; 78:969-979.

165. Bigger JT Jr, La Rovere MT, Steinman RC, et al. Comparison of baroreflex sensitivity and heart period variability after myocar-

dial infarction. J Am Coll Cardiol 1989; 14:1511-1518.

166. Kollai M, Jokkel G, Bonyhay I, et al. Relation between baroreflex sensitivity and cardiac vagal tone in humans. Am J Physiol 1994; 266:H21-27.

167. McCallister BD, Christian TF, Gersh BJ, et al. Prognosis of myocardial infarctions involving more than 40% of the left ventricle after acute reperfusion therapy. Circulation 1993; 88:1470-1475.

168. ISIS-2 (Second International Study of Infarct Survival) Collaborative Group: randomised trial of intravenous streptokinase, oral aspirin, both or neither among 17,187 cases of suspected acute myocardial infarction: ISIS-2. Lancet 1988; 2(8607):349-360.

169. Goldberg RJ, Gorak EJ, Yarzebski J, et al. A communitywide perspective of sex differences and temporal trends in the incidence and survival rates after acute myocardial infarction and out-of-hospital deaths caused by coronary heart disease. Circulation 1993; 87:1947-1953.

170. Volpi A, De Vita C, Franzosi MG, et al. Determinant of 6-month mortality in survivors of myocardial infarction after thrombolysis. Results of the GISSI-2 data base. Circulation 1993; 88:416-429.

171. Shechter M, Rabinowitz B, Beker B, et al. Additional ST segment evaluation during the first hour of thrombolytic therapy: an electrocardiographic sign predicting a favorable clinical outcome. J Am Coll Cardiol 1992; 20:1460-1464.

172. Cerqueira MD, Maynard C, Ritchie JL, et al. Long-term survival in 618 patients from the Western Washington streptokinase in myocardial infarction trials. J Am Coll Cardiol 1992; 20:1452-1459.

173. Malik M, Kulakowski P, Odemuyiwa O, et al. Effect of thrombolytic therapy on the predictive value of signal-averaged electrocardiography after myocardial infarction. Am J Cardiol 1992; 70:21-25.

174. Dorado M, Gonzalez-Hermosillo JA, Garcia-Arenal F, et al. Influence of the permeability of the artery responsible for the infarction on the variability of heart rate and late potentials. Its importance in the risk stratification after myocardial infarction. Rev Esp Cardiol 1993; 46:71-83.

175. Zabel M, Klingenheben T, Hohnloser SH. Changes in autonomic tone following thrombolytic therapy for acute myocardial infarction: assessment by analysis of heart rate variability. J Cardiovasc Electrophysiol 1994; 5:211-218.

Chapter 30

Practicality of Postinfarction Risk Assessment Based on Time-Domain Measurement of Heart Rate Variability

Marek Malik, Katerina Hnatkova, A. John Camm

The potential of reduced heart rate variability (HRV) to identify patients who are at high risk of cardiac complications after acute myocardial infarction has been well documented. Reduced HRV assessed from 24-hour electrocardiograms (ECGs) has been shown to predict early cardiac mortality independently of other recognized risk factors[1] (see Chapter 25) and to predict arrhythmic events (sudden death and/or symptomatic sustained ventricular tachycardia) more powerfully than reduced left ventricular ejection fraction.[2]

Nevertheless, direct clinical application of these findings is limited because of several factors. One of the major limitations is the requirement to assess HRV using error-free and artifact free measurement of individual sinus rhythm RR intervals. The most frequently used methods for both statistical and frequency-domain measurement of HRV have been shown to depend crucially on the quality of analyzed sequences of RR intervals.[3,4] Automatic quality check, eg, prematurity filters, can be performed on the long-term sequences of RR intervals,[1] but their general performance is poor,[5] and careful visual checks and manual corrections of the RR interval sequence are required. However, meticulous manual editing of long-term ECGs is impractical in a typical clinical setting.

In principle, there are two possible solutions to this problem. Either, risk stratification relevant assessment of HRV might be obtained from recordings substantially shorter than 24 hours, or an equally predictive value of 24-hour HRV might be obtained by methods independent of the recognition artifact. The idea of assessing HRV from short-term recordings is very appealing.[6] However, it has been suggested that HRV assessed from randomly selected short portions of long-term ECGs has a substantially lower predictive power compared to

From: Malik M., Camm AJ (eds.): *Heart Rate Variability*. Armonk, NY. Futura Publishing Company, Inc., © 1995.

evaluations of total 24-hour recordings[7] (See Chapter 26).

The degree to which different time- and frequency-domain methods depend on the noise and imprecision of long-term RR interval sequences has only been compared at a technical level of numerical reproduction of HRV measurement from edited and unedited Holter records[3,4] (see Chapter 8). Here, we shall report on the influence of the imprecision of automatic recognitions of long-term ECGs on the predictive power of HRV assessed by several recognized time-domain methods.

Methods

Patient Population

During June 1987 to October 1991, 780 patients aged ≤75 years who were admitted to our hospital with acute myocardial infarction (AMI) survived to discharge. AMI had been diagnosed using previously published standard criteria.[2]

The population of the present study consisted of 545 patients (353 men; mean age: 57.1, range: 25 to 75 years; mean left ventricular ejection fraction: 49.1, range 10% to 89%; 243 patients with anterior infarctions) from whom a technically suitable (see next section) predischarge 24-hour ECG record was available. These records were recorded on days 5 to 12 (median day: 7) after the admission for AMI. The population of the study did not include patients with atrial fibrillation or permanent pacemaker implant who were not suitable for HRV assessment, and patients with other significant disease which was likely to influence life expectancy. Patients were also excluded if they were unable to participate in the follow-up research program of our institution.

All patients in the study population have been followed for at least 24 months (range: 24 months to 6 years). During the first 2 years after admission, 55 patients died in 7 of these, the cause of death was clearly not associated with cardiovascular morbidity. Of the 48 patients who suffered cardiac death during the first 2 years of follow-up, 35 and 26 died during the first year and first 6 months after the admission respectively; 25 patients died suddenly (according to the standard criteria),[8] 19 and 15 of these sudden cardiac deaths occurred during the first year and first 6 months respectively.

Analysis of Holter Recordings

Long-term ECGs were recorded using either a Reynolds Tracker TRl or Marquette 8500 3 channel recorder. The analysis of each record was performed on the Marquette 8000 Laser Holter system. The standard equipment was used to download the sequence of RR intervals to a personal computer; the sequence included the duration of each RR interval measured in technical units of 7.8125 milliseconds (1/128 seconds) and morphological classification of each QRS complex.

Two sequences of RR intervals were obtained for each long-term ECG record: one after fully automatic analysis of the tape by the commercial software of the Holter system accepting the automatic initial classification of QRS morphologies, and one after careful visual inspection of the results of the automatic analysis and manual correction of each misrecognized ECG pattern and misclassified QRS complex. These two RR interval files were subsequently converted into three sequences of 'normal-to-normal' intervals (see the following section). The Holter record was considered technically suitable for the study if the fully automatic analysis of the tape resulted in at least 1000 RR intervals between QRS complexes of normal supraventricular morphology. On this basis, 34 patients were excluded who were otherwise eligible (4 of these patients died during the first 2 years of follow-up, all suffered from cardiac death, 2 died suddenly. The incidence of cardiac death in this group did not differ from the studied population: 11.8% versus 8.8%; p = 0.534, Fisher's exact test). The threshold of 1000 RR intervals was taken arbitrarily and

Table 1
Methods for HRV Assessment

Method	Description
(1) SDNN	Standard deviation of durations of RR intervals between QRS complexes of 'normal morphology' (NN intervals)
(2) HRV index	Proportion N/M where N is the total number of NN intervals, and M is the height of their distribution histogram
(3) TINN	Baseline width of the minimum square difference triangular interpolation of the distribution histogram of NN interval durations
(4) SDANN	Standard deviation of 5-minute means of NN interval durations
(5) pNN50	Relative number of NN intervals which were longer than the immediately preceding NN interval by more than 50 ms
(6) SDNN index	Mean of 5-minute standard deviations of NN interval durations
(7) rMSSD	Square root of the mean of squares of differences between durations of neighboring NN intervals

Methods (1–3) express an overall measure of HRV, method (4) enhances long-term components of HRV, method (6) medium term components, and methods (5) and (7) short term components of HRV. Several different definitions of 'normal QRS complexes' were used in the study (see the text for details).

introduced because some of the methods for HRV assessment do not work correctly when analyzing too sparse RR interval sequences which are unsuitable for the construction of an RR interval histogram.

Heart Rate Variability Assessment

The study utilized seven different methods for HRV assessment which are summarized in Table 1. These methods included all those time-domain methods which have been previously used in studies aimed at risk stratification among survivors of AMI. Each of these methods has been applied to the long-term ECG in three different ways which differ in the definition of 'normal' QRS complexes and 'normal-to-normal' (NN) RR intervals:

1. (RRa) The manually edited sequence of RR intervals was used, and only QRS complexes related to sinus rhythm were considered;
2. (RRb) The unedited sequence of RR intervals was used, but only those nonpremature QRS complexes which the automatic recognition

classified as of supraventricular morphology were used; and
3. (RRc) The unedited sequence of RR intervals was used and all QRS complexes, regardless of their automatic morphological classification, were used.

In cases RRb and RRc, those 'normal-to-normal' intervals which were longer than 2000 milliseconds, and those which differed by more than 20% from the immediately preceding 'normal-to-normal' interval were excluded from the analysis. In total, 21 time-domain measures of HRV (seven methods applied to three sequences of RR intervals) were obtained for each patient.

Statistics

Three different major endpoints were used: cardiac death within the first 6 months, within 1 year, and within 2 years after hospital admission. For each of these endpoints, the study compared the measures of HRV of patients with the endpoint (Groups P6, P12, and P24, respectively) and without the endpoint (Groups N6, N12, and N24, respectively). Specifically, patients who died later than 6, 12, and 24 months after the admission were considered as belonging to groups N6, N12, and N24, respectively.

The association of each of the 21 HRV measures with 6-month, 1-year and 2-year cardiac mortality was tested with the standard nonparametric Wilcoxon test. A level of p >0.05 was considered as nonsignificant. For each of the 21 measures and for each pair of P6-N6, P12-N12, and P24-N24 groups of patients, the positive predictive characteristics (ie, the curve assigning the maximum achievable positive predictive accuracy to each level of sensitivity)[9] was computed for the identification of the patients with the endpoint.

The differences between the predictive power of individual HRV methods were tested separately when using sequences RRa, RRb, and RRc of RR intervals. These tests were based on the sign test comparing the stratification of the population at 25% and 40% sensitivity for the identification of all endpoints. The details of this statistical procedure are presented in the Appendix. In a similar way, the influence of the differences between the precision of sequences RRa, RRb, and RRc on the mortality predicting performance of individual HRV methods was tested (see the Appendix).

Results

Heart Rate Variability Measures in Individual Groups

The statistical comparison of individual measures of HRV for 2-year cardiac mortality is presented in Table 2. Similar comparisons for 6-month and 1-year mortality are not shown here. However, the overall image of these comparisons was the same as that of Table 2.

All methods for HRV assessment applied to manually edited recognitions of Holter tapes resulted in statistically significant or nearly significant distinctions between positive and negative patients. How-

ever, using NN interval sequences which were obtained without manual editing, only the methods HRV index, TINN, and pNN50 distinguished between the two groups.

When using the manually edited NN intervals (sequence RRa), the highest significance of differences between the positive and negative patients was achieved with methods addressing the total overall HRV, while the lowest significance was achieved with methods enhancing short-term components of HRV (see Table 2).

Positive Predictive Characteristics

The positive predictive characteristics of individual HRV measures for 2-year mortality are shown in Figure 1. Similar characteristics have also been computed for 6-month and 1-year mortality, but are not presented here since they are similar to those shown in Figure 1.

Part A of the figure which shows the characteristics of HRV measures using manually edited Holter data is in good agreement with the statistical comparison of these measures presented in Table 2. It can be clearly seen that the measures characterizing total HRV (SDNN, HRV index, and TINN) have a higher predictive power than other HRV measures.

Among all measures, only HRV index and TINN preserved a predictive value when applied to unedited Holter data (sequences RRb and RRc). Note that when using all RR intervals irrespective of their morphological classification (RR interval category RRc, part C of the figure), the predictive accuracy of the SDNN, pNN50, and rMSSD methods corresponded to the overall incidence of the endpoints for most of the practical levels of sensitivity, suggesting that these methods were not valuable in this setting.

The values of positive predictive accuracy achieved at 25% and 40% sensitivity level with different methods when using edited and unedited Holter data (sequences RRa and RRc) are shown in Table 3 together

Table 2

Comparison of HRV Measures in Patients Who Did and Did Not Suffer From Cardiac Death Within 2 Years After Hospital Admission

Measure	NN Interval Sequence	Positive Pts (n = 48)	Negative Pts (n = 497)	p =
SDNN	RRa	70.83 ± 51.25	96.06 ± 39.10	0.0001
[ms]	RRb	194.25 ± 133.58	208.54 ± 130.06	0.3611
	RRc	205.32 ± 127.27	219.25 ± 127.33	0.4619
HRV index	RRa	18.05 ± 12.06	28.20 ± 10.63	0.0001
	RRb	17.91 ± 11.50	27.29 ± 10.41	0.0001
	RRc	19.48 ± 12.29	29.04 ± 11.09	0.0001
TINN	RRa	269.37 ± 190.02	429.75 ± 169.54	0.0001
[ms]	RRb	249.67 ± 172.35	400.48 ± 164.02	0.0001
	RRc	269.53 ± 191.66	416.62 ± 176.96	0.0001
SDANN	RRa	70.60 ± 49.06	86.37 ± 36.97	0.0001
[ms]	RRb	107.67 ± 66.43	123.75 ± 82.19	0.2077
	RRc	113.49 ± 68.89	131.50 ± 88.36	0.2988
pNN50	RRa	3.31 ± 4.63	5.00 ± 6.27	0.0310
[%]	RRb	2.25 ± 4.60	4.14 ± 6.30	0.0003
	RRc	3.12 ± 4.53	4.61 ± 6.22	0.0683
SDNN index	RRa	39.90 ± 30.65	48.89 ± 23.88	0.0001
[ms]	RRb	81.96 ± 73.91	86.48 ± 62.31	0.1057
	RRc	94.31 ± 75.75	96.68 ± 65.61	0.2997
rMSSD	RRa	27.65 ± 15.39	31.99 ± 19.11	0.0778
[ms]	RRb	27.11 ± 16.92	32.46 ± 20.25	0.0283
	RRc	33.03 ± 17.04	34.93 ± 20.18	0.8174

The values are presented as mean ± standard deviation. The HRV measures are explained in Table 1; the categories of NN intervals are explained in the text. Note the huge differences in mean values of statistical methods applied to edited and unedited Holter data. These differences were caused by the overwhelming influence of the artifact in the Holter data on the results of the statistical methods.

with the corresponding dichotomy 'normality' limits. Thus, for instance, dichotomizing the HRV index method using edited Holter data at 12.5 units (ie, taking the HRV result ≤12.5 as test positive) resulted in 40% sensitivity and 44.4% positive predictive accuracy for the prediction of 2-year mortality.

Differences Between Predictive Power of Individual Heart Rate Variability Methods

The statistical differences between the performance of individual HRV measures applied to manually edited Holter data and to all RR intervals irrespective of their morphological classification are shown in Tables 4 and 5, respectively. The same comparison was also performed for the HRV measures using NN interval sequence RRb but the re-sult is not presented here since it closely resembles the results with the sequence RRc (Table 5).

Table 3 confirms in statistical terms what can be seen in Figure 1A. Applied to manually edited data, there are no significant differences between the predictive power of SDNN, HRV index, and TINN. However, these methods were statistically significantly more powerful than all other measures. In addition, the SDANN and SDNN index methods were significantly more powerful than the pNN50 and rMSSD measures.

The pattern changes dramatically when applying the methods to unedited Holter data (Table 5). Then, HRV index and TINN were signifcantly more powerful than the other measures. Although the table shows

A Positive Predictive Accuracy

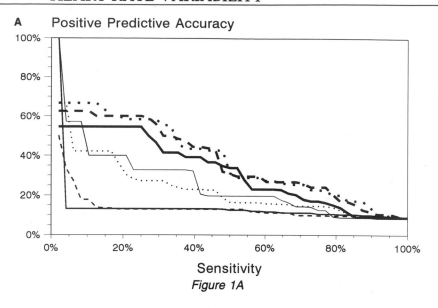

Sensitivity

Figure 1A

B Positive Predictive Accuracy

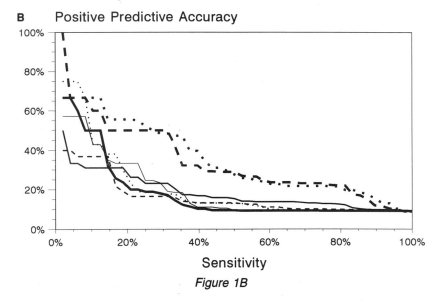

Sensitivity

Figure 1B

some significant differences between the remaining five methods, these are not systematic and, as shown in Figure 1C, of no practical value because the overall performance of all of these methods was poor.

Influence of the Quality of RR Interval Recognition on Individual Heart Rate Variability Methods

Table 6 shows the statistical differences between the performance of SDNN, SDANN TINN, and pNN50 methods when applying them to edited and unedited Holter data. Similar computations were performed for the remaining three methods, but the results are not presented here.

The results of the statistical tests were in good agreement with the results shown in Tables 4 and 5 and in Figure 1. The performance of SDNN, SDANN, and SDNN index methods was seriously worsened when applying them to the unedited rather than edited Holter data. The methods HRV index

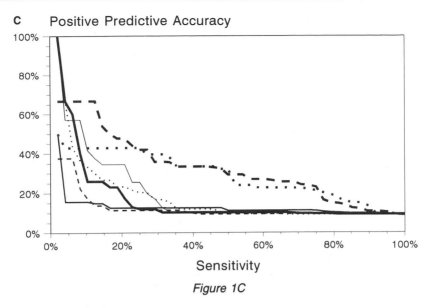

C   Positive Predictive Accuracy

Figure 1C

Figures 1A-C. Different HRV assessment methods used to predict 2-year cardiac mortality. The figure shows positive predictive characteristics (curves assigning the maximum achievable positive predictive accuracy to each level of sensitivity) for different HRV assessment methods (explained in Table 1) operating with edited Holter data (NN interval sequence RRa: **part A**) and unedited data (NN interval sequences RRb and RRc: **parts B and C, respectively**). The curves of the characteristics are smoothed, ie, they show the maximum positive predictive accuracy achievable for a given or higher level of sensitivity. Bold solid lines correspond to the SDNN method; bold dashed line: HRV index; bold dotted line: TINN; medium solid line: pNN50; medium dashed line: rMSSD; medium dotted line: SDNN index; fine solid line: SDANN.

and TINN performed similarly with all sets of data; their performance with edited Holter data was only marginally better. The methods pNN50 and rMSSD did not exhibit significantly worse performance with unedited data compared to edited data. This, as shown in Figure 1, was the consequence of their poor performance in all settings.

Discussion

Limitations of the Study

The major limitation of this study was the exclusive use of the Marquette Laser Holter 8000 system. If we had used another Holter system, the detailed results might have changed. Nevertheless, this particular Holter system is not only widely used, but the performance of its algorithms may be taken as a reasonable representation of automatic processing of Holter tapes. The

principal results of the study would have been different only if another Holter system had a substantially different performance.

We did not perform a comparison of fully edited Holter data with partially edited RR sequences (eg, with a limitation of 1 hour of manual editing time). Such an approach would possibly be closer to clinical reality but would be biased because the amount of the manual work is very difficult to control and depends on the number of ventricular premature beats which are more frequent in the records of high-risk patients.[10] It is possible that the difference between fully and partially edited data subjected to some methods (eg, SDNN or SDANN) would be less expressed than the difference between fully edited and completely unedited data. Nevertheless, the striking difference between the positive predictive accuracy achieved with these methods operating on edited and unedited data suggests that all the standard deviation

Table 3

Dichotomy Limits of Individual Measures of HRV Assessed from Manually Edited and Unedited Holter Data

	Cardiac Mortality up to 6 Months							
Method	NN category RRa				NN category RRc			
	25% sensitivity		40% sensitivity		25% sensitivity		40% sensitivity	
	PPA	dichotomy	PPA	dichotomy	PPA	dichotomy	PPA	dichotomy
SDNN	35.0	34.8	26.8	43.5	4.4	134	4.8	170
HRV index	43.7	9.64	36.7	11.4	43.7	9.78	24.4	13.6
TINN	46.6	132	44.0	164	33.3	125	31.4	148
SDANN	15.9	42.2	11.3	53.3	8.5	64.9	5.4	88.6
pNN50	10.3	3.43	7.6	10.6	8.7	3.58	7.3	8.82
SDNN index	38.9	16.8	11.4	28.3	7.8	44.8	5.8	60.5
rMSSD	6.6	18.5	6.3	22.3	6.1	21.6	4.9	26.9

	Cardiac Mortality up to 24 Months							
Method	NN category RRa				NN category RRc			
	25% sensitivity		40% sensitivity		25% sensitivity		40% sensitivity	
	PPA	dichotomy	PPA	dichotomy	PPA	dichotomy	PPA	dichotomy
SDNN	54.5	35.2	39.2	46.4	12.0	110	9.0	166
HRV index	60.0	10.2	44.4	12.5	40.0	11.6	32.3	14.6
TINN	54.5	156	43.4	187	42.9	140	32.8	187
SDANN	30.0	41.8	20.6	53.3	25.5	55.6	9.9	88.6
pNN50	11.4	5.95	12.5	11.6	11.6	4.90	11.9	10.4
SDNN index	23.5	23.2	22.9	27.4	20.3	36.0	11.4	58.6
rMSSD	113	18.5	11.4	22.3	10.4	21.6	8.9	26.8

For each HRV assessment method (see Table 1) and for the NN categories RRa and RRc of RR interval data (see the text for detail) the table lists the values of positive predictive accuracies (PPA: values in percent) achieved at sensitivity levels of 25% and 40% together with the corresponding dichotomy 'normality' limits. The normality limits of SDNN, TINN, rMSSD, SDNN index, and SDANN methods are in ms, the normality limits of pNN50 method in percent, and the normality limits of HRV index method in technical dimensionless units.

based methods are very sensitive to the quality of Holter analysis.

The study investigated only positive predictive accuracy and omitted similar considerations of negative predictive accuracy. It is likely that all HRV methods applied to standard quality data will have a reasonable negative predictive accuracy which will enable their use in negative screening. However, the methods performing with best positive predictive accuracy along the whole range of sensitivity will also have, for simple mathematical reasons, the best negative predictive characteristics.

The study involved a high number of individual statistical tests. We did not per-

form any correction for the multiplicity of the tests because the data investigated in repeated tests were not mutually independent. For the same reasons, the multiplicity of statistical tests was not likely to influence the results of the study.

Interpretation of Results

First of all, this study confirmed the high predictive power of HRV for identifying those survivors of AMI who were at high risk of an early death. With a retrospective adjustment of the dichotomy limits, we were able to identify the 24-month mortality with a predictive positive accuracy of 60.0%

Table 4

Comparison of the Predictive Power of Individual Methods Assessing HRV in Manually Edited Holter Data

Method	Sen	SDNN			HRV i			TINN			pNN50			rMSSD			SDNN i			SDANN		
		6m	1y	2y	6m	1y	2y	6m	1y	2y	6m	1y	2y	6m	1y	2y	6m	1y	2y	6m	1y	2y
SDNN	25%										8	9	9	8	9	9		4	2	4	3	3
	40%										9	9	9	9	9	9	9	7	4	9	9	7
HRV i	25%										9	9	9	9	9	9		6	3	5	4	3
	40%	2									9	9	9	9	9	9	9	9	6	9	9	8
TINN	25%										9	9	9	9	9	9		5	3	5	3	3
	40%	2									9	9	9	9	9	9	9	7	5	9	9	7
pNN50	25%														3							
	40%																					
rMSSD	25%																					
	40%																					
SDNN i	25%										9	9	7	9	9	9				4		
	40%										2	9	9	5	9	9					2	
SDANN	25%										2	9	5	2	9	9						
	40%										2	3	5	2	3	5						

The table shows the results of statistical comparisons of the positive predictive accuracy of individual methods for predicting mortality during the first 6 months (6m), 12 months (1y), and 24 months (2y), at 25% and 40% sensitivity (Sen). If the method listed in a horizontal line was significantly superior to the method listed in the vertical column, a mark has been put into the table corresponding to the level of statistical significance ($2\text{--}10^{-2}$, $3\text{--}10^{-3}$, $4\text{--}10^{-4}$, $5\text{--}10^{-5}$, $6\text{--}10^{-6}$, $7\text{--}10^{-7}$, $8\text{--}10^{-8}$, $9\text{--}10^{-9}$). The methods for HRV measurement are explained in Table 1.

and 44.4%, at 25% and 40% sensitivity, respectively (HRV index method applied to manually edited Holter data).

Previously, it has been reported by Bigger et al[11] that different spectral components of HRV had different predictive power in a population similar to ours. Thus, it is not surprising that we found different values of predictive power using different time-domain methods for HRV assessment. In this respect, our fndings are in good agreement with those of Bigger et al.[11] Those methods assessing the overall total HRV were the most predictive; the methods addressing medium term components were somewhat less predictive; and the methods which emphasize the fastest components of HRV were the least predictive. In this respect, we have not confirmed the suggestions that the results of SDANN are equally predictive as those of SDNN. Perhaps, the formula for calculating SDANN might be adversely influenced by a higher number of ectopic beats or short segments of the Holter tape which have to be excluded because of recording artifact. In such cases, the mean NN interval calculated over a 5-minute period might be based on too few samples to be representative for the whole 5-minute segment.

The major result of this study is the fact that the predictive power of some HRV methods is less affected by recognition noise and artifact of the automatic Holter analysis than that of others. This has already been suggested by an earlier investigation looking at the numerical reproducibility of HRV measures taken from different sequences of RR intervals.[3] However, this study is the

Table 5

Comparison of the Predictive Power of Individual Methods Assessing HRV in Unedited Holter Data

Method	Sen	SDNN			HRV i			TINN			pNN50			rMSSD			SDNN i			SDANN		
		6m	1y	2y	6m	1y	2y	6m	1y	2y	6m	1y	2y	6m	1y	2y	6m	1y	2y	6m	1y	2y
SDNN	25%																					
	40%														2						2	
HRV1	25%	9	9	9							9	9	9	9	9	9	9	6	4	9	9	4
	40%	9	9	9							9	9	9	9	9	9	9	9	9	9	9	9
TINN	25%	9	9	9							9	9	9	9	9	9	9	6	3	9	9	4
	40%	9	9	9							9	9	9	9	9	9	9	9	9	9	9	9
pNN50	25%	2	3											4		2						
	40%	6	5												9	8					9	2
rMSSD	25%		3																			
	40%	4																				
SDNN i	25%	9	9	7								5	4	7	8	9					2	9
	40%	8	9												9	4						9
SDANN	25%	3	3	2										2		4						
	40%	4																				

Abbreviations and table layout as in Table 3.

first showing this difference in the power of predicting risk post-AMI.

The study was performed with a set of tapes which excluded those of poorest technical quality. The arbitrary criterion which required at least 1000 automatically recognized normal-to-normal intervals excluded 5.9% of all eligible tapes. It is very likely that casual manual editing of the Holter tapes which is, in the majority of cases, performed anyway for other reasons (such as diagnosis of arrhythmia or of ST segment changes) will mostly ensure sequences of RR intervals suitable for HRV assessment with the robust methods. The arbitrary exclusion criterion applied in this study could be used as a rough estimate of the suitability of a Holter tape for HRV analysis and of the quality of its analysis.

We did not confirm our previous suggestion that the TINN method might be superior to the HRV index method.[12] In this study, both methods performed equally well and no statistical differences were observed between their predictive powers.

We did not observe any significant differences or marked trends between HRV values of patients who suffered sudden and nonsudden cardiac death. The methods which were found useful for identification of patients at high risk of an early cardiac death (ie, SDNN, HRV index, and TINN with edited Holter data and HRV index, and TINN with unedited data) stratified the patients who died suddenly and nonsuddenly without any significant differences. This finding might have several explanations. First, the standard definition of sudden death[8] does not necessarily distinguish between patients who die because of arrhythmia and those who die because of heart failure. It is likely that the proportion of patients with an arrhythmia related death will be higher among the sudden death group, but sudden death is also a common mode of death in pump failure. It is also

Table 6

Comparison of the Predictive Power Achieved from Manually Edited and Unedited Holter Data by Selected Methods of HRV Assessment

SDNN

	Sen	RRa 6m	RRa 1y	RRa 2y	RRb 6m	RRb 1y	RRb 2y	RRc 6m	RRc 1y	RRc 2y
RRa	25%				2	9	7	9	9	5
RRa	40%				9	9	9	9	9	9
RRb	25%							9	9	9
RRb	40%							3		3
RRc	25%									
RRc	40%									

pNN50

	Sen	RRa 6m	RRa 1y	RRa 2y	RRb 6m	RRb 1y	RRb 2y	RRc 6m	RRc 1y	RRc 2y
RRa	25%							2		2
RRa	40%							3	3	
RRb	25%	3	6	3				6	8	6
RRb	40%	9	2	3				9	6	5
RRc	25%									
RRc	40%									

SDANN

	Sen	RRa 6m	RRa 1y	RRa 2y	RRb 6m	RRb 1y	RRb 2y	RRc 6m	RRc 1y	RRc 2y
RRa	25%					8		9		5
RRa	40%				4	9	9	9	9	9
RRb	25%							5	7	4
RRb	40%							5		
RRc	25%									
RRc	40%									

TINN

	Sen	RRa 6m	RRa 1y	RRa 2y	RRb 6m	RRb 1y	RRb 2y	RRc 6m	RRc 1y	RRc 2y
RRa	25%									2
RRa	40%						3	2	3	
RRb	25%									3
RRb	40%									
RRc	25%									
RRc	40%									

The table shows the results of statistical comparisons of the positive predictive accuracy achieved by selected HRV methods applied to RR interval categories RRa, RRb, RRc (details in the text) for predicting mortality during the first 6 months (6m), 12 months (1y), and 24 months (2y), at 25% and 40% sensitivity (Sen). If the particular method applied to the RR interval category listed in a horizontal line was significantly superior to the same method applied to the RR interval category listed in the vertical column, a mark has been put into the table corresponding to the level of statistical significance (the meaning of the marks is as in Table 3). The methods for HRV measurement are explained in Table 1.

possible that depressed HRV has a different physiological background in patients with high risk of arrhythmic complications and in patients with impaired ventricular performance. The time-domain methods for HRV assessment used in this study are unlikely to distinguish between depressed HRV due to primary parasympathetic withdrawal which may carry a risk of arrhythmia and depressed HRV because of saturated sympathetic tone which may be directly linked to heart failure. Similarly, standard spectral analysis of HRV is not very likely to distinguish between primary parasympathetic withdrawal and sympathetic overdrive. Thus the distinction between patients at high risk of arrhythmic and nonarrhythmic death should probably be multifactorial, eg, combining depressed HRV as a general marker with depressed left ventricular ejection fraction, which demonstrates pumping failure, and with reduced baroreflex sensitivity, which documents impaired cardiac parasympathetic reflexes.

Conclusion

This study showed that a clinically relevant assessment of HRV in survivors of AMI can be obtained from data which are very easily obtainable in clinical settings. Robust geometrical methods (such as HRV index and TINN), when applied to data which have been obtained automatically, gave results which were comparable to those provided by any time-domain method applied to Holter data which have been very carefully edited.

For the edited data, the results were in agreement with the previously published SDNN normality threshold of 50 milliseconds[1] (sensitivity: 46% and positive predictive accuracy: approximately 34% for the prediction of 24-month cardiac mortality). The optimum normality limit of the HRV index method (applicable to Holter systems measuring the RR intervals with the 1/128 second precision) seems to be between 10 and 15 units (sensitivity: 25% to 40%, positive predictive accuracy: 33% to 60%) and might be taken as independent of the editing of Holter data. The population stratified in this way contains approximately the same number of patients who will suffer from sudden and nonsudden cardiac death.

Appendix

The differences between the predictive power of individual HRV measures were based on statistical comparison of positive predictive characteristics and utilized the following procedure. In order to compare the HRV measures A and B for the identification of patients with endpoint Px among patients with the endpoint Nx, a sensitivity level σ was selected and the dichotomy limits α and β were obtained, which lead to sensitivity σ of identification of patients of Px based on values of measures A and B, respectively. In other words, taking the measure A $\leq\alpha$ (and B $\leq\beta$, respectively) as test positive, the group Px was identified with sensitivity σ. Then, the group of patients Z for which the methods A and B disagreed, was identifed, ie, group Z was composed of those patients for which A $\leq\alpha$ and B $>\beta$ or A $>\alpha$ and B$\leq\beta$. This group Z was further divided into two subgroups Zα and Zβ of those patients for which the classification based on methods A and B, respec-

tively, was correct; ie, the subgroup Zα was composed of those patients of Px for who A $\leq\alpha$ and of those patients of Nx for who A $>\alpha$, while the subgroup Zβ was composed of those patients of Px for whom B $\leq\beta$ and of those patients of Nx for whom B $>\beta$. The sizes of subgroups Zα and Zβ were compared using the standard sign test. If the number of patients in the group Zα was significantly higher than the number of patients in group Zβ, the measure A performed significantly better than the measure B at sensitivity level σ.

This procedure was used to compare the performance of different methods for HRV assessment applied to the same category of RR interval sequences, and to compare the performance of the same method applied to different categories of RR interval sequences. Each of such comparisons was performed six times: for each pair of endpoint groups P6-N6, P12-N12, and P24-N24 using sensitivity levels σ of 25% and 40%. However, as the possible levels of sensitivity depend on the number of positive patients, the exact levels of 25% and 40% were not achievable in all cases. Then, the nearest levels were used in the tests.

References

1. Kleiger RE, Miller JP, Bigger JT Jr, et al. Decreased heart rate variability and its association with increased mortality after acute myocardial infarction. Am J Cardiol 1987; 59:256-262.
2. Odemuyiwa O, Malik M, Farrell T, et al. A comparison of the predictive characteristics of heart rate variability index and left ventricular ejection fraction for all-cause mortality, arrhythmic events and sudden death after acute myocardial infarction. Am J Cardiol 1991; 68:434-439.
3. Malik M, Xia R, Odemuyiwa O, et al. Influence of the recognition artefact in the automatic analysis of long term electrocardiograms on time-domain measurement of heart rate variability. Med Biol Eng Comput 1993; 31:539-544.
4. Xia R, Odemuyiwa O, Gill J, et al. Influence of recognition errors of computerised analysis of 24-hour electrocardiograms on the measurement of spectral components of

heart rate variability. Int J Biomed Comput 1993; 32:223-235.

5. Malik M, Cripps T, Farrell T, et al. Prognostic value of heart rate variability after myocardial infarction—a comparison of different data processing methods. Med Biol Eng Comput 1989; 27:603-611.

6. Malik M, Farrell T, Camm AJ. Circadian rhythm of heart rate variability after acute myocardial infarction and its influence on the prognostic value of heart rate variability. Am J Cardiol 1990; 66:1049-1054.

7. Bigger JT, Fleiss JL, Rolnitzky LM, et al. The ability of several short-term measures of RR variability to predict mortality after myocardial infarction. Circulation 1993; 88:927-934.

8. Greene H, Richardson D, Barker A, et al. Classification of death after myocardial infarction as arrhythmic or nonarrhythmic. Am J Cardiol 1989; 63:1-6.

9. Hnatkova K, Poloniecki J, Camm AJ, et al. Computation of multifactorial receiver operator and predictive accuracy characteristics. Comput Methods Programs Biomed 1994; 42:147-156.

10. Bigger JT Jr, Fleiss JL, Kleiger RE, et al. The relationship among ventricular arrhythmias, left ventricular dysfunction and mortality in the 2 years after myocardial infarction. Circulation 1984; 69:250-258.

11. Bigger JT Jr, Fleiss JL, Steinman RC, et al. Frequency domain measures of heart period variability and mortality after myocardial infarction. Circulation 1992; 85:164-171.

12. Malik M, Farrell T, Cripps T, et al. Heart rate variability in relation to prognosis after myocardial infarction—selection of optimal processing techniques. Eur Heart J 1989; 10:1060-1074.

Chapter 31

Interventions Changing Heart Rate Variability After Acute Myocardial Infarction

Peter J. Schwartz, G.M. De Ferrari

Introduction

The rationale for trying to modify heart rate variability (HRV) after myocardial infarction (MI) stems from the multiple observations indicating that cardiac mortality is higher among those post-MI patients who have a more depressed HRV.[1-3] The logical inference is that interventions that augment vagal activity may be protective against cardiac mortality and sudden cardiac death. This concept has been recently reviewed in detail[4] and is supported by data indicating that the risk for ventricular fibrillation during acute myocardial ischemia is markedly reduced by interventions that increase vagal activity.[5] Specifically, antifibrillatory activity has been documented for direct stimulation of the right cervical vagus in conscious post-MI dogs,[6] for pharmacological stimulation of cholinergic receptors by oxotremorine in conscious dogs[7] and in anesthetized cats,[8] and for exercise training in conscious dogs with[9] and without[10] an MI. Conversely, among conscious post-MI animals the risk for ventricular fibrillation increases after block of the effects of vagal tone and reflexes by atropine.[11]

The evidence listed above indicates that the rationale for changing HRV is sound. However, it also contains an inherent danger; namely, to lead many investigators to the unwarranted assumption that modification of HRV translates directly in cardiac protection. This may or may not be the case. It is essential to remember that the true target is the improvement of cardiac electrical stability and that HRV is just a marker of autonomic activity.

The hard lesson of what happened to the time honored 'premature beats hypothesis' after publication of the results of CAST[12] should not be forgotten; that hypothesis had its solid background too. There had been studies galore showing that the greater the number of premature beats, the greater the risk for sudden cardiac death,[13,14] and many investigators have centered their hopes on the idea that if a drug was effective in eliminating premature ventricular beats it had to

From: Malik M., Camm AJ (eds.): *Heart Rate Variability*. Armonk, NY. Futura Publishing Company, Inc., © 1995.

be effective also in reducing sudden death. We now know that it is not as simple as that. Similarly, we should be prepared for the possibility that mere improvement of HRV may not be sufficient to reduce the risk of ventricular fibrillation.

A critical issue is represented by the fact that even though there seems to now be a consensus that increases in vagal activity can be beneficial, we really do not know how much vagal activity (or its markers) have to increase in order to provide adequate protection. On the other hand, it should not be forgotten that excessive vagal stimulation may also be harmful. The facilitation of atrioventricular (AV) block, or of sinus node pauses may be of concern in patients with advanced heart failure[15] or with a new episode of MI.

Given the current incomplete knowledge and keeping in mind the caveats expressed above, it is fair to examine with healthy skepticism and without excessive enthusiasm the possible ways to increase HRV. In this chapter we will briefly review the results obtained with the following interventions: β-adrenergic blockade, antiarrhythmic drugs, scopolamine, thrombolysis, and exercise training.

Beta-Adrenergic Blockade and Heart Rate Variability

Clinical Studies

Medical literature is an endless source of surprises. Given the demonstration beyond any doubt that β-adrenergic blockade reduces the post-MI incidence of cardiac mortality and sudden death,[16] one would have expected an abundance of studies on the effect of β-blockers on HRV in post-MI patients. Incredibly enough, at the time of writing this chapter only one such study has just been published[17] and another one is in press.[18]

The brief report by Molgaard et al[17] is difficult to evaluate because it does not even indicate the number of patients! Patients with a first MI were randomly allocated to either placebo or metoprolol (100 mg/day); a 24-hour Holter recording was made at discharge (2 weeks post-MI) and after 4 weeks of treatment. Mean age in the placebo and in metoprolol group were 59 and 53 years and left ventricular ejection fraction was 49% in both groups. The strongest feature of this study is the fact that the comparison between metoprolol and placebo allowed to assess the potential importance of time as a confounding factor. The SD of the RR intervals with placebo increased by 17 milliseconds, a change that fell just short of statistical significance (p = 0.06); this confirms previous observations,[19] and calls for caution in the interpretation of studies that are not placebo-controlled. After metoprolol, the SD of the RR intervals increased daytime and nighttime. This change was statistically significant; however, the average values of SDNN were within normal limits (110±27 milliseconds) and increased by only 18 milliseconds. It is difficult to assess the biological significance and impact of such a modest change. A somewhat greater change seemed to occur after propranolol when the measure considered was pNN50; however, this may have been largely due to the prolongation of the RR intervals. It is unfortunate that in most studies the investigators do not apply the necessary correction for the heart rate (HR) changes; this is easily done by using the coefficient of variance (this is obtained by dividing the SD of the mean RR interval by the mean RR interval and multiplying by 100) and provides a normalization of HRV for the level of HR.

Sandrone et al very recently assessed the effects of 8- to 10-days treatment with either atenolol (100 mg/day) or metoprolol (150 mg/day) in patients after a first and uncomplicated MI.[18] This is a small size study, but at least the number of patients is specified (n = 20). The mean age of the patients was 50 years and their mean left ventricular ejection fraction was 51%. The β-blockers increased significantly the 24-hour RR variance, from 13,886 to 16,728 milliseconds^2. However, when one calculates the

SD of the RR interval (not reported in the article) it appears that the actual change was of a mere 11 milliseconds (from 118 to 129 milliseconds). It is very difficult to attribute some biological significance to such a small change; even more so given the fact that the starting point is within the normal values for low-risk post-MI patients.[1] This point is clear to the authors who correctly conclude 'the potential clinical relevance of the increase in RR variance remains to be established.'

These investigators also reported a significant reduction in the low-frequency (LF) component and an increase in the high-frequency (HF) component; they also noted that the increase in overall HRV involved primarily the so-called very low-frequency (VLF) component (<0.03 Hz). This component has attracted recent attention because of the reported association with post-MI mortality,[20] but its physiological meaning remains uncertain. A potentially interesting twist, in light of the reported circadian occurrence of MI and sudden death,[21] was the finding that β-blockers greatly reduce the early morning increase in the LF component. A limitation of this study is the absence of a placebo controlled group. Despite the relatively short time interval between recordings (10 days), the early post-MI phase is one characterized by upward changes in all markers of vagal activity[19,22,23] and, particularly when dealing with small absolute changes, it becomes necessary to ensure that part of these changes is not simply due to the passage of time.

The decrease in the LF component reported by Sandrone et al[18] is opposite to what was reported by Cook et al in healthy young subjects.[24] Besides the inappropriateness of comparing healthy young subjects to much older patients who have suffered an MI, an additional complexity originates from the fact that one group[18] used normalized units, whereas the other[24] used absolute units. Most readers would appreciate if investigators using the same technique would express their results using the same parameters and the same units,

otherwise comparisons become very difficult and tentative; reviewers and journal editors could very much help here. The unfortunate bottom line is that while Sandrone et al used their results on the LF component of the power spectrum to confirm their opinion that this component reflects sympathetic activity, Cook et al used their own results to confirm their opinion that 'this variable is also an indicator of tonic vagal activity.' Thus, the average nonexpert reader is left in the middle of nowhere.

Experimental Studies

Several factors contribute to make complex the interpretation of interventions on HRV post-MI. The effectiveness of any intervention that aims at increasing HRV after an MI has to be judged keeping into account the spontaneous tendency toward recovery of all markers of vagal activity, that manifests itself already during the first few weeks and months post-MI.[19,22,25,26] There is considerable interindividual variability in measures of HRV in the absence of an MI.[27] Furthermore, there are large differences in HRV among post-MI patients;[19] this indicates the inclusion of subjects who were probably at different levels of recovery. Accordingly, it may not be unreasonable to surmise that the effect of β-blockade on HRV post-MI may, in part, be related to the level of sympathetic and vagal activity prior to the index infarction and to how large or small the change has been in HRV produced by the infarction itself. Related issues are the relationships between post-MI survival, recovery of HRV post-MI, and the effect of β-blockade on HRV.

Since these questions are not easily addressed by clinical studies, we performed a longitudinal study in high- and low-risk conscious dogs before and after an MI.[28] Arrhythmia risk was determined based on the development of ventricular fibrillation during exercise and transient ischemia 30 days post-MI, according to a well-established and clinically relevant animal model for sudden cardiac death.[29] In 22 animals, HRV was measured before and periodically during the first 30 days after an anterior wall MI. Each HRV measurement was made before and after β-blockade with atenolol. Preinfarction measurements were not different between the low- and high-risk animals, confirming a previous observation,[30] but HRV increased much more in response to β-blockade in animals destined to survive the exercise and ischemia test ("resistant") compared to those destined to develop ventricular fibrillation ("susceptible"). Indeed, the standard deviation of the RR intervals increased by 28% from 289±26 to 369±35 milliseconds among the resistant dogs, and by only 5% from 270±36 to 283±34 milliseconds among the susceptible dogs (Figure 1). Immediately after the infarction, HRV decreased markedly in all dogs, but in the resistant animals it recovered to the preinfarction level within 10 days (Figure 2). In the post-MI state, β-blockade no longer increased HRV in either group of animals. Among the susceptible dogs, HRV remained attenuated throughout the entire first month post-MI (Figure 3).

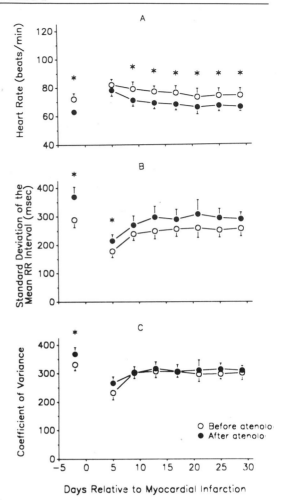

Figure 2. HR (beats/min, **panel A**), standard deviation of the mean RR interval (ms, **panel B**), and the coefficient of variance (standard deviation/mean RR interval X 1,000) before (open circles) and after (closed circles) 1 mg/kg intravenous atenolol in 12 conscious dogs shown to be resistant to ventricular fibrillation. Measurements were made 3 days before and periodically after an anterior wall MI. * indicates a significant difference when the baseline value is compared to the measurement after atenolol (p <0.01). From Adamson et al.[28]

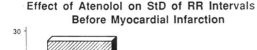

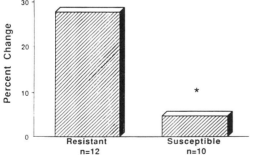

Figure 1. Percent change in the standard deviation of the mean RR interval in response to 1 mg/kg of intravenous atenolol before MI in 12 dogs shown to be resistant (**left**) to ventricular fibrillation and 10 dogs shown to be susceptible (**right**) to ventricular fibrillation during an exercise and ischemia test performed 30 days after myocardial infarction. Data shown are group means. * p <0.01 when resistant and susceptible values are compared. From Adamson et al.[28]

This study provides a longitudinal analysis on the evolution of HRV after an MI with two features not readily available in clinical investigations. One is the comparison of HRV after MI with values prior to the infarction, which allows a correct assessment of the extent of recovery; the other is the comparison between animals at low and

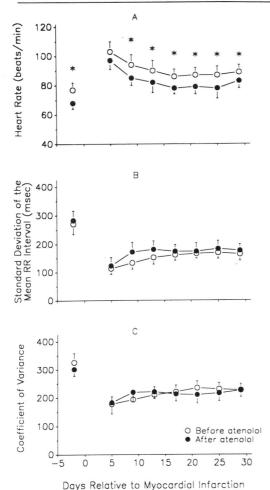

Figure 3. HR (beats/min, **panel A**), standard deviation of the mean RR interval (ms, **panel B**), and the coefficient of variance (standard deviation/mean RR interval X 1,000) before (open circles) and after (closed circles) 1 mg/kg intravenous atenolol in 10 conscious dogs shown to be susceptible to ventricular fibrillation. Measurements were made 3 days before and periodically after an anterior wall MI. * indicates a significant difference when the baseline value is compared to the measurement after atenolol (p <0.01). From Adamson et al.[28]

at high risk for sudden cardiac death, which allows a refined assessment of the prognostic value of HRV. Three main findings emerged, and they all have significant clinical implications.

The first is that MI produces a depression in HRV which shows a strikingly different temporal evolution between low- and high-risk animals. Among resistant dogs, the depression is quite transient as HRV returns to pre-MI values within 10 days. In contrast, HRV in susceptible dogs remains significantly depressed at 1 month after the infarction.

The second finding is that after MI, β-adrenergic blockade, highly effective in preventing ventricular fibrillation in this animal model,[7,31] does not alter HRV. Specifically, the expected increase in HRV after β-adrenergic blockade is absent in all dogs following MI. Thus, treatment with β-blockers would not be a confounding factor in the analysis of HRV.

The third finding is the unexpected and intriguing observation that, prior to MI, β-blockade increases HRV only in the animals destined to be at low risk for lethal arrhythmias after the infarction. This raises the possibility that individuals at high risk for arrhythmic death after an MI can be identified very early, even before the infarction.

Antiarrhythmic Drugs and Heart Rate Variability

Part of the detrimental effect on survival observed in the CAST study may have been due to an unfavorable interaction of the Na channel blockers utilized with the autonomic nervous system (ANS).[12] This hypothesis would be in agreement with the capability of β-adrenergic blockade to reverse the proarrhythmic effect of flecainide, both at clinical[32] and experimental[33] level. Accordingly, the evaluation of the effects of antiarrhythmic drugs on HRV, as an index of sympatho-vagal balance after MI, could be of clinical relevance. However, it is important to underline that antiarrhythmic drugs may theoretically cause a change in HRV not only via an interaction with the ANS but also because of two other mechanisms.

The first is a direct electrophysiological effect. Although most of the current antiarrhythmic drugs should have only a small effect on sinus node automaticity, such a depressant effect has been reported for several drugs, particularly in patients with some degree of preexisting sinus node dysfunction.[34,35] A marked effect on sinoatrial conduction, which may vary at different cycle lengths, would also cause an interference between the real signal (sinus node cycle) and the measured variable (RR interval).

The second potential mechanism is related to the presence of arrhythmia itself. Besides the problem of the identification of the best fitting estimate for the dropped sinus beats, very often patients treated with antiarrhythmic drugs have a marked reduction of premature beats compared to the drug-free state. Even a single premature ventricular complex may cause a brief burst of sympathetic activity.[36,37] Thus, the finding of a different autonomic balance after antiarrhythmic treatment may be caused not only by the direct 'autonomic' effect of the drug, but also by the concurrent change in the frequency of premature beats and of the attendant reduction in sympathetic reflexes.

Despite these limitations, the potential interest of assessing the effects of different antiarrhythmic drugs on HRV is significant. Although to date no study has specifically addressed this issue in post-MI patients, two related papers deserve discussion.

We have assessed the effects of flecainide, propafenone and amiodarone in patients with chronic ventricular arrhythmia.[38]

Ischemic heart disease (either angina or an MI older than 8 weeks) was present in 74% of the patients. HRV was quantitatively assessed by the number of RR intervals differing from the preceding one more than 50 milliseconds, during a 24-hour Holter recording. This number of counts was significantly reduced both by flecainide (n = 22) and propafenone (n = 17) but was not modified by amiodarone (n = 17); the overall results are shown in Figure 4. The effect on HRV appeared to be reversible after treatment discontinuation and was not related to the presence or absence of arrhythmias. These results, by suggesting a decrease in cardiac vagal activity with flecainide and propafenone, may contribute to understand

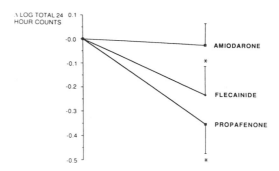

Figure 4. Effect of three antiarrhythmic agents on total 24-hour counts in 56 patients with ventricular arrhythmias. * indicates significant decreases in total 24-hour counts from baseline values in patients treated with flecainide and propafenone. From Zuanetti et al.[38]

the mechanism(s) underlying the atypical proarrhythmic effects not related to the early phase of therapy as suggested also by the Task Force document on CAST.[12]

Lombardi et al[39] have studied the effects of propafenone on HRV, assessed in a 20-minute recording, in 15 patients, 8 of whom had a remote MI, and reached somewhat different conclusions. They suggested that propafenone, because of its β-blocking effect[40] and despite a marked reduction in RR variance, exerted an antiadrenergic effect since it decreased the LF power spectral component much more than the HF one, thus resulting in a significantly smaller LF/HF ratio.

Scopolamine and Heart Rate Variability

Low-dose muscarinic receptor blockers may produce a paradoxical increase in vagal efferent activity, as suggested by a decrease in HR. For atropine, this phenomenon has been recognized since the beginning of the century,[41] but the precise mechanism has not yet been fully clarified.[42] A central effect has been suggested by the increase in vagal efferent activity recorded at cervical level.[43] A peripheral effect is likely to also play a significant role, as compounds that do not cross the blood brain barrier produce a similar bradycardia.[44] At any rate, the vagomimetic effect has been shown to consist in the modulation of neural activity, since it is present in the recipient innervated sinus node but not in the donor, noninnervated, sinus node in patients with a transplanted heart.[45]

Scopolamine has a more prominent central effect compared to atropine.[42] Its transdermal application in healthy, young (22 to 34 years) volunteers, increased mean RR interval by 13% and mean SD by 31%.[46]

Four different articles examining the effects of transdermal scopolamine on indices of vagal activity in patients with a recent MI have recently been published.[47-50] All studies have utilized the same, commercially available, scopolamine patch and none have measured plasma levels of the drug.

Casadei et al[47] have randomized patients to either a scopolamine (n = 17) or a placebo (n = 19) patch 4 days after MI. HRV was derived from 512 normal consecutive RR intervals. The standard deviation of the mean RR interval increased significantly in the scopolamine as compared with the placebo group, as did the power in the HF spectral component, whereas the LF power was not different in the two groups.

We have studied 20 patients (mean age: 59±11 years) in pharmacological washout 14±3 days after MI.[48] HRV was measured during a 15-minute rest ECG recording in baseline conditions, 24 hours after the application of a scopolamine patch and 24 hours after the application of a placebo patch. Whereas placebo had no effect, all the time-domain indices of HRV were significantly increased by scopolamine. Figure 5 shows an example of the time-domain results in one patient, and Figure 6, the mean values observed in the three experimental conditions. The ratio of LF to HF areas of the power spectral analysis was also significantly reduced.

Pedretti et al[49] have administered transdermal scopolamine to 28 patients 2 to 3 weeks after MI, and have compared this effect to that observed in 20 patients subsequently given a placebo patch. Although

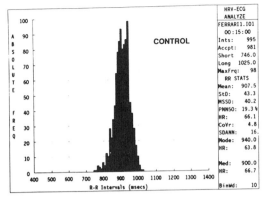

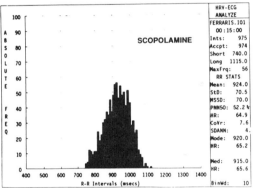

Figure 5. Example of frequency (FREQ) histogram and related time-domain measures in one patient during control conditions (**upper panel**), and scopolamine treatment (**lower panel**). In this patient there was a very modest effect on mean RR interval (Mean) but a marked effect on standard deviation (StD) (+63%), mean squared successive difference (MSSD) (+74%) and pNN50 (+170%). Also shown is: the total number of intervals that occurred during the recording (Ints); the number of those accepted for the analysis (Accpt); the duration of the shortest (Short) and longest (Long) interval; the frequency of occurrence of the most common class of beats (MaxFrq), according to the selected bin width (BinWd, in the example 10 ms); the mode and median (Med) of the distribution; the coefficient of variance (CoVr) and the standard deviation of the 5-min average normal to normal (NN) intervals (SDANN). From De Ferrari et al.[48]

standard deviation of the 24-hour RR interval did not change, MSSD, pNN50 and both LF and HF areas of power spectral analysis significantly increased after scopolamine.

Vybiral et al[50] have randomized 61 male patients to either a scopolamine or a placebo patch and have compared time-domain

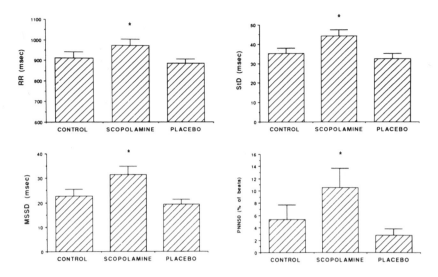

Figure 6. Effect of scopolamine and placebo on the mean sinus cycle (RR), its standard deviation (StD), the mean squared successive interval (MSSD) and pNN50. Bars represent mean ± SEM for each variable. * Analysis of variance for repeated measures for RR (p <0.002), StD (p <0.001) and MSSD (p<0.001), and the Kruskal Wallis test for pNN50 (p <0.001). From De Ferrari et al.[48]

variables derived from the Holter recording during treatment with those derived from the baseline recording. A significant increase was observed in the variables analyzed in the scopolamine group, but not in the placebo group.

The conclusion, derived from the HRV results, of an increased vagal activity induced by scopolamine is strengthened by the study of baroreceptor reflex sensitivity performed in the first three of these four studies. This index of vagal reflexes was uniformly and significantly increased by scopolamine by an extent ranging from 42% to 98%. Table 1 summarizes the main characteristics and results of the studies with scopolamine after MI. Notable is the very limited incidence of side effects observed in the studies. No patches had to be removed before the termination of the study.

These four studies indicate that pharmacological modulation of neural activity with scopolamine may effectively increase vagal activity shortly after MI. Although this is a stimulating area of investigation in the search of new strategies for the prevention of sudden death, neither the efficacy during a long-term treatment, nor the relation between the increase in indices of vagal activity and the actual decrease in susceptibility to malignant arrhythmias have been assessed.

The need for caution, before excessive expectations are generated on the basis of moderate increases in HRV, comes from experiments performed in a post-MI animal model for sudden death[29] in which several potentially antifibrillatory interventions have been tested.[6,7,31,51] Intravenous scopolamine, at a dose shown to increase significantly HRV, was unable to provide protection from ventricular fibrillation in six of the seven dogs tested.[51a] This suggests that the acute neural modulation by scopolamine is insufficient to protect from ventricular fibrillation induced by acute myocardial ischemia during exercise.

Table 1

	Casadei	De Ferrari	Pedretti	Vybiral
Pts studied with scopolamine	17	20	18	28
Age (yrs)	59 ± 8	59 ± 11	55 ± 9*	58 ± 10
Days after MI	4 ± 1	14 ± 3	15–21*	6 (median)
Anterior MI	76%	40%	58%*	47%
LVEF	n.a.	52 ± 12%	45 ± 13%*	45 ± 16%
Pharmacological washout	no	yes	from BB/Dig/Ca ant/AA	no
ECG recording	15 min°	15 min	24 hours	24 hours
Mean RR change	+13%	+7%	+4%	+6%
Mean SD change	+72%	+25%	+3% (ns)	+34%
Mean MSSD change	n.a.	+38%	+16%	+26%
Mean pNN50 change	n.a.	+100%	+40%	n.a.
LF	+72% (ns)	n.a.	+7%**	n.a.
HF	+370%	n.a.	+6%**	n.a.
LF/HF ratio	n.a.	−24%	n.a.	n.a.
Mean BRS change	+98%	+42%	+67%	n.a.

n.a. = data not available from the manuscript; ° = 512 beats were analyzed

*These data refer to a wider group composed of 41 patients

**Log units

All the changes were statistically significant (p < 0.05), except where "ns" is marked.

BB = Beta-blockers; Dig = Digoxin; Ca ant = Calcium antagonists; AA = Antiarrhythmic drugs

Thrombolysis and Heart Rate Variability

Thrombolysis is nowadays performed in the majority of post-MI patients, as indicated by the growing percentages observed in ongoing clinical trials; as an example, 71% of the patients enrolled in EMIAT (European Myocardial Infarction Amiodarone Trial) have undergone thrombolysis.[52] It becomes, therefore, necessary to know if this almost routine intervention alters a parameter with elevated prognostic value such as HRV.

Very recently, Zabel et al reported the effect of thrombolysis on HRV, measured as the proportion of adjacent RR intervals different by more than 50 milliseconds (pNN50), in 95 patients with acute MI.[53] Coronary angiography for assessment of the status of coronary perfusion was performed in all patients 90 minutes after onset of thrombolytic therapy and repeated after 24 hours. Patency of the infarct-related artery was observed in 74 (78%) patients, whereas in 21 patients the infarct-related artery was occluded; accordingly, the analysis was made separately for the two groups. For patients with coronary artery patency after 90 minutes, pNN50 was 13±12% for the first hour compared to 7±7% for patients without successful reperfusion; despite considerable overlap, this difference reached statistical significance (p = 0.024). However, this difference was no longer significant when the entire first 24 hours were analyzed and was actually reversed, as pNN50 was somewhat greater among the patients with an occluded infarct-related artery (11±11% versus 9±8%, NS). The effect of thrombolysis on pNN50 was independent of infarct location.

These results were interpreted by Zabel et al as suggesting that successful thrombolysis results in a higher vagal tone during the early hours of MI as compared to failed reperfusion. An alternate explanation would be that the relief from acute myocardial ischemia produced by successful thrombolysis is accompanied not only by reflex increases in vagal activity, but also by a cessation of reflex sympathetic excitation[54] and that this facilitates the appearance of longer cycles resulting in an increase in pNN50. We also believe that the lack of difference in pNN50 1-day post-MI between patients with and without successful reperfusion suggests strongly that the prognostic value of HRV in post-MI patients is not influenced by thrombolysis.

Exercise Training and Heart Rate Variability

Exercise training has been suggested to decrease cardiovascular mortality and sudden cardiac death.[55] In addition to improving cardiovascular performance, regular exercise training is also thought to be capable of modifying the autonomic balance toward a condition of relative parasympathetic dominance.

Clinical Studies

There is an amazing paucity of clinical studies on the effect of exercise training on HRV after an MI. La Rovere et al[56] randomized 22 patients with a recent MI to enter or not in a 4-week exercise training program. In resting conditions, patients of both groups showed a clearly predominant LF component at spectral analysis. Head-up tilt was associated with a reduction in mean RR, but with no change in the spectral profile. After the intervention, no difference was observed in the two groups of patients in resting conditions, while a puzzling difference was reported in response to tilting. While the untrained patients did not modify their spectral profile, the trained ones increased the LF component and decreased the HF component. Although, at first glance this may appear the opposite of what one would have expected. The authors suggest that the different response to tilt may indicate a restoration toward a normal autonomic reflex function. They also propose that the absence of an effect in resting conditions may be related to an insufficient duration or intensity of the training program, a suggestion that raises questions on the entire study.

The modesty of the effect observed on HRV is in contrast with the marked changes reported a few years ago by La Rovere et al[57] when the parameter under study was a marker of vagal reflexes, ie, baroreflex sensitivity (BRS). Seventy patients were studied 1 month post-MI, and a case-control study was formed by matching them for BRS, left ventricular ejection fraction, and site of infarction. The patients were randomized to enter or not a 4-week endurance program. At 2 months after infarction, BRS had increased by 27% (from 7.8±4.0 to 10.4±5.3 ms/mm Hg, p <0.001) among the trained patients, whereas it did not change (+1.5%) among the controls. This study showed that in man a nonpharmacological intervention, such as exercise, can improve the autonomic balance as indicated by the increase in BRS.

In patients with chronic heart failure, eight weeks of exercise training produced an overall increase of both SD of the RR interval and HF component, and a decrease of the LF component in 10 of the 15 subjects.[57a]

Experimental Studies

A very recent experimental study, designed to assess the effects of exercise training on markers of vagal activity, is highly relevant because it simultaneously provides information on changes in cardiac electrical stability. Seven conscious dogs, without MI but documented to be at high risk by the occurrence of ventricular fibrillation during acute myocardial ischemia were randomly assigned to 6 weeks of either daily exercise training or cage rest followed by exercise training.[10] After 6 weeks of training, HRV (standard deviation of 25 minutes of RR interval recording) increased by 74% and BRS increased by 69%. These significant changes in markers of vagal activity were accompanied by a 44% increase in the repetitive ex-

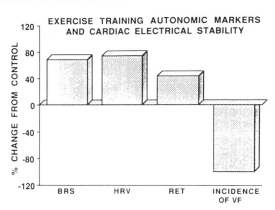

Figure 7. Bar graph illustrating the percent change observed after exercise training in BRS (HRV, standard deviation of the mean RR intervals), repetitive extrasystole threshold (RET), and incidence of ventricular fibrillation (VF) during the exercise and ischemia test in seven dogs. Exercise training produced a concomitant increase in BRS, HRV, and RET and protected all animals from recurrence of VF. From Hull et al.[10]

trasystole threshold, a marker of ventricular electrical stability and, more importantly, by the disappearance of ventricular fibrillation during a new trial of acute myocardial ischemia during an exercise stress test (Figure 7).

This study suggested, for the first time, that regular exercise, even in individuals with a normal heart, may reduce the risk of malignant arrhythmias should they undergo acute myocardial ischemia. The results are in full agreement with what we had previously demonstrated in post-MI dogs using only BRS as a marker of vagal activity.[9]

The importance of this finding, as this chapter is concerned, lies in the fact that at this time it is the only documentation of an increase in HRV induced by an intervention which is actually accompanied by a simultaneous decrease in the susceptibility to ventricular fibrillation.

Conclusion

The rationale for the attempts to increase HRV in post-MI patients rests on the multiple evidence that the risk for cardiac mortality and sudden death is higher among individuals with signs of decreased vagal activity. A major limitation is represented by the fact that the degree of increase in vagal activity that may produce antifibrillatory effects is still unknown. So far, only one study has provided the simultaneous documentation of an increase in HRV associated with protection from ventricular fibrillation.[10] Too many of the existing reports describe, with variable degrees of enthusiasm, modest changes in HRV without any evidence that these variations are accompanied by a truly protective effect.

We have been early proponents[58-60] of the efforts to augment vagal activity with the goal of reducing ischemia-induced malignant arrhythmias, and we still share[5,61] this nowadays fashionable concept.[62] However, just for this reason it seems appropriate to call for caution before attributing excessive importance to changes in 'markers' of vagal activity in the absence of clearcut evidence for a causal relationship with an antifibrillatory effect.

References

1. Kleiger RE, Miller JP, Bigger JT Jr, et al. Decreased heart rate variability and its association with increased mortality after acute myocardial infarction. Am J Cardiol 1987; 59:256-262.
2. Farrell TG, Bashir Y, Cripps T, et al. Risk stratification for arrhythmic events in postinfarction patients based on heart rate variability, ambulatory electrocardiographic variables and the signal-averaged electrocardiogram. J Am Coll Cardiol 1991; 18:687-697.
3. Algra A, Tijssen JGP, Roelandt JRTC, et al. Heart rate variability from 24-hour electrocardiography and the 2-year risk for sudden death. Circulation 1993; 88:180-185.
4. Levy MN, Schwartz PJ. Vagal Control of the Heart: Experimental Basis and Clinical Implications. Armonk, NY: Futura Publishing Co., 1994; 644.
5. De Ferrari GM, Vanoli E, Schwartz PJ. Vagal activity and ventricular fibrillation. In: Levy MN, Schwartz PJ (eds). Vagal Control of the Heart: Experimental Basis and Clinical Implications. Armonk, NY: Futura Publishing Co., 1994; 613-636.
6. Vanoli E, De Ferrari GM, Stramba-Badiale M, et al. Vagal stimulation and prevention of sudden death in conscious dogs with a healed myocardial infarction. Circ Res 1991; 68:1471-1481.
7. De Ferrari GM, Salvati P, Grossoni M, et al. Pharmacologic modulation of the autonomic nervous system in the prevention of sudden cardiac death. A study with propranolol, methacholine and oxotremorine in conscious dogs with a healed myocardial infarction. J Am Coll Cardiol 1993; 22:283-290.
8. De Ferrari GM, Vanoli E, Curcuruto P, et al. Prevention of life-threatening arrhythmias by pharmacologic stimulation of the muscarinic receptors with oxotremorine. Am Heart J 1992; 124:883-890.
9. Billman GE, Schwartz PJ, Stone HL. The effects of daily exercise on susceptibility to sudden cardiac death. Circulation 1984; 69:1182-1189.
10. Hull SS Jr, Vanoli E, Adamson PB, et al. Exercise training confers anticipatory protection from sudden death during acute myocardial ischemia. Circulation 1994; 89:548-552.
11. De Ferrari GM, Vanoli E, Stramba-Badiale M, et al. Vagal reflexes and survival during acute myocardial ischemia in conscious dogs with a healed myocardial infarction. Am J Physiol 1991; 261:H63-H69.
12. Task Force of the Working Group on Arrhythmias of the European Society of Cardiology (Akhtar M, Breithardt G, Camm AJ, et al). CAST and beyond. Implications of the Cardiac Arrhythmia Suppression Trial. Eur Heart J 1990; 11:194-199 and Circulation 1990; 81:1123-1127.
13. Bigger JT Jr, Fleiss JL, Kleiger J, et al. The relationship among ventricular arrhythmias, left ventricular dysfunction, and mortality in the two years after myocardial infarction. Circulation 1984; 69:250-258.
14. Ruberman W, Weinblatt E, Goldberg JD, et al. Ventricular premature beats and mortality after myocardial infarction. N Engl J Med 1977; 297:750-757.
15. Luu M, Stevenson WG, Stevenson LW, et al. Diverse mechanisms of unexpected cardiac arrest in advanced heart failure. Circulation 1989; 80:1675-1680.
16. Yusuf S, Peto R, Lewis J, et al. Beta blockade during and after myocardial infarction. An overview of the randomized trials. Prog Cardiovasc Dis 1985; 27:335-371.
17. Molgaard H, Mickley H, Pless P, et al. Effects of metoprolol on heart rate variability in survivors of acute myocardial infarction. Am J Cardiol 1993; 71:1357-1359.
18. Sandrone G, Mortara A, Torzillo D, et al. Effects of β-blockers (atenolol or metoprolol)

on heart rate variability after acute myocardial infarction. Am J Cardiol 1994; 74:340-345.

19. Bigger JT, Fleiss JL, Rolnitzky LM, et al. Time course of recovery of heart period variability after myocardial infarction. J Am Coll Cardiol 1991; 18:1643-1649.

20. Bigger JT Jr, Fleiss JL, Rolnitzky LM, et al. Frequency domain measures of heart period variability and mortality after myocardial infarction. Circulation 1992; 85:164-171.

21. Muller JE, Stone PH, Turi ZG, et al. Circadian variation in the frequency of onset of acute myocardial infarction. N Engl J Med 1985; 313:1315-1322.

22. Schwartz PJ, Zaza A, Pala M, et al. Baroreflex sensitivity and its evolution during the first year after a myocardial infarction. J Am Coll Cardiol 1988; 12:629-636.

23. Osculati G, Grassi G, Giannattasio C, et al. Early alterations of the baroreceptor control of heart rate in patients with acute myocardial infarction. Circulation 1990; 81:939-948.

24. Cook JR, Bigger JT, Kleiger RE, et al. Effect of atenolol and diltiazem on heart period variability in normal persons. J Am Coll Cardiol 1991; 17:480-484.

25. Lombardi F, Sandrone G, Pernpruner S, et al. Heart rate variability as an index of sympathovagal interaction after acute myocardial infarction. Am J Cardiol 1987; 60:1239-1245.

26. Mazzuero G, Lanfranchi P, Colombo R, et al. Long-term adaptation of 24-h heart rate variability after myocardial infarction. Chest 1992; 101:304S-308S.

27. Kleiger RE, Bigger JT, Bosner MS, et al. Stability over time of variables measuring heart rate variability in normal subjects. Am J Cardiol 1991; 68:626-630.

28. Adamson PB, Huang MH, Vanoli E, et al. Unexpected interaction between β-adrenergic blockade and heart rate variability before and after myocardial infarction: a longitudinal study in dogs at high and low risk for sudden death. Circulation 1994; 90:976-982.

29. Schwartz PJ, Billman GE, Stone HL. Autonomic mechanisms in ventricular fibrillation induced by myocardial ischemia during exercise in dogs with a healed myocardial infarction. An experimental preparation for sudden cardiac death. Circulation 1984; 69:780-790.

30. Hull SS Jr, Evans AR, Vanoli E, et al. Heart rate variability before and after myocardial infarction in conscious dogs at high and low risk of sudden death. J Am Coll Cardiol 1990; 16:1475-1480.

31. Vanoli E, Hull SS Jr, Foreman RD, et al. Alpha₁ adrenergic blockade and sudden cardiac death. J Cardiovasc Electrophysiol 1994; 5:76-89.

32. Myerburg RJ, Kessler KM, Cox MM, et al. Reversal of proarrhythmic effects of flecainide acetate and encainide hydrochloride by propranolol. Circulation 1989; 80:1571-1579.

33. Stramba-Badiale M, Lazzarotti M, Facchini M, et al. Malignant arrhythmias and acute myocardial ischemia: interaction between flecainide and autonomic nervous system. Am Heart J 1994. In press.

34. Benditt DG, Milstein S, Goldstein M, et al. Sinus node dysfunction: pathophysiology, clinical features, evaluation, and treatment. In: Zipes DP, Jalife J. Cardiac Electrophysiology. From Cell to Bedside. Philadelphia, Pa: W.B. Saunders Co, 1990; 708-734.

35. Josephson ME. Sinus node function. In: Josephson ME (ed). Clinical Cardiac Electrophysiology. Philadelphia, Pa: Lea & Febiger, 1993; 71-95.

36. Herre JM, Thames MD. Responses of sympathetic nerves to programmed ventricular stimulation. J Am Coll Cardiol 1987; 9:147-153.

37. Lombardi F, Gnecchi-Ruscone T, Malliani A. Premature ventricular contraction and reflex sympathetic activation in cats. Cardiovasc Res 1989; 23:205-212.

38. Zuanetti G, Latini R, Neilson JMM, et al. Heart rate variability in patients with ventricular arrhythmias: effect of antiarrhythmic drugs. J Am Coll Cardiol 1991; 17:604-612.

39. Lombardi F, Torzillo D, Sandrone G, et al. Beta-blocking effect of propafenone based on spectral analysis of heart rate variability. Am J Cardiol 1992; 70:1028-1034.

40. Malfatto G, Pessano P, Zaza A, et al. Experimental evidence for beta-adrenergic blocking properties of propafenone and for their potential clinical relevance. Eur Heart J 1993; 14:1253-1257.

41. Wilson FN. The production of atrioventricular rhythm in man after the administration of atropine. Arch Intern Med 1915; 16:989-1007.

42. De Ferrari GM, Zaza A. Drugs acting on cholinergic receptors. In: Singh BN, Dzau VJ, Van Houtten P, et al (eds). Cardiovascular Pharmacology and Therapeutics. New York, NY: Churchill Livingstone, 1993; 125-144.

43. Katona PG, Lipson D, Dauchot PJ. Opposing central and peripheral effects of atropine on parasympathetic cardiac control. Am J Physiol 1977; 232:H146-H151.

44. Kottmeier CA, Gravenstein JS. The parasympathomimetic activity of atropine and atropine methylbromide. Anesthesiology 1968; 29:1125-1133.

45. Epstein AE, Hirschowitz BI, Kirklin JK, et al. Evidence for a central site of action to explain the negative chronotropic effect of atropine: studies on the human transplanted heart. J Am Coll Cardiol 1990; 15:1610-1617.

46. Dibner-Dunlap ME, Eckberg DL, Magid NM, et al. The long-term increase of baseline and reflexly augmented levels of human vagal-cardiac activity induced by scopolamine. Circulation 1985; 71:797-804.

47. Casadei B, Pipilis A, Sessa F, et al. Low doses of scopolamine increase cardiac vagal tone in the acute phase of myocardial infarction. Circulation 1993; 88:353-357.

48. De Ferrari GM, Mantica M, Vanoli E, et al. Scopolamine increases vagal tone and vagal reflexes in patients after myocardial infarction. J Am Coll Cardiol 1993; 22:1327-1334.

49. Pedretti R, Colombo E, Sarzi Braga S, et al. Influence of transdermal scopolamine on cardiac sympathovagal interaction after acute myocardial infarction. Am J Cardiol 1993; 72:384-392.

50. Vybiral T, Glaeser DH, Morris G, et al. Effects of low-dose transdermal scopolamine on heart rate variability after myocardial infarction. J Am Coll Cardiol 1993; 22:1320-1326.

51. Vanoli E, Hull SS Jr, Adamson PB, Foreman RD, Schwartz PJ: K+ channel blockade in the prevention of ventricular fibrillation due to acute ischemia and enhanced sympathetic activity. J Cardiovasc Pharmacol (In press).

51a. Hull SS Jr, Vanoli E, Adamson PB, De Ferrari GM, Foreman RD, Schwartz PJ: Do increases in markers of vagal activity imply protection from sudden death? The case of scopolamine. Circulation (In press).

52. Schwartz PJ, Camm AJ, Frangin G, et al. Does amiodarone reduce sudden death and cardiac mortality after myocardial infarction? The European Myocardial Infarct Amiodarone Trial (E.M.I.A.T.). Eur Heart J 1994; 15:620-624.

53. Zabel M, Klingenheben T, Hohnloser SH. Changes in autonomic tone following thrombolytic therapy for acute myocardial infarction: assessment by analysis of heart rate variability. J Cardiovasc Electrophysiol 1994; 5:211-218.

54. Malliani A, Schwartz PJ, Zanchetti A. A sympathetic reflex elicited by experimental coronary occlusion. Am J Physiol 1969; 217:703-709.

55. O'Connor GT, Buring JE, Yusuf S, et al. An overview of randomized trials of rehabilitation with exercise after myocardial infarction. Circulation 1989; 80:234-244.

56. La Rovere MT, Mortara A, Sandrone G, et al. Autonomic nervous system adaptations to short-term exercise training. Chest 1992; 101:299S-303S.

57. La Rovere MT, Mortara A, Cobelli F, et al. Baroreflex sensitivity improvement after physical training in post myocardial infarction patients. Eur Heart J 1989; 10(suppl):126. Abstract.

57a. Coats AJS, Adamopoulos S, Radaelli A, McCance A, Meyer TE, Bernardi L, Solda PL, Davey P, Ormerod O, Forfar C, Conway J, Sleight P: Controlled trial of physical training in chronic heart failure. Circulation 1992; 85:2119-2131.

58. Schwartz PJ, Stone HL. The analysis and modulation of autonomic reflexes in the prediction and prevention of sudden death. In: Zipes DP, Jalife J (eds). Cardiac Electrophysiology and Arrhythmias. Orlando, Fla: Grune & Stratton, Inc., 1985; 165-176.

59. Schwartz PJ. Manipulation of the autonomic nervous system in the prevention of sudden cardiac death. In: Brugada P, Wellens HJJ (eds). Cardiac Arrhythmias: Where to Go From Here? Mount Kisco, NY: Futura Publishing Co., Inc., 1987; 741-765.

60. Schwartz PJ. Cardiac innervation and sudden death: new strategies for prevention. In: Rosen MR, Palti Y (eds). Lethal Arrhythmias Resulting From Myocardial Ischemia and Infarction. Boston, Ma: Kluwer Academic Publishers, 1989; 293-309.

61. Schwartz PJ, La Rovere MT, Vanoli E. Autonomic nervous system and sudden cardiac death. Experimental basis and clinical observations for post-myocardial infarction risk stratification. Circulation 1992; 85(suppl I):I77-I91.

62. Sneddon JF, Bashir Y, Ward DE. Vagal stimulation after myocardial infarction: accentuating the positive. J Am Coll Cardiol 1993; 22:1335-1337.

Chapter 32

Changes of Heart Rate Variability Preceding Ventricular Arrhythmias

Tomas Vybiral, Donald H. Glaeser

Sudden cardiac death accounts for over 500,000 fatalities each year in the United States with ventricular fibrillation being the main cause.[1] Recent studies have pointed out that a decrease in heart rate variability (HRV) is an independent long-term statistical predictor of overall and sudden arrhythmic mortality after myocardial infarction (MI).[2-4] The prevailing hypothesis is that because HRV is dependent on intact neurocardiac autonomic regulation, a decrease in HRV may reflect the autonomic dysfunction associated with cardiac electrical instability. Adrenergic hyperactivity and/or lack of presumably protective parasympathetic autonomic tone are the purported pathophysiological mechanisms of such lethal arrhythmogenesis.[5,6] However, while decreased HRV may represent a long-term predictor of adverse outcome, it remains unclear whether in fact the same holds true with regard to short-term prediction. In other words, the ability of HRV measures to identify the single patient who will in fact suffer ventricular arrhythmia and sudden death is

poorly defined, and more importantly, none of the HRV measures has consistently been shown to forecast the exact time of sudden death. It is the aim of this chapter not only to summarize the current body of knowledge on the subject of HRV and ventricular arrhythmias, but also to point out avenues for potential future investigation on this important clinical subject.

The relationship between HRV and ventricular arrhythmias has been studied extensively in the post-MI population. In a series of reports since 1987, Kleiger, Bigger and their coworkers have not only established the independent value of time-domain indices of HRV to predict *overall mortality* after MI, but have also suggested that alterations at the very low-frequency (VLF) end of the 24-hour interbeat interval power spectrum may, in fact predict *arrhythmic death*.[2,7] Similarly, Odemuyiwa and colleagues proposed that their nonspectral HRV index may also predict important postinfarction arrhythmic complications.[8] More recently, Algra and coworkers have

From: Malik M., Camm AJ (eds.): *Heart Rate Variability*. Armonk, NY. Futura Publishing Company, Inc., © 1995.

essentially confirmed these observations in a large, independent patient cohort.[4] Bigger and colleagues subsequently defined the long-term natural history of HRV after MI and demonstrated that, even when measured at least 1 year after an MI, HRV was still predictive of adverse outcome.[9-11] Van-Hoogenhuyze and his coworkers have independently observed during long-term follow-up of cardiac patients that HRV was declining to very low values in those subjects who also ultimately suffered premature, presumably sudden, arrhythmic cardiac death.[12] In applying these observations to the ultimately highest risk patient population, Vybiral and colleagues evaluated a cohort of 24 subjects who suffered ventricular fibrillation while they had their heartbeat monitored with a Holter monitor.[13] Based upon the previous observations, they hypothesized that conventional, time-domain indices of HRV decrease significantly during the hours preceding ventricular fibrillation, and that HRV is lower in patients with imminent ventricular fbrillation as compared to clinically matched patients with only nonsustained ventricular tachycardia. Global standard deviation, standard deviation over 5-minute data segments and the mean of 5-minute standard deviations were calculated for all recordings. Somewhat surprisingly, HRV parameters did not differ between the ventricular fibrillation patient group and the control group. Specifically, the median global standard deviation was, at 76 milliseconds, considerably higher than the value of 50 milliseconds shown by Kleiger[2] to distinguish post-MI patients with poor and good long-term survival. Figure 1 compares 1-hour, 5-minute normal-to-normal interval means during the first (A) and the last (B) hour of the Holter ambulatory electrocardiographic recording of subjects with ventricular fibrillation. This comparison shows that there was no consistent downward trend in HRV during the hour preceding ventricular fibrillation (p = 0.49). Based upon the observation of Bigger and colleagues, it may be argued that the likeliest changes in HRV ought to be ex-

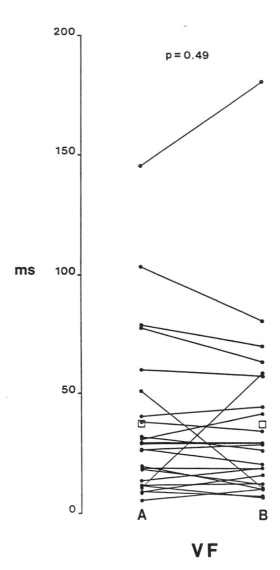

Figure 1. Comparison of 1-hour, 5-minute normal-to-normal interbeat interval means (HRV) during the first (A) and the last (B) hour of the Holter ambulatory electrocardiographic recording in patients with ventricular fibrillation (VF). Data are given as median values (25th, 75th percentile). There is no difference in HRV between an early (A = 0.3 [0.1] hour from the beginning of the recording) and a late episode (B = 1.8 [1.15, 3.1] hour immediately preceding ventricular fibrillation). A: 27.9[13,49] ms; B: 27.2[15,54] ms. Median difference = 0.7 ms (95% confidence limits, -3.88, 5.8: p = 0.49, Wilcoxon signed rank-sum test). Boxes indicate median values.

pected by applying frequency-domain analysis.[7] Specifically, they had shown that a decrease in the VLF power band (0.003 to 0.04 Hz) in postinfarction Holter recordings was strongly predictive of arrhythmic death. In support of this hypothesis, Huikuri and coworkers have examined HRV in the frequency domain of patients with coronary artery disease and ventricular arrhythmias, and found that all spectral components of HRV are decreased during the hour preceding spontaneous episodes of sustained ventricular tachycardia on Holter recordings.[14] They hypothesized that such decline may reflect subtle neuro-autonomic perturbations that can facilitate the perpetuation of these arrhythmias. In contrast, Cerquetani and colleagues have performed frequency analysis of HRV in eight patients with chronic ischemic heart disease and heart failure and found that the VLF power significantly *increased* immediately preceding nonsustained ventricular tachycardia episodes, while other parts of the spectrum remained stable.[15] Palacios and colleagues have similarly applied frequency-domain analysis in the coronary care unit and demonstrated that decreased low-frequency (LF) power, measured over 1-hour data periods, is predictive of ventricular tachyarrhythmias in the coronary care unit during acute myocardial infarction.[16] In contrast, Ben-Haim and coworkers demonstrated in dogs that increased LF power of interbeat intervals (as measured in 30-minute data segments) precedes ventricular fibrillation in an acute ischemic model.[17] In a series of elegantly designed animal studies, Hull and coworkers demonstrated (by spectral and nonspectral techniques) that intact HRV—presumably representing preserved cardiac sympatho-vagal equilibrium—is of paramount importance to the electrical stability of the canine heart.[18,19] Finally, in a recent case report, Carter and colleagues pointed out increased sympathetic activity as assessed by frequency-domain analysis of HRV preceding an episode of Torsades de Pointes.[20] Interestingly, and in accord with the findings of Vybiral and colleagues,[13] the

corresponding time-domain analysis again did not reach the very low values suggested by Kleiger and collegues to represent the highest risk (<50 milliseconds).[2] Nevertheless, and in spite of its apparent promise, the application of spectral analysis to Holter ambulatory ECG data remains problematic because of unresolved questions relative to optimal data set size, nonstationariness, the type of algorithm and, most importantly, the presence of ectopic beats.

Skinner and Vybiral, in a novel approach, recognized that nonstationarities in the interbeat-interval time series may mask subtle and short-lived autonomic transients that may be important to arrhythmogenesis. They developed an algorithm for the correlation dimension PD2 of the heartbeat that is sufficiently sensitive for the detection of nonlinear and transient fluctuations within the heartbeat time series. This algorithm was initially applied to the study of neurocardiac reflex behavior in the conscious pig during experimental MI. After occlusion of the left anterior descending coronary artery, the mean PD2 of the interbeat intervals rapidly declined to very low values (1.0 dimensions) minutes before ventricular fibrillation. Occlusions that did not result in ventricular fibrillation did not produce the low dimensional shifts.[21] Applying this dimensional analysis of HRV to human data, Skinner and Vybiral demonstrated similar findings in 34 cardiac patients who suffered ventricular fibrillation while their heartbeat was monitored with a Holter recorder. The average lowest PD2 value of patients who suffered ventricular fibrillation reached 0.8 dimensions, while the control subjects (cardiac patients without ventricular fibrillation) did not exhibit PD2 values below 1.3 dimensions (p = 0.001). Figure 2 shows a composite of RR intervals (top) and PD2 (bottom) in a subject who suffered ventricular fibrillation (VF) at the end of the recording. Note that the tracing is a composite of three 13-minute data segments from the beginning, the middle and the end of the Holter tape. A downward drift of PD2 preceding ventricular fibrillation toward the

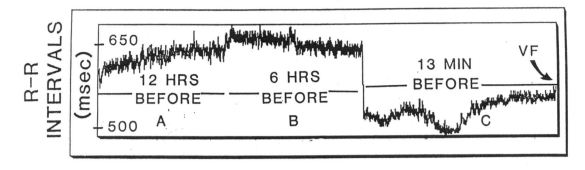

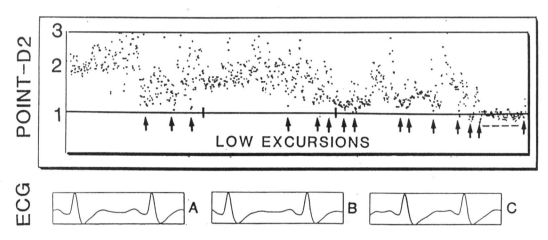

Figure 2. Interbeat (RR) intervals **(upper panel)** and corresponding PD2 series **(lower panel)** for three time-epochs (A,B, and C) from a subject who died of ventricular fibrillation (VF: large arrow) at the end of epoch C, while wearing a Holter electrocardiographic monitor. Small arrows indicate low PD2 excursions that occur throughout all three time-epochs, hours preceding VF.

value of 1.0 dimensions is apparent. However, and more importantly, not only did PD2 tend to decline to very low values immediately preceding ventricular fibrillation in the majority of the subjects, but transient low dimensional shifts in heart rate behavior were already detectable at the beginning of the recording (mean tape length: 12 hours).[22,23] Figure 3 illustrates continuous interbeat intervals and PD2 in a Holter recording of another subject with ventricular fibrillation at the end of the recording. Again, note the transient low dimensional shifts in PD2 (marked by arrows) throughout the entire recording, hours before ventricular fibrillation. These results thus suggest that not only may PD2 serve as a predictor of sudden cardiac death, but that, for the first time, such dimensional analysis of HRV may provide important insight into the *exact time of occurrence of impending ventricular fibrillation in a specifc subject*.

Interestingly, HRV appears to exert predictive power only in the setting of established heart disease, as illustrated by Gill and colleagues who examined 20 patients with apparently normal hearts and ventricular tachycardia, and found HRV values not substantially different from those measured in healthy individuals.[24] Also, investigators have come to recognize that, while HRV may be a predictor of mortality and ventric-

24–HR STUDY OF PD2

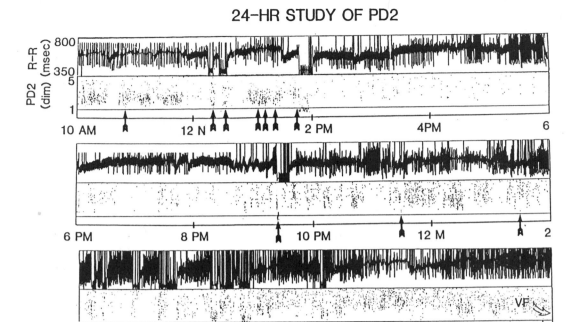

Figure 3. Full-length disclosure of interbeat intervals **(upper panel)** and corresponding PD2 series **(lower panel)** derived from a Holter electrocardiographic recording of another subject with ventricular fibrillation at the end of the recording **(large arrow)**. Black arrows indicate low PD2 excursions throughout the hours preceding VF.

ular arrhythmias after MI, its individual predictive accuracy is not substantially better than that of more conventional indicators of risk, such as left ventricular function, rate and complexity of ventricular arrhythmias and extent of coronary artery disease. Farrell, Odemuyiwa, Pedretti and colleagues have pointed out that probably the best predictive accuracy after MI may be achieved by combining HRV measures with left ventricular ejection fraction and signal-averaged electrocardiography.[25-27] In a preliminary study, Vybiral and coworkers measured short-term time- and frequency-domain parameters of HRV parameters in 53 cardiac patients referred for evaluation of symptomatic ventricular tachycardia.[28] Figure 4 illustrates that in their cohort the probability of inducing sustained ventricular tachycardia during invasive programmed ventricular stimulation decreased

with higher values in high-frequency (HF) power of the interbeat-interval spectrum (P1535: 0.15 to 0.35 Hz band of the RR interval power spectrum, calculated from 5-minute recordings). Since the HF end of the spectrum is largely controlled by the input of the vagus nerve on the heart, these findings are consistent with an important role of the cardiac parasympathetic nervous system in the electrical stabilization of the heart. In this study, the diagnosis of coronary artery disease, age, and left ventricular ejection fraction were the strongest univariate predictors of inducibility of monomorphic ventricular tachycardia during programmed electrical stimulation, but their individual and combined predictive accuracy did not exceed 90%. However, by including them with the HRV measures into a multivariate regression model, complete separation of inducible from noninducible

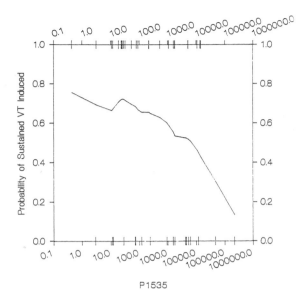

Effect of .15-.35 on Inducibility
Nonparametric Regression Curve

P1535

Figure 4. Cummulative power within the 0.15 to 0.35 Hz spectral band of a 5-minute interbeat interval data segment (acquired in the supine position during resting condition) (P1535, abscissa, arbitrary units on logarhythmic scale) correlates inversely with the calculated probability of inducibility of sustained ventricular tachycardia during programmed ventricular stimulation (ordinate).

subjects was achieved. Figure 5 illustrates these findings by plotting classification accuracy (ordinate) as a function of cutpoint probability (abscissa). The probability of being inducible for ventricular tachycardia is calculated for each individual based upon the regression equation.[28] For each cutpoint along the probability scale (ranging from 0.0 to 1.0), the classification accuracy with respect to predicting VT inducibility was determined. Inducible (top) and noninducible (bottom) subjects are listed separately. A probability range between 0.35 and 0.52 yields 100% separation of inducible and noninducible subjects, since no subject had a probability between 0.35 to 0.52. These findings are in accord with the observations of Magid, Ahmed and colleagues, that long-term prognosis, as assessed by inducibility of monomorphic ventricular tachycardia in high-risk subjects, parallels the assessment of prognosis based upon HRV alone.[29,30] In contrast, Farrell and coworkers, and Pedretti and colleagues failed to derive any additional benefit from HRV analysis, as compared to baroreflex sensitivity in the risk stratification of postinfarction patients with regard to inducibility of sustained ventricular tachycardia.[31,32]

In summary, in light of the recent emphasis on *noninvasive management* of high-risk cardiac patients with ventricular arrhythmias and mindful of our era of cost containment, the potential clinical importance of the young field of HRV analysis in its various applications lies in the exciting prospect for *identifying and better defining such high-risk subjects noninvasively*.

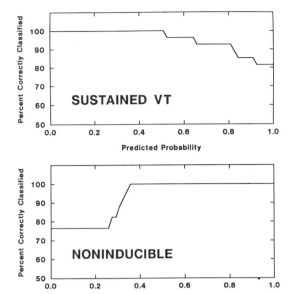

Figure 5. Classification accuracy (ordinate) as a function of Cutpoint in predicted probability (abscissa). The probability of being inducible for sustained monomorphic ventricular tachycardia (SUSTAINED VT, **top graph**), and no being inducibile (NONINDUCIBLE, **bottom graph**) is calculated for each individual based upon a regression equation. For each cutpoint along the preducted probability scale (ranging from 0.0 to 1.0), the classification accuracy with respect to predicting inducibility/noninducibility is determined. Inducible **(top graph)** and noninducible **(bottom graph)** subjects are listed separately. A probability range between 0.35 and 0.52 yields 100% separation of inducible and noninducible subjects, since no subject had a probability between 0.35 and 0.52.

References

1. Rapaport E. Sudden cardiac death. Am J Cardiol 1988; 62(suppl):3-6.
2. Kleiger RE, Miller JP, Krone RJ, et al. Decreased heart rate variability and its association with increased mortality after myocardial infarction. Am J Cardiol 1987; 59:256-262.
3. Cripps TR, Malik M, Farrell TG, et al. Prognostic value of reduced heart rate variability after myocardial infarction: clinical evaluation of a new analysis method. Br Heart J 1991; 64:14-19.
4. Algra A, Tijssen JGP, Roelandt JRTC, et al. Heart rate variability from 24-hour electrocardiography and the 2-year risk for sudden death. Circulation 1993; 88:180-185.
5. Pagani M, Lombardi F, Guzzetti S, et al. Power spectral analysis of heart rate and blood pressure variabilities as a marker of sympatho-vagal interaction in man and conscious dog. Circ Res 1986; 59:178-193.
6. Schwartz PJ, La Rovere MT, Vanoli E. Autonomic nervous system and sudden cardiac death. Circulation 1992; 85(suppl):I77-91.
7. Bigger JT, Fleiss JL, Steinman RC, et al. Frequency domain measures of heart period variability and mortality after myocardial infarction. Circulation 1992; 85:164-171.
8. Odemuyiwa O, Malik M, Farrell T, et al. Comparison of the predictive characteristics of heart rate variability index and left ventricular ejection fraction for all-cause mortality, arrhythmic events and sudden death after acute myocardial infarction. Am J Cardiol 1991; 68:434-439.
9. Bigger JT, Fleiss JL, Rolnitzky L, et al. Stability over time of heart period variability in patients with previous myocardial infarction and ventricular arrhythmias. Am J Cardiol 1992; 69:718-723.
10. Bigger JT, Fleiss JL, Rolnitzky LM, et al. Time course of recovery of heart period variability after myocardial infarction. J Am Coll Cardiol 1991; 18:1643-1649.
11. Bigger JT, Fleiss JL, Rolnitzky L, et al. Frequency domain measures of heart period variability to assess risk late after myocardial infarction. J Am Coll Cardiol 1993; 21:729-736.
12. VanHoogenhuyze D, Martin G, Weiss J, et al. Spectrum of heart rate variability. Comp Cardiol 1989; 65.
13. Vybiral T, Glaeser D, Goldberger A, et al. Conventional heart rate variability analysis of ambulatory electrocardiographic recordings fails to predict imminent ventricular fibrillation. J Am Coll Cardiol 1993; 22:557-565.
14. Huikuri HV, Valkama JO, Airaksinen J, et al. Frequency domain measures of heart rate variability before the onset of nonsustained and sustained ventricular tachycardia in patients with coronary artery disease. Circulation 1993; 87:1220-1228.
15. Cerquetani E, Volterrani M, Ponikowski, et al. The very low frequency component of heart rate variability is increased in patients with chronic heart failure prior to episodes ofnon-sustained ventricular tachycardia. J Am Coll Cardiol 1994; (suppl):66A.
16. Palacios F, Ruiz R, Vila J, et al. Application of heart rate variability analysis in the stratification of arrhythmia risks in acute myocardial infarction. Comp Cardiol 1992; :265-268.
17. Ben-Haim SA, Harel T, Scherf M, et al. Immediate ventricular fibrillation and heart rate

variability in dogs with acute ischemia. Comp Cardiol 1991; :463-466.

18. Hull SS, Evans AR, Vanoli E, et al. Heart rate variability before and after myocardial infarction in conscious dogs at high and low risk of sudden death. J Am Coll Cardiol 1990; 16:978-985.

19. Hull SS, Vanoli E, Adamson P, et al. Exercise training confers anticipatory protection from sudden death during myocardial infarction. Circulation 1994; 89:548-552.

20. Carter JE, Childers RW. Torsade de pointes complicating acute myocardial infarction: the importance of autonomic dysfunction as assessed by heart rate variability. Clin Cardiol 1992; 15:769-772.

21. Skinner JE, Carpeggiani C, Landisman CE, et al. The correlation-dimension of the heartbeat is reduced by myocardial ischemia in conscious pigs. Circ Res 1991; 68:966-976.

22. Skinner JE, Pratt CM, Vybiral T. A reduction in the corelation dimension of heartbeat intervals precedes imminent ventricular fibrillation in human subjects. Am Heart J 1993; 125:731-743.

23. Vybiral T, Skinner JE. The point correlation dimension of R-R intervals predicts sudden cardiac death among high-risk patients. Comp Cardiol 1993; :257-260.

24. Gill JS, Farrell T, Baszko D, et al. RR variability and baroreflex sensitivity in patients with ventricular tachycardia associated with normal heart and patients with ischemic heart disease. PACE 1991; 14:2016-2021.

25. Farrell TG, Bashir Y, Cripps T, et al. Risk stratification for arrhythmic events in postinfarction patients based on heart rate variability, ambulatory electrocardiographic vari-ables and the signal-averaged electrocardiogram. J Am Coll Cardiol 1991; 18:687-697.

26. Odemuyiwa O, Malik M, Farrell T, et al. Multifactorial prediction of arrhythmic events after myocardial infarction. Combination of heart rate variability and left ventricular ejection fraction with other variables. PACE 1991; 14:1986-1994.

27. Pedretti R, Etro MD, Laporta A, et al. Prediction of late arrhythmic events after acute myocardial infarction from combined use of noninvasive prognostic variables and inducibility of sustained monomorphic ventricular tachycardia. Am J Cardiol 1993; 71:1131-1141.

28. Vybiral T, Knight C, Hess K, et al. Noninvasive, heart-rate variability-based index predicts inducibility of sustained monomorphic ventricular tachycardia by programmed electrical stimulation. J Am Coll Cardiol 1993; 21:459A.

29. Magid NM, Martin GJ, Kehoe RF, et al. Diminished heart rate variability in sudden cardiac death. Circulation 1985; 72(suppl):III241.

30. Ahmed M, Fintel D, Zhang F, et al. Survival post-sudden cardiac death: predictive value of heart rate variability vs. inducibility. J Am Coll Cardiol 1992; 19:167A.

31. Farrell TG, Paul V, Cripps TR, et al. Baroreflex sensitivity and electrophysiological correlates in patients after acute myocardial infarction. Circulation 1991; 83:945-952.

32. Pedretti R, Colombo E, Braga S, et al. Influence of transdermal scopolamine on cardiac sympathovagal interaction after acute myocardial infarction. Am J Cardiol 1993; 72:384-392.

Chapter 33

Changes in Heart Rate Variability Associated with Sudden Cardiac Death

Donald H. Singer, Zsolt Ori

Introduction

Paroxysmal dysrhythmias, principally ventricular tachyarrhythmias,[1-5] represent the leading cause of sudden death in the western world. In the United States, such disturbances claim about 400,000 lives annually, usually in the setting of chronic coronary disease. Death due to this cause, designated 'sudden cardiac death' (SCD), usually strikes in the prime of life, frequently without prior warning and outside the hospital. Economic and social costs are, therefore, high. Early identification of patients at high risk of SCD is a key need.

The pathophysiology of SCD may be viewed as an interaction between an abnormal anatomic substrate, eg, myocardial scarring associated with coronary artery disease, left ventricular hypertrophy, cardiomyopathy, AV nodal bypass tracts, etc. *and* transient functional disturbances which serve to trigger the terminal dysrhythmia, eg, ischemia, early premature beats, abrupt rate increases, electrolyte imbalance, and

fluctuations in autonomic balance.[6] Numerous investigators have sought to identify reliable predictors of SCD[7-13] from among the factors known to contribute to the pathophysiology. Many have been proposed,[13,14] but none have proven sufficiently specific or reliable.

Cobb et al[15] pointed out the importance of ventricular dysfunction manifested by low ejection fraction (EF), wall motion abnormalities and left ventricular aneurysm. Frequency and complexity of ventricular ectopy also have been suggested.[16-19] However, other investigators have found complex ventricular ectopy to be more a manifestation of the severity of the underlying heart disease than an independent risk factor.[20,21] Ineffectiveness of antiarrhythmic agents in protecting against SCD[20,22] further detracts from this possibility. More recently, interest has focused on findings of late potentials (LP) in the signal-averaged ECG as an index of risk of ventricular tachycardia and SCD in postmyocardial infarction (MI) patients.[13,23,24] However, this too is contro-

From: Malik M., Camm AJ (eds.): *Heart Rate Variability*. Armonk, NY. Futura Publishing Company, Inc., © 1995.

versial. It does, however, seem fair to say that the absence of LP is associated with lesser degrees of risk of future sustained VT or VF in this population.[13]

Suggestive evidence that SCD survivors at high risk of a second episode could be distinguished on the basis of their response to programmed ventricular stimulation, ie, whether or not they developed sustained runs of rapid, monomorphic ventricular tachycardia,[25-29] has served to focus attention on this methodology for risk stratification purposes. The method also has been used to distinguish benign from potentially lethal ventricular dysrhythmias and to assist in directing antiarrhythmic drug and other types of therapy.[25,27-30] Programmed ventricular stimulation represents the current 'gold standard' for determination of risk of SCD. However, the inducibility criterion may be of uncertain utility in a number of clinical settings, including recent MI[11] and cardiomyopathy.[31-33] In addition, invasive electrophysiological studies are costly and are not risk free.

Combinations of the aforementioned indices may be a more potent indicator of risk of SCD than any individual measure.[34] Kuchar et al[24] and Gomes et al[23] showed that the combination of an LP and low ejection fraction served to identify subjects at high risk of ventricular tachycardia, ventricular fibrillation, and SCD with a remarkably high degree of sensitivity (80% to 100%)[24] and specificity (89% to 50%).[23] In contrast, Farrel et al[35] found the combination LP and low heart rate variability (HRV), a measure of autonomic function (see below), to be the best predictor of a major cardiac event after MI (sensitivity: 58%, specificity: 93%, positive predictive accuracy: 33%, negative predictive accuracy: 93%). The combination of LP and low left ventricular ejection fraction ranked second best in their hands (sensitivity: 25%, specificity: 94%, positive predictive accuracy: 19%, negative predictive accuracy: 94%).[35]

However, alone or in combination, use of the aforementioned parameters for prediction of risk of SCD still leaves much to be desired. This probably reflects the fact that development of malignant ventricular dysrhythmias is almost certainly due to multiple causes. In addition, these factors are nonspecific and may not provide an adequate insight into the unique mechanism underlying SCD in any given individual.

The Autonomic Nervous System and Sudden Cardiac Death

Fluctuations in autonomic neural activity have been receiving increased attention both for their role in the initiation of ventricular tachyarrhythmias and SCD *and* for their potential utility as a marker of subgroups of patients at high risk of SCD.[36-44] Experimental and clinical studies dating back many years[36-38,45] suggest that the autonomic nervous system, particularly an imbalance between its sympathetic and parasympathetic components, represents an important determinant of the predisposition to ventricular tachycardia and ventricular fibrillation.[46-49] Lown and Verrier[48] have shown that sympathetic activity decreases fibrillation threshold and predisposes to ventricular fibrillation.

The report by Coumel and associates[49a] of catecholamine dependent ventricular tachycardia / fibrillation represents another case in point, as does the known relationship between the hereditary form of the prolonged QT syndrome and autonomic imbalance. Findings that psychologic and emotional stress can trigger ventricular tachyarrhythmias and SCD are also pertinent. Voodoo death syndromes in primitive cultures probably represent an example in this regard.[49b,49c] More pertinent to Western culture, is the occurrence of SCD in individuals, many young, without evidence of structural cardiovascular abnormalities. A neural trigger also would seem reasonable in these cases. In contrast, vagal activity increases the threshold and appears to protect against malignant ventricular tachyarrhythmias.[46-49] In conscious dogs with healed MI, it was found that direct vagal stimulation after onset of acute ischemia prevented ventricular fibrillation,[50] conversely, atropine caused worsening of susceptibility to ventricular fibrillation.[51] Findings that patients with heart disease exhibit defective parasympathetic control mechanisms[41] further support this hypothesis.

Findings that cardioactive drugs with strong anti-adrenergic and reflex vagal activity, for example, beta adrenergic blocking agents, appear to protect against SCD, whereas drugs with predominant parasympatholytic actions, for example, standard antiarrhythmic agents, are often pro-arrhythmic, are also pertinent in this regard.

The mechanisms underlying the protective effect of vagal activity are unclear. Findings[52,53] that specimens of ischemic and diseased heart contain large numbers of partially depolarized, slow response type ventricular muscle and Purkinje fibers, many exhibiting spontaneous diastolic depolarization, a characteristic which confers pacemaker capabilities on the involved cells (abnormal automaticity).[52] Such cells would be expected to predispose to slow conduction, fragmentation of excitation, and dysrhythmia due to reentry and abnormal automaticity.[52] Conversely, normalization of the diastolic potential would be expected to be antiarrhythmic.[52] The finding by Bailey et al[54] that acetylcholine hyperpolarizes partially depolarized Purkinje cells in an ischemia model is of interest in this regard, since such an action could provide one possible explanation for the 'protective' effects of vagal activity against ventricular tachyarrhythmias. There also is evidence that the vagal influence may be indirect, serving to oppose the effects of increased sympathetic tone on ventricular vulnerability.[55]

Heart Rate Variability

Quantitative measures of autonomic activity thus may have the potential to serve as predictors of risk of SCD and possibly also of risk of mortality due to other causes. Systematic investigation of this hypothesis requires clinically utilizable measures of sympathetic and parasympathetic activity. Direct determination of efferent vagal activity is not yet possible in conscious humans. Indirect measures are, however, available. Attention has focused on the spontaneous cyclical changes in heart rate (HR) and in hemodynamic parameters, including arterial blood pressure (BP) and stroke volume.[56,57] These have been known since ancient times and have been systematically examined at least since the 18th century.[58] The cyclical change in sinus rate over time is termed HRV.[44]

Current thinking holds that HRV is attributable to cyclical fluctuations in autonomic tone, virtually disappearing following combined sympathetic and parasympathetic blockade[59] and cardiac transplantation.[60,60a] The initial view, based on experimental animal studies[61,62] and on time-domain HRV studies on man,[63] held that the spontaneous respiratory fluctuations in sinus rate were mediated solely by efferent vagal activity. More recently, frequency-domain studies have provided strong suggestive evidence that HRV reflects oscillations in sympathetic-parasympathetic balance[64] associated with a variety of factors[65-67] including respiration, baroreceptor reflexes, vasomotor control, and thermoregulatory processes. Akselrod in his now classic 1982 report[68] confirmed the contribution of these factors and also noted the role of the renin-angiotensin system. Since these early studies there has been increasing recognition of the importance of HRV as an index of autonomic function.[5,56,66,69-78]

Determinations of baroreflex sensitivity (BRS) also may be used to assess parasympathetic influences on the heart.[43] BRS is expressed by the slope of the regression line correlating the degree of RR interval prolongation occurring in response to BP increases induced by a pressor agent.[12] The correlation between HRV and BRS is high but not perfect.[12] This reflects the fact that the two methodologies explore different aspects of the autonomic control of the heart: HRV is a direct measure of cardiac vagal tone, whereas BRS measures reflex vagal activity. Determinations of BRS also have been used to predict risk of ventricular tachycardia and SCD in the post-MI population.[79]

Heart Rate Variability: Methods of Analysis

There are two major approaches to HRV analysis: time-domain analysis and frequency-domain analysis.

Time-Domain Analysis[66,80]

A number of methods have been proposed.[10,35,56,66,73,80-82] These fall into two general classes:

1. RR Interval Analysis. Simply stated, this approach assesses HRV in terms of fluctuations in sinus rate about the mean by delineating the standard deviation of an RR interval series for a given time block, usually 5 minutes. Subsequent computation of the mean of the standard deviations of all sequential 5-minute time blocks included in the total recording period allows assessment of HRV changes over prolonged periods, usually 24 hours for Holter monitor based recordings. This measure, designated the standard deviation (SD) measure,[81] is also referred to as the SDNN Index.[80] A variant of this method is to determine the mean of the RR interval series for each 5-minute time block and then to calculate the standard deviation of all 5-minute interval means in the recording (SDANN measure).[73,80,83] These measures are broad based and subject to diurnal and other long-term trends which affect HR;

2. RR Interval Difference Analysis[80]: This class of indices, which measures differences in duration be-

tween adjacent RR intervals, includes the rMSSD measure (the root mean square of successive RR interval differences) and the PNN50 measure (the proportion of the differences between adjacent RR intervals that exceed an arbitrary limit, usually 50 milliseconds). In contrast to indices computed from sequential RR interval measurements, this group of measures is only minimally, if at all, affected by long-term trends, and is thought to reflect primarily alterations in parasympathetic activity.

Frequency-Domain (Power Spectrum) Analysis[44,84-86]

This decomposes the HR signal into its frequency components and quantifies them in terms of their relative intensity, termed 'power.'[22,44] The review by Ori et al[44] provides a detailed discussion of the potential clinical application of the methodology, particularly with respect to cardiovascular disease. A principal attraction of the method is that, in addition to measuring parasympathetic activity, it also provides insights concerning sympathetic activation and sympatho-vagal balance. The power spectrum encompasses at least three major frequency bands ranging from 0.01 to 0.35 Hz. Band boundaries are defined differently by different authors. The bands, together with the most commonly employed boundaries are:

1. High-frequency (HF) band (0.2 to 0.35 Hz), associated with parasympathetic activity. Peak frequency varies with respiration but approximates 0.25 Hz.[56] We have noted still higher frequency components (0.35 to 0.50 Hz), which comprise a very HF band. This may reflect nonrespiration related parasympathetic function.

2. Low-frequency band (LF) (0.04 to 0.2 Hz) which is ill-defined but has been attributed to thermoregulatory processes,[66] peripheral vasomotor activity and the renin-angiotensin system.[68] This band currently encompasses the intermediate frequency baroreceptor band (0.05 to 0.15 Hz). The LF band, including its baroreceptor component, is modulated by both sympathetic and parasympathetic activity, but predominantly by the latter.[68,75,87] The ratio of LF to HF power (LF/HF power content ratio) is considered a measure of sympatho-vagal balance, a conclusion supported by many experimental[56,68,87] and clinical[65,69,75,88-92] studies.

3. Very low-frequency band (VLF) (0.01 to 0.04 Hz) also has been identified and proposed as a marker of sympathetic activity.[76,89] However, recent pharmacological and physiological testing of sympathetic modulation of HRV power spectrum[93] suggests that VLF power cannot be viewed simply as a measure of sympathetic modulation.

4. The heart may fluctuate at still longer periodicities ranging from 10^{-2} to 10^{-5} Hz, designated the ultra-low frequency band (ULF). Physiological significance of the ULF band is unknown.

Correlations between all currently used time-domain and frequency-domain measures have been defined.[80] These have shown that all time-domain measures primarily reflect parasympathetic activity.[63,73,94,95]

Frequency-domain measures are generally much more sensitive to technical artifacts such as timing error due to differences in taping speed, or missing data due to ectopic beats, than are frequency-domain measures. For optimum reliability and reproducibility, the HR signal must meet a number of conditions which are prerequisites for meaningful power spectrum analyses[44]: ideally the signal should be random,[1] stationary,[2] and sufficiently long.[3] Since, in reality, these conditions are not always met or even monitored, power spectral determinations may be subject to unpredictable variations, particularly at lower frequencies.[96]

Heart Rate Variability: A Powerful Predictor of All Cause Mortality

Numerous studies, carried out using a variety of methodologies, have found low HRV to be a powerful predictor of all cause mortality.[73] Early studies made use of relatively simple time-domain measures, eg, observations of beat-to-beat variability, the presence or absence of sinus arrhythmia, and measurements of maximum - minimum PP intervals or the standard deviation of mean sinus PP intervals obtained from short rhythm strips. Perhaps the earliest description of the relationships between HR fluctuations and mortality is contained in a 1965[97] report on fetal monitoring showing that diminished beat-to-beat variability in HR signified fetal distress and a need for rapid delivery. Subsequent reports have confirmed this relationship.[3,77,98]

Another early study relating HRV to mortality was that reported by Wolf et al in 1978[99] for a population of soldiers admitted to an army hospital for acute MI. HRV was defined in terms of the presence or absence of sinus arrhythmia in 60-second rhythm strips obtained on admission to the hospital. After controlling for such factors as infarct location and initial sinus rate, they found that patients with acute MI who did not

---

1. sequences which cannot be determined/defined by a unique mathematical expression or rule.
2. the probability function of the signal does not change over time.
3. assuming constant stationarity, the consistency of power spectral estimates improves with an increase in the duration of the signal.

exhibit sinus arrhythmia on the initial ECG had a much greater chance of dying during the hospitalization (15.5%) compared with those exhibiting sinus arrhythmia (4.1%).

Masaoka et al[100] used similarly simple measures to examine the association between HRV, aging and diabetes. Subjects were told to breathe as deeply as possible at a rate of six times per minute for 1 minute and HRV, defined as maximum minus minimum bpm, was measured. HRV was found to decrease with aging and the duration and severity of diabetes, being most severe in insulin dependent diabetics with autonomic neuropathy. Insofar as relationships to mortality are concerned, it has been shown that diabetic patients with clinical signs of autonomic neuropathy and abnormal tests of autonomic function (Valsalva maneuver and handgrip test) have disproportionately high mortality rates relative to similar type patients with normal test results.[101] Relationships between normal aging and mortality are self evident and require no comment.

The advent of Holter monitoring and computer technology has greatly facilitated HRV analysis by making possible long-term measures of HRV, usually 24 or 48 hours, and detailed statistical analysis of the data. Kleiger et al[73,83,102] used time-domain HRV analysis of 24-hour ambulatory ECG recordings to extend Wolf's observations on the relationships between this parameter and mortality in the post-MI state in a group of 850 patients followed for 3 years after acute infarction. Low HRV, defined in terms of the standard deviation of the mean of all 'normal' RR intervals (ie, interval between two sequential sinus beats without contained ectopic beats) was found to be a powerful independent predictor of long-term mortality in survivors of MI. Similar observations have been reported by others.[35,103,104] Indeed, low HRV may be a more powerful predictor of mortality than such standard determinants as left ventricular ejection fraction, wall motion abnormalities, frequency and complexity of ventricular ectopy, standard ECG indices, exercise capacity, and the signal averaged ECG.[35,73] Pilot studies by Van Hoogenhuyze et al[82] and Singer et al[105] showing that mortality in a mixed group of congestive heart failure patients was associated with the lowest levels of HRV (SD measure) for the group, underscore its potential utility for risk stratification in the noncoronary, as well as coronary, population.

The protective effects of beta-adrenergic blocking agents in reducing risk of SCD in the post-MI population[106] are pertinent to considerations of the autonomic contribution to SCD and the predictive value of HRV with respect to mortality. These agents are among the small handful of cardioactive drugs known to simultaneously depress adrenergic activity and reflexly increase vagal tone.[107] As might be expected, they also increase HRV.[108] In view of this, it is tempting to think that, to the extent that the beneficial effects of this group of drugs stem from their indirect autonomic actions as opposed to their weak direct antiarrhythmic (membrane stabilizing) activity, and/or nonspecific membrane effects,[109] HRV can be used as a simple tool for monitoring therapeutic effectiveness.

It follows from the foregoing that agents which depress parasympathetic activity might be pro-arrhythmic and increase risk of SCD. Class IA and Class IC antiarrhythmic agents, including quinidine and procainamide, represent a case in point. These agents, which are well known for pro-arrhythmic activity, also exhibit strong indirect atropine-like effects and are well known for pro-arrhythmic activity. In addition, Zuanetti et al[109a] compared the autonomic effects of a Class IC agent (flecanide) with those of propafenone and amiodarone on HRV. They found that amiodarone, which generally does not exhibit major pro-arrhythmia, did not modify HRV. In contrast, flecanide and propafenone, both of which have been shown to increase mortality,[34] decreased HRV (pNN50) significantly, a finding interpreted as reflecting depressive effects on parasympathetic activity. There was no information concerning possible sympathetic effects.

Correlations between HRV and mortality also have been made for a number of noncardiac disease states, including diabetes[110] and alcoholic neuropathy.[111] Early studies by Masaoka on diabetics[100] have been previously alluded to. Findings by Ewing et al[110] that diabetics with autonomic neuropathy exhibited a 5-year mortality rate (56%) that was three times higher than for patients with normal autonomic function are of particular interest in that of those who died, almost 30% experienced SCD. In addition, there was a surprising absence of coronary artery disease. In a similar vein, Johnson and Robinson[111] found that depressed vagal activity in chronic alcoholics was associated with an increased risk of mortality, particularly due to cardiovascular causes.

Heart Rate Variability: Sudden Cardiac Death

Time-domain studies showing that HRV (SD and SDANN measures) was significantly lower in SCD survivors[112] and in patients experiencing SCD during ambulatory monitoring than for nonSCD patients with structural heart disease[3] and normal controls,[81] respectively, support suggestions that this method may be useful in identifying individuals at high risk of sudden death. The fact that HRV was comparable for both SCD groups (SCD during ambulatory monitoring and SCD survivors) is important in that it indicates that the low level of HRV in the SCD survivors was not due to physiological changes associated with the cardiac arrest. Additional findings of a progressive reduction in HRV, defined in terms of 24-hour mean LF and HF power, in individuals who died during Holter monitoring also are pertinent in this regard.[113]

To test the hypothesis that HRV could correctly discriminate between inducible and noninducible SCD survivors, inducible and noninducible 'asymptomatic VEA' patients (patients with complex ventricular ectopy but without syncope or SCD) and normal controls,[10,112,114] all subjects were Holter monitored for 24 hours prior to programmed ventricular stimulation and while off antiarrhythmic drugs. Suspected covariates were controlled for by means of a stepwise discriminant analysis. Univariate analysis showed that inducible and noninducible patients did not differ with respect to age, sex, mean RR interval, ejection fraction, cardiac drugs (digitalis or beta-blocking agents), and frequency or complexity of ventricular ectopy. HRV in inducible SCD survivors was found to be markedly decreased as compared with normal.[114] Preliminary observations indicate that HRV of inducible SCD survivors also was decreased as compared to noninducible SCD survivors, although differences were not as pronounced (unpublished data, 1989). Inducible 'asymptomatic VEA' patients also were found to exhibit low HRV, thus further underscoring the relationship between HRV, inducibility, and risk of sudden death. HRV of noninducible 'asymptomatic VEA' patients also appeared diminished, but differences did not reach statistical significance when compared with normal controls.[114] Combining low HRV (SD measure <30 milliseconds) and inducibility correctly identified all SCD survivors who died during a 100-month follow-up.[93] Correlations between low HRV and inducibility in SCD survivors suggest the potential utility of HRV as a predictor of SCD and as a possible screen for programmed ventricular stimulation studies. Findings in a study of 59 patients referred for routine electrophysiological study in which the 28 inducible patients exhibited significantly lower HRV than did the 31 noninducible patients[114a] are supportive.

Despite the putative importance of sympathetic activity to considerations of SCD, only very little power spectral information is available. The paucity of such studies may be due, at least in part, to the fact that time-domain determinations are easier to make and also provide excellent correlations with mortality.[94] However, Meyers et al[81] suggested that power spectral analysis may be even more useful, changes in the HF component providing the best separation between SCD survivors, nonSCD patients with chronic structural heart disease, and normal controls. LF power did not distinguish SCD and nonSCD heart disease patients but was significantly lower in both groups than in normals.

Most studies of the relationship between HRV and SCD have been carried out in the coronary population. However, studies[115] on seven patients with primary ventricular fibrillation and three cardiomyopathy patients with ventricular fibrillation confirm significantly lower HRV for SCD survivors in noncoronary populations than for healthy age and gender matched controls. Interestingly enough, in this study SCD patients and controls differed significantly with respect to power spectral determinations but not with respect to time-domain measures. In addition, hourly HRV analysis showed that minimum observed HRV values were significantly lower in the SCD patients than in the normal controls, whereas maximum hourly HRV remained unchanged, suggesting that this mode of analysis may provide additional information relevant to considerations of risk.

HRV methodology also has been applied to the sudden infant death syndrome (SIDS). Gordon et al[116] compared the HR and respiratory power spectra during quiet sleep of infants who subsequently died from SIDS with those of healthy controls. They found significant enhancement of LF, but not HF, power in the HR power spectrum and a widened HF band in the respiratory spectra, in SIDS infants. However, in a second study on a larger population, the same investigators reported that these characteristics did not adequately distinguish SIDS infants from controls.[117] In a subsequent similar type of investigation, Kluge et al[118] found HF power to be significantly lower in the SIDS children than in controls, a finding consistent with parasympathetic withdrawal and comparable with findings in adult SCD cases.

Heart Rate Variability: Aging and Sudden Cardiac Death

Time-domain studies have clearly shown that HRV decreases with increasing age,[77,100,119,120] the decline being generally attributed to age-related reduction in parasympathetic activity.[61,121] Sympathetic activity also declines with age, but at a slower rate.[122-124] Since, as noted above, development of chronic heart disease per se[63] and SCD[7,77,125,126] also have been associated with declining vagal activity, it is necessary to define areas of HRV overlap between SCD patients, patients with organic heart disease but without SCD, and the healthy elderly. Cutoff points to separate these groups need to be established. Preliminary observations suggest that it may be possible to define cutoff points for time-domain measures which separate SCD survivors from nonSCD patients with heart disease with an 80% sensitivity and a 66% specificity.[127]

Distinctions between low HRV due to heart disease and risk of SCD due to aging, are more complex. Our own data suggest that SCD patients over age 60 often exhibit substantially lower 24-hour mean HRV (SD measure) than do younger SCD patients.[128] Findings by Odemuyiwa et al[129] that arrhythmic death is a more common mode of dying and is more reliably predicted by HRV in postinfarct patients younger than 60 years than in those over 60 underscore the influence of aging on HRV.

Observations by Monir et al[130,131] concerning differences between cycle length (CL) dependence of HRV of normal individuals and patients with symptomatic heart disease, could prove useful in distinguishing low HRV due to aging from that due to disease and risk of SCD. More specifically, normal individuals of all ages exhibit a linear relationship between cycle length (HR) and HRV: HRV increases with increases in cycle length to a maximum at CL 1000 milliseconds. In contrast, in patients with symptomatic heart disease, the strength of the relationship was variably decreased. In patients with high-grade, complex ventricular ectopy and severe congestive failure, the slope of the relationship was markedly depressed and in some individuals was almost flat. The possibility that the relationship may cease to hold in patients with end stage disease and at high risk of SCD needs to be investigated in SCD survivors and patients who develop ventricular fibrillation during Holter monitoring. If further documented, marked depression or disappearance of the cycle length dependence of HRV could represent another potential indicator of risk of SCD.

This type of analysis also provides a potential tool for distinguishing previously alluded to 'normal outliers,' ie, normal individuals with lower than expected HRV for age, since such individuals, in contrast to those in whom low HRV indicates heart disease and high risk of SCD, should exhibit normal cycle length dependence of HRV. In addition, application of the concept of cycle length dependence of HRV could allow one to distinguish 'normal outliers' who exhibit low HRV in relation to high mean HRs from patients with heart disease at increase risk of SCD. Clearly, further study is indicated. One additional focus of such new studies would be to compare HF and LF power at comparable cycle lengths in normal individuals and SCD survivors to assess the extent to which these differ.

Heart Rate Variability, Circadian Rhythms and Sudden Cardiac Death

The increased incidence of acute cardiovascular events, including sudden cardiac death,[132] MI,[37] transient myocardial ischemia,[133] and arrhythmias [134] during the early morning hours, particularly in patients with heart disease, suggests a possible relationship to altered circadian fluctuations in autonomic tone.

Studies on normal subjects and patients without organic heart disease have shown that HRV exhibits circadian variation, the lowest values occurring upon awakening in the morning.[56] In a study of 44 patients with coronary disease complicated by MI, of whom 22 were SCD survivors, HRV (SD measure) was found to be significantly lower in the SCD group. The 24-hour mean HF spectral area also was lower in the SCD patients. However, the circadian variation in time- and frequency-domain measures of HRV did not differ between the two groups. Thus, survivors exhibited very low HRV in the morning immediately on awakening, corresponding to the time period at which the incidence of SCD is highest.[135] These observations support conclusions that autonomic imbalance contributes to the increased prevalence of SCD during the morning hours and underscores potential utility of HRV determinations as a marker of increased risk.

Heart Rate Variability and Sudden Cardiac Death: Long-Term Predictive Value

The potential utility of low HRV as a predictor of risk of SCD has been most extensively examined with respect to long-term survival after MI.[7,8,35,77,126,129, 136,137] In general, both experimental and clinical studies indicate that HRV is a powerful long-term predictor of risk of SCD.

Experimental studies by Hull et al[136] showed that low HRV distinguishes dogs at increased risk of development of SCD in response to exercise and transient ischemia 1 month postexperimental MI (sensitivity: 88%; specificity: 80%). A large scale clinical epidemiologic survey of 6693 consecutive Holter monitoring patients followed for periods of up to 2 years corroborated low HRV as a risk predictor in that patients with HRV (SD measure)<25 milliseconds had an increased risk for SCD independent of other factors.[7] Dougherty and Burr[55] compared baseline 24-hour HRV determinations on SCD patients who were alive 1 year after the event with those from patients who died of a subsequent episode of SCD during the follow-up period. Baseline HRV was significantly lower in those who died than in survivors. Preliminary analysis of data from long-term (to 8 years) follow-up of SCD survivors with mortality as the endpoint confirms the strong predictive value of low HRV (SD<30 milliseconds) for recurrence of major arrhythmic events: of seven patients exhibiting two or more major arrhythmic events, five died during the observation period. Of these, four exhibited very low HRV (SD:<20 milliseconds).[105] Odemuyiwa et al[126] found low HRV to be the single best predictor of major arrhythmic events after MI, superior to such powerful variables as ventricular ejection fraction, HR, late potentials, and frequency and complexity of ectopic beats. Optimum risk stratification was achieved using a combination of HRV with late potentials or ventricular ectopy.

Most studies of the association between low HRV and SCD have been based on determinations from 24-hour Holter monitoring records. Recently, because of considerations of convenience and cost, there has been a surge of interest in HRV determinations from short-term records. In a study of 715 patients, power spectral measures (VLF, LF, HF, LF/HF) of HRV determined 2 weeks after MI proved to be powerful predictors of SCD and all cause mortality during a 2.5-year follow-up period regardless of whether HRV was determined calculated from short (2 to 15 minutes) or long (24-hour) recordings.[8] Predictive value was even further improved when HRV was used in combination with New York Heart Association functional class criteria. The combination of HF power and New York Heart Association criteria provided the highest positive predictive accuracy underscoring the protective effect of parasympathetic activity in this population. A preliminary to the effect that risk of death following MI could be successfully predicted using HRV determinations calculated from 2- to 15-mi-

nute electrocardiographic records also is pertinent in this regard.[138]

During the past year, we have had the opportunity to examine short-term ECG machine[4] based time- and frequency-domain HRV determinations derived from analysis of 1,027 beats and to make comparisons with conventional Holter based measurements. To date, records from approximately 100 patients have been accumulated. Preliminary evaluation suggests that, in general, HRV determinations appear more or less comparable for the two techniques provided that the mean HRs for the time blocks studied approximate each other. As might be expected, comparability appeared to be closest when the cycle length distribution in ECG machine and Holter based records was similar. The relationship between mean HR and comparability of the HRV determinations using the two methods is being investigated in detail. If confirmed, it would underscore the potential importance of cycle length dependence analysis to short-term HRV studies. Reproducibility of short-term HRV determinations also is being assessed. The half dozen comparisons made to date suggest that baseline measurements show a high degree of reproducibility 1 to 6 months after initial study in the absence of intervening changes in clinical state or mean HR.

Heart Rate Variability and Sudden Cardiac Death, Short-Term Predictive Value

Since substrate conditions thought to predispose to SCD may be present for prolonged time periods prior to the event, the question arises as to the nature of the changes which trigger the onset of ventricular fibrillation at a particular point in time. As noted earlier, acute alterations in autonomic balance, more specifically, increases in sympathetic and/or decreases in para-

---

4. data were collected using a Cardiovit AT-10 machine, which was graciously provided by Schiller AG, Baar, Switzerland.

sympathetic activity with resultant accentuation of sympathetic dominance, represent one possible trigger.

Coumel,[139] in a 1990 report on HRV changes associated with the onset of ectopic tachyarrhythmias, concluded that paroxysmal ventricular, as well as supraventricular, tachyarrhythmias may be triggered by autonomic changes. In support, he showed a case of paroxysmal ventricular tachycardia and one of atrial fibrillation in which the onset of these dysrhythmias was immediately preceded by changes in HR and HR oscillations consistent with increased sympathetic and parasympathetic activity, respectively. Insofar as ventricular tachyarrhythmias are concerned, this conclusion is tempered by inferences that in individuals at highest risk, the degree of sympathetic increase required to trigger the dysrhythmia may be so small as to defy ready definition, possibly because of high baseline levels of sympathetic activity.

Analysis of time- and frequency-domain changes in patients who experienced SCD during Holter monitoring, particularly changes occurring during the few minutes preceding the terminal event, might be expected to yield important clues. Early observations from our own laboratory by Magid et al[10] were encouraging. They compared HRV (standard deviation measure) determined during the 5 minutes immediately preceding the onset of ventricular fibrillation with that obtained during the preceding 5-minute period for 11 SCD patients. HRV decreased between the two time periods (p = <.02). Similarities in mean HR between the two periods indicated that the decrease in HRV was not a function of change in rate.

Early 24-hour time- and frequency-domain HRV records from eight patients with coronary disease who experienced SCD during Holter monitoring are also pertinent.[105] HF (0.15 to .50 Hz) and LF (baroreceptor) (0.05 to 0.15) power, indices of parasympathetic and sympathetic activity respectively, were measured. Crude assessments of sympathetic/parasympathetic balance also were made by comparing the areas under the HF and LF components of the power spectrum.

Time-domain measures of 24 hours of HRV were very low in all eight subjects, SD <30 milliseconds, a level consistent with that previously reported for SCD patients.[3,10,77,81,112,114] HF power also was extremely low. LF (baroreceptor) power, although much reduced as compared with normal, was nevertheless much greater than the power in the HF bands. Given the virtual disappearance of HF activity, it seems reasonable to assume that the residual power in the LF (baroreceptor) band largely reflected nonvagal (sympathetic) activity. To the extent that this holds, the records are indicative of sympathetic dominance throughout the monitoring period. The generally fast sinus rates, which these patients also exhibited, support this interpretation.

In all eight patients, a detailed analysis of frequency-domain and vagal/sympathetic balance changes during the 15 minutes preceding the onset of ventricular fibrillation showed virtually unopposed LF (baroreceptor) activity. Sympathetic/parasympathetic balance studies showing an increase in the LF/HF ratio further highlighted sympathetic dominance during this period. Six of the eight patients also appeared to exhibit an additional surge in LF (baroreceptor) power just prior to the terminal event, suggesting the possibility of a sympathetic trigger for SCD.

Findings by others[140] that time- and frequency-domain HRV measures were significantly lower prior to the onset of sustained, as compared with nonsustained, ventricular tachyarrhythmias, and that the LF/HF ratio increases significantly just prior the onset of sustained ventricular tachyarrhythmias, are supportive. Recent reports that episodes of ventricular tachycardia were preceded by increases in LF power (a marker of sympathetic activity) during the 5 minutes before the event[141] also are supportive. Further findings that episodes of ischemia were immediately preceded by increases in indices of sympathetic tone, ie, increases in HR[142] and in LF power,[143] also are pertinent in that this condition is frequently associated with ventricular dysrhythmias.

However, as Coumel has commented[125,139], delineation of specific patterns of autonomic change which serve to trigger lethal ventricular tachyarrhythmias is complex and difficult. For example, in our own experience, two of six patients experiencing preterminal increases in baroreceptor power also exhibited comparable increases earlier during the monitoring period. These early increases appeared grossly comparable to those observed preterminally, although they were not associated with ventricular fibrillation. In addition, two of the eight patients in the group did not exhibit clear-cut increases in baroreceptor power prior to the onset of ventricular fibrillation. Rather, in these individuals, the few minutes just prior to SCD were characterized by small surges in both HF and baroreceptor band power. Findings by Vybiral et al[144] further highlight difficulties in defining the specific pattern of changes which trigger SCD. This study, in which HRV was evaluated on an hour-by-hour basis during the monitoring period with special attention in the hour just prior to SCD, did not show consistent patterns of autonomic change of the type which might be expected to trigger ventricular fibrillation. Studies utilizing power changes in the LF and VLF bands as indices of sympathetic activity would help clarify the nature of autonomic triggers of ventricular dysrhythmias. However, even these may not be adequate for the purpose for the reason that the high levels of ectopy which characterize the preterminal period may markedly distort time- and frequency-domain HRV determinations, particularly the latter. In addition, high-base levels of sympathetic dominance in SCD patients may make it difficult to precisely define additional, possibly small, changes in autonomic activity needed to trigger lethal ventricular tachyarrhythmias, at least using current methods. Use of new and more sophisticated indices of HRV may facilitate a better understanding of patterns of HRV

change associated with SCD.[131,145] Application of 'chaos theory'[146-149] also shows promise.

Summary and Conclusions

1. The weight of evidence indicates that cardiac parasympathetic function is markedly depressed in patients prone to development of SCD and that this, and possibly other, alterations in autonomic balance contribute importantly to the development of electrical instability in such individuals. Major risk factors for SCD, including coronary artery disease, MI, congestive heart failure, and hypertension, all have been associated with reduced parasympathetic activity or attenuation of parasympathetic reflexes. The reasons for the deleterious effects of reduced parasympathetic activity are not known. Perhaps vagal withdrawal reduces or abolishes ability to counter the potentially arrhythmogenic effects of sympathetic activity.[52]

2. The available data also strongly support the view that HRV measurements provide information pertinent to the identification of individuals at increased risk of SCD, which is independent of that afforded by other risk factors:

a. low HRV has been shown to be a powerful independent predictor of all cause mortality in the post-MI population, as well as in patients with a number of noncardiac disease states.[100,110,111] Indeed, low HRV may be a more powerful predictor than left ventricular ejection fraction, wall motion abnormalities, frequency and complexity of ventricular ectopy, standard ECG and exercise ECG indices, and findings of late potentials in the SAECG[35,73];

b. low HRV also was found to be the best single predictor of major arrhythmic events, including ventricular fibrillation and SCD in post-MI patients, optimum risk stratification being achieved using a combination of HRV with SAECG or ventricular ectopy indices.[35] Although increases in ventricular ectopy just prior to the onset of the terminal dysrhythmia severely hamper analysis, records obtained during this period provide suggestive evidence that HRV may decrease still further,[10,77,114,139] suggesting that short-term HRV changes may prove significant with respect to delineation of near-term risk of ventricular tachyarrhythmias and SCD. Improved methods of compensating for the confounding effects of the preSCD surges in ectopy are needed;

c. HRV is markedly depressed in SCD survivors compared with normal controls,[112] particularly in patients found to have inducible ventricular tachyarrhythmias at invasive electrophysiological study.[10,114] This patient population appears to be at very high risk of a second episode of SCD. The combination of low HRV and inducibility correctly identified all SCD survivors who subsequently died during a 100-month follow-up[93];

d. HRV also may be low in patients with asymptomatic, complex ventricular ectopy who develop sustained ventricular tachycardia during programmed ventricular stimulation, the degree of reduction paralleling that in inducible SCD survivors. In contrast, noninducible asymptomatic complex ventricular ectopy patients exhibited somewhat diminished HRV, but at a level which did not differ statistically from normal.[114] To the extent that this is documented by large scale prospective studies, it would suggest that HRV measurements have the potential for serving as an independent predictor of inducibility and for providing a noninvasive

screen for patients referred for evaluation of risk of SCD; and

e. HRV exhibits circadian variation, the lowest values occurring during the morning hours.[56] This parallels the increased morning incidence of MI[37] and SCD,[135] and underscores the importance of the autonomic contribution to these conditions.

3. However, despite the foregoing, we agree with Malik and Camm that HRV changes may lack sufficient specificity with respect to considerations of SCD.[151] The autonomic contribution to SCD cannot be viewed simplistically, ie, vagal withdrawal and/or sympathetic surges = loss of protection against evolution of lethal arrhythmia and SCD. In part, this undoubtedly reflects the multicausality of SCD. For example:

a. observations that not all recorded SCD events are preceded by the same sequence of autonomic changes represents one important example. Evidence that apparently healthy individuals, particularly the elderly, as well as some patients with severe structural heart disease, may exhibit very low levels of HRV for prolonged periods without necessarily developing major arrhythmic events, represents another example. With respect to the healthy elderly with low HRV, autonomic activity, but particularly parasympathetic activity, is known to decrease with aging.[77,100,119,120] The overlap between low HRV values exhibited by some healthy elderly individuals and the values exhibited by patients with a number of pathophysiologic states, including SCD survivors[7,77,121,125,126,127] underscores the need to distinguish reduction in HRV due to normal aging[79] from that associated with disease and increased risk of SCD. The frequent occurrence of organic SA nodal disease in the elderly, with resultant restrictions in sinus rate variability, compounds the problem. Evaluation of HRV, in light of reported differences in the cycle length dependence of HRV between normal individuals and those with heart disease, could prove helpful. In this regard, it also would be of interest to determine whether impending SCD or development of conditions associated with increased risk of SCD, eg, inducibility by programmed ventricular stimulation, are associated with changes in the autonomic contribution to the HR power spectrum, particularly at long cycle lengths with a normally high vagal content;

b. observations by Bigger et al,[150] that the predictive power of the lowest frequency components of the HR, ie, VLF and ULF of the power spectral bands appears substantially greater than that of conventional indices of reduced vagal activity, represent another confounding example. The controversy reflects the fact that the physiological basis of all of the component frequencies of the HR power spectrum, but particularly that of the VLF and ULF bands, still are not well defined. Clarification of the nature of these bands is urgently needed.

4. Assuming low HRV to be an index of increased risk of SCD, the question arises as to whether subsequent increases in this variable in response to different types of therapeutic interventions are associated with decreased risk of arrhythmic death. The beneficial effects of beta-blocking drugs in the post-MI population are encouraging in this regard. However, the effects of other major therapeutic modalities on risk of SCD and on HRV need to be assessed. Although we and others have tried to control for such covariants as age, gender, cardiovascular drug use, complexity and frequency of ven-

tricular ectopy, etc., systematic prospective studies are clearly required.

5. Despite these and other caveats, the data support conclusions that HRV determinations represent an independent predictor that greatly facilitates the identification of individuals at increased risk of SCD. Given the human and economic costs of SCD and the potential benefits to be gained by early identification of patients at increased risk, intensive study and large scale patient trials to clarify the outstanding questions and ready the methodology for clinical use are clearly warranted.

Acknowledgments: The authors acknowledge and thank Ms. Ruth H. Singer for her critical comments and outstanding editorial assistance, and Marcus Moritz of Schiller AG for his support of this work.

References

1. Kempf FC, Josephson ME. Cardiac arrest recorded on ambulatory electrocardiograms. Am J Cardiol 1984; 53:1577.
2. Liberthson R, Nagel E, Hirschman J, et al. Pathophysiologic observations in pre-hospital ventricular fibrillation and sudden cardiac death. Circulation 1974; 49:790.
3. Martin GJ, Magid NM, Myers G, et al. Heart rate variability and sudden death secondary to coronary artery disease during ambulatory ECG monitoring. Am J Cardiol 1987; 60:86-89.
4. Milner PG, Platia EV, Reid PR, et al. Ambulatory electrocardiographic recordings at the time of fatal cardiac arrest. Am J Cardiol 1985; 56:588.
5. Panidis IP, Morganroth J. Holter monitoring and sudden cardiac death. Cardiovasc Rev Rep 1984; 5(3):283-304.
6. Myerburg JR, Kessler KM, Castellanos A. Sudden cardiac death. Structure, function, and time-dependence of risk. Circulation 1992; 85(suppl I):I2-I10.
7. Algra A, Tijssen JPG, Roelandt JCTR, et al. Heart rate variability from 24-hour electrocardiography and the 2-year risk for sudden death. Circulation 1993; 88:180-185.
8. Bigger JT, Fleiss JL, Rolnitzky LM, et al. The ability of several short-term measures of RR variability to predict mortality after myo-

cardial infarction. Circulation 1993; 88:927-934.

9. Cupples AL, Gagnon DR, Kannel WB. Long- and short-term risk of sudden coronary death. Circulation 1992; 85(suppl I):I11-I18.

10. Magid NM, Martin GJ, Kehoe RF, et al. Diminished heart rate variability in sudden cardiac death. Circulation 1985; 72(suppl III):241. Abstract.

11. Marchlinski FE, Buxton AE, Waxman HL, et al. Identifying patients at risk of sudden death after myocardial infarction: value of the response to programmed stimulation, degree of ventricular activity, and severity of left ventricular dysfunction. Am J Cardiol 1983; 52:1190.

12. Schwartz JP, La Rovere T, Vanoli E. Autonomic nervous system and sudden cardiac death, experimental basis and clinical observations for post-myocardial infarction risk stratification. Circulation 1992; 85(suppl I):I77-91.

13. Simson MB. Noninvasive identification of patients at high risk for sudden cardiac death. Circulation 1992; 85(suppl I):I145-I151.

14. Josephson ME. Sudden Cardiac Death. Philadelphia, Pa: F.A. Davis Company, 1985.

15. Cobb LA, Baum RS, Alvarez H, et al. Resuscitation from out-of-hospital ventricular fibrillation: four year follow-up. Circulation 1975; 52(suppl 3):223.

16. Bigger JT, Fleiss JL, Kleiger R, et al. The relationships among ventricular arrhythmias, left ventricular dysfunction, and mortality in the two years after myocardial infarction. Circulation 1984; 69:250.

17. Holmes J, Kubo SH, Cody RJ, et al. Arrhythmias in ischemic and non-ischemic dilated cardiomyopathy: prediction of mortality by ambulatory electrocardiography. Am J Cardiol 1985; 55:146.

18. Lown B, Calvert AF, Armington R, et al. Monitoring for serious arrhythmias and high risk of sudden death. Circulation 1975; 52(suppl III):189.

19. Ruderman W, Weinblatt E, Goldberg JD, et al. Ventricular premature complexes and sudden death after myocardial infarction. Circulation 1981; 64:297.

20. Moss AJ, Davis HT. Clinical significance of ventricular arrhythmias in patients with and without coronary artery disease. Prog Cardiovasc Dis 1980; 23:33.

21. Moss AJ, Davis HT, DeCamilla J, et al. Ventricular ectopic beats and their relation to sudden death and non-sudden cardiac death after myocardial infarction. Circulation 1979; 60:998.

22. Vlay SE, Reid PR. Ventricular ectopy: etiology, evaluation and therapy. Am J Med 1982; 73:899.

23. Gomes AJ, Winters LS, Stewart D, et al. A new noninvasive index to predict sustained ventricular tachycardia and sudden death in the first year after myocardial infarction: based on signal-averaged electrocardiogram, radionuclide ejection fraction and holter monitoring. J Am Coll Cardiol 1987; 10:349-357.

24. Kuchar LD, Thorburn WC, Sammel LN. Prediction of serious arrhythmic events after myocardial infarction: signal averaged electrocardiogram, holter monitoring and radionuclide ventriculography. J Am Coll Cardiol 1987; 9:531-538.

25. Josephson ME, Horowitz L, Spielman SR, et al. Electrophysiologic and hemodynamic studies in patients resuscitated from cardiac arrest. Am J Cardiol 1980; 46:948.

26. Kehoe R, Tommaso C, Zheutlin T, et al. Factors determining programmed stimulation responses and long-term arrhythmic outcome in survivors of ventricular fibrillation with ischemic heart disease. Am Heart J 1988; 116:355.

27. Mason JW, Winkle RA. Electrode catheter arrhythmia induction in the selection and assessment of antiarrhythmic drug therapy for recurrent ventricular tachycardia. Circulation 1978; 58:971.

28. Ruskin JN, D'Marco JP, Garan A. Out-of-hospital cardiac arrest: electrophysiologic observations and selection of long-term antiarrhythmic therapy. N Engl J Med 1980; 303:607.

29. Zheutlin TA, Roth H, Chua W, et al. Programmed electrical stimulation to determine the need for antiarrhythmic therapy in patients with complex ventricular ectopic activity. Am Heart J 1986; 111:860.

30. Gomes AJ, Hariman RI, Kang PS, et al. Programmed electrical stimulation in patients with high grade ventricular ectopy: electrophysiologic findings and prognosis for survival. Circulation 1984; 70:43.

31. Milner PG, DiMarco JP, Lerman BB. Electrophysiological evaluation of sustained ventricular tachyarrhythmia in idiopathic dilated cardiomyopathy. PACE 1988; 11:562-568.

32. Poole JE, Mathisen TL, Kundenchuk PJ, et al. Long-term outcome in patients who survive out of hospital ventricular fibrillation and undergo electrophysiologic studies: evaluation by electrophysiologic subgroups. J Am Coll Cardiol 1990; 16:657-665.

33. Stevenson WG, Stevenson LW, Weiss J, et al. Inducible ventricular arrhythmias and

sudden death during vasodilator therapy of severe heart failure. Am Heart J 1988; 116:1447-1454.

34. Multicenter Post-infarction Research Group. Risk stratification and survival after myocardial infarction. N Engl J Med 1983; 309:331.

35. Farrel TG, Bashir Y, Cripps T, et al. Risk stratification for arrhythmic events in post-infarction patients based on heart variability, ambulatory electrocardiographic variables and signal averaged electrocardiogram. J Am Coll Cardiol 1991; 8:687-697.

36. Campese VM, Romoff MS, Levitan D, et al. Mechanisms of autonomic nervous system dysfunction in uremia. Kidney Int 1981; 20:246-253.

37. Muller JE, Stone PH, Turi ZG, et al. Circadian variation in the frequency of onset of acute myocardial infarction. N Engl J Med 1985; 313:1315-1322.

38. Cerati D, Schwartz PJ. Single cardiac vagal fiber activity, acute myocardial ischemia, and risk for sudden death. Circ Res 1991; 69:1389-1401.

39. Comi G, Sora MGN, Bianchi A, et al. Spectral analysis of short-term heart rate variability in diabetic patients. J Auton Nerv Syst 1990; 30:S45-S50.

40. Dangman KH, Miura DS (eds). Proarrhythmic effects of antiarrhythmic drugs. In: Electrophysiology and Pharmacology of the Heart. New York, NY: Marcel Dekker, Inc., 1991; 375-395.

41. Eckberg DL, Drabinsky M, Braunwald E. Defective cardiac sympathetic control in patients with heart disease. N Engl J Med 1971; 285:877.

42. Ewing DJ, Neilson JM, Shapiro CM, et al. Twenty four hour heart rate variability: effects of posture, sleep and time of day in healthy controls and comparison with bedside tests of autonomic function in diabetic patients. Br Heart J 1991; 65:239-244.

43. Kjellgren O, Gomes JA. Heart rate variability and baroreflex sensitivity in myocardial infarction. Am Heart J 1993; 125(1):204-215.

44. Ori Z, Monir G, Weiss J, et al. Heart rate variability: frequency domain analysis. Cardiol Clin 1992; 10(3):499-537.

45. Campbell BC, Sturani A, Reid JL. Evidence of parasympathetic activity of the angiotensin converting enzyme inhibitor, captopril, in normotensive man. Clin Sci 1985; 68:49-56.

46. Corr PB, Gillis RA. Autonomic neural influences on the dysrhythmias resulting from myocardial infarction. Circ Res 1978; 43:1.

47. Kolman B, Verrier R, Lown B. The effect of vagus nerve stimulation upon vulnerability of the canine ventricle: role of sympathetic parasympathetic interactions. Circulation 1975; 52:578.

48. Lown B, Verrier R. Neural activity and ventricular fibrillation. N Engl J Med 1976; 294(21):1165.

49. Rabinowitz S, Verrier R, Lown B. Muscarinic effects of vagosympathetic trunk stimulation on the repetitive extrasystole (RE) threshold. Circulation 1976; 53:622.

49a. Coumel P, Rosengarten MD, Leclercq JF, Attuel P: Role of sympathetic nervous system in nonischemic ventricular arrhythmias. Br Heart J 47:137, 1982.

49b. Cannon WB: "Voodoo" death. Psychosom Med 1957; 19:182.

49c. Burrell RJW: The possible bearing of curse death and other factors in Bantu culture in the etiology of myocardial infarction. In James TN and Keyes JW (eds.): The Etiology of Myocardial Infarction. (Boston) Little Brown, 1963.

50. Vanoli E, De Ferrari MG, Stramba-Badiale M, et al. Vagal stimulation and prevention of sudden death in conscious dogs with a healed myocardial infarction. Circ Res 1991; 68:147-181.

51. De Ferrari MG, Vanoli E, Stramba-Badiale M, et al. Vagal reflexes and survival during acute ischemia in conscious dogs with healed myocardial infarction. Am J Physiol 1991; 261:H63-H69.

52. Singer DH, Baumgarten CM, Ten Eick RE. Cellular electrophysiology of ventricular and other dysrhythmias: studies on diseased and ischemic heart. Prog Cardiovasc Dis 1981; 24:97-156.

53. Ten Eick RE, Singer DH, Solberg LE. Coronary occlusion: effect on cellular electrical activity of the heart. Med Clin North Am 1976; 60:49-67.

54. Bailey JC, Greenspan K, Elizari MV, et al. Effects of acetylcholine on automaticity and conduction in the proximal portion of the His-Purkinje specialized conduction of the dog. Circ Res 1972; 30:210-216.

55. Dougherty CM, Burr RL. Comparison of heart rate variability in survivors and non-survivors of sudden cardiac arrest. Am J Cardiol 1992; 70(4):441-448.

56. Furlan R, Guzzetti S, Crivellaro W, et al. Continuous 24-hour assessment of neural regulation of systemic arterial pressure and RR variabilities in ambulant subjects. Circulation 1990; 81:537-547.

57. Malliani A, Pagani M, Lombardi F, et al. Cardiovascular neural regulation explored

in the frequency domain. Circulation 1991; 84(2):482-492.

58. Hales S. Statical Essays. Vol 2, Haemostaticks. London, England: Innings Manby Woodward, 1733.

59. Jose AD. Effect of combined sympathetic and parasympathetic blockade on heart rate and cardiac function in man. Am J Cardiol 1966; 18:476-478.

60. Sands KEF, Appel ML, Lilly LS, et al. Power spectrum analysis of heart rate variability in human cardiac transplant recipients. Circulation 1989; 79:76-82.

60a. Bernardi L, Rossi M, Soffiantino F, et al. Cross relation of heart rate and respiration versus deep breathing. Diabetes 1990; 38:589-596.

61. Katona P, Poitras JW, Barnett GO, et al. Cardiac vagal efferent and heart period in the carotid sinus reflex. Am J Physiol 1970; 218(4):1030-1037.

62. Katona P, Jih F. Respiratory sinus arrhythmia: non-invasive measure of parasympathetic cardiac control. J Appl Physiol 1975; 39(5):801-805.

63. Eckberg DL. Human sinus arrhythmia as an index of vagal cardiac outflow. J Appl Physiol 1983; 54(4):961-966.

64. Malliani A, Schwartz PJ, Zanchetti A. Neural mechanisms in life-threatening arrhythmias. Am Heart J 1980; 100(5):705-715.

65. Hyndman BW, Gregory JR. Spectral analysis of sinus arrhythmia during mental loading. Ergonomics 1975; 18(3):255-270.

66. Kitney RI, Rompelman O. The Study of Heart Rate Variability. Oxford, England: Clarendon Press, 1980.

67. Sayers B McA. Analysis of heart rate variability. Ergonomics 1973; 16(1):17-32.

68. Akselrod S, Gordon D, Ubel FA, et al. Power spectrum analysis of heart rate fluctuation: a quantitative probe of beat-to-beat cardiovascular control. Science 1981; 213:210-222.

69. Binkley PF, Nunziata E, Haas GJ, et al. Parasympathetic withdrawal is an integral component of autonomic imbalance in congestive heart failure: demonstration in human subjects and verification in a paced canine model of ventricular failure. J Am Coll Cardiol 1991; 18(2):464-472.

70. Ewing DJ, Martyn CN, Young RJ, et al. The value of cardiovascular autonomic function tests: Ten years experience in diabetes. Diabetes Care 1985; 8:491-498.

71. Guzetti S, Piccaluga E, Casati R, et al. Sympathetic predominance in essential hypertension: a study employing spectral analysis of heart rate variability. J Hypertens 1988; 6:711-717.

72. Hayano J, Sakakibara Y, Yamada M, et al. Decreased magnitude of heart rate spectral components in coronary artery disease: its relation to angiographic severity. Circulation 1990; 81:1217-1224.

73. Kleiger RE, Miller JP, Bigger JT, et al. Decreased heart rate variability and its association with increased mortality after acute myocardial infarction. Am J Cardiol 1987; 59(4):256-262.

74. Lombardi F, Sandrone G, Pernpruner S, et al. Heart rate variability as an index of sympathovagal interaction after acute myocardial infarction. Am J Cardiol 1987; 60:1239-1245.

75. Pagani M, Malfatto G, Pierini S, et al. Spectral analysis of heart rate variability in the assessment of autonomic diabetic neuropathy. J Auton Nerv Syst 1988; 23:143-153.

76. Saul JP, Arai Y, Berger RD, et al. Assessment of autonomic regulation in chronic congestive heart failure by heart rate spectral analysis. Am J Cardiol 1988; 61:1292-1299.

77. Singer DH, Martin GJ, Magid N, et al. Low heart rate variability and sudden cardiac death. J Electrocardiol 1988; S46-55.

78. Webb SW, Adgey AAJ, Pantridge JF. Autonomic disturbance at onset of acute myocardial infarction. Br Med J 1972; 3:89-92.

79. Farrel TG, Paul V, Cripps TR, et al. Baroreflex sensitivity and electrophysiological correlates in patients after acute myocardial infarction. Circulation 1991; 83:985-952.

80. Kleiger RE, Stein PK, Bosner MS et al. Time domain measurements of heart rate variability. Cardiol Clin 1992; 10(300):487-498.

81. Myers GA, Martin GJ, Magid NM, et al. Power spectral analysis of heart rate variability in sudden cardiac death: comparison to other methods. IEEE Trans Biomed Eng 1986; 33(12):1149-1156.

82. Van Hoogenhuyze D, Weinstein N, Martin GJ, et al. Reproducibility and relation to mean heart rate variability in normal subjects and in patients with congestive heart failure secondary to coronary artery disease. Am J Cardiol 1991; 68:1668-1676.

83. Kleiger RE, Miller JP, Bigger JT Jr, et al. Heart Rate variability: a variable predicting mortality following acute myocardial infarction. JACC 1984; 3(2):547. Abstract.

84. Bloomfield P. Fourier Analysis of Time Series: An Introduction. New York, NY: John Wiley & Sons, 1976.

85. Makhoul J. Linear prediction: a tutorial review. Proc IEEE 1975; 63:561-580.

86. Shiavi R. Introduction to Applied Statistical Signal Analysis. Homewood, Ill: Aksen Associates Inc, 1991.

87. Chess GF, Tam RMK, Calaresu FR. Influences of cardiac neural inputs on rhythmic variations of heart rate period in the cat. Am J Physiol 1975; 228(3):775-780.

88. Pagani M, Lombardi F, Guzetti S, et al. Power spectral analysis of heart rate and arterial pressure variabilities as a marker of sympatho-vagal interaction in man and conscious dog. Circ Res 1986; 59:178-193.

89. Perini R, Orizio C, Baselli G, et al. The influence of exercise intensity on power spectrum of heart rate variability. Eur J Appl Physiol 1990; 61(1-2):143-148.

90. Pomeranz B, Macaulay RJB, Caudill MA, et al. Assessment of autonomic function in humans by heart rate spectral analysis. Am J Physiol 1985; 248(Heart Circ Physiol)17:H151-H153.

91. Saul JP, Rea RF, Eckberg DL, et al. Heart rate and muscle sympathetic nerve variability during reflex changes of autonomic activity. Am J Physiol 1990; 258(Heart Circ Physiol)27:H713-H721.

92. Vybiral T, Bryg RJ, Maddens ME, et al. Effect of passive tilt on sympathetic and parasympathetic components of heart rate variability in normal subjects. Am J Cardiol 1989; 63:1117-1120.

93. Ahmed M, Fintel D, Zhang F, et al. Survival post-sudden cardiac death: predictive value of heart rate variability vs. inducibility. J Am Coll Cardiol 1992; 3:167A.

94. Bigger JT, Albrecht P, Steinman RC, et al. Comparison of time and frequency domain-based measures of cardiac parasympathetic activity in holter recordings after myocardial infarction. Am J Cardiol 1989; 64:536-538.

95. Coker R, Koziell A, Oliver C, et al. Does the sympathetic nervous system influence sinus arrhythmia in man? Evidence from combined autonomic blockade. J Physiol 1984; 356:459-464.

96. Xia R, Odemuyiwa O, Gill J, et al. Influence of recognition errors of computerized analysis of 24-hour electrocardiograms on the measurement of spectral components of heart rate variability. Int J Biomed Comput 1993; 32(3-4):223-235.

97. Hon EH, Lee ST. Electronic evaluation of the fetal heart rate patterns preceding fetal death, further observations. Am J Obstet Gynecol 1965; 87:814-826.

98. Gaziano EP, Freeman DW. Analysis of heart rate patterns preceding fetal death. Obstet Gynecol 1977; 50:578-582.

99. Wolf MM, Varigos GA, Hunt D, et al. Sinus arrhythmia in acute myocardial infarction. Med J Aust 1978; 2:52.

100. Masaoka S, Lev-Ran A, Hill LR, et al. Heart rate variability in diabetes: relationship to age and duration of the disease. Diabetes Care 1985; 8(1):64-68.

101. Ewing DJ, Campbell IW, Clarke BF. Mortality in diabetic autonomic neuropathy. Lancet 1976; 1:601.

102. Kleiger RE, Miller JP, Krone RJ, et al. Independent effect of heart rate variability controlling for exercise testing predicting mortality of 808 patients after myocardial infarction. JACC 1987; 9:241a. Abstract.

103. Cripps TR, Malik M, Farrell TS, et al. Prognostic value of reduced heart rate variability after myocardial infarction: clinical evaluation of a new analysis method. Br Heart J 1991; 65:14.

104. Malik M, Cripps TR, Farrell TS, et al. Prognostic value of heart rate variability after myocardial infarction: a comparison of different data-processing methods. Med Biol Eng Comput 1989; 29:603.

105. Singer DH, Van Hoogenhuyze D, Monir G, et al, unpublished observation.

106. Yusuf S, Peto R, Lewis J, et al. Beta blockade during and after myocardial infarction: an overview of the randomized trials. Prog Cardiovasc Dis 1985; 27:335-371.

107. Gilman AG, Rall TW, Nies AS, et al (eds). Goodman and Gilman's The Pharmacological Basis of Therapeutics. New York: Pergamon Press, 1990.

108. Cook JR, Bigger JT, Kleiger RE, et al. Effect of atenolol and diltiazem on heart period variability in normal persons. J Am Coll Cardiol 1991; 17:480-484.

109. Hoffman B, Singer D. Appraisal of the effects of catecholamines on cardiac electrical activity. In: New adrenergic blocking drugs: Their pharmacological, biochemical and clinical actions. Ann NY Acad Sci 1967; 139:914-939.

109a. Zuanetti G, Latini R, Neilson JMM, Schwartz PJ, Ewing DJ and the Antiarrhythmic Drug Evaluation Group (ADEG): Heart rate variability in patients with ventricular arrhythmias: Effect of antiarrhythmic drugs. J Am Coll Cardiol 1991; 17(3):604-612.

110. Ewing DJ, Campbell IW, Clarke BF. Assessment of cardiovascular effects in diabetic autonomic neuropathy and prognostic implications. Ann Intern Med 1980; 92(part 2):308-311.

111. Johnson RH, Robinson BJ. Mortality in alcoholics with autonomic neuropathy. J Neurol Neurosurg Psychiatry 1988; 51:476-480.

112. Martin GJ, Magid NM, Valentini V, et al. Heart rate variability and the evaluation of risk of sudden cardiac death. Clin Res 1987; 35(3):302A.

113. Nakagawa M, Saikawa T, Ito M. Progressive reduction of heart rate variability with eventual sudden death in two patients. Br Heart J 1994; 71(1):87-88.

114. Martin GJ, Magid NM, Eckberg DL, et al. Heart rate variability and sudden cardiac death during ambulatory monitoring. Clin Res 1987; 35:302a. Abstract.

114a. Kjellgren O, Ip J, Suh K, et al. The role of parasympathetic modulation of the reentrant arrhythmic substrate in the genesis of sustained ventricular tachycardia. PACE 1994; 17(7):1276-1287.

115. Fei L, Anderson MH, Katritsis D, et al. Decreased heart rate variability in survivors of sudden cardiac death not associated with coronary artery disease. Br Heart J 1994; 71(1):16-21.

116. Gordon D, Cohen RJ, Kelly D, et al. Sudden infant death syndrome: abnormalities in short term fluctuations in heart rate and respiratory activity. Pediatr Res 1984; 18:921-926.

117. Gordon D, Southall DP, Kelly DH, et al. Analysis of heart rate and respiratory patterns in sudden infant death syndrome victims and control infants. Pediatr Res 1986; 20:680-684.

118. Kluge KA, Harper RM, Schechtman VL, et al. Spectral analysis assessment of respiratory sinus arrhythmia in normal infants who subsequently died of sudden infant death syndrome. Pediatr Res 1988; 24:677-682.

119. Hellman JB, Stacy RW. Variations of respiratory sinus arrhythmia with age. J Appl Physiol 1976; 41(5):734-738.

120. Hrushesky WJ, Fader D, Schmitt O, et al. Respiratory sinus arrhythmia: a measure of cardiac age. Science 1984; 224:1001-1004.

121. Shannon DC, Carley DW, Benson H. Aging of modulation of heart rate. Am J Physiol 1987; 253(Heart Circ Physiol)22:H874-H877.

122. Finley JP, Nugent ST, Hellenbrand W. Heart rate variability in children. Spectral analysis of developmental changes between 5 and 24 years. Can J Physiol Pharmacol 1987; 65:2048-2052.

123. Korkushko OV, Shatilo VB, Plachinda YuI, et al. Autonomic control of cardiac chronotropic function in man as a function of age: assessment by power spectral analysis of heart rate variability. J Auton Nerv Syst 1991; 32:191-198.

124. Lipsitz LA, Mietus J, Moody GB, et al. Spectral characteristics of heart rate variability before and during postural tilt relation to aging and risk of syncope. Circulation 1990; 81:1803-1810.

125. Coumel P, Deschams J. Lessons from recordings of sudden death by holter monitoring. In: Bayes de Luna A, Brugada P, Cosin Aguilar J, et al (eds). Sudden Cardiac Death. Dordrecht and Boston: Kluwer Academic Publishers, 1991; 191-207.

126. Odemuyiwa O, Malik M, Farrell TG, et al. Multifactorial prediction of arrhythmic events after myocardial infarction. Combination of heart rate variability and left ventricular ejection fraction with other variables. PACE 1991; 14(11):1986-1991.

127. Van Hoogenhuyze D, Martin GJ, Weiss JS, et al. Heart rate variability. An update. J Electrocardiol 1989; 22(suppl):204-208.

128. Suleiman M, Monir G, Sahyouni N, et al. Age modulation of heart rate variability in normal and sudden cardiac death patients. PACE 1992; 15(4):526.

129. Odemuyiwa O, Farrell TG, Malik M, et al. Influence of age on relation between heart rate variability, left ventricular ejection fraction, frequency of ventricular extrasystoles, and sudden death after myocardial infarction. Br Heart J 1992; 67(5):387-391.

130. Monir G, Fintel D, Yarnold P, et al. Cycle length dependence of heart rate variability. J Am Coll Cardiol 1992; 19(3):167A.

131. Monir G, Fintel D, Yarnold P, et al. Heart rate variability: focus on defined cycle lengths. J Am Coll Cardiol 1992; 19(3):166A.

132. Muller JE, Ludmer PL, Willich SN, et al. Circadian variation in the frequency of sudden cardiac death. Circulation 1987; 75(1):131-138.

133. Rocco MB, Barry J, Cambell S, et al. Circadian variation of transient myocardial ischemia in patients with coronary artery disease. Circulation 1987; 75:395-400.

134. Lucente M, Rebuzzi AG, Lanza GA, et al. Circadian variation of ventricular tachycardia in acute myocardial infarction. Am J Cardiol 1988; 62:670-674.

135. Huikuri HV, Linnaluoto MK, Sepannen T, et al. Circadian rhythm of heart rate variability in survivors of cardiac arrest. Am J Cardiol 1992; 70:610-615.

136. Hull SS, Evans AR, Vanoli E, et al. Heart rate variability before and after myocardial infarction in conscious dogs at high and low risk of sudden death. J Am Coll Cardiol 1990; 16(4):978-985.

137. Bigger JT, Fleiss JL, Steinman RC, et al. Frequency domain measures of heart period

variability and mortality after myocardial infarction. Circulation 1992; 85:164-171.

138. Bigger JT Jr, et al. Prediction of death after myocardial infarction with RR variability calculated from 2 to 15-minute ECGs. JACC 1993; 21:271A.

139. Coumel P. Modification of heart rate variability preceding the onset of tachyarrhythmias. Cardiologia 1990; 35:(suppl):7-12.

140. Huikuri HV, Valkama JO, Airaksinen KEJ, et al. Frequency domain measures of heart rate variability before the onset of nonsustained and sustained ventricular tachycardia in patients with coronary artery disease. Circulation 1993; 87:1220-1228.

141. Yoshida A, et al. Heart rate variability before spontaneous episodes of ventricular tachycardia originating from right ventricular outflow tract (RVOT) in patients without organic heart disease. Circulation 1992; 86(suppl):I660.

142. Pelliccia F, et al. Transient impairment in cardiac parasympathetic activity precedes myocardial ischemia in variant angina. Circulation 1992; 86(suppl):I730.

143. Bernardi L, Lumina C, Ferrari MR, et al. Relationship between fluctuations in heart rate and asymptomatic nocturnal ischemia. Int J Cardiol 1980; 20:399-351.

144. Vybiral T, Glaeser DH, Goldberger AL, et al. Conventional heart rate variability analysis of ambulatory electrocardiographic recording fails to predict imminent ventricular fibrillation. J Am Coll Cardiol 1993; 22(2):557-565.

145. Skinner JE, Pratt CM, Vybiral T. A reduction in correlation dimension of heartbeat intervals precedes imminent ventricular fibrillation in human subjects. Am Heart J 1993; 125(3):731-743.

146. Goldberger AL, Rigney DR, Mietus J, et al. Nonlinear dynamics in sudden cardiac death syndrom: heart rate oscillations and bifurcations. Experientia 1989; 44:983-987.

147. Goldberger AL, Rigney D. Sudden death is not chaos. In: Kelso JAS, Mandell AJ, Shlesinger MF (eds). Dynamic Patterns in Complex Systems. Singapore and New Jersey: World Scientific Publishers, 1988.

148. Goldberger AL, West BJ. Chaos in physiology: Health or disease? In: Degn H, Holden AV, Olsen LF (eds). Chaos in Biological Systems. New York, NY: Plenum Press, 1987; 1.

149. Goldberger AL, West BJ. Fractals in physiology and medicine. Yale J Biol Med 1987; 60:421.

150. Bigger JT Jr, Fleiss JL, Steinman RC, et al. Frequency domain measures of heart period variability and mortality after myocardial infarction. Circulation 1992; 85:164-171.

151. Malik M, Camm AJ. Heart variability: from facts to fancies. J Am Coll Cardiol 1993; 22(2):566-568.

Chapter 34

Heart Rate Variability in Patients with Heart Failure

Gian Carlo Casolo

Introduction

It is now generally accepted that heart rate variability (HRV) is reduced in patients with heart failure.[1-3] Both time-domain and frequency-domain measures of HRV are in fact decreased in heart failure patients when compared to normal individuals. Normal subjects are able to modulate heart rate (HR) in a wide range of different levels. Furthermore, these levels can be modified very rapidly. This ability can be viewed as a 'variability reserve' that characterizes the normal heart. Heart failure patients, on the contrary, are not able to modify HR to the same extent and as rapidly as normal subjects. Sometimes their ability to vary HR in time is so altered that they appear to have lost this property.[4] Their 'variability reserve' is therefore greatly reduced.

Because HRV depends on the activity of the autonomic nervous system (ANS) and on its integrity, one is tempted to relate the HRV changes taking place in heart failure patients with the degree and kind of neuro-humoral control. This issue is particularly interesting if we consider that exercise capacity and prognosis of heart failure patients are weakly related to the extent of left ventricular dysfunction,[5-7] while neurohumoral mechanisms, and particularly the activity of the ANS, appear to possess a relevant independent weight.[8-10] Unfortunately, there are no simple means to characterize the degree of neurohumoral activation in heart failure. Thus, HRV can represent a very important parameter to collect in heart failure patients. To date, we do not have a definite idea of how HRV is related to the neurohumoral activation in heart failure, although some available information can provide the basis for at least a few hypotheses.

An interesting issue is also offered by the demonstration of decreased HRV in heart failure on one side and the relationship between death and decreased HRV on the other. In fact, decreased HRV is a powerful independent predictor of mortality (particularly sudden death) and arrhythmic events after myocardial infarction.[11-14] It is

From: Malik M., Camm AJ (eds.): *Heart Rate Variability*. Armonk, NY. Futura Publishing Company, Inc., © 1995.

also well known that heart failure patients represent a high-risk group for death. Up to 80% of heart failure patients die suddenly with an average 60% survival at 4 years.[15,16] Such a relationship cannot be casual, but unfortunately at this moment there are no prospective studies on the ability of HRV as a predictor of outcome in heart failure.

It should be stressed how, for the purposes of this chapter, the definition of heart failure is crucial. Heart failure includes, in the broadest sense, all those patients both symptomatic and asymptomatic having left and/or right ventricular failure, and systolic and/or diastolic dysfunction.[15] The main information available on this subject has been obtained in symptomatic patients with left ventricular dysfunction due to loss of muscle mass available to bring about contraction, usually secondary to coronary artery disease. This chapter mainly deals with the HRV changes observed in this subset of heart failure patients, that are also usually described as having congestive heart failure.[16] Information on HRV in acute with respect to chronic heart failure, systolic versus diastolic heart failure, and heart failure due to different mechanisms can only be indirectly derived from some investigations.

The following points will be addressed: the evidence of low HRV in heart failure; the relationship between HRV and etiology of heart failure; the effect of left ventricular function on HRV; the HRV behavior with the increasing severity of heart failure; the effect of therapy on HRV; and the physiopathologic mechanisms underlying decreased HRV in heart failure.

Decreased Heart Rate Variability in Heart Faillure

The demonstration of decreased HRV in heart failure is now reported by several authors.[1-3,17] It is somewhat surprising how this evidence was found only recently. This can be, in part, explained by problems with patients' selection, methods of analysis employed, and the desire to study patients with other clinical signs of distinction (ie, previous myocardial infarction, and/or ventricular arrhythmias) that are also frequently present in heart failure. The increasing interest of the medical community toward heart failure, the large proportion of these patients, the ability to modify the natural history of this disease by the use of new drugs, and the awareness of the importance to recognize patients in the early stages of heart failure, are important factors in the evolution of this field.[18,19]

A few years ago the difficulty of studying HR for long periods of time and the lack of computer assisted techniques prevented a systematic approach to the study of HRV in heart failure. However, if we consider the changes of the RR intervals determined by an external challenge as a measure of HRV in heart failure patients, much information was available in the past indicating an abnormal (usually reduced) control of HR by studying baroreflex responses to external stimuli.[20-24]

The introduction of Holter monitoring allowed the study of long periods of HR. We were thus able to show how there is an abnormal 24-hour behavior of HR in patients with heart failure and impaired left ventricular function due to coronary artery disease.[25] The main abnormality found was the lack of nocturnal decline in HR of the patients' group as compared to controls (Figure 1). Furthermore, when HR measured at 5 am was plotted against left ventricular ejection fraction we could demonstrate a significant inverse linear correlation (r = 0.7, p <0.001). This result, which can be viewed as a first demonstration of reduced HR variation in heart failure, was subsequently confirmed by others with striking similarities.[26,27]

The advent of computerized methods to analyze HR allowed to evaluate more sensitive measure of HRV other than the daily HR excursion. We were therefore able to show a marked difference in HRV between normal subjects and heart failure patients that was evident throughout the day

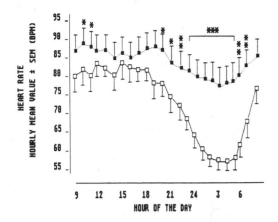

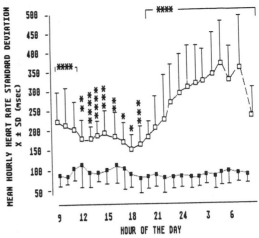

Figure 1. 24-hour HR behavior in normal subjects (white dots) and in heart failure patients (black dots). Note the higher HR values and greatly reduced slowing of HR at night of heart failure patients. (* = p <0.01, ** = p <0.005, *** = p<0.001). From Casolo et al[1] with permission.

Figure 2. Mean hourly HR standard deviation in control subjects (white squares) and heart failure patients (dark squares). Note the markedly reduced HRV in heart failure patients compared to normal individuals. (* = p <0.05, ** = p <0.01 , *** = p <0.005, **** = p <0.0001). From Casolo et al[1] with permission.

(Figure 2).[1] We studied 20 heart failure patients due to both coronary artery disease and primary cardiomyopathy. We used several indices of HRV: mean 24 hourly HR standard deviation, mean hourly HR standard deviation, and the width of the frequency distribution of the 24-hour RR intervals at its base, and at 10% and 50% of its height (Figure 3). All the measures used were significantly smaller in heart failure patients with respect to controls (Figure 4). Three patients with very low HRV values died within 4.3 months, suggesting a possible prognostic significance of HRV in this group of patients.

Spectral techniques have also been applied to the study of heart failure. Saul et al studied 3 to 6 HR segments of 15 minutes from 25 patients with severe chronic heart failure.[28] They found a marked reduction of the HR spectral power at all frequencies examined (Figure 5). Spectral power was virtually absent at frequencies >0.04 Hz, while fluctuations of HR at very low frequencies (VLF) were still present, although to a lesser extent with respect to normal individuals.

A similar behavior for spectral composition of HR was subsequently obtained by our group when studying the entire day.[4]

We studied 15 patients belonging to advanced NYHA functional classes. Spectral analysis was repeated every hour for the entire 24-hour period on a 1024 point data series. The low-frequency (LF) (0.04 to 0.12 Hz) and the high-frequency (HF) (0.22 to 0.32 Hz) power were almost absent throughout the day (Figure 6). Compared to normal subjects, in heart failure patients the power under the LF and HF area was 10 times smaller (Figure 7). Furthermore, while spectral composition of HR during the day appeared to be very different both quantitatively and qualitatively in normal subjects, it did not vary significantly in heart failure patients.

Several other authors have subsequently confirmed these early observations by using either similar or different measures of HRV. When HRV is examined in patients with overt heart failure, it appears to be almost invariably decreased in spite of different methods in the processing of data, techniques of analysis, and length of the HR recording (Figure 8 and Figure 9). Furthermore, these measures appear to be reproducible as they do not show significant day-to-day variations.[29]

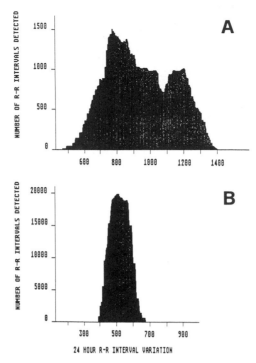

Figure 3. Frequency distribution of the 24-hour RR variation in a normal subject (A) and in a heart failure patient (B). Note the different shape and RR variation of the two patients. From Casolo et al[1] with permission.

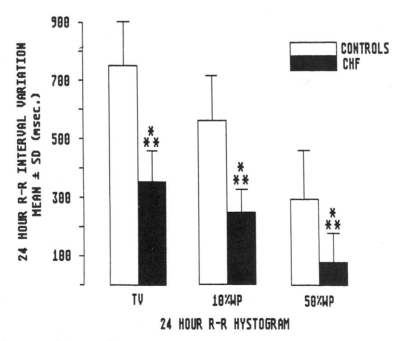

Figure 4. Measures of HRV in heart failure patients as compared to controls. TV, 10%WP, 50%WP represent the 24-hour RR variation as assessed at the base (TV), at 10% of the height of the histogram (10%WP), and at 50% of the height of the histogram). Note the smaller HRV of heart failure patients as compared to controls. *** = p <0.001. From Casolo et al[1] with permission.

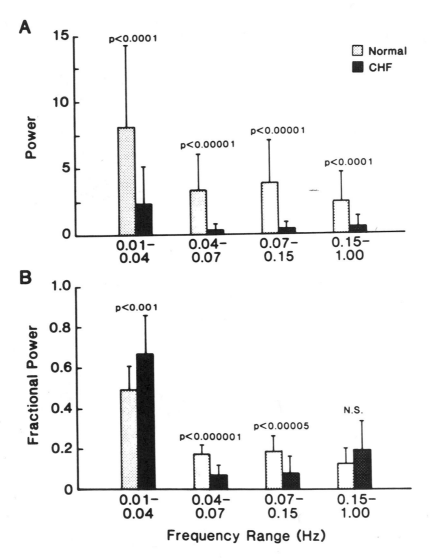

Figure 5. HR spectral power in four frequency bands for control subjects and patients expressed as absolute power in (beats/min)^2, (A), and normalized by the power from 0.01 to 1 Hz, (B). The fractional power (%) allows insight into the typical spectral appearance for each group. When using this approach, the 0.01 to 0.04 power is significantly increased in heart failure patients meaning that while HRV is reduced in absolute terms, the residual variation is qualitatively altered. From Saul et al[28] with permission.

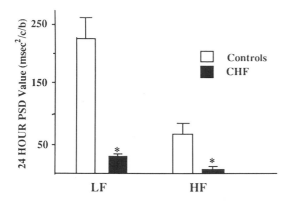

Figure 6. Mean and standard deviation 24-hour value of the LF and HF components in normal persons (controls) and in patients with heart failure (CHF). Note the markedly reduced spectral compositions of heart failure patients as compared to normal subjects. (* = p <0.001). From Casolo et al[4] with permission.

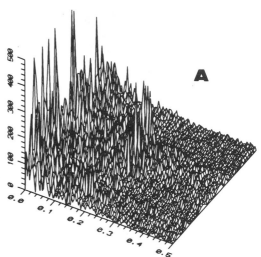

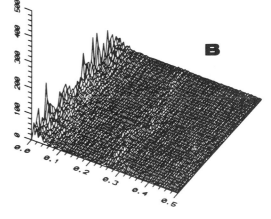

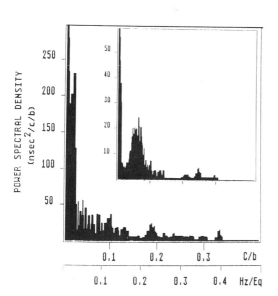

Figure 7. Spectral analysis of HR in a heart failure patient. The use of a vertical scale comparable to that used in normal subjects does not allow to recognize any component. By using a scale 10 times smaller, the two main bandwidths of interest are seen. From Casolo et al[4] with permission.

Figure 8. Three-dimensional plot of the 24-hour spectral composition in a normal subject (A) and in a NYHA Class IV heart failure patient (B). Each segment represents the results of an FFT-based algorithm computed on 256 nonoverlapping segments. Amplitude is calculated in $msec^2/Hz$. The HR recordings started at 9 am. The first spectra of each subject is the lowest of the series. Note the greater HR variation of (A) with respect to (B). Also note the increase of the the high frequency components (A) at night as compared to (B). Patient in (B) almost does not exhibit any HR variation during the whole 24 hours.

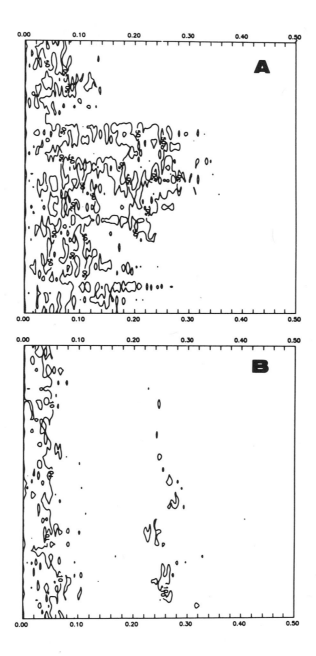

Figure 9. Two-dimensional plot of the 24-hour spectral composition in a normal subject (A) and in a NYHA Class IV heart failure patient (B). Same data as in Figure 8. The third-dimension (the amplitude of the signal) is indicated by the numbers inside the drawing. The amplitude scale in (A) was set to 50 ms^2/Hz, while it was set to 10 ms^2/Hz in (B). Note the very scarce amount of spectral components at all the frequencies examined. Also note the evident presence of the HF (0.2 to 0.35 Hz) components in (A) at the time corresponding to sleep.

Etiology of Heart Failure and Heart Rate Variability

It is reasonable to speculate whether decreased HRV depends from, or is affected by the disease causing heart failure. In other words, depressed HRV may reflect the severity of the disease underlying heart failure rather than being the effect of heart failure itself.

As an example, it has been shown how HRV may be affected by several risk factors for coronary artery disease or the simple presence of a coronary lesion. Smoking and lack of physical activity may decrease HRV in normal subjects,[30] while diabetes is known to be associated with a low RR variation. It has also been reported how coronary artery disease by itself is associated with a decrease in the HF spectral power and how this decrease correlates with the angiographic severity.[31]

Unpublished data from our previous investigation[1] showed how HRV did not differ in patients with primary cardiomyopathy and coronary artery disease. Similar results can also be derived from the investigation of Stefenelli et al who also studied HRV in heart failure.[32] Sixteen out of their 21 heart failure patients had primary cardiomyopathy, but all patients had a low HRV count. Recently, Gang et al and Dadoun et al addressed this subject and could not find any significant difference in HRV between patients whose heart failure was of ischemic etiology versus those with cardiomyopathy.[33,34]

Therefore, in spite of the fact that some conditions may alter, per se, HRV, once heart failure is present HRV is low without any difference based on the etiology of heart failure.

Heart Rate Variability and Left Ventricular Function

It is reasonable to assume that the abnormal HR variation present in heart failure is related to the degree of left ventricular function. Indeed, heart failure patients have both depressed left ventricular function and a low RR variability count. Nevertheless, such a relationship is not very strict.

In the study of Saul et al,[28] only the absolute power in the 0.04 to 0.07 Hz was directly related to the cardiac index (r = 0.466, p <0.05) and inversely to pulmonary capillary wedge pressure (r = -0.545, p <0.01). No other commonly measured index of left ventricular function was related to HRV.

On the contrary, in the investigation of Nolan et al, who used the count of RR intervals exceeding 50 milliseconds as a measure of HRV, they found a significant inverse linear correlation (r = 0.49, p <0.05) with the radionuclide determined left ventricular ejection fraction.[17]

Kienzle et al, studying 23 heart failure patients, analyzed both spectral measures of HRV and the 24-hour standard deviation of HR (SDNN).[35] They related these measures to left ventricular ejection fraction, pulmonary wedge pressure, and cardiac output. Left ventricular ejection fraction and pulmonary wedge pressure did not correlate with any measure of HRV. They only found a significant relationship between the 0.05 to 0.15 Hz and the 0.2 to 0.5 Hz spectral components of HR and cardiac output (r = 0.49 and 0.42, p <0.02 and 0.045, respectively).

Adamopoulos et al analyzed the ability of different methods of HRV to characterize the autonomic tone in 25 congestive heart failure patients.[36] In this investigation, no significant relationship between spectral and nonspectral measures of HRV and left ventricular ejection fraction was found.

It can be concluded that there is not a clear demonstration of the relationship between left ventricular function and HRV in heart failure. This relationship, however, is nevertheless present as previously described. Furthermore, HRV and left ventricular ejection fraction are closely related in other conditions such as during acute myocardial infarction and in the few following days.[11,37] Differences in the selection of patients as well as in processing techniques of HRV analysis may account for the observed differences in the above mentioned investigations. Also the small number of patients examined may have masked a weak correlation. It should also be stressed how, when studying heart failure patients, the degree of left ventricular dysfunction is usually severe and similar between patients. This fact may again mask a relationship between variables. In a recent investigation we studied 80 patients with different degrees of heart failure secondary to coronary artery disease.[38] They were divided in four equal groups of 20 patients according to the New York Heart Association functional class. When left ventricular ejection fraction was plotted versus SDNN we observed a significant relationship (Figure 10) (r = 0.77, p <0.001). Such a relationship could not be found either in each of the heart failure groups or in the control group.

Measures of HRV and left ventricular function may also not be related for other reasons. In the first place, left ventricular dysfunction may not be easy to characterize with only a few parameters. It is well known that ejection fraction may not represent an

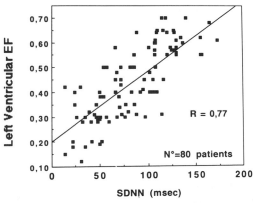

Figure 10. Plot of the 24-hour standard deviation of HR (SDNN) versus the echocardiographically determined left ventricular ejection fraction (EF) in 80 coronary artery disease patients. These patients were divided in four equal groups of 20 according to the NYHA functional classification. Note that a strong correlation between EF and SDNN is present (r = 0.77, p<0.001). Such a relationship is not present when each group is considered separately.

adequate mean to evaluate left ventricular function in several conditions. Also, at the same level of left ventricular dysfunction two patients may have a markedly different exercise capacity due to different compensatory mechanisms.[5,39]

It should also be stressed how if heart failure is far from being described only by depressed left ventricular function, HRV also depends from many factors, some of which are known to be altered in heart failure. It would not be surprising if HRV were related to both depressed left ventricular function and the presence, degree, and adequacy of compensatory mechanisms, rather than to depressed left ventricular function alone.

Heart Rate Variability and Severity of Heart Failure

A very important issue is the possible role of measures of HRV as indicators of the severity of heart failure. If HRV reflects the presence and severity of heart failure, then it can be used to follow up and identify patients who are at greater risk of death or complications, and/or to monitor therapeutic interventions. There is now evidence for significant neuroendocrine activation in patients with left ventricular dysfunction and no heart failure.[40] The potential ability of HRV to detect such an abnormality could be of great clinical importance.

There are few data on this subject. In a prospective study performed in 21 heart failure patients, HRV (measured by using the 24-hour RR interval histogram) at baseline and after 6 months was related to the severity of heart failure according to the NYHA Functional Class.[32] Patients belonging to different NYHA Classes had different HRVs: the higher the functional class, the lower the HRV values. Also, the clinical deterioration of three patients was associated with a further decrease in HRV, while patients who improved did not show any significant change.

We also observed, by studying 80 coronary artery disease patients how with the increasing severity of heart failure all the measures of HRV (both spectral and nonspectral) decreased progressively. HRV ranged from a normal behavior such as in NYHA Class I patients to a severely reduced or absent HRV variation in NYHA Class IV patients.[38]

In a recent investigation, Gibelin et al showed a significant relationship between spectral and nonspectral measures of HRV and severity of symptoms in heart failure.[41] Patients with more severe forms of heart failure had the lowest values of LF power of the spectra and the lowest values of total spectral power. There are two main studies that were designed to evaluate the effects of treatment with angiotensin enzyme (ACE) inhibitors on HRV in heart failure.[42,43] In both of these investigations, HRV increased after treatment. In one of these investigations, the clinical status was also recorded.[42] The increased HRV count (+50%) was also associated with clinical amelioration (mean NYHA Class before treatment: 2.4+0.4 versus NYHA Class after zofenopril: 1.8+0.8, p<0.007) thus indirectly demonstrating that different HRV characteristics reflect the severity of heart failure.

It can be concluded that HRV can identify patients with different severity of heart failure. Both spectral and nonspectral measures of HRV show a progressive decrease with the increasing severity of symptoms as assessed by the NYHA Class. Because of these observations, measures of HRV can be used for follow-up purposes in heart failure patients.

Effect of Therapeutic Interventions

HRV can be modified in heart failure by a variety of therapeutic measures. In order to evaluate the effect of physical training on HRV in heart failure patients, Coats et al studied prospectively 17 patients belonging to NYHA Class II to III.[3] After 8 weeks of physical training at home they observed an increase in the SDNN (+19%, p <0.05), and in the HF component of the spectra (+53%, p <0.05), while the LF component decreased significantly (-21.2%, p <0.07). In a similar investigation, Adamopoulos et al evaluated the effect of physical training on 25 patients with stable heart failure and obtained similar results.[36]

The effect of the use of captopril on heart failure was evaluated by Flapan et al in 32 heart failure patients.[43] They measured HRV as the number of successive RR intervals >50 milliseconds from tapes obtained in two separate occasions. Their index showed a significant increase in the majority of the treated patients (group mean count: 482 before treatment versus 1032 after treatment, p <0.002) while no change was observed in a control group.

Binkley et al evaluated the effect of the ACE-inhibitor zofenopril in a double blind randomized placebo-controlled trial.[42] Patients and controls were balanced at baseline study in terms of functional class, ventricular performance and spectral composition of HRV. After 3 months they observed a significant increase in the total power of the spectra (+50%, p <0.09), and in the HF component (+100%, p <0.03) of the treated group. No significant increase was found for the LF component.

There are several other investigations designed to evaluate the effect of some drugs on HRV in heart failure. Carvedilol (a new beta-blocking agent) has been found to significantly increase the HF power of the spectra, pNN50, and r-MSSD after 3 to 4 months of treatment in spite of the concomitant use of digitalis and ACE-inhibitors.[44] Scopolamine has also been reported to increase several indices of HRV in some patients (13/20) with end-stage heart failure.[45] Digoxin, a drug able to improve the neurohumoral status in heart failure patients,[46] has been found to significantly increase the power under the HF area of the spectra and the r-MSSD,[47] the SDNN, pNN50, and the SDANN.[48] Pimobedan has been reported to improve symptoms of heart failure but does not increase HRV.[32] Ibopamine does not seem to induce any significant HRV change in heart failure.[48]

Physiopathology of Heart Rate Variability in Heart Failure

Although there is a general agreement on the presence of decreased HRV in heart failure, it is not clear how and why these changes take place.

It is well known that the autonomic control of the cardiovascular system is deranged in heart failure. The activity of the sympathetic nervous system is augmented as reflected by increased plasma catecholamine levels and neural sympathetic traffic as evaluated by microneurographic techniques.[49,50] On the other side, this increased adrenergic drive is associated with depletion of catecholamine stores in the failing myocardium and also with a reduction of density and affinity of beta-adrenergic receptors.[51-53] Besides the alterations of the sympathetic control, there is also evidence for decreased vagal traffic to the heart.[20,21] Thus, a complex abnormality of the autonomic control to the heart is present. It should also be outlined how these abnormalities are only a part of a more complex neurohumoral activation involving several other mechanisms (ie, the renin-angiotensin-aldosterone system, the atrial natriuretic peptide, the antidiuretic hormone, etc.)[16] whose effects on HRV are not known.

HR and HRV are strictly dependent on both the sympathetic and parasympathetic activity to the heart.[54] Therefore, depressed HRV in heart failure may have different causes.

Relating Heart Rate Variability and Autonomic Activity in Heart Failure

In order to consider HRV as an index of vagal traffic to the heart, it is important to extract from the total variability of the RR interval the one that is controlled by the parasympathetic activity. This is not an easy task because parasympathetic activity can affect the RR variability over a wide range of levels. The study of those variations that can be modulated only by the vagal outflow to the heart (ie, HF spectral components, pNN50, r-MSSD) may represent a reasonable method to assess vagal activity to the sinus node. Nevertheless, this approach leaves out some information whose relevance cannot be stated precisely. Modulated vagal activity may result decreased or absent in at least three different situations: cardiac denervation,[55] parasympathetic blockade, and tonic stimulation of vagal activity.[56] To further complicate things one should also keep in mind the complex interplay at different levels of the ANS. The modulation of HRV is, in fact, a complex mechanism with a continuous interplay between vagal and sympathetic activity.[57] It is therefore not entirely correct to interpret decreased HRV in heart failure as the isolated effect of reduced vagal outflow to the heart. The demonstration that parasympathetic blockade abolishes respiratory sinus arrhythmia and the HF component of the spectra does not necessarily imply that every time we observe a decrease of these two measures there is a reduced vagal activity to the heart. It is nevertheless widely accepted that decreased HRV in heart failure represents the demonstration of decreased vagal outflow to the heart.

Although there are some investigations indicating that vagal activity is reduced in heart failure, there is no doubt that increased adrenergic activity is a well-known feature of this condition. It represents a compensatory mechanism that has been found to adversely influence prognosis and symptoms.[6,19,58] It would be quite surprising if HRV would not reflect these changes. However, the association of decreased HRV and increased sympathetic outflow to the heart is difficult to be explained. Increased sympathetic activity has been found to augment the LF component of the HR spectrum. One may expect a qualitative change of the HR spectrum in heart failure, with an increase of the LF component and a decrease of the HF component with little or no change in the total variance. As previously reported, we observe instead a decrease of all the spectral components of HRV and a marked reduction in the variance. The LF component of HRV is usually considered an index of sympathetic activation. However, vagal activity also contributes to this component of the spectra. Therefore, the LF/HF ratio has been proposed as a pure index of sympathetic activity to the heart. No data are currently available that provide a clinical validation for this assumption in heart failure. Preliminary data from our group indicate a progressive decrease of the LF (0.04 to 0.12 Hz) component of the spectra

from NYHA Class II to Class IV patients with no consistent change in the LF to HF ratio.

There are some studies relating plasma levels of norepinephrine, norepinephrine spill-over and/or muscle sympathetic nerve activity with measures of HRV in heart failure. Saul et al found a significant and positive relationship between plasma levels of catecholamines and the ratio of the power in the spectral bands 0.01 to 0.04/0.04 to 0.07.[28] Kienzle et al found a strongly significant inverse relationship between spectral and nonspectral measures of HRV and plasma norepinephrine and sympathetic nerve activity (norepinephrine versus

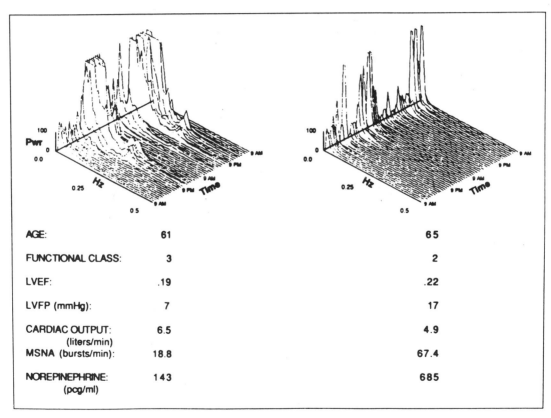

AGE:	61	65
FUNCTIONAL CLASS:	3	2
LVEF:	.19	.22
LVFP (mmHg):	7	17
CARDIAC OUTPUT: (liters/min)	6.5	4.9
MSNA (bursts/min):	18.8	67.4
NOREPINEPHRINE: (pcg/ml)	143	685

Figure 11. Three-dimensional plots of HR power spectrum during a 48-hour period from two heart failure patients. Note the relative lower spectral composition of the patient on the right as compared to the patient on the left. As shown, these patients have comparable values of left ventricular ejection fraction (EF) and age. However, the patient on the right has a more pronounced hemodynamic impairment as indicated by a higher end-diastolic left ventricular pressure (LVFP) and a lower cardiac output. This patient also shows signs of increased adrenergic activity as indicated by higher levels of plasma norepinephrine and a significantly increased muscle sympathetic nerve activity (MSNA). From Kienzle et al[35] with permission.

SDNN r = -0.68, p <0.008; muscle sympathetic nerve activity versus SDNN r = -0.76, p<0.001) (Figure 11).[35] By contrast, in the study of Adamopoulos et al, radionuclide norepinephrine whole-body spill over was not related to any measure of HRV.[36] Their patients, however, were all taking drugs that may have influenced results.

Plasma levels of catecholamines were found to be significantly related to several measures of HRV in the investigations of Gibelin et al and Mortara et al.[41,59]

Why is Heart Rate Variability Reduced in Heart Failure?

In spite of the available investigations and large amount of information on the physiopathology of heart failure, the explanation for reduced HRV in heart failure at this moment can only be speculative.

A simple explanation that can be inferred by the analysis of spectral composition is that both vagal and sympathetic control of HR are deranged in heart failure. However, if it is easy to accept that vagal activity is decreased in heart failure, it is far less acceptable that the sympathetic control is absent or near so. Vagal outflow is considered to modulate the cardiovascular activity with negative chronotropic and inotropic effects. Thus, decreased parasympathetic control can even be viewed as providing favorable effects on heart failure.

On the other hand, evidence for decreased, rather than increased, adrenergic drive to the sinus node is less obvious. In fact, increased sympathetic activity represents a major compensatory mechanism to the failing heart although it is still debated if increased adrenergic drive may, in some instances, play a detrimental role.[6,19,58] In spite of the signs and measures of increased overall sympathetic drive in heart failure, the contemporary presence of depressed HRV suggests impaired sympathetic neural discharge to the sinus node. Thus, while adrenergic activity is greatly enhanced in heart failure and plays a major role in supporting the heart and circulation, the neural drive to the sinus node seems to be greatly reduced and sometimes even to be lost.

Several experimental investigations show that cardiac neurotransmitter activity is altered in heart failure. Cardiac norepinephrine content has been repeatedly reported to be greatly reduced,[51,52] probably because of an increase in sympathetic discharge and release of norepinephrine into the coronary sinus.[60] Other investigation have not confirmed evidence of increased norepinephrine release by the failing heart and some data even suggest that such release is less than normal.[61-63] Decreased norepinephrine content in heart failure has been found to be associated with a decrease of sympathetic neural endings.[64] Thus, there is evidence for a neural sympathetic damage at the cardiac level in heart failure. Such a noradrenergic nerve terminal damage can be reproduced in the dog by the chronic infusion of norepinephrine.[64] These data suggest that a chronic excess of plasma catecholamines may play a primary role in the damage to the neural sympathetic endings.

Decreased HRV in heart failure may reflect a neural damage rather than the effect of an increased sympathetic stimulation and decreased vagal activity. Indeed patients with severe heart failure show aspects of HRV comparable to those observed in diabetics with autonomic dysfunction,[65] or following heart transplantation.[55] Therefore, a low HRV count may indicate the presence of a cardiac denervation.

However, as previously described, depressed HRV may increase after treatment: the alteration responsible for the low HR variation in heart failure is at least partially reversible and should be viewed as a functional autonomic denervation. Such a functional denervation has been reported to be present also for the baroreceptor control of circulation.[46,66] Both the vagal and sympathetic response associated with the baroreceptor activity are, in fact, impaired in heart failure[21,22,67] but are at least partially reversible after treatment.

Investigations designed to evaluate the behavior of HRV during exercise have shown that increased norepinephrine concentrations in plasma are associated with a decrease in HRV.[68,69] These results indicate a negative feedback of circulating catecholamines on the sympathetic control of HR. Also, it has been shown how increased plasma levels of catecholamines do not augment the LF component of the HR spectrum.[70]

Therefore, low HRV in heart failure may simply reflect the progressive loss of the neural modulation of HR that is caused by the progressive increase of plasma catecholamine levels.

Future Directions

Several issues have to be addressed in evaluating HRV in heart failure. It is still not clear whether spectral measures of HRV in heart failure have the ability to offer adjunctive information to nonspectral indices. It may well be that during the early phases of heart failure and possibily even during the asymptomatic phase, spectral analysis of HR may identify those patients with increased sympathetic tone or neurohumoral activation but who are clinically silent.

The relationship between HRV and left ventricular dysfunction in heart failure is still an open issue. Depressed left ventricular function promotes all the alterations that ultimately bring to decreased HRV; nevertheless, we know very little about the links existing between these two variables. We know, for example, that chronic heart failure patients may have different levels of left ventricular impairment and yet have the same symptoms. Vice versa, they may have a large variety of different functional impairments and yet have similar values of left ventricular function. It may be interesting to evaluate HRV in these subgroups.

The relationship between the severity of heart failure, altered neurohumoral activity and HRV requires further investigation in order to correctly use this parameter for follow-up purposes. In spite of some hypothetical explanations, we cannot be certain of the reason for depressed HRV during heart failure. It may well indicate the responsiveness of the heart to all the neurohormonal stimula instead of reflecting the effect of one in particular. As HRV represents the integrated response of the ANS to the heart from different stimuli, it may also be that this parameter is also linked to symptoms and mortality in heart failure in a more strict manner than that offered by other more commonly used parameters.

Although the are now several investigations on HRV in heart failure, a large scale trial relating HRV to survival in heart failure patients is still not available at the moment. Such an investigation would be particularly important, as it may provide the clinical validation to such a theorically interesting parameter.

Finally, the effect of therapeutic interventions indicate that HRV increases with some drugs, while not increasing with others. Such a behavior may simply indicate that some drugs are able to favorably modify the neurohumoral activation of heart failure patients while others, albeit improving symptoms, do not have the same property.

In conclusion, the link existing between HRV, left ventricular function, sympathetic activation, and degree of functional impairment highlights the importance of this parameter and suggests a more widespread use of HRV analysis in the management of HF patients.

References

1. Casolo GC, Balli E, Taddei T, et al. Decreased spontaneous heart rate variability in congestive heart failure. Am J Cardiol 1989; 64:1162-1167.
2. Coumel P, Hermida S, Wennerblom B, et al. Heart rate variability in left ventricular hypertrophy and heart failure, and the effects of beta blockade. Eur Heart J 1991; 12:412-422.
3. Coats AJS, Adamopoulos S, Radaelli A, et al. Controlled trial of physical training in

chronic heart failure. Exercise performance, hemodynamics, ventilation, and autonomic function. Circulation 1992; 85:2119-2131.

4. Casolo GC, Balli E, Fazi A, et al. Twenty-four-hour spectral analysis of heart rate variability in congestive heart failure secondary to coronary artery disease. Am J Cardiol 1991; 67:1154-1158.

5. Litchfield RL, Kerber RE, Benge JW, et al. Normal exercise capacity in patients with severe left ventricular dysfunction: compensatory mechanisms. Circulation 1982; 66:129-134.

6. Packer M, Lee WH, Kessler PD, et al. Role of neurohumoral mechanisms in determining survival in patients with severe chronic heart failure. Circulation 1987; 75:IV80-IV92.

7. Rouleau JL, Kortas C, Bichet D, et al. Neurohumoral and hemodynamic changes in congestive heart failure: lack of correlation and evidence of compensatory mechanisms. Am Heart J 1988; 116:746-757.

8. Cohn JN, Levine TB, Olivari MT, et al. Plasma norepinephrine as a guide to prognosis in patients with chronic congestive heart failure. N Engl J Med 1984; 311:819-823.

9. Cohn JN, Johnson GR, Shabetai R, et al. Ejection fraction, peak exercise oxygen consumption, cardiothoracic ratio, ventricular arrhythmias, and plasma norepinephrine as determinants of prognosis in heart failure. Circulation 1993; 87:VI5-VI16.

10. Swedberg K, Eneroth P, Kjekshus J, et al. Hormones regulating cardiovascular function in patients with severe congestive heart failure and their relation to mortality. Circulation 1990; 82:1730-1736.

11. Kleiger RE, Miller JP, Bigger JT, et al. Decreased heart rate variability and its association with increased mortality after acute myocardial infarction. Am J Cardiol 1987; 59:256-262.

12. Farrell TG, Paul V, Cripps TR, et al. Baroreflex sensitivity and electrophysiological correlates in patients after acute myocardial infarction. Circulation 1991; 83:945-952.

13. Cripps TR, Malik M, Farrell TG, et al. Prognostic value of reduced heart rate variability after myocardial infarction: clinical evaluation of a new analysis method. Br Heart J 1991; 65:14-19.

14. Bigger JT, Fleiss JL, Rolnitzky LM, et al. The ability of short term measures of r-r variability to predict mortality after myocardial infarction. Circulation 1993; 88:927-934.

15. Poole-Wilson PA. Future perspectives in the management of congestive heart failure. Am J Cardiol 1990; 66;462-467.

16. Packer M. Physiopathology of chronic heart failure. Lancet 1992; ii:88-95.

17. Nolan J, Flapan AD, Capewell S, et al. Decreased cardiac parasympathetic activity in chronic heart failure and its relation to left ventricular function. Br Heart J 1992; 67:482-485.

18. Swedberg K. Reduction in mortality by pharmacological therapy in congestive heart failure. Circulation 1993; 87:IV126-IV129.

19. Packer M. The neurohumoral hypothesis: a theory to explain the mechanism of disesase progression in heart failure. JACC 1992; 20:248-254.

20. Eckberg DL, Drabinsky M, Braunwald E. Defective cardiac parasympathetic control in patients with heart disease. N Engl J Med 1971; 285:877-883.

21. Higgins CB, Vatner JF, Eckberg DL, et al. Alterations in the baroreceptor reflex in conscious dogs with heart failure. J Clin Invest 1972; 51:715-724.

22. Goldstein RE, Beiser GD, Shampfer M, et al. Impairment of automatically mediated heart rate control in patients with cardiac dysfunction. Circ Res 1975; 36:571-578.

23. Levine TB, Francis GS, Goldsmith SR, et al. The neurohumoral and haemodynamic response to orthostatic tilt in patients with congestive heart failure. Circulation 1983; 67:1070-1075.

24. Olivari MT, Levine TB, Cohn JN. Abnormal neurohumoral response to nitroprusside infusion in congestive heart failure. JACC 1982; 3:411-417.

25. Casolo GC, Fazi A, Boddi M. Twenty-four-hour heart rate behavior in patients with impaired left ventricular function due to coronary artery disease. Cardiology 1987; 74:116-123.

26. Caruana MP, Lahiri A, Cashman PMM, et al. Effects of chronic congestive heart failure secondary to coronary artery disease on the circadian rhythm of blood pressure and heart rate. Am J Cardiol 1988; 62:755-759.

27. van de Borne P, Abramowicz M, Degre S, et al. Effects of chronic congestive heart failure on 24-hour blood pressure and heart rate patterns: a hemodynamic approach. Am Heart J 1992; 123:998-1004.

28. Saul J, Arai Y, Berger R, et al. Assessment of autonomic regulation in chronic congestive heart failure by heart rate spectral analysis. Am J Cardiol 1988; 61:1292-1299.

29. VanHoogenhuyze D, Weinstein N, Martin G, et al. Reproducibility and relation to mean heart rate of heart rate variability in normal subjects and in patients with congestive heart failure secondary to coronary artery disease. Am J Cardiol 1991; 68:1668-1676.

30. Molgaard H, Sorensen K, Bjerregaard P. Circadian variation and influence of risk fac-

tors on heart rate variability in healthy subjects. Am J Cardiol 1991; 68:777-784.

31. Hayano J, Sakakibara Y, Yamada M, et al. Decreased magnitude of heart rate spectral components in coronary artery disease. Its relation to angiographic severity. Circulation 1990; 81:1217-1224.

32. Stefenelli Th, Bergler-Klein J, Globits S, et al. Heart rate behavior at different stages of congestive heart failure. Eur Heart J 1992; 13:902-907.

33. Gang Y, Keeling PJ, Fei L, et al. An analysis of heart rate variability in patients with congestive heart failure. Br Heart J 1993; 69:273. Abstract.

34. Dadoun M, Morand PG. Heart rate variability in heart failure as a function of etiology. J Heart Failure 1993; 1:197. Abstract.

35. Kienzle MG, Ferguson DW, Birkett CL, et al. Clinical, hemodynamic and sympathetic neural correlates of heart rate variability in congestive heart failure. Am J Cardiol 1992; 69:761-767.

36. Adamopoulos S, Piepoli M, McCance A, et al. Comparison of different methods for assessing sympathovagal balance in chronic congestive heart failure secondary to coronary artery disease. Am J Cardiol 1992; 70:1576-1582.

37. Casolo GC, Stroder P, Signorini C, et al. Heart rate variability during the acute phase of myocardial infarction. Circulation 1992; 85:2073-2079.

38. Casolo GC, Stroder P, Sulla A, et al. Heart rate variability and severity of congestive heart failure secondary to coronary artery disease. J Heart Failure 1993; 1:507. Abstract.

39. Judge KW, Pawitan Y, Caldwell J, et al. Congestive heart failure symptoms in patients with preserved left ventricular systolic function: analysis of the CASS Registry. JACC 1991; 18:377-382.

40. Francis GS, Benedict C, Johnstone DE, et al. Comparison of neuroendocrine activation in patients with left ventricular dysfunction with and without congestive heart failure. Circulation 1990; 82:1724-1729.

41. Gibelin P, Dybal-Dadoun M, Morand P. Is heart rate variability a good marker of the severity of chronic heart failure? Eur Heart J 1993; 14:90. Abstract.

42. Binkley PF, Haas GJ, Starling RC, et al. Sustained augmentation of parasympathetic tone with angiotensin-converting enzyme inhibition in patients with congestive heart failure. JACC 1993; 21:655-661.

43. Flapan AD, Nolan J, Neilson JMM, et al. Effect of captopril on cardiac parasympathetic activity in chronic cardiac failure secondary to coronary artery disease. Am J Cardiol 1992; 69:532-535.

44. Goldsmith RL, Krum H, Bigger JT, et al. Beta blockade increases parasympathetic activity in chronic heart failure. Circulation 1993; 88(suppl I):I103. Abstract.

45. LaRovere MT, Mortara A, Pantaleo P, et al. Manipulation of the autonomic nervous system by scopolamine in end stage congestive heart failure. Circulation 1993; 88(suppl I):I108. Abstract.

46. Georghiade M, Ferguson D. Digoxin. A neurohormonal modulator in heart failure? Circulation 1991; 84:2181-2186.

47. Krum H, Bigger JT, Goldsmith R, et al. Long term therapy with digoxin reduces sympathetic and enhances parasympathetic nervous system activity in chronic heart failure. Circulation 1993; 88(suppl I):I108. Abstract.

48. Brouwer J, van Veldhuisen DJ, Man in't Veld AJ, et al. Relation between heart rate variability and neurohumoral status in patients with heart failure. Effects of neurohumoral modulation by digoxin and ibopamine. Circulation 1993; 88:4, I108.

49. Mancia G. Sympathetic activation in congestive heart failure. Eur Heart J 1990; II(A):3-11.

50. Leimbach WN, Wallin BG, Victor RG, et al. Direct evidence from intraneuronal recordings for increased central sympathetic outflow in patients with heart failure. Circulation 1986; 73:913-919.

51. Chidsey CA, Braunwald E, Morrow AC. Catecholamine excretion and cardiac stores of norepinephrine in congestive heart failure. Am J Med 1965; 39:442-451.

52. DeQuattro V, Nagatsu T, Mendez A, et al. Determinants of cardiac noradrenaline depletion on human congestive heart failure. Cardiovasc Res 1973; 7:344-350.

53. Bristow MR, Ginsburg R, Minobe W, et al. Decreased catecholamine sensitivity and beta adrenergic receptor density in failing human hearts. N Engl J Med 1982; 307:205-211.

54. Levy MN, Martin PL. Neural regulation of the heart beat. Ann Rev Physiol 1981; 43:443-453.

55. Sands KEF, Appel ML, Lilly LS, et al. Power spectrum analysis of heart rate variability in human cardiac transplant recipients. Circulation 1989; 79:76-82.

56. Malik M, Camm J. Components of heart rate variability. What they really mean and what we really measure. Am J Cardiol 1993; 72:821-822.

57. Wurster RD. Central nervous system: regulation of the heart. An overwiew. In: Randall WC (ed). Nervous Control of Cardiovascular

Function. New York, NY: Oxford University Press, 1984; 307-320.

58. Massie BM, Swedberg K, Cohn YN. Is neurohumoral activation deleterious to the long-term outcome of patients with congestive heart failure? JACC 1988; 12:547-558.

59. Mortara A, La Rovere MT, Pantaleo P, et al. Can spectral analysis of heart rate variability identify congestive heart failure patients with more pronounced neurohormonal activation? Eur Heart J 1993; 14:9. Abstract.

60. Hasking GJ, Esler MD, Jennings GL, et al. Norepinephrine spillover to plasma in patients with congestive heart failure: evidence for increased overall and cardiorenal sympathetic nervous activity. Circulation 1986; 73:615-621.

61. Rutenberg HL, Spann JF. Alterations of cardiac sympathetic neurotransmitter activity in congestive heart failure. Am J Cardiol 1973; 32:472-480.

62. Spann JF, Chidsey Ca, Pool PE, et al. Mechanism of norepinephrine depletion in experimental heart failure produced by aortic constriction in the guinea pig. Circ Res 1965; 17:312-321.

63. Rose CP, Burgess JH, Cousineau D. Tracer norepineprine kinetics in coronary circulation of patients with heart failure secondary to chronic pressure and volume overload. J Clin Invest 1985; 76:1740-1747.

64. Himura Y, Felten S, Kashiki M, et al. Cardiac noradrenergic nerve terminal abnormalities in dogs with experimental congestive heart failure. Circulation 1993; 88:1299-1309.

65. Lishner M, Akselrod S, Avi VM, et al. Spectral analysis of heart rate fluctuations. A noninvasive, sensitive method for the early diagnosis of autonomic neuropathy in diabetes mellitus. J Auton Nerv Sys 1987; 19:119-125.

66. White CW. Reversibility of abnormal arterial baroreflex control of heart rate in heart failure. Am J Physiol 1981; 241:H778-782.

67. White CW. Abnormalities in baroreflex control of heart rate in canine heart failure. Am J Physiol 1981; 240:H793-799.

68. Perini R, Orizio C, Comande A, et al. Plasma norepinephrine and heart rate dynamics during recovery from submaximal exercise in man. Eur J Appl Physiol 1989; 58:879-883.

69. Breuer H-W, Skyschally A, Schulz, et al. Heart rate variability and circulating catecholamine concentrations during steady state exercise in healthy volunteers. Br Heart J 1993; 70:144-149.

70. Yamamoto Y, Hugson RL, Peterson JC. Autonomic control of heart rate during exercise studied by heart rate variability spectral analysis. J Appl Physiol 1991; 71:1136-1142.

Chapter 35

Heart Rate and Blood Pressure Variability and Their Interaction in Hypertension

Gianfranco Parati, Marco Di Rienzo, Antonella Groppelli,
Antonio Pedotti, Giuseppe Mancia

Introduction

The interest to the analysis of heart rate variability (HRV) in hypertensive patients, often associated with the analysis of the concomitant variations in blood pressure (BP), has been stimulated by a number of observations which have suggested the possibility to obtain, by this approach, a deeper knowledge of the alterations in cardiovascular control mechanisms which may characterize essential hypertension. In this chapter, a selection of the observations made both by laboratory studies and by means of ambulatory monitoring techniques will be briefly discussed.

Baroreflex Modulation of Heart Rate: Evaluation by Laboratory Studies

Among the first studies which addressed the features of heart rate (HR) varia-

tions in hypertensive patients were those investigating the reflex control of HR exerted by arterial baroreflexes. Bristow et al[1] and Gribbin et al[2] showed that the reflex lengthening in RR interval, which accompanies the increase in systolic blood pressure (SBP) induced by IV phenylephrine bolus injection, was progressively reduced, as compared to normotensive subjects, going from mild to more severe hypertension (Figure 1). These observations were confirmed and extended by other studies.[3-6] Further evidence was provided that the RR interval lengthening induced by baroreceptor stimulation is reduced in secondary, as well as in primary, hypertension,[7] and characterizes also borderline hypertension.[8-11]

Not only the reflex bradycardia which accompanies baroreceptor stimulation, but also the reflex tachycardia associated to baroreceptor deactivation by IV injection of vasodilator drugs (eg, nitroglycerine) is reduced in hypertension.[12] This implies that the sensitivity of the reflex arterial barore-

From: Malik M., Camm AJ (eds.): *Heart Rate Variability.* Armonk, NY. Futura Publishing Company, Inc., © 1995.

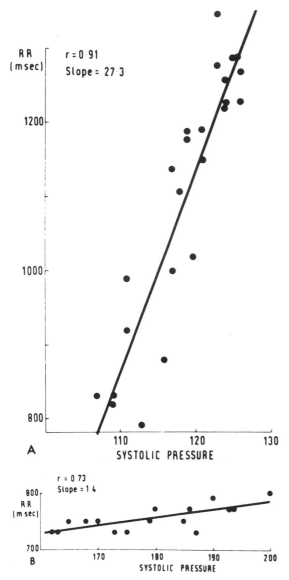

Figure 1. Slope of the linear regression between increases in SBP (mm Hg) induced by IV injection of angiotensin and the resulting reflex lengthening of RR interval. Data from a normal subject (A) and a hypertensive patients are separately shown. From Bristow et al[1] (B) with permission.

ceptor control of the sinus node is impaired in human hypertension along its whole stimulus-response curve, at variance from the baroreflex control of BP which is largely preserved (see below).[13,14]

Another technique to evaluate baroreflex control of HR in humans is based on the selective stimulation or deactivation of carotid baroreceptors by a neck chamber device.[15-17] When this technique was used in hypertensive patients, it documented a reduction in the sensitivity of carotid baroreflex HR modulation similar to that observed by manipulating the whole baroreceptor population via injection of vasoactive drugs.[13] This supports the hypothesis that in hypertensive patients, at variance from normotensive subjects,[18] the residual reflex HR control is predominantly exerted by carotid rather than by aortic baroreflexes.

A peculiar advantage of the neck chamber technique over the techniques based on the injection of vasoactive drugs is that it also allows baroreflex control of BP to be assessed.[16,17] By means of this technique, Mancia et al have been able to show that hypertensive patients, in spite of the above mentioned impairment of their baroreflex control of HR, do not display any reduction in the sensitivity of carotid baroreflex control of BP.[13,14,17]

This finding, combined with the observation that the elevated BP of hypertensive patients is not accompanied by a reduction in baseline HR, suggests that essential hypertension is also characterized by a resetting of the baroreflex towards the higher BP values reached in this condition. This is associated with a displacement of the set point of the carotid-baroreceptor reflexes from near saturation (as found in normotensive individuals) to near threshold of the stimulus-response curve.[13,14] Such a reading is reflected by the greater BP response to baroreceptor stimulation than to baroreceptor deactivation in hypertension, at variance from what can be observed in normotensive subjects (Figure 2).

The different effects of hypertension on baroreflex control of BP and HR may be partly explained by differences in the effects of hypertension on the responsiveness of the sinus node and the peripheral vessels.[14] An alternative explanation is the possible occurrence of differences in baroreflex con-

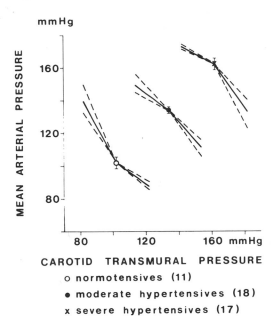

mmHg

Figure 2. Carotid baroreceptor effects on mean arterial pressure in 11 normotensive (O), 18 moderately hypertensive (●) and 17 severely hypertensive (X) subjects. Data are shown as mean values ±SE for each group. Solid lines represent regression lines for mean individual regression coefficients between changes in mean arterial pressure (intra-arterial catheter) and changes in carotid transmural pressure with respect to control values; dashed lines indicate standard errors of regressions. Data are shown for steady-state effects of varying the air pressure within a neck chamber, with carotid transmural pressure calculated as the difference between mean arterial pressure and the tissue pressure outside carotid sinuses. The latter was calculated from variations in the value of neck chamber pressure after application of a correction factor for loss of pressure transmission through the neck tissues. From Mancia et al[13] with permission.

trol of parasympathetic and sympathetic activity. Baroreflex control of HR primarily involves parasympathetic mechanisms, whereas control of vascular resistance mainly reflects sympathetic activity.[17] The impairment of HR control and the preservation of vascular and BP control observed in hypertensive patients might thus be accounted for by the greater impairment of baroreflex control of parasympathetic than of sympathetic activity produced by hyper-

tension.[19] The differences in the baroreflex control of parasympathetic and sympathetic activity in hypertension may involve efferent, central neural or afferent mechanisms.[17]

Blood Pressure and Heart Rate Variability Over the 24 Hours

The availability of techniques for continuous HR and BP recordings in ambulant subjects over the 24 hours has allowed a detailed description of the changes of both BP and HR throughout the day and night.[20,21]

Both in normotensive and hypertensive individuals, these changes seem to be determined to a substantial extent by neural influences originating within the central nervous system.[22] This is supported by the observation that over the 24 hours half-hour changes in BP are paralleled by changes in HR in the same direction (Figure 3).[21,22] As shown in Figure 3, this is particularly evident for circadian BP and HR fluctuations, which are characterized by a comparable magnitude in subjects with normal BP and in patients with mild to moderate essential hypertension.[23]

That these parallel changes in half-hour BP and HR values reflect the parallel modulation of cardiac and vascular targets by central influences and do not imply a causal interaction between these two variables was clearly shown by the demonstration that, when HRV was reduced by administration of atropine, BP variability did not fall but, at least in ambulant individuals, rather displayed a tendency to increase (Figure 4).[24] These findings support the concept that daily BP variability cannot just be considered as the result of variations in HR and cardiac output. Actually, evidence in animals and man rather seems to suggest the opposite, ie, in most cases, short-term HRV is reflexly modulated to oppose rather than to produce BP variations.[24-26]

HR and BP variability over 24 hours can also be assessed by means of spectral analysis. This was done by applying, in a

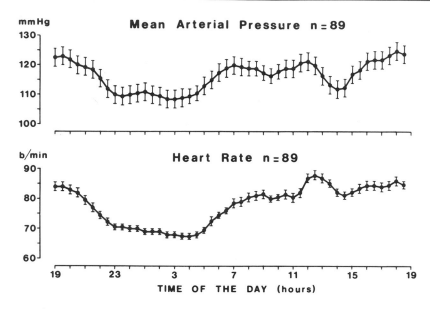

Figure 3. Plots show mean arterial pressure and HR in 89 ambulant subjects with untreated essential hypertension. Data are shown as mean ±SEM for each half-hour. BP was measured intra-arterially by the Oxford method all over the 24 hours in ambulatory conditions. From Mancia et al[23] with permission.

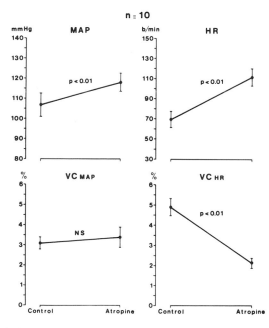

Figure 4. Mean arterial pressure (MAP) and HR mean and variability (standard deviations) before and after intravenous administration of atropine (0.04 mg/kg body weight). Data are shown as means ± for 10 subjects in whom BP was recorded intra-arterially for 2 hours before and for 2 hours after atropine injection. From Parati et al[24] with permission.

sequential fashion, Fast Fourier Transform (FFT) or autoregressive modeling techniques to 24-hour intra-arterial ambulatory BP recordings, after subdividing the signal into consecutive 256 or 512 beat segments and removing those segments containing nonstationarities.[27-29] In the study by Di Rienzo et al[27] stationary segments could be identified over more than 70% of day and night segments (Figure 5). BP and pulse-interval (the reciprocal of heart rate) spectral powers were integrated over three frequency bands, defined as low frequency (LF, 0.025 to 0.07 Hz), mid-frequency (0.07 to 0.14 Hz) and high frequency (HF, 0.14 to 0.35 Hz), respectively. All together, these powers accounted for 20% to 25% of the 24-hour BP or pulse-interval variance.[28] In both normotensive and mild essential hypertensive patients, the powers of the above mentioned components underwent marked day and night changes that did not invariably correlate with changes in overall variance (Figure 6). In particular, a marked reduction at night in the powers of systolic and diastolic BP fluctuations near 0.1 Hz and an increase in HF pulse-interval powers were

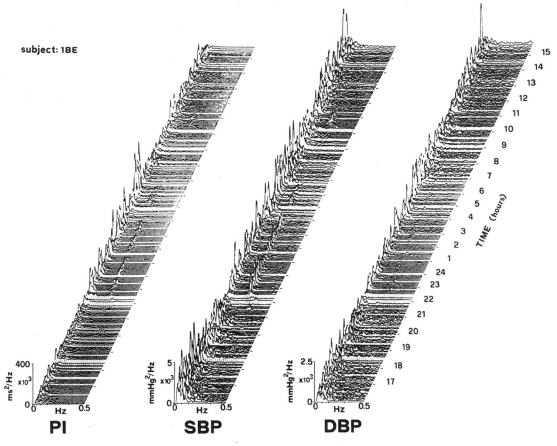

subject: 1BE

PI

SBP

DBP

Figure 5. Sequential power spectral densities of SBP, diastolic blood pressure (DBP) and pulse-interval (PI) throughout the 24 hours. The dotted lines refer to segments in which power spectral densities could not be estimated because of the occurrence of nonstationarities. From Di Rienzo et al[27] with permission.

observed. The reduction in 0.1 Hz BP powers was similarly evident in normotensive and mild hypertensive patients,[28] while the nocturnal increase in HF HR (or pulse-interval) powers was less evident in hypertensive as compared to normotensive individuals.[28,29] The diurnal changes in these spectral components may reflect the reported decrease in sympathetic and increase in parasympathetic activity which occur during night sleep,[30] although spectral powers in these frequency regions cannot always be regarded as specific autonomic markers but rather seem to have a multifactorial origin.[23,31-35]

Dynamic Assessment of Baroreflex Sensitivity by Computer Analysis of Blood Pressure and Pulse-Interval Variability

Surgical deafferentation of arterial baroreceptors by sinoaortic denervation is responsible in conscious animals for a pronounced increase in BP variability (Figure 7).[32,36,37] Studies carried out in man have clearly shown that baroreflex sensitivity (BRS), as assessed by traditional laboratory techniques, is inversely related to BP variability and positively related to HRV, quan-

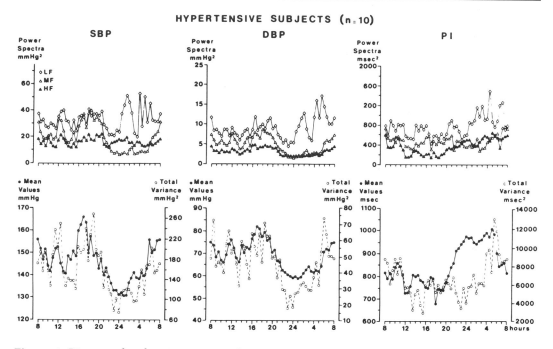

Figure 6. Line graphs showing mean values and variances (lower panels) and power spectrum densities of (LF), mid-frequency (MF) and (HF) oscillations (upper panels) of SBP, DBP and PI. Data are shown as absolute average values for each half hour of recording in 10 mild hypertensive patients. From Parati et al[28] with permission.

tified by the respective 24-hour standard deviations (Figure 8).[38]

The existence of such a relationship between BRS and BPV and HRV has spurred the development of techniques to dynamically assess the sensitivity of baroreflex control of HR based on the evaluation of the interaction between spontaneous variations in SBP and HR. To this aim both time-domain and frequency-domain analysis methods have been proposed.[39]

In the frequency domain, the sensitivity of baroreflex control of the heart can be assessed by the ratio between the spectral powers of SBP and pulse-interval in the frequency regions where these two signals are coherent (usually around 0.1 and 0.3 Hz).[40-42]

In the time domain, dynamic quantification of BRS can be obtained by computer identification of the sequences of heartbeats characterized by progressive spontaneous increase in SBP associated with a linearly

related reflex lengthening in pulse-interval, or by progressive reduction in SBP and shortening in pulse-interval. Similarly to what is done when BRS is measured by evaluating the reflex changes in pulse-interval artificially induced in the laboratory by injection of vasoactive drugs (see above), the slope of the regression line between SBP and pulse-interval changes is taken as an index of the sensitivity of baroreflex control of HR (Figure 9).[43-44] The baroreflex nature of these sequences was shown in animals by their almost complete disappearance after sinoaortic denervation.[43]

The latter method was applied to the analysis of 24-hour intra-arterial ambulatory BP recordings obtained from a group of normotensive and a group of hypertensive subjects.[44]

In normotensive subjects the number of both hypertension/bradycardia and hypotension/tachycardia sequences was more than one thousand over the 24 hours, ie, it was more than enough to provide a dynamic characterization of BRS all over the different behavioral conditions of daily life. In normotensive subjects, the slope of these sequences (ie, the index of BRS provided by this method) was characterized by a pronounced variability at the time of the different behaviors occurring during the 24 hours. In particular, it showed a marked diurnal fluctuation, with a pronounced night time increase.[44] In hypertensive patients, the number and, more importantly, the slope of these sequences were reduced (Figure 10).[44] These data support, by an innovative approach, the finding by previous laboratory studies of an impairment of baroreflex control of HR in hypertensive patients (see above). They also offer new information on this issue, however, by providing the first demonstration that such an impairment characterizes the whole 24-hour period and is variably evident under the different activities of the day and night. In particular, hypertensive patients are characterized not only by a reduction in the 24-hour mean sequence slope, but also by a marked impairment of its nocturnal increase as it can be physiologically observed in normotensive individuals (Figure 11).[44,45]

Similar results were also obtained by applying to the analysis of 24-hour intra-arterial recordings obtained in normotensive and hypertensive subjects, the frequency-domain approach based on the calculation of the so-called alpha coefficient (Figure 12).[39]

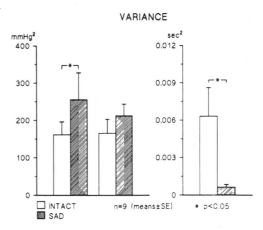

Figure 7. SBP, DBP and PI mean values (top) and variances (bottom) in control condition (intact) and after sinoaortic denervation (SAD). Data are shown as averages (±SE) for nine cats. Asterisks refer to the statistical significance of differences before and after SAD. From Di Rienzo[32] with permission.

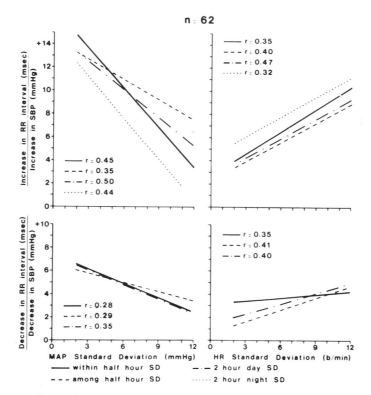

Figure 8. Regression lines of mean arterial pressure (MAP) and HR standard deviations and BRS measured by the changes in RR interval induced by increasing and reducing SBP through phenylephrine and nitroglycerine injections. Only the regression lines achieving statistical significance are shown. From Mancia et al[38] with permission.

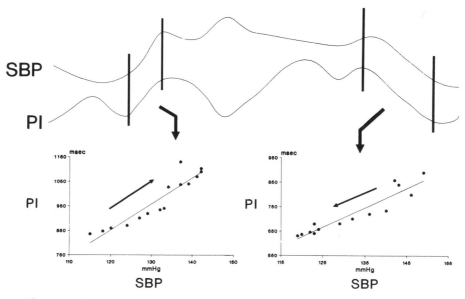

Figure 9. Schematic drawing illustrating the hypertension/bradycardia and hypotension/tachycardia sequences automatically identified by the computer to quantify BRS. The corresponding regression lines between changes in SBP and changes in PI are also shown. From Parati et al[39] with permission.

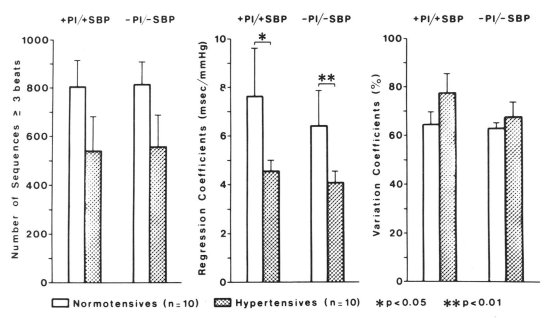

Figure 10. Histograms illustrate the number of sequences characterized by a progressive increase (+PI/+SBP) or by a progressive decrease (-PI/-SBP) in PI and SBP during 24 hours (left panel), their mean 24-hour slopes or regression coefficients (middle panel) and the 24-hour variation coefficients of these slopes (right panel). Data represent means ±SE for normotensive and hypertensive subjects. From Parati et al[44] with permission.

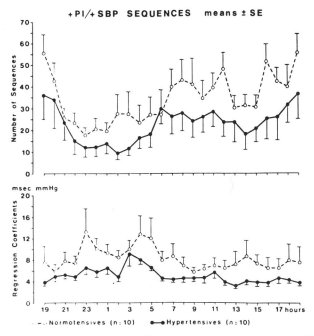

Figure 11. Number and mean regression coefficients (or slopes) of +PI/+SBP sequences during each hour of the 24-hour recording. Data are separately shown as means ±SE for normotensive and hypertensive subjects. Sequences of different duration are pooled. From Parati et al[44] with permission.

SPECTRAL TECHNIQUE
24 HOUR ASSESSMENT OF BAROREFLEX SENSITIVITY

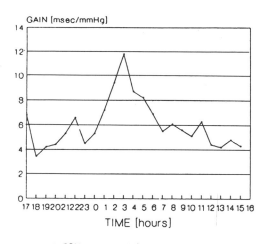 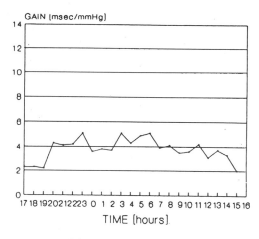

Figure 12. Average hourly values of the "alpha" coefficient (gain) in one normotensive (BON) and in one hypertensive (COR) subject over a 24-hour time. These coefficients were obtained by cross-spectrum analysis of SBP and PI fluctuations in the frequency region between 0.07 and 0.14 Hz, where the SBP and PI signals were coherent. From Parati et al[39] with permission.

Conclusions

The assessment of HRV, alone or in combination with the analysis of BP variability, offers valuable information on the mechanisms responsible for cardiovascular regulation.

In particular, when such an assessment is extended over the 24 hours, a unique dynamic picture of cardiovascular regulation can be obtained. This approach may turn out to be extremely useful in different physiological and pathophysiological conditions, where it may allow to more sharply characterize the features of cardiovascular regulation and may offer a tool for an early diagnosis of alterations in autonomic control of the heart and peripheral circulation, before they become clinically evident. The prognostic relevance of the information on the specific features of autonomic cardiovascular modulation explored by the analysis of BPV and HRV decribed in the previous sections remains to be evaluated.

References

1. Bristow JD, Honour AJ, Pickering GW, et al. Diminished baroreflex sensitivity in high blood pressure. Circulation 1969; 39:48-54.
2. Gribbin B, Pickering TG, Sleight P, et al. Effect of age and high blood pressure on baroreflex sensitivity in man. Circ Res 1971; 29:424-431.
3. Randall OS, Esler MD, Bullock GF, et al. Relationship of age and blood pressure to baroreflex sensitivity and arterial compliance in man. Clin Sci Mol Med 1976; 51:357s-360s.
4. Simon G, Kiowski W, Julius S. Effect of beta adrenoceptor antagonists on baroreceptor reflex sensitivity in hypertension. Clin Pharmacol 1977; 22:293-298.
5. Simon ACH, Safar ME, Weiss YA, et al. Baroreflex sensitivity and cardiopulmonary blood volume in normotensive and hypertensive patients. Br Heart J 1977; 39:799-805.
6. Watson RDS, Stallard TS, Littler WA. Effects of beta-adrenoceptor antagonists on sinoaortic baroreflex sensitivity and blood pressure in hypertensive man. Clin Sci 1979; 57:241-247.
7. Pickering TG, Gribbin B, Oliver DO. Baroreflex sensitivity in patients on long-term haemodialysis. Clin Sci 1972; 43:645-657.

8. Eckberg DL. Carotid baroreflex function in young men with borderline blood pressure elevation. Circulation 1979; 59:632-636.

9. Julius S, Esler MD, Randall OS. Role of the autonomic nervous system in mild human hypertension. Clin Sci Mol Med 1975; 48:2435-2525.

10. Takeshita A, Tanaka S, Kuroiwa A, et al. Reduced baroreceptor sensitivity in borderline hypertension. Circulation 1975; 51:738-742.

11. Takeshita A, Tanaka S, Nakamura M. Effects of propanolol on baroreflex sensitivity in borderline hypertension. Cardiovasc Res 1978; 12:148-151.

12. Mancia G, Ferrari A, Gregorini L, et al. Blood pressure variability in man: its relation to age, high blood pressure and baroreflex sensitivity. Clin Sci 1980; 59:401s-403s.

13. Mancia G, Ludbrook J, Ferrari A, et al. Baroreceptor reflexes in human hypertension. Circ Res 1978; 43:170-177.

14. Mancia G, Ferrari A, Gregorini L, et al. Control of blood pressure by carotid sinus baroreceptors in human beings. Am J Cardiol 1979; 44:895-902.

15. Eckberg DL, Cavanaugh MS, Mark AL, et al. A simplified neck suction device for activation of carotid baroreceptors. J Lab Clin Med 1975; 85:167-173.

16. Ludbrook J, Mancia G, Ferrari A, et al. The variable-pressure neck-chamber method for studying the carotid baroreflex in man. Clin Sci Mol Med 1977; 53:165-171.

17. Mancia G, Mark AL. Arterial baroreflexes in humans. In: Shepard JT, Abboud FM (eds). Handbook of Physiology. The Cardiovascular System III. Bethesda, Md: American Physiological Society, 1983; 755-793.

18. Mancia G, Ferrari A, Gregorini L, et al. Circulatory reflexes from carotid and extracarotid baroreceptor areas in man. Circ Res 1977; 41:309-315.

19. Guo GB, Thames MD, Abboud FM. Preservation of baroreflex control of lumbar sympathetic nerve activity in renal hypertensive rabbits. Clin Res 1981; 29:751A. Abstract.

20. Bevan AT, Honour AJ, Stott FD. Direct arterial pressure in unrestricted man. Clin Sci 1969; 36:328-344.

21. Mancia G, Ferrari A, Gregorini L, et al. Blood pressure and heart rate variabilities in normotensive and hypertensive human beings. Circ Res 1983; 53:96-104.

22. Mancia G, Zanchetti A. Blood pressure variability. In: Zanchetti A, Tarazi R (eds). Handbook of Hypertension. Pathophysiology of Hypertension, Cardiovascular Aspects. Volume 7. Amsterdam: Elsevier, 1986; 125-152.

23. Mancia G, Di Rienzo M, Parati G. Ambulatory blood pressure monitoring use in hypertension research and clinical practice. Hypertension 1993; 21:510-524.

24. Parati G, Pomidossi G, Casadei R, et al. Role of HRV in the production of blood pressure variability in man. J Hypertens 1987; 5:557-560.

25. Conway J, Boon N, Davies C, et al. Neural and humoral mechanisms involved in blood pressure variability. J Hypertens 1984; 2:203-208.

26. Ferrari AU, Daffonchio A, Albergati F, et al. Inverse relationship between heart rate and blood pressure variabilities in rats. Hypertension 1987; 10:533-537.

27. Di Rienzo M, Castiglioni P, Mancia G, et al. 24 hour sequential spectral analysis of arterial blood pressure and pulse interval in free-moving subjects. IEEE Trans Biomed Eng 1989; 36:1066-1075.

28. Parati G, Castiglioni P, Di Rienzo M, et al. Sequential spectral analysis of 24-hour blood pressure and pulse interval in humans. Hypertension 1990; 16:414-421.

29. Furlan R, Guzzetti S, Crivellaro W, et al. Continuous 24-hour assessment of the neural regulation of systemic arterial pressure and RR variabilities in ambulant subjects. Circulation 1990; 81:537-547.

30. Mancia G, Zanchetti A. Cardiovascular regulation during sleep. In: Orem J, Barnes CD (eds). Physiology in Sleep. New York, NY: Academic Press, 1980; 1-55.

31. Berger RD, Saul PJ, Cohen RJ. Transfer function analysis of autonomic regulation. I. Canine atrial rate response. Am J Physiol 1989; 256:H142-H152.

32. Di Rienzo M, Parati G, Castiglioni P, et al. Role of sinoaortic afferents in modulating BP and pulse interval spectral characteristics in unanaesthetized cats. Am J Physiol 1991; 261:H1811-H1818.

33. Daffonchio A, Franzelli C, Di Rienzo M, et al. Effect of sympathectomy on blood pressure variability in the conscious rat. J Hypertens 1991; 9(suppl 6):S70-S71.

34. Kaye DM, Esler M, Kingwell B, et al. Functional and neurochemical evidence for partial cardiac sympathetic reinnervation after cardiac transplantation in humans. Circulation 1993; 88:1110-1118.

35. Mancia G, Grassi G, Parati G, et al. Evaluating sympathetic activity in human hypertension. J Hypertens 1993; 11(suppl 5):S13-S19.

36. Cowley AW, Liard LF, Guyton AC. Role of the baroreceptor reflex in daily control of arterial blood pressure and other variables in dogs. Circ Res 1973; 32:564-576.

37. Ramirez AJ, Bertinieri G, Belli L, et al. Reflex control of blood pressure and heart rate by arterial baroreceptors and by cardiopulmonary receptors in the unanaesthetized cat. J Hypertens 1985; 3:327-335.

38. Mancia G, Parati G, Pomidossi G, et al. Arterial baroreflexes and blood pressure and heart rate variabilities in humans. Hypertension 1986; 8:147-153.

39. Parati G, Omboni S, Frattola A, et al. Dynamic evaluation of the baroreflex in ambulant subjects. In: Di Rienzo M, Mancia G, Parati G, et al (eds). Blood Pressure and Heart Rate Variability. Amsterdam: IOS Press, 1992; 122-137.

40. De Boer RV, Karemaker JM, Strackee J. Relations between short-term blood pressure fluctuations and heart rate variability in resting subjects. I. A spectral analysis approach. Med Biol Eng Comput 1985; 23:352-358.

41. Robbe HWJ, Mulder LJM, Ruddel H, et al. Assessment of baroreceptor reflex sensitivity by means of spectral analysis. Hypertension 1987; 10:538-543.

42. Cerutti S, Baselli G, Civardi S, et al. Spectral anlysis of heart rate and arterial blood pressure variability signals for physiological and clinical purposes. Proceedings Comp Cardiol IEEE 1987; 435-438.

43. Bertinieri G, Di Rienzo M, Cavallazzi A, et al. Evaluation of baroreceptor reflex by blood pressure monitoring in unanaesthetized cats. Am J Physiol 1988; 254:H377-H383.

44. Parati G, Di Rienzo M, Bertinieri G, et al. Evaluation of the baroreceptor-heart rate reflex by 24-hour intra-arterial blood pressure monitoring in humans. Hypertension 1988; 12:214-222.

45. Smyth HS, Sleight P, Pickering GW. Reflex regulation of arterial pressure during sleep in man: a quantitative method of assessing baroreflex sensitivity. Circ Res 1969; 24:109-121.

Chapter 36

Heart Rate Variability After Cardiac Transplantation

J. Philip Saul, Luciano Bernardi

Introduction

As attested to by the many chapters in this book, heart rate variability (HRV) is an integral part of cardiovascular regulatory physiology, reflecting the response of the heart to ongoing perturbations throughout the cardiovascular system. Analysis of beat-to-beat variations in heart rate (HR) can provide specific quantitative information about modulation of cardiac vagal and sympathetic efferent activity.[1-3] Thus, the study of HRV in the denervated heart provides an excellent model for understanding cardiovascular regulatory physiology when neural control of the heart is impaired or absent. Elimination of cardiac innervation leaves the heart dependent on other non-neural regulatory mechanisms. In addition, analysis of HR variations after human cardiac transplantation may provide an excellent model for this study of autonomic reinnervation.

Heart Rate Control After Transplantation

In the resting supine position after cardiac transplantation, the beating of the heart is essentially metronomic, giving a fixed stable HR. However, under conditions of increased cardiovascular demand, HR is able to change, presumably because of changes in the level of circulating catecholamine.[4] These changes occur considerably more slowly than in the normal heart, generally over a period of seconds to minutes. In addition, the return to the fixed metronomic HR at rest takes considerably longer because of the need for elimination of the circulating catecholamine.

Resting HR is higher than in normal subjects,[5] closely resembling what has been described as the intrinsic HR in normal subjects after pharmacological denervation with atropine and propranolol.[6] Although earlier reports showed that the transplanted

From: Malik M., Camm AJ (eds.): *Heart Rate Variability*. Armonk, NY. Futura Publishing Company, Inc., © 1995.

heart had an increased sensitivity[7-9] and density[10] of myocardial adrenergic receptors, more recent studies have indicated that beta-receptor density is not significantly different from normal in the transplanted heart,[11] and that the sensitivity of the transplanted sinus node to beta-adrenergic stimulation with isoproterenol is also normal.[12] Although most of the HR changes which occur with activity and exercise in heart transplant patients have been ascribed to changing levels of circulating catecholamines, there is also evidence of non-neurohumoral mechanisms contributing to the HR increases with exercise and standing, and to rapid decreases postexercise.[13-16] Interestingly, regardless of the mechanism, the pattern of HR changes during exercise in transplant patients is similar to that seen in normals (Figure 1).[17] However, the maximum HR achieved, the absolute change in HR, and the rate of increase and decrease in HR are all significantly less than normals, and even slightly less than those seen in patients with severe congestive heart failure.[17] In fact, the time constant tau of the best fit exponential decay of HR during early recovery after exercise was 28.2 minutes in a group of transplant patients, compared to 24.8 minutes for heart failure subjects and 9.6 minutes for normals.[17]

Heart Rate Variability After Transplantation

As noted above, short-term variability in most patients after cardiac transplantation is typically much less than that seen in the normal heart. However, as will be discussed in more detail below, short-term HR variations coincident with respiration are present early after transplantation, suggesting a nonautonomic mechanism for HR control.[18-20] In addition, short-term variations at lower frequencies reappear in some patients late after transplantation, suggesting reinnervation.[21] Of note, although total HRV over 24 hours is considerably re-

duced in the transplanted heart, the slowest fluctuations associated with wide swings and activity appear to be relatively preserved.[22]

Long-Term Variability

By 7 months after transplantation, a circadian rhythm can be found in both the HR and blood pressure (BP) of most patients.[23] Although the amplitude of the HR variation is lower 1 month after transplantation than at 7 months, at both stages it is more than 50% of that seen in normal controls.[23,24] In fact, as shown for the single patients in Figure 2, long-term variations in HR over 24 hours have similar spectral characteristics in subjects after transplantation to those seen in both normal subjects and patients with congestive heart failure.[22]

Short-Term Variability Patterns

Early clinical observations based on visual inspection or on low precision computerized data described a fixed metronomic HR and an absence of respiratory sinus arrhythmia (RSA) after cardiac transplantation. Although this observation was certainly correct when compared to the amplitude of RSA in normal subjects, more accurate measurements made with direct computer acquisition of the electrocardiogram (ECG) at sampling rates of 256 to 1,000 Hz (time resolution 1 to 4 milliseconds) have found that HR is usually not fixed in these patients. The most common finding, which can be observed immediately after transplantation and persist though long-term follow-up, is a very low amplitude RSA at higher frequencies greater than 0.15 Hz, with a peak-to-peak range of RR intervals between 5 and 20 milliseconds (Figure 3).[3,17,18,15-18] Most of these investigators used a frequency-domain technique such as autoregressive or FFT base spectral analysis or, in one case, a single cosinor method.[25] As

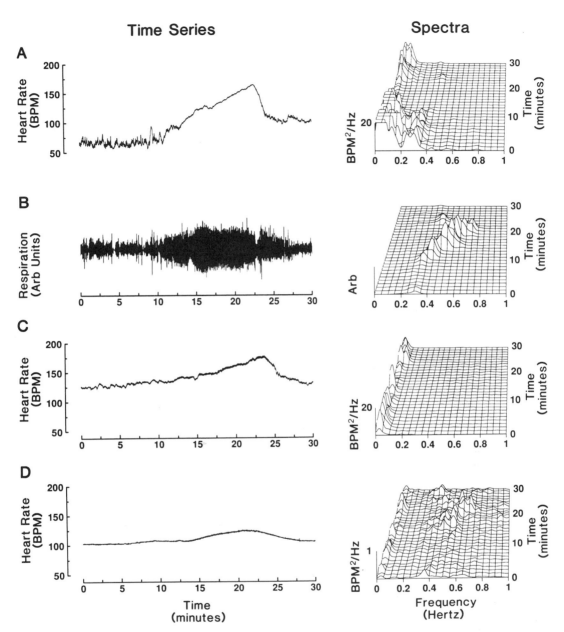

Figure 1. Time series and three dimensional spectra of the complete excercise protocol for one normal subject **(3A and B)**, one subject with congestive heart failure **(C)** and one subject status-postcardiac transplantation **(D)**. Slope of increase and decrease in HR, as well as % change in HR is higher in normal subjects than in two subjects with cardiac pathology. Z-axis on spectra displays time between 0 and 30 min of consecutive spectra computed each minute on overlapping 2-min segments of data. Differences in variability patterns are demonstrated by spectra. For respiratory signal in **B**, the frequency (respiratory rate) and amplitude (tidal volume) increase throughout exercise and decrease to levls just abovve baseline during recovery. At *time 0*, a peak at respiratory frequency (-0.3 Hz) can be seen in **A**, which diminishes with exercise, is too small to be seen after 13 min, and reappears near 0.4 Hz at 22 min. Spectra in **C** are on same Y-scale as in **A**, but no significant activity is visible >0.15 Hz. Finally, in **D**, spectra are on a scale 20 times as large as in **A** or **C** and reveal somewhat random, very low amplitude activity throughout. Respiratory signals and spectra were similar for all three groups. From Arai et al[17] with permission.

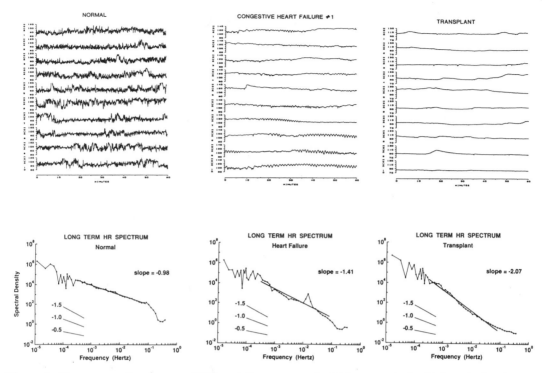

Figure 2. Ten consecutive hours of HR and the spectra of a 24-hour period which includes the 10 hours shown for a normal subject **(A, D)**, a patient with severe CHF **(B, E)**, and a transplant recipient **(C, F)**. The HR is displayed over a 60 bpm range for all three cases—normal 60 to 126 bpm, CHF: 80 to 140 bpm, transplant: 70 to 130 bpm. Spectral slopes are calculated over the range where the regression lines are shown and are typical for the three groups. Note the peak just above 0.01 Hz in **E**.

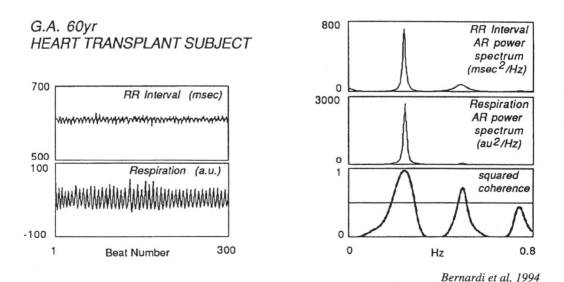

Bernardi et al, 1994

Figure 3. RR interval and respiratory time series with autoregressive spectra and squared coherence function in a heart transplant subject. Notice the presence of low amplitude but clear RR interval fluctuations at the respiratory frequency.

Figures 3 and 4 show, the respiratory related component of the HRV is much easier to identify if the breathing is kept at a constant frequency.[26-28] When respiratory activity has broader frequency components (Figure 4), the RR interval variability also has broader frequency content. Sands et al[29] also used spectral techniques and identified a small respiratory component in some patients, but were less willing to describe it as RSA, questioning whether small variations in beat timing may have resulted from changes in the cardiac electrical axis rather than true RR interval variability. A number of mechanisms have been proposed to explain the RSA in cardiac transplantation, including small changes in cardiac electric axis,[29,30] sinoatrial stretch reflexes,[18-20] and autonomic reinnervation.[25] These will be discussed in detail below. Of note, a residual RSA has also been observed in animals and humans after complete combined sympathetic and parasympathetic blockade of the SA node receptors.[2,25,30-34]

Low-frequency (LF) fluctuations of HR at frequencies between 0.001 and 0.15 Hz have also been observed after cardiac transplantation.[21,22,35] Although these LF fluctuations have sometimes been associated with respiratory activity (Figure 4),[35] they are at times of much higher amplitude than the respiratory frequency variability (Figure 5),[22] and are seen almost exclusively late after transplantation (Figure 6).[21] This observation is in direct contrast to the high-frequency (HF) RSA with an amplitude unrelated to the time after transplantation (Figure 5).[21] As will be discussed below, these observations suggest the possibility of autonomic reinnervation as the basis for the late LF variability.

Finally, Sands et al[29] identified a non-rhythmic pattern of HRV which was associated with rejection episodes in the transplanted heart (Figure 7). The pattern was low amplitude compared to normal variability, and did not have clearly identifiable peaks similar to those seen during spontaneous respiration in normals.

M.M. 22 yr HEART TRANSPLANT 25W EXERCISE LOAD

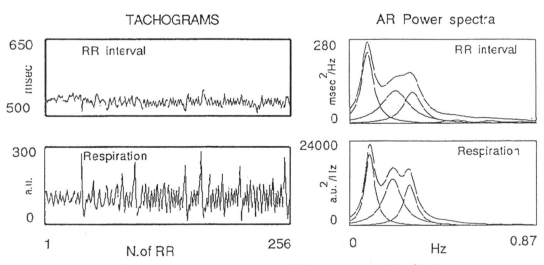

Figure 4. Similar to Figure 1, but the respiratory and RR interval variability has frequency content at both HF and LF. Notice the correlation between the peaks of the respiratory and RR interval spectra.

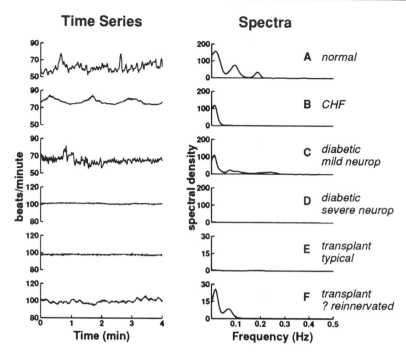

Figure 5. Examples of 4-min segments of HR and corresponding spectra from a normal subject **(A)** and patients with CHF **(B)**, diabetes **(C and D)**, and cardiac transplants **(E and F)**. Although range of HRs in bpm on y-axis is different for subjects A-C than for subjects D-F, scale of 40 bpm is the same for all tracings. Note that spectral density scale is the same in tracings A-D (0 to 200 bpm ^{2}/Hz) for comparison with data from the normal subject, but is changed to 0 to 20 bpm ^{2}/Hz for the two transplant subjects to better demonstrate the unusual finding of low amplitude but frequency-specific HR fluctuations in trace **(F)**. Also note similarities between data for the diabetic subject with severe neuropathyy and the 'typical' transplant subject. From Saul[3] with permission.

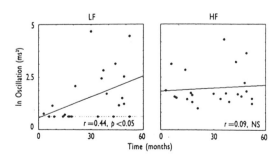

Figure 6. Relationship between time since transplantation and RR interval fluctuations, obtained in the supine position. There is no correlation between the HF components, with higher values present even at few months since transplantation, suggesting the nonautonomic origin of these fluctuations. Notice the presence of a significant correlation between time since transplantation and LF components. Notice also the particular shape of the scattergram, indicating that immediately after transplantation, all subjects have almost no LF components, while with progression of time and trend diverges; after approximately 20 months, the LF fluctuations are fairly common and tend to be higher with longer time, but still remain low or absent in other subjects even after 52 months. NS: not significant. From Bernardi et al[21] with permission.

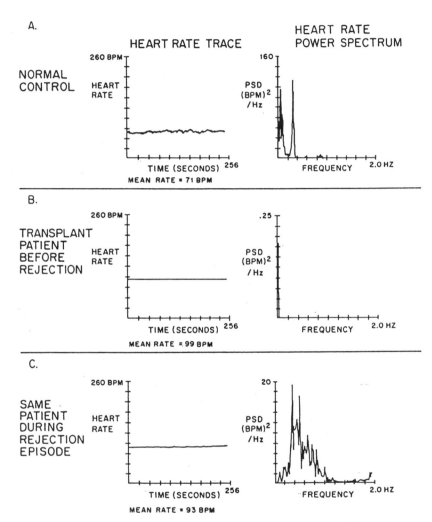

Figure 7. HR tachograms and power spectra from a healthy contral **(2A)**, a transplant patient without rejection **(2B)**, and the same patient during a subsequent rejection episode **(2C)**. Note the different y-axis scales for power spectral density (PSD). From Sands et al[29] with permission.

Mechanism of Respiratory Sinus Arrhythmia—High Frequencies

As noted above, a number of mechanisms could be responsible for the HF respiratory related HRV seen after transplantation. These include QRS complex variations, sinus node stretch, intra-atrial reflexes, and autonomic reinnervation. Due to changes in the cardiac electrical axis with respiration, the QRS morphology does change during normal respiration. In fact, the mean cardiac electrical axis can be used as a nonquantitative ECG derived measure of respiratory activity.[36] These changes in QRS morphology could result in slight variations of the fiducial point used to mark the timing of each QRS complex, leading to artifactual modulation of the RR interval. Sands et al[29] hypothesized that this mechanism might explain most of the residual variability observed after transplantation, and after denervation in animals.[30] Bernardi et al[18] used the simple method shown in Figure 8 to clearly demonstrate that changes in QRS morphology are very unlikely to explain the RSA typically observed after cardiac transplant. By aligning the QRS complexes of beats, and observing those at beat n+1, one can see that there is a rhythmic displacement of the entire QRS complex at the respiratory frequency. The authors also found that changes in the QRS axis due to respiratory activity have minimal or no effect during physical exercise when increased ventilatory activity should cause a much larger change in QRS morphology.

The HF RSA in normal controls is due primarily to modulation of cardiac vagal activity.[1,22,37] In addition, modulation of cardiac sympathetic activity occurs at higher respiratory frequencies; however, the response of the sinus node to modulation of that activity is very small above 0.15 Hz.[38] Thus, one might hypothesize that RSA after transplantation could be due to either a small degree of vagal reinnervation or virtually complete sympathetic reinnervation. However, if either of these were true, one would expect the small amplitude of the HF RSA observed in the transplanted heart to first appear at least a few weeks after transplantation, and probably increase in amplitude with the time elapsed. In fact, Bernardi et al[20,21] have observed RSA in the first few weeks after transplantation and have found no correlation between RSA and time since transplantation over a period from 2 to 52 months. These findings favor a nonautonomic mechanism for the HF component of RSA in transplants. In addition, as noted above, a nonautonomic RSA has been described in both animals and humans after a complete pharmacological autonomic blockade of the sinus node.[2,30,31,34]

A number of observations have linked this respiratory related variability to intracardiac stretch. In 1920 Bainbridge[38] first hypothesized that some of the respiratory related HR fluctuations he observed were due to the effects of changing intrathoracic pressure on the diastolic filling of the heart. Since intrathoracic pressure is related to both total lung volume and the rate of change of lung volume, one might expect to find both a tidal volume and respiratory frequency dependence of this nonautonomic RSA. In fact, using the peak of the cross-correlation function between the respiratory signal and the RR signal to quantify RSA, Bernardi[18] found that RSA in trans-

HEART TRANSPLANT SUBJECT (25W EXERCISE)

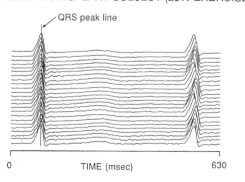

Bernardi et al, JAP, 1989

Figure 8. Plot of sequential pairs of QRS complexes from a heart transplant subject during physical exercise. Notice the presence of small but clear changes in RR interval. From Bernardi et al[18] with permission.

plant patients increased with both breathing frequency and tidal volume. In agreement with many other investigators,[2,39-41] their observations in normal controls showed that RSA decreases with increasing breathing frequency and demonstrates a smaller dependence on tidal volume. The decrease in RSA with respiratory frequency in normal subjects begins at frequencies near 0.1 Hz and is quite marked after that. Saul et al[2] used the broad-band transfer function between respiration and HR to obtain nearly identical results after combined autonomic blockade with atropine and propranolol in normal volunteers (Figure 9). In addition, they were able to identify that the transfer magnitude increased nearly linearly with frequency above 0.15 Hz, and the phase was very close to 90° at the same frequencies. Importantly, despite the relatively small magnitude compared to normal controls, the stand and errors for both the magnitude and phase indicated that the response was

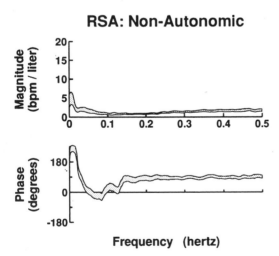

RSA: Non-Autonomic

Figure 9. ILV-HR relations (blockade). Group average transfer function magnitude and phase between ILV and HR (PSA nonautonomic) after combined autonomic blockade in supine position. At frequencies above 0.15 Hz, magnitude is small, but increases linearly with frequency while phase is very close to 90°. Together these findings are consistant with nonautonomic changes in HR, which are proportional to derivative of instantaneous lung volume (respiratory flow). Gray area includes mean ±SE. From Saul et al[2] with permission.

consistent among the subjects and suggested a common mechanism. The specific transfer characteristics were actually very similar to those of a positive derivative function, suggesting that the nonautonomic RSA is closely related to the rate of change lung volume or respiratory flow. Such a mechanism would also account for the frequency and tidal volume dependence observed by Bernardi.[18] The hypothesis is also in agreement with the observation that steady-state changes in intrathoracic pressure, such as those elicited by either the Valsalva or Mueller maneuvers, lead to only minor changes in RR interval, while a single large and rapid deep breath leads to the greatest variations in RR interval.[18]

The importance of stretch of the isolated right atrium in changing HR has been demonstrated in a number of studies which were extensively reviewed by Pathak.[42] This mechanism has been documented in the isolated perfused heart,[43] where it was found that an increase in atrial stretch increased HR, consistent with the positive differentiator mechanism discussed above. Brooks et al[44] observed similar findings in the dog, and Solda[32] showed that the rate of change in right atrial pressure is related to RSA in the vagotomized, anesthetized rabbit. Thus, there is a clear experimental basis to support the observation of a nonautonomic RSA after cardiac transplant in humans.

Mechanism of Respiratory Sinus Arrhythmia—Low Frequencies

As noted above, LF fluctuations of HR (0.03 to 0.15 Hz) have also been observed after transplantation. Interpretation of this LF variability is generally more difficult than that of the HF variability for a number of reasons. First, autonomic mediation of LF variability occurs through both vagal and sympathetic cardiac efferent activity.[1,2,37,38] Second, most physiological control mechanisms act as low-pass filters. Thus, as one goes down in frequency, more and more mechanisms begin to have significant amplitude and may be capable of modulating HR and other physiological variables. Third, a wide range of physiological variables have been observed to spontaneously fluctuate in this frequency band, including both respiratory frequency and tidal volume,[2,39-41,45] sympathetic nerve activity,[46] PCO2 and PO2,[47,48] and perhaps most importantly, arterial BP.[46] In addition, the nonautonomic atrial stretch mechanism described above for HF variability will be clearly present at lower frequencies when respiration occurs in that range. Of note, because of the differentiator effect, the amplitude of the nonautonomic mechanism decreases considerably at lower frequencies. As shown in Figure 4, spontaneous respiratory variability in transplant subjects may both contain significant energy at low frequencies and be strongly correlated to the LF variability in RR interval.[35] Thus, accurate interpretation of LF HRV is considerably enhanced through a careful analysis of other physiological signals such as respiration or arterial pressure.

Nonetheless, the intriguing data of Figure 6, demonstrating that significant levels of LF variability are observed almost exclusively at an interval of more than 20 months after transplantation suggests the possibility that autonomic reinnervation occurs in some subjects.[21] Since HF variability does not increase with the time after transplantation, there is no evidence for vagal reinnervation, suggesting that the autonomic reinnervation is almost certainly sympathetic. In support of such a hypothesis, the LF variability observed in heart transplants subjects is not always associated with LF respiratory activity, and many of the same subjects who demonstrate this variability have significant responses to amyl nitrite inhalation (Figure 7). The hypothesis of sympathetic reinnervation is further supported by the study of Wilson et al[49] demonstrating cardiac release of norepinephrine in response to both tyramine administration and sustained handgrip in 39 of 50 patients studied more than 1 year after cardiac transplantation. These observations have now been confirmed by other groups. Thus, it seems likely that the reappearance of LF variability late after cardiac transplant (Figures 5 and 6) is causally related to the sympathetic reinnervation which has been observed in similar patient groups.

Heart Rate Variability With Physiological Manipulations

Exercise

In normal subjects, exercise produces profound respiratory, hemodynamic, and neurohumoral changes. Specifically, there is an early withdrawal of vagal activity which is associated with a marked decrease in HF respiratory related vagal modulation of HR.[17,19] There is also a large increase in ventilation, manifest as an increase in both respiratory rate and total volume. Thus, if RSA in heart transplant subjects during exercise were due to vagal modulation of HR, one would expect it to decrease as it does in normal subjects. However, if RSA were due to the mechanical effects of respiration on atrial stretch, one would expect that the increase in ventilation would lead to an increase in RSA. In fact, two studies of RSA during exercise in cardiac transplant subjects have found that RSA increases during the early phases of exercise when ventilation increases are more pronounced and then plateaued at the higher levels of exercise when ventilation was more constant (Figure 1).[17,19] In one, there was also a significant but somewhat weak correlation between HF respiratory variability and both VO2 consumption (R = 0.21, P <0.05) and HR (R = −0.45, P <0.001).[35] A multiple regression analysis showed a significant independent contribution of both VO2 and HR to the HF variability measure. Thus, it seems that as with transplant subjects at rest, during exercise RSA is not due to modulation of vagal activity. Because both sympathetic activity and ventilation are significantly increased during exercise, it is difficult to know whether sympathetic modulation plays a small role in the transplant subjects.

Tilt

In normal subjects, passive tilt virtually always leads to a decrease in HF HRV and an increase in LF variability.[1,22,37,41] These changes are probably due to a reduction in vagal and an increase in sympathetic modulation of HR. Although it is less clear what the hemodynamic or reflex effect is that leads to these changes, there is clearly an associated decrease in central venous volume with tilt. In contrast, Bernardi et al[20] found that passive tilting did not reduce HF variability (RSA) in nine subjects studied 18 months after cardiac transplantation. RR interval variability was coherent with respiration in both the supine and tilt positions. These data again suggest that RSA in transplants is not due to vagal modulation of HR, but more likely due to changes in atrial stretch which may not be as significantly effected by the change in posture.

Arterial Baroreflexes

To further evaluate potential autonomic modulation of HR after cardiac transplantation, one can look at the responses of RR interval to baroreflex stimuli. These stimuli should have an absent or minimal effect on changes in atrial stretch, but should be able to indirectly evaluate the ability of cardiac autonomic efferent activity to modulate HR. Using a neck suction technique similar to that described by Cross,[50] Bernardi and colleagues evaluated the response of RR interval to simultaneous sinusoidal changes in neck suction and fixed rate breathing, with each stimulus at a separate frequency. The frequencies were selected to be as close as possible to each other to avoid the confounding frequency dependence of sinus node responses to vagal and sympathetic activity. Respiration was fixed at 0.25

Hz (15 breaths per minute) and the sinusoidal neck suction was fixed at 0.20 Hz (12 cycles per minute) with an amplitude from 0 to -30 mmHg neck chamber pressure. A normal subject had two discrete peaks in the RR interval spectra, one at the respiratory frequency and one at the neck chamber frequency (Figure 10, left), while a subject with a recent heart transplant had only the respiratory peak at 0.25 Hz (Figure 5, right). The lack of an autonomically mediated response to the sinusoidal neck chamber variations is consistent with the respiratory related fluctuations of RR interval being nonautonomically mediated. Another baroreflex stimuli inhalation of amyl nitrite also failed to induce a reflex tachycardia in recently transplanted subjects (636 ± 22 milliseconds preinhalation versus 629 ± 22 milliseconds post).[20] However, as noted above, some subjects later after transplant have both the reappearance of LF HRV, and amyl nitrite responses (Figure 11), consistent with sympathetic reinnervation. It appears then that the sympathetic reinnervation is able to modulate both respiratory related LF HRV and baroreflex related LF HRV.

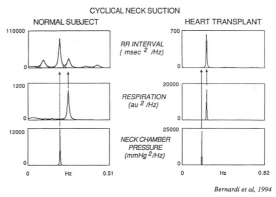

Bernardi et al, 1994

Figure 10. Effect of 0.2 Hz sinusoidal neck suction in a normal (left panel) and in a heart transplant subject (right panel) with controlled respiration at 0.25 Hz. Notice two HF peaks (baroreflex and respiratory) in the RR interval spectrum of the normal subject and the single peak (respiratory only) in the RR spectrum of the transplant subject, indicating absence of baroreflex HR modulation.

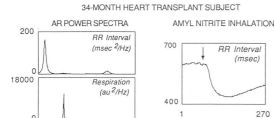

34-MONTH HEART TRANSPLANT SUBJECT

AR POWER SPECTRA   AMYL NITRITE INHALATION

Figure 11. LF fluctuation which are not correlated with respiratory activity in a subject who was transplanted 34 months earlier. The RR interval spectrum (in the upright position) shows a LF component which is not related to respiration (upper panel left). The same subject was able to decrease RR interval slowly but with a large magnitude after inhalation of amyl nitrite, suggesting the presence of sympathetic modulation of HR due to reinnervation.

1/f Heart Rate Variability

To understand the link between global HRV and neurohumoral modulation of HR, the 24-hour spectra shown in Figure 2 were computed from Holter monitor recordings in normal, congestive heart failure, and cardiac transplant subjects. The normal subjects had significantly more total variability than both the other groups (p <0.05), but there were no differences between the heart failure and transplant subjects.[22] Interestingly, variability at very low frequencies (0.00003 to 0.01 Hz) reached similar levels and was responsible for more than 75% of the total power in all three groups. In addition, for all three groups, the spectral characteristics below 0.1 Hz scaled as $1/f\alpha$, where f is frequency and alpha was 1.02 ±0.05 (range 0.93 to 1.07) for the normals, 1.31 ±0.43 (range 0.87 to 1.7) for the heart failure patients, and 1.95±0.35 (range 1.7 to 2.2) for the transplant patients. As Figure 2 shows, the slope of these spectra were nearly linear over 4 decades of frequency. Although the slope has not been correlated with any clinical parameters, there is recent data suggesting that it is the VLF power which is most predictive of death in the postmyocardial infarction group.[51,52] The consistent 1/f relation found in these three groups of subjects and the similar power at the lowest frequencies probably reflects some fundamental property of HR regulation on a time scale of seconds to hours which is different in the three groups.

Rejection

Two studies have examined the potential use of HRV parameters to detect graft rejection in the transplanted heart. In 1988, Zbilut el al[26] reported that the peak spectral power of the HF peak in the HR power spectrum (called PSP-RSA) was a sensitive but nonspecific predictor of graft rejection. There was no clear explanation for their findings; however, they did note that without a measure of respiratory activity, it was difficult to know what effect varying respiratory activity may have had. Sands et al[29] reported a different finding that broad-band (in frequency) changes in HR spectral power tracked biopsy proven rejection in some transplant recipients. They suggested that the findings were due to involvement of the sinoatrial node or supraventricular conduction system in the rejection process which then lead to erratic beat-to-beat variations in R wave location. Although there was a significant difference between spectral power in rejection and nonrejection episodes for all subjects, the spectral measures only tracked the biopsies in some of the subjects. Thus, limitations in both of these studies suggest that they should serve as preliminary data for further investigation.

Summary

Given the current data from HRV and baroreflex response studies, there is no evidence that heart transplant subjects up to

52 months after transplantation have any vagally mediated HRV. Alternatively, there is evidence that between 12 and 20 months after transplantation, some subjects develop HRV patterns and baroreflex responses consistent with sympathetic reinnervation. Thus, HF respiratory related variations of HR in transplant subjects appear to be mediated solely by nonautonomic mechanisms such as respiratory related atrial stretch. In contrast to vagally mediated RSA, these nonautonomic variations are increased with increasing respiratory rate, consistent with a direct relation to respiratory flow. LF HR variations may also be related to respiration, but probably often serve as an indicator of late functional sympathetic reinnervation. An understanding of these nonautonomic and autonomic mechanisms of HR control in heart transplant patients is necessary when designing, performing and analyzing studies of cardiovascular control in these patients.

References

1. Pomeranz B, Macauley RJB, Caudill MA, et al. Assessment of autonomic function in humans by heart spectral analysis. Am J Physiol 1985; 248:H151-H153.
2. Saul JP, Berger RD, Albrecht P, et al. Transfer function analysis of the circulation: unique insights into cardiovascular regulation. Am J Physiol 1991; 261:H1231-1245.
3. Saul JP. Beat-to-beat variations of heart rate reflect modulation of cardiac autonomic outflow. News in Physiologic Sciences 1990; 5:32-37.
4. Kent KM, Cooper T. The denervated heart. A model for studying autonomic control of the heart. N Engl J Med 1974; 291:1017-1021.
5. Kavanagh T, Yacoub MH, Mertens DJ, et al. Cardiorespiratory response to exercise training after orthotopic cardiac transplantation. Circulation 1988; 77:162-171.
6. Jose DA, Taylor RR. Autonomic blockade by propranalol and atropine to study intrinsic myocardial function in man. J Clin Invest 1969; 48:2019.
7. Dempsey PJ. Supersensitivity of the chronically denervated feline heart. Am J Physiol 1966; 211:703-711.
8. Vanter ED. Mechanism of supersensitivity to sympathomimetic amines in the chronically denervated heart of the conscious dog. Circ Res 1963; 13:39-47.
9. Yusuf S, Theodoropulos S, Mathias CJ, et al. Increased sensitivity of the denervated transplanted human heart to isoprenaline both before and after beta adrenergic blockade. Circulation 1987; 74:696-704.
10. Lurie KG, Bristow MR, Reitz BA. Increased beta-adrenergic receptor density in a experimental model of cardiac transplantation. J Thorac Cardiovasc Surg 1983; 86:195.
11. Denniss AR, Marsh JD, Quigg RJ, et al. Beta-adrenergic receptor number and adenylate cyclase function in denervation transplanted and cardiomyopathic human hearts. Circulation 1989; 79:1028-1034.
12. Quigg RJ, Rocco MB, Gauthier DF, et al. Mechanisms of attenuated peak heart rate response to exercise following orthotopic cardiac transplantation. J Am Coll Cardiol 1989; 14:338-344.
13. Rudas L, Pflugfelder PW, Menkis AH, et al. Evolution of heart rate responsiveness after orthotopic cardiac transplantation. Am J Cardiol 1991; 68:232-236.
14. Donald DE, Shepherd JT. Response to exercise in dogs with cardiac denervation. Am J Physiol 1963; 205:393-400.
15. Bexton RS, Milne JR, Cory Pearce R, et al. Effect of beta blockade on exercise response after cardiac transplantation. Br Heart J 1983; 49:584-588.
16. Epstein SE, Robinson BF, Kahler RL, et al. Effects of beta-adrenergic blockade on the cardiac response to maximal and submaximal exercise in man. J Clin Invest 1965; 24:1745-1753.
17. Arai Y, Saul JP, Albrecht P, et al. Modulation of cardiac autonomic activity during and immediately after exercise. Am J Physiol 1989; 256:H132-H141.
18. Bernardi L, Keller F, Sanders M, et al. Respiratory sinus arrhythmia in the denervated human heart. J Appl Physiol 1989; 67:1447-1455.
19. Bernardi L, Salvucci F, Suardi R, et al. Evidence for an intrinsic mechanism regulating heart rate variability in the transplanted and the intact heart during submaximal dynamic exercise? Cardiovasc Res 1990; 24:968-981.
20. Bernardi L, Leuzzi S, Valle F, et al. Respiratory sinus arrhythmia in recently heart transplanted subjects is caused by a non-autonomic mechanism. Eur Heart J 1993; 14:207. Abstract.
21. Bernardi L, Valle F, Leuzzi S, et al. Non-respiratory components of heart rate variability in heart transplant recipients: evi-

dence of autonomic reinnervation? Clin Sci 1994; 86:537-545.

22. Saul JP. Heart rate variability during congestive heart failure: observations and implications. In: DiRienzo M, Mancia G, Parati G, et al (eds). Blood Pressure and Heart Rate Variability: Computer Analysis, Methodology and Clinical Applications. Amsterdam: IOS Press, 1993; 266-275.

23. Van de Borne P, Leeman M, Primo G, et al. Reappearance of normal circadian rhythm of blood pressure after cardiac transplantation. Am J Cardiol 1992; 69:794-801.

24. Cugini P, Lucia P, di Palma L, et al. Ritmo circadiano della pressione arteriosa e della frequenza cardiac in pazienti con trapianto di cuore: studio longitudinale prima e dopo l'impianto. Cardiology 1991; 36:765-775.

25. Hrusheska WJ. Quantitative respiratory sinus arrhythmia analysis. Ann NY Acad Sci 1984; 24:1001-1004.

26. Zbilut JP, Murdock DK, Lawson L, et al. Use of power spectral analysis of respiratory sinus arrhythmia to detect graft rejection. J Heart Transplant 1988; 7:280-288.

27. Emdin M, Carpeggiani C, Balocchi R, et al. La variabilita' della frequenz cardiaca nel cuore normale e nel cuore trapiantato, "Il punto su sistema neurovegetativo e cuore". L'Abbate A and Schwartz P, Florence: OIC Medical Press, 1990; 81-95.

28. Zeuzem S, Olbrich HG, Seeger C, et al. Beat to beat variation of heart rate in diabetic patients with autonomic neuropathy and in completely cardiac denervation patients following orthotopic heart transplantation. Int J Cardiol 1991; 33:105-114.

29. Sands KEF, Appel ML, Lilly LS, et al. Power spectrum analysis of heart rate variability in human cardiac transplant recipients. Circulation 1989; 79:76-82.

30. Raeder EA, Berger R, Kenet R, et al. Assessment of autonomic cardiac control by power spectrum of heart rate fluctuations. J Appl Cardiol 1987; 2:283-300.

31. Ferrari AU, Daffonchio A, Albergati F, et al. Inverse relationship between heart rate and blood pressure variabilities in rats. Hypertension 1987; 10:533-537.

32. Solda PL, Perlini S, Valdata S, et al. Determinants of respiratory sinus arrhythmia in the vagotomized rabbit heart. Eur Heart J 1991; 12(suppl):419.

33. Hayano J, Sakakibara Y, Yamada A, et al. Accuracy of assessment of cardiac vagal tone by heart rate variability in normal subjects. Am J Cardiol 1991; 67:199-204.

34. Perlini S, Bernardi L, Calciati A, et al. Parasympathetic and ventilatory contributions to blood pressure and heart rate variabilities in unanesthetized rats. J Hypertens 1992; 10:S36.

35. Radaelli A, Bernardi L, Falcone C, et al. Factors modulating respiratory sinus arrhythmia during physical exercise in heart transplanted patients. Eur Heart J 1991; 12(suppl):226.

36. Moody GB, Mark RG, Zoccola A, et al. Derivation of respiratory signals from multi-lead ECGs. Comp Cardiol 1986; 12:113-116.

37. Malliani A, Pagani M, Lombardi F, et al. Cardiovascular neural regulation explored in the frequency domain. Circulation 1991; 84:482-492.

38. Berger RD, Saul JP, Cohen RD. Tranfer function analysis of autonomic regulation. I. Canine atrial rate response. Am J Physiol 1989; 25:H142-H152.

39. Hirsch JA, Bishop B. Respiratory sinus arrhythmia in humans: how breathing pattern modulates heart rate. Am J Physiol 1981; 241:H620-H629.

40. Angelone A, Coulter NA. Respiratory sinus arrhythmia: a frequency dependent phenomenon. J Appl Physiol 1964; 19:479-482.

41. Saul JP, Berger RD, Chen MH, et al. Transfer function analysis of autonomic regulation. II. Respiratory sinus arrhythmia. Am J Physiol 1989; 25:H153-H161.

42. Pathak CL. Autoregulation of chronotropic response of the heart through pacemaker stretch. Cardiology 1973; 58:45-64.

43. Blinks JR. Positive chronotropic effect of increasing right atrial pressure in the isolated mammalian heart. Am J Physiol 1956; 186:299-303.

44. Brooks C, Lu HH, Lange G, et al. Effects of localized stretch of sinoatrial node region of the dog heart. Am J Physiol 1966; 211:1197-1202.

45. Eckberg DL. Human sinus arrhythmia as an index of vagal cardiac outflow. J Appl Physiol 1983; 54:961-966.

46. Preiss G, Iscoe S, Polosa C. Analysis of a periodic breathing pattern associated with Mayer waves. Am J Physiol 1975; 228:768-774.

47. Goldberger AL, Findley LJ, Blackburn MR, et al. Nonlinear dynamics in heart failure: implications of long-wavelength cardiopulmonary oscillations. Am Heart J 1984; 107:612-615.

48. Sayers B. Analysis of heart rate variability. Ergonomics 1973; 16:17-32.

49. Wilson RF, Christensen BV, Olivari MT, et al. Evidence for structural sympathetic reinnervation after orthotopic cardiac transplantation in humans. Circulation 1991; 83:1210-1220.

50. Cross SJ, Crowe MR, Rowles JM. Mutual interactions of respiratory sinus arrhythmia and the carotid baroreceptor-heart rate reflex. Clin Sci 992[82]:139-145.

51. Kleiger RE, Miller JP, Bigger JT, et al. Decreased heart rate variability and its association with increased mortality after acute myocardial infarction. Am J Cardiol 1987; 59:256-262.

52. Bigger JT, Fleiss JL, Steinman RC, et al. Frequency domain measures of heart period variability and mortality after myocardial infarction. Circulation 1992; 85:164-171.

Chapter 37

Heart Rate Variability in Patients With Other Cardiovascular Diseases

Josef Kautzner

Heart rate variability (HRV) assessment has become a widely used technique for noninvasive study of sympatho-vagal modulation of heart rate (HR) in a broad spectrum of cardiovascular disorders. In this chapter, we attempt to summarize the results of studies evaluating HRV in less frequent cardiac diseases not covered by other chapters in the book. To date, clinical studies in this area are limited both in number as well as in small sample size and thus, only suggestions on potential clinical utility can be made. For easier orientation, a brief summary of these studies is listed in Table 1.

Hypertrophic Cardiomyopathy

Hypertrophic cardiomyopathy is known to be associated with an increased risk of sudden cardiac death. However, identification of those individuals at high risk still remains a major problem in clinical cardiology.[1] Based on preliminary data suggestive of abnormal peripheral vascular response and autonomic dysfunction in patients with hypertrophic cardiomyopathy,[2] Counihan et al studied various time- and frequency-domain indices of HRV in 104 adult patients during a drug-free period.[3] Although they found that both global and high-frequency (HF) components of HRV were reduced in those with symptoms and supraventricular or ventricular arrhythmias on Holter monitoring, neither relation of HRV to syncope nor its association with occurrence of sudden cardiac death during period of follow-up was observed. The association of potential autonomic disturbances to syncope was also studied by Gillingan et al who, using simple autonomic function tests, demonstrated that patients with hypertrophic cardiomyopathy presented with lower variation in HR as compared to healthy subjects, but this finding was not associated with the occurrence of syncopal episodes.[4]

These observations probably reflect a broad variety of potential mechanisms initiating sudden cardiac death in patients

From: Malik M., Camm AJ (eds.): *Heart Rate Variability.* Armonk, NY. Futura Publishing Company, Inc., © 1995.

Table 1

List of Clinical Studies Using Sophisticated Methods of HRV Assessment in Other Cardiovascular Diseases

Study (Reference)	Clinical Condition	Subjects	Major Conclusions	Suggested Clinical Utility
Couniham et al 1993[3]	Hypertrophic cardiomyopathy	104 patients	Reduction of global and HF components in symptomatic patients without predictive value for risk stratification	Not apparent
Ajiki et al 1993[5]		15 patients 18 controls	Decreased HF components and increase of LF/HF ratio during night, independent of the degree of LV hypertrophy	
Guzzetti et al 1994[6]		18 patients 18 controls	Reduction of total power and increase in LF/HF during night; day/night difference in LF/HF ratio blunted and related to myocardial beta-receptor density	
Ajiki et al 1993[5]	Dilated cardiomyopathy	14 patients 18 controls	Lowered HF components and increase in LF/HR ratio related to LV ejection fraction	Not apparent
Mbaissouroum et al 1993[9]		20 patients 15 controls	Decreased overall HRV measures with strong correlation to LV filling time	
Mandawat et al 1993[11]	Myocardial hypertrophy (aortic valve disease in 43 patients)	99 patients 49 controls	Decreased overall measures, their reverse relationship with LV mass index and association with high grade ventricular arrhythmias	Potential prognostic value
Stein et al 1993[12]	Chronic mitral regurgitation	38 patients	Overall HRV measures correlate with RV and LV performance and predict development of atrial fibrillation, mortality or progression to surgery	Potential prognostic value
Kozlowski et al 1992[16]	Mitral valve prolapse	29 patients 21 controls	Increased HF components and decrease in LF/HF ratio both in recumbent and supine position	Not apparent
Frisinghelli et al 1992[17]		41 patients 36 controls	Increase in HF with decrease LF components in supine position, increase LF components during tilt apparent only in 27 patients with mitral regurgitation	
Marangoni et al 1993[18]		39 patients 24 controls	Lower HF components; no difference between patients with and without syncope	

(Table 1-continued)

Finley et al 1989	Atrial septal defect (children)	10 patients 10 controls	Decreased SDNN and HF components with a tendency to normalisation after surgical closure	Not apparent
Guzzetti et al 1991[24]	Chronic Chagas' disease (without heart failure)	19 patients 7 controls	Lack of increase in LF component during tilt test or handgrip, reduced changes in HF components during standing and Valsalva manoeuvre	Potential for early diagnostic capability, prognostic value unknown
Fei et al 1993[26]	Idiopathic ventricular tachycardia	27 patients 20 controls	Decrease in HF components and lost correlation between spectral measures and QT interval	No apparent
Leenhardt 1994[27]		14 patients	Decreased overall HRV measures and predominantly HF components, increased LF/HF ratio	
Morillo et al 1994[28]		10 patients 20 controls	Decrease in LF and HF components, lower LF/HF ratio both in supine and upright position	
Frey et al 1993[30]	Postablation sinus tachycardia	16 patients 7 controls	Increased SDANN and HF components following modification of AV node or ablation of left lateral and right posteroseptal pathways, and its correlation with RF current energy	Not apparent
Kocovic et al 1993[91]		64 patients 21 controls	Decreased SDNN, pNN$_{50}$, rMSSD and HF spectral components following modification of AV node or ablation of left lateral and posteroseptal pathways with resolution within 1 month period	

with hypertrophic cardiomyopathy, for example, like primary arrhythmia, hemodynamic events and/or ischemia. Therefore, HRV does not seem to be of value for risk stratification in patients with hypertrophic cardiomyopathy.

More detailed description of autonomic milieu in hypertrophic cardiomyopathy was obtained by power spectral analysis. Ajiki et al showed a significantly increased ratio between the low-frequency (LF) and HF power of HRV with a corresponding decrease in HF components during nighttime (Figure 1), and thus, blunted day-to-night variation.[5] These data were subsequently confirmed by Guzzetti et al, who additionally observed a positive correlation of day-to-night LF/HF ratio changes with myocardial density of beta-adrenergic receptors measured by positron emission tomography.[6] Of importance also is that density of beta-adrenergic receptors correlated

A: Spectral power at night

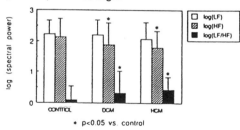

B: Spectral power in daytime

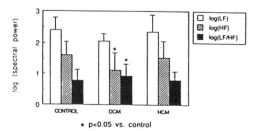

Figure 1. Comparison of HF power components and LF/HF ratio in logarithmic scale in patients with hypertrophic cardiomyopathy (HCM) and idiopathic dilated cardiomyopathy (DCM). Panel **A** shows values at night and panel **B** those in the daytime; bars represent mean value ±SD. Reproduced with permission from Ajiki et al.[5]

with echocardiographic index of left ventricular diastolic function.

Both studies are compatible with the hypothesis of increased sympathetic output to the heart with shift of sympatho-vagal balance towards sympathetic predominance. The second observation may also question whether impaired diastolic function, which is a hallmark of hypertrophic cardiomyopathy, plays a role in the modulation of HRV. However, further studies focused on the potential relationship of HRV and parameters of diastolic function are essential.

Dilated Cardiomyopathy

Clinical use of HRV in patients with dilated cardiomyopathy corresponds to a great extent with its use in cardiac failure (see Chapter 34) because the clinical manifestation is analogous and usually mixed populations are studied. On the other hand, it may not always be appropriate, since the cause of congestive heart failure may influence the time-course or magnitude of sympathetic activation in these patients.[7] Thus, we will restrict our analysis to studies exploring HRV specifically in dilated cardiomyopathy with reference to left ventricular function. In this respect, Ajiki et al investigated spectral measures of HRV in 14 patients and observed significant decrease in HF spectral power, as well as increase in the LF/HF ratio regardless of day or night period (Figure 1), and these changes were correlated with ejection fraction.[5]

This might suggest that autonomic imbalance is related to severity of left ventricular dysfunction. However, large scale study involving a great proportion of patients with dilated cardiomyopathy did not confirm this relationship.[8]

A more detailed study focusing predominantly on the diastolic function of the left ventricle in relation to HRV was conducted by Mbaissouroum et al in patients with dilated cardiomyopathy.[9] Using standard time-domain indices of HRV, they re-

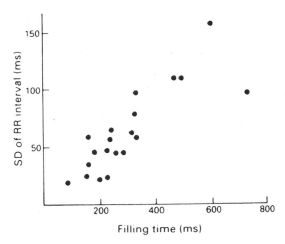

Figure 2. Correlation between left ventricular filling time and the standard deviation of the normal RR intervals (SDNN) in patients with dilated cardiomyopathy. It is apparent that the shorter filling periods are associated with the more reduced HRV. Reproduced with permission from Mbaissouroum et al.[9]

vealed that overall measures like SDNN or SDANN were significantly reduced as compared with normal controls and, more importantly, were strongly correlated to left ventricular filling time assessed by Doppler echocardiography (r = 0.81 and r = 0.79, respectively). Further, the most striking correlation of these indices of HRV was found with mean RR interval (r = 0.82 and r = 0.81, respectively) (Figure 2).

This observation is interesting from a pathophysiological point of view, since it emphasizes the importance of short filling time as a mechanical restraint for HRV. Certain minimum filling time needs to be maintained in order to preserve cardiac output and thus, variation of RR interval in faster rhythm is limited.

Aortic Stenosis

Increased risk of sudden cardiac death in hemodynamically significant aortic stenosis is well established, but the exact mechanism remains unknown. Only isolated attempts to evaluate autonomic influences to the heart by means of HRV have been reported so far. In the study of Airaksinen et al, significant decrease of HRV during deep breathing was observed with its weak correlation (r = 0.41, p <0.05) to the left ventricular end-diastolic pressure.[10] HRV was also found to be decreased in a large group of patients with left ventricular hypertrophy, of which almost 50% were diagnosed with aortic valve disease.[11] Of interest is an inverse relationship between HRV measures and left ventricular mass index, and association of low HRV with higher grade of ventricular arrhythmias on Holter monitoring.

These preliminary data might indicate that depressed HRV reflects degree of left ventricular hypertrophy in aortic stenosis. At present, there is no information on the usefulness of HRV for detection of those at risk of sudden cardiac death in aortic stenosis.

Mitral Regurgitation

Natural history of chronic mitral regurgitation varies in different patients, and timing of cardiac surgery may be a difficult clinical decision. The prognostic value of HRV in severe nonischemic mitral regurgitation has recently been reported by Stein et al.[12] In their study, both time- and frequency-domain measures of HRV were used in 38 patients. Heart rate, SDANN, total spectral power and LF power predicted mortality and total events. However, the most powerful predictor of subsequent events proved to be SDANN. Patients with reduced SDANN were significantly more likely to progress to valvular surgery (Figure 3), develop atrial fibrillation or die. Furthermore, SDANN correlated with resting right and left ventricular ejection fraction and with HR.

Strong inverse relationship of SDANN, which is believed to correspond mainly to the ultra-low component of HRV to prognosis is of important value, but the pathophysiological mechanism is unclear. The correlation of this parameter to mean RR interval may indicate again, as in dilated cardiomyopathy, its partial dependence on short dia-

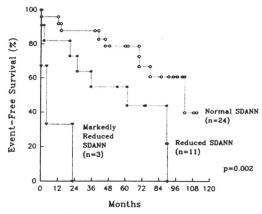

Figure 3. The life-time curve for survival free of mitral valve surgery and other events stratified by the standard deviation of the 5-minute mean RR intervals (SDANN) in patients with chronic mitral regurgitation. Normal SDANN represents value >100 ms, reduced values range between 50 and 100 ms, and markedly reduced SDANN is characterized by value <50 ms. Significance is estimated as a univariate continuous variable in a proportional-hazards model. Reproduced with permission from Stein et al.[12]

stolic filling time. It may also reflect reduced physical activity in patients with more advanced disease. Similarly, the relationship to ejection fraction seems to represent a higher degree of hemodynamic impairment. The clinical use of HRV in chronic mitral regurgitation may advance the optimal timing of cardiac surgery. However, these observations need further confirmation.

Mitral Valve Prolapse

Suggestions that mitral valve prolapse accounts for clinical manifestations previously attributed to neurocirculatory asthenia, panic disorder and autonomic dysfunction led to the definition of mitral valve prolapse syndrome. However, controlled studies have not supported the relationship between mitral valve prolapse and most of these allegedly associated signs or symptoms.[13] Yet, the problem has not been solved and similarly, the degree of risk of sudden cardiac death in patients with mitral valve prolapse needs further evaluation.[14] In this

respect, it is rather surprising that HRV has not been applied more extensively for studies of potential autonomic dysfunction. Early studies by Weissman et al compared simple measures of autonomic function in response to deep breathing, postural stress and Valsalva maneuver, and urine catecholamine excretion in patients with mitral valve prolapse and patients with panic attacks.[15] No signs of adrenergic hyperactivity were found in those with mitral prolapse. Furthermore, they exhibited decreased effectiveness of response to orthostatic stress and loss of the normal decrease with age in HRV during breathing. In another study, Kozlowski et al revealed significantly higher values of spectral power for HF components together with decrease in LF/HF ratio in supine, as well as in the standing, position in patients with mitral valve prolapse and history of syncope.[16] These results were subsequently reproduced, albeit in patients with concomitant mitral regurgitation.[17] Thus, the studies seem to strongly indicate increased parasympathetic modulation of HR in mitral valve prolapse. However, quite opposite changes in LF/HF ratio and decrease in HF power components in patients with mitral valve prolapse as compared to normal subjects were reported, both at rest and during tilt test.[18] Moreover, there were no significant differences between patients with syncope and without syncope in terms of HRV parameters in this study.

The inconsistent results may either indicate different types of autonomic dysfunction in mitral valve prolapse populations as suggested by Coghlan et al,[19] or merely random coincidence of various degree of autonomic dysfunction and the presence of prolapsing mitral valve. Therefore, the clinical utility of HRV in mitral valve prolapse appears to be doubtful.

Atrial Septal Defect

Based on earlier observation of decreased respiratory sinus arrhythmia in adult patients with atrial septal defect,[20] Finley et al employed SDNN and power spectrum analysis of HRV to evaluate the analogous relationship in children.[21] Both SDNN and HF components of HRV were significantly depressed in those with atrial septal defect as compared with normals, and the difference was more pronounced in the supine position. The fact that HRV parameters were significantly improved after surgical closure of defect (Figure 4), suggests a relationship of HRV to hemodynamic changes in the heart. In other words, it appears that increased mechanical stretch of volume-overloaded right atrium may directly influence HRV. This suggestion is in accord with recent experimental observation of the relationship of mechanical stretch applied on the sinoatrial (SA) nodal area to HRV.[22] Stretching the SA node led to significant decrease of SDNN and HF components of HRV.

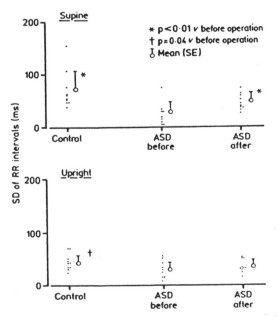

Figure 4. Values of the standard deviation of the RR intervals (SDNN) during supine and upright position in control subjects, and in children before and after surgical closure of an atrial septal defect. Reproduced with permission from Finley et al.[21]

These presumably mechanically induced changes in HRV could be a consequence of either a direct effect on diastolic depolarization within SA node via stretch-activated channels or reflex-mediated response on afferent signals from atrial stretch receptors. The extent to which this mechanism may influence HRV is unknown and this is an attractive area for further research.

Chronic Chagas' Disease

Chagas' disease, which is responsible for most of the cases of sudden cardiac death in Latin America, represents almost a paradigm of cardiac intrinsic denervation.[23] In this respect, the disease may serve as an unique experimental model for the assessment of the cardiac autonomic control in man. From a clinical point of view, the improvement in risk stratification of patients at risk of sudden cardiac death is of great importance. So far, only a preliminary study by Guzzetti et al has been published addressing the application of HRV in chagasic patients without an overt heart failure.[24] Using spectral power analysis they observed reduced capability to activate sympathetic responses (lack of response of LF components to tilt or handgrip) (Figure 5), together with signs of impairment of vagal modulatory activity (decreased changes in HF components during standing or deep breathing). However, the total spectral power remained unchanged during these procedures.

In summary, the initial findings suggest a simultaneous effect on both sympathetic and parasympathetic modulations and are in accordance with clinical and morphological studies. Nevertheless, the potential for early diagnosis of cardiac involvement and/or the prognostic impact of observed changes in HRV remains to be established.

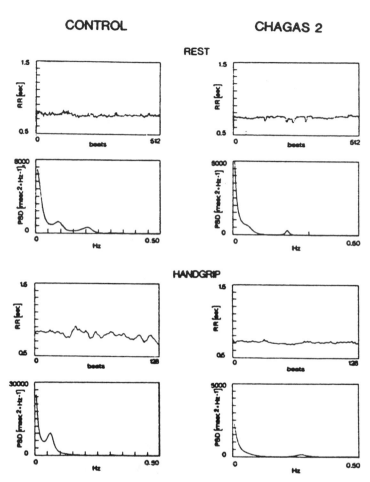

Figure 5. Representative power spectra of HR derived at rest and during handgrip test in a control subject (left panels) and in patient with Chagas' disease (right panels). The LF components, which are predominant in control subject during handgrip exercise, are absent in chagasic patient during the same exercise. Reproduced from Guzzetti et al[24] with permission.

Idiopathic Ventricular Tachycardia

Ventricular tachycardia or ventricular fibrillation can occur in patients with a structurally normal heart, accounting for roughly 10% of all patients with ventricular tachyarrhythmias.[25] It is a rather nonhomogeneous group of arrhythmias presumably with different pathophysiological mechanisms. Autonomic imbalance is supposed to play a role in some of them. Accordingly, impaired cardiac vagal efferent activity was found in a series of 27 patients with idiopathic ventricular tachycardia, but this fact had no discriminant value for identification of patients who presented with syncope.[26] A

low day/night ratio of the HR, and overall decreased HRV with depressed vagal activity as compared to sympathetic was revealed in a specific group of patients with short-coupled variant of torsades de pointes tachycardia in the setting of a normal QT interval.[27] Markedly reduced sympatho-vagal response with decrease in both LF and HF power in the supine position and also during orthostatic stress was observed in survivors of sudden cardiac death without structural heart disease.[28]

The lack of consistency in clinical studies reflect probable heterogeneity of pathogenic mechanisms in this particular group of arrhythmias and also the fact that we are not often able to diagnose subtle structural heart disease. This precludes formulation of any conclusions about the role of sympatho-vagal dysbalance in idiopathic ventricular arrhythmias.

Inappropriate Postablation Sinus Tachycardia

Recently, several reports have been published about persistent inappropriate sinus tachycardia following catheter modification of the atrioventricular node for atrioventricular junctional reentrant arrhythmias.[29] In an attempt to characterize pathophysiological mechanisms, HRV was analyzed in a series of 16 patients following radio frequency ablation of fast atrioventricular nodal or accessory pathways.[30] Surprisingly, increased HRV was found and its measures correlated with the amount of radio frequency energy applied, except in four patients after right lateral pathway ablation. A far-field effect on the sinus node or enhanced vagal modulation were proposed as potential mechanisms. However, these results were not confirmed in a subsequent more comprehensive study where HRV was evaluated before and immediately after RF ablation in 64 patients with supraventricular tachycardia.[31] Inappropriate sinus tachycardia was observed only in five patients (7.8%). Nevertheless, compared to control patients who underwent diagnostic study only, postablation HRV was significantly lower among the 17 individuals who had atrioventricular nodal modification (in 14 of them, the slow pathway was ablated) (Figure 6). Similarly, patients undergoing ablation of posteroseptal accessory pathway had a significant decrease in the time-domain indices of HRV and decrease in the HF components of spectral analysis. The resolution of HRV abnormalities over a time (up to 6 months after ablation) was suggestive of reinnervation.

Thus, the occurrence of inappropriate sinus tachycardia after radio frequency modification of the atrioventricular node or

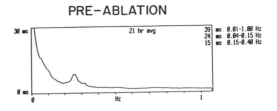

PRE-ABLATION

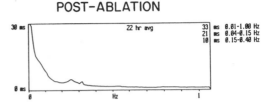

POST-ABLATION

Figure 6. Frequency-domain analysis of HRV obtained from ambulatory 24-hour Holter recording before **(upper panel)** and 24 hours after ablation **(bottom panel)** of the slow atrioventricular nodal pathway in a patient with typical form of atrioventricular reentrant supraventricular tachycardia. HF component of the spectrum (0.15 to 0.40 Hz) is significantly reduced after ablation. Reproduced from Kocovic et al[31] with permission.

accessory pathways seems to be mostly prevalent in fast pathway ablation or posteroseptal accessory pathway ablation and the underlying mechanism is supposed to be destruction of the parasympathetic ganglia or postganglionic fibers in the region of the low atrial septum. It still remains unanswered whether a lesser degree of parasympathetic denervation becomes a common consequence of radio frequency ablation in this region.

Conclusion

At present, only limited data exists on the potential diagnostic or prognostic value of HRV in less frequent cardiovascular diseases and this technique remains an investigational tool only. However, given HRV is considered to be a clinically useful marker of the cardiac response to parasympathetic and sympathetic activity, its broader application in patients with less frequent cardiovascular diseases may substantially improve our understanding of the pathophysiology of these disorders. On the other hand, the use of HRV in a broad spectrum of different conditions allows us to understand more thoroughly the background of its depression. Hopefully, this will make further clinical utility more fruitful.

References

1. McKenna WJ, Camm AJ. Sudden death in hypertrophic cardiomyopathy. Assessment of patients at high risk. Circulation 1989; 80:1489-1492.
2. Counihan PJ, Haywood GA, McKenna WJ. Cardiovascular reflexes in hypertrophic cardiomyopathy: association with clinical features. J Am Coll Cardiol 1991; 17:183A.
3. Counihan PJ, Fei L, Bashir Y, et al. Assessment of heart rate variability in hypertrophic cardiomyopathy. Association with clinical and prognostic features. Circulation 1993; 88:1682-1690.
4. Gillingan DM, Chan WL, Sbarouni E, et al. Autonomic function in hypertrophic cardiomyopathy. Br Heart J 1993; 69:525-529.
5. Ajiki K, Murakawa Y, Yanagisawa-Miwa A, et al. Autonomic nervous system activity in idiopathic dilated cardiomyopathy and in hypertrophic cardiomyopathy. Am J Cardiol 1993; 71:1316-1320.
6. Guzzetti S, Choudhury L, Mezzetti S, et al. Enhanced sympathetic activity identified by heart rate variability analysis in hypertrophic cardiomyopathy. J Am Coll Cardiol 1994; 23:47A. Special Issue.
7. Floras JS. Clinical aspects of sympathetic activation and parasympathetic withdrawal in heart failure. J Am Coll Cardiol 1993; 22(suppl A):72A-84A.
8. Kienzle MG, Ferguson DW, Birkett CL, et al. Clinical, hemodynamic and sympathetic neural correlates of heart rate variability in congestive heart failure. Am J Cardiol 1992; 69:761-767.
9. Mbaissouroum M, O'Sullivan C, Brecker SJ, et al. Shortened left ventricular filling time in dilated cardiomyopathy: additional effects on heart rate variability? Br Heart J 1993; 69:327-331.
10. Airaksinen KEJ, Ikaheimo MJ, Koistinen MJ, et al. Impaired vagal heart rate control in aortic valve stenosis. Eur Heart J 1988; 9:1126-1130.
11. Mandawat MK, Wallbridge DR, Pringle SD, et al. Heart rate variability in left ventricular hypertrophy. Eur Heart J 1993; 14(suppl):207. Abstract.
12. Stein KM, Borer JS, Hochreiter C, et al. Prognostic value and physiological correlates of heart rate variability in chronic severe mitral regurgitation. Circulation 1993; 88:127-135.
13. Devereux RB, Kramer-Fox R, Kligfield P. Mitral valve prolapse: causes, clinical manifestations, and management. Ann Intern Med 1989; 111:305-317.
14. Kligfield P, Levy D, Devereux RB, et al. Arrhythmias and sudden death in mitral valve prolapse. Am Heart J 1987; 113:1298-1307.
15. Weissman NJ, Shear MK, Kramer-Fox R, et al. Contrasting patterns of autonomic dysfunction in patients with mitral valve prolapse and panic attacks. Am J Med 1987; 82:880-888.
16. Kozlowski JW, Trzos S, Rozentryt P, et al. Spectral analysis of heart rate variability in patients with mitral valve prolapse. Eur Heart J 1992; 13(suppl):407. Abstract.
17. Frisinghelli A, Turiel M, Milletich A, et al. The role of mitral regurgitation in the neurovegetative regulation of mitral valve prolapse. Cardiologia 1992; 37:781-783.
18. Marangoni S, Scalvini S, Mai R, et al. Heart rate variability assessment in patients with mitral valve prolapse syndrome. Am J Noninvas Cardiol 1993; 7:210-214.
19. Coghlan CH. Autonomic dysfunction in the mitral valve prolapse syndrome: the brain-heart connection and interaction. In: Boudoulas H, Wooley CF (eds). The Mitral Valve Prolapse and the Mitral Valve Prolapse Syndrome. Mount Kisco, NY: Futura Publishing Company, 1988; 389-426.
20. Davies LG, Fotiades B. Sinus arrhythmia: observations in atrial septal defect and normal subjects. Br Heart J 1960; 22:301.
21. Finley JP, Nugent ST, Hellenbrand W, et al. Sinus arrhythmia in children with atrial septal defect: an analysis of heart rate variability before and after surgical repair. Br Heart J 1989; 61:280-284.
22. Homer SM, Murphy CF, Dick DJ, et al. The effect of stretch on the SA node: a physiological mechanism contributing to heart rate variability? Br Heart J 1994; 71(suppl):P90
23. Oliveira JSM. A natural human model of intrinsic heart nervous system denervation: chagas' cardiopathy. Am Heart J 1985; 110:1092-1098.
24. Guzzetti S, Iosa D, Pecis M, et al. Impaired heart rate variability in patients with chronic chagas' disease. Am Heart J 1991; 121:1727-1734.
25. Klein LS, Miles WM. Ventricular tachycardia in patients with normal hearts. Drugs or ablation. Cardiol Rev 1993; 1:336-343.
26. Fei L, Gill JS, Katritsis D, et al. Abnormal autonomic modulation of QT interval in pa-

tients with idiopathic ventricular tachycardia associated with clinically normal hearts. Br Heart J 1993; 69:311-314.

27. Leenhardt, Glaser E, Burguera M, et al. Short-coupled variant of torsade de pointes. A new electrocardiographic entity in the spectrum of idiopathic ventricular tachyarrhythmias. Circulation 1994; 89:206-215.

28. Morillo CA, Li HG, Zardini M, et al. Sympatho-vagal balance in sudden death survivors with and without heart disease. Circulation 1993; 88:I605.

29. Ehlert FA, Goldberger JJ, Brooks R, et al. Persistent inappropriate sinus tachycardia after radiofrequency current catheter modification of the atrioventricular node. Am J Cardiol 1992; 69:1092-1095.

30. Frey B, Heinz G, Kreiner G, et al. Increased heart rate variability after radiofrequency ablation. Am J Cardiol 1993; 71:1460-14ol.

31. Kocovic DZ, Harada T, Shea JB, et al. Alterations of heart rate and of heart rate variability after radiofrequency catheter ablation of supraventricular tachycardia. Delineation of parasympathetic pathways in the human heart. Circulation 1993; 88:1671-1681.

Chapter 38

Heart Rate Variability in Patients With Diabetes and Other Noncardiological Diseases

Federico Bellavere

Since the early 1970s, tests based on heart rate variability (HRV) have been proposed and used in diabetes.[1,2] This is because diabetes is known to be complicated by a dreadful disease, autonomic neuropathy (DAN), which affects about 40% of all diabetic patients and, in its severe form, offers a very poor prognosis.

As HRV reflects the degree of autonomic control of the heart, it is widely used for the diagnosis of autonomic dysfunctions in noncardiological patients on the assumption that, if such a dysfunction in the heart is identified, it is a sign of a more widespread autonomic neuropathy affecting all organs. In the case of a systemic disease, such as diabetes, this assumption is usually justified.

Other important reasons why diabetologists have chosen tests based on HRV as markers for DAN are: they are noninvasive, generally reproducible, and easy to perform.

The clinical importance of HRV tests is easy to appreciate if one considers the high incidence of diabetes in the normal population and the high incidence of DAN among diabetics.

In this chapter, HRV tests are divided into three main groups according to how widely they are used, which, of course, is related to how easy they are to use. The three groups are:

1. traditional cardiovascular reflex maneuvers;
2. HRV tests on time domain; and
3. HRV tests on frequency domain.

Traditional Cardiovascular Reflex Maneuvers

Of all the tests proposed for the diagnosis of DAN in the last 20 years, five have met with success among diabetologists.

From: Malik M., Camm AJ (eds.): *Heart Rate Variability*. Armonk, NY. Futura Publishing Company, Inc., © 1995.

These five tests are usually performed at a single session and are grouped into what is commonly called Ewing's Battery.[3] In this battery, three tests are based on HRV analysis and two on blood pressure (BP) variation analysis (which will not be commented upon here). The three HRV tests, which are thought to detect parasympathetic activity provide the evaluation of HRV during:

1. Valsalva maneuver;
2. deep breathing; and
3. lying to standing.

Valsalva Maneuver

Valsalva maneuver is usually performed by the patient sitting and blowing into a manometer against a resistance of 40 mm Hg for a period of 15 seconds, followed by complete rest. The complex autonomic reflex pattern elicited by this maneuver is treated elsewhere[4,5] and is illustrated in Figure 1.

Briefly, (after phase 1 which is not commented on here) the pattern consists of progressive tachycardia during strain (phase 2), further tachycardia after strain (phase 3), followed by pronounced bradycardia (phase 4). The reflex pathways involve almost all autonomic fibers linked to the heart and their connections with the baroreceptor system which is stimulated to maintain constant BP during all the phases mentioned.

On the contrary, in autonomic patients, dramatic variations in BP can be observed even while there are few variations in heart rate (Figure 1).

This maneuver can offer several parameters for the interpretation of autonomic interactions, but within the routine diagnosis of DAN, the Valsalva ratio, ie, the simple ratio between the longest RR interval after the strain and the shortest within the strain, is used as a marker for parasympathetic activity.

The Deep Breathing Maneuver

The deep breathing maneuver is performed by the patient sitting and breathing deeply, with a constant rate of one breath cycle per second, for 1 minute. In normals, this results in the amplification of respiratory arrhythmia which reflects the level of vagal activity in the heart.[1] The routine measurement taken by this HRV test is the simple evaluation of the[1] difference between the average of 3 hour maximums and 3 hour minimums, or the ratio between the maximal and minimal RR intervals obtained.[6] No variations in HR occur in autonomic patients (Figure 1).

Lying to Standing Maneuver

The patient is asked to stand up, and the ratio between the longest RR interval around the 30th beat and the shortest RR interval around the 15th beat, after standing, is calculated. This provides a further parameter of parasympathetic activity as the relative bradycardia, observed around the 30th beat after standing, has been proved to be dependent on vagal activation (Figure 1).[7]

A further, complementary test that we have proposed, is based on the evaluation of the maneuver carried out in reverse: standing to lying.[8] Here normal subjects show a characteristic dual phase: the first, which consists of a short, rapid cardiac acceleration has been shown to be due to vagal withdrawal, while the second, consisting of a gradual cardiac deceleration has been shown to be mainly due to sympathetic withdrawal. Hence, a simple calculation of the ratio between the longest RR interval within the 20th to 25th beat and the shortest RR interval within the first 5 beats after lying, offers a partial evaluation of sympathetic activity. It also provides a unique opportunity for evaluating sympathetic activity while using traditional cardiovascular reflex maneuvers.

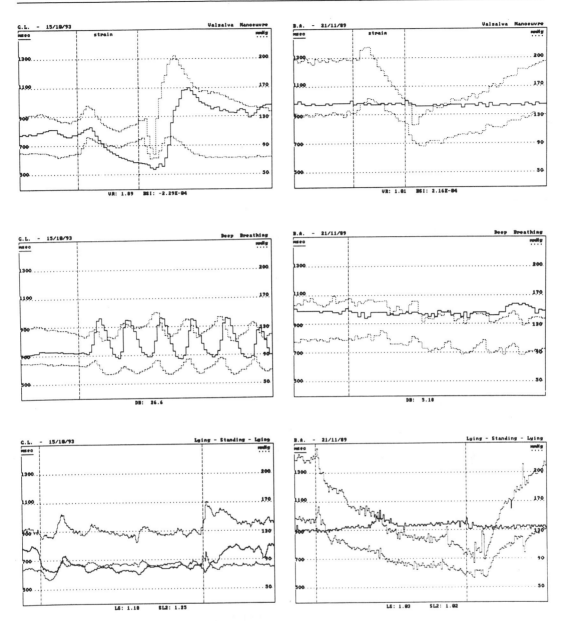

Figure 1. Cardiovascular autonomic patterns in Ewing's battery maneuvers: normal subject **(left side)** and neuropathic subject **(right side)** responses. The continuous line shows RR interval variations; the dotted lines show systolic and diastolic BP variations.

Although we recognize the limitations of cardiovascular reflex tests, which offer only a rough guide in the study of the state of the autonomic nervous system, it should be remembered that these are the diagnostic tools most widely used in clinical practice today. Indeed, cardiovascular reflex tests have enabled important diagnoses of autonomic dysfunctions to be made, not only in diabetes but also in a variety of other diseases such as alcholism,[9,10] ocular hypertension,[11,12] uremia,[13] Chagas' disease,[14,15] obesity,[16] lipomatosis,[17] multiple sclerosis,[18] Parkinson's disease,[19] rheumatoid arthritis,[20] hypothyroidism,[21] and many other pathologies.

Moreover, for most investigators, cardiovascular reflex tests have long represented only a preliminary procedure, from which they move on to use more sophisticated diagnostic tools and, furthermore, these tests are still considered reliable enough to be used as a standard of comparison and validation of the more advanced diagnostic techniques.[22-26]

Heart Rate Variability Tests on Time Domain

Resting HRV tests are characterized by the application of various well-known statistical parameters for the analysis of RR variations. Despite their being simple to use, they have not met with the same sort of enthusiasm from diabetologists as did cardiovascular reflex tests, perhaps because they are somewhat less specific, less reproducible, and they do not add much to the traditional cardiovascular reflex maneuvers.

In a 24-hour electrocardiogram (ECG) recording study, carried out in the early 1980s, it was clearly shown that the greater the autonomic dysfunction, the more a diabetic patient will show enhanced cardiac rhythm, reduced HRV, and a progressive loss of nychtomeral HR differences due to impaired nocturnal HR lengthening. Thus, DAN was resulted to be mainly characterized by vagal deficiency which leads to a tendency to fixed tachycardia, as well as to a reduced number of supraventricular ectopic beats.[27]

Quantification of the reduced HRV in DAN, described above, was first attempted in the early 1970s by applying the simple measurement of standard deviation (SD) to an RR interval series recorded over a period of 5 minutes.[28]

Shortly after, a new approach was tried, which focused on the analysis of the real beat-to-beat variation through measurement of the mean square of successive RR interval differences (MSSD)[29] or, more simply, by measuring the mean of successive RR differences (MSD).[30]

In the early 1980s, a paper published by Ewing offered some valuable indications which can help in the choice of method to be adopted for clinical purposes: HRV SD, MSSD, MSD and Max-Min HR Variation were compared using an ECG recording technique.[30] The results showed that Max-Min HR and HRV SD but not HRV MSD and MSSD could reliably identify patients with differing degrees of autonomic involvement. Moreover, HRV SD, but not HRV MSD or MSSD correlate with other traditional cardiovascular tests. However, HRV SD was shown to be affected by the value of resting HR, while HR Max-Min was not. Thus, the study suggested using HRV SD and, particularly, HR Max-Min as parameters for the detection of autonomic neuropathy in clinical practice.

More recently, in a 24-hour ECG recording, Malpas adopted a method of measuring the standard deviation of RR successive differences (SDSD). He found that this method was more sensitive than traditional cardiovascular reflex tests for detecting early autonomic involvement in diabetics.[31] It should be remembered though, that the above methodology was, in this case, applied in long-term recording acquisition (24 hours) hence, when a comparison is made with the previous methodologies based on short-term recording (5 to 20 minutes), it becomes clear that the increase in sensitivity is mainly due to the far greater amount of data gathered.

Another approach using long-term ECG recording was proposed by Ewing when he applied what he called the 'counts' method (Figure 2).[32] This consists of counting how many RR intervals per hour exceed, by either ±50 milliseconds, the directly preceding RR length. Thus, this method could be considered to be a "threshold" system as ±50 milliseconds is the real threshold each RR interval must pass in order to be "counted." The rationale behind this method is that in normal people there are many 'brisk' changes in the sequence of RR intervals which are greater than ±50 milliseconds, but that these brisk changes do not occur either in surgically denervated (transplanted) hearts or in diabetics affected by DAN. Moreover, as the Edinburgh group stated, the rapid RR changes are not necessarily related to respiratory activity, although they do depend on parasympathetic activity in the heart. The parasympathetic dependency of these brisk RR changes is strongly suppported by evidence of their circadian pattern: their major increase coincides with the well-known night-time parasympathetic overactivity.

The Edinburgh group also maintains that this 'counts' method is more sensitive than any of the traditional cardiovascular tests for the detection of DAN.

Although this method is very interesting, and has met with success in cardiological applications, it is not yet widely used by diabetologists, perhaps because it requires ECG Holter monitoring which is not easy to carry out due to the large number of patients affected by diabetes mellitus.

From the above it can be argued that there is no real agreement about which is the best test to use for the diagnosis of autonomic dysfunctions in diabetes or other noncardiological pathologies. A critical comparison of these methods does not lie within the scope of this short chapter, but can be found elsewhere.[25,30,31,33] Here, it should simply be remembered that the choice of tests is influenced by some elementary variables which reflect what the investigators wish to show, how many patients they seek to study and which technologies they have available.

From the theoretical point of view, as far as the target of the investigation is concerned, it has been said that the measure-

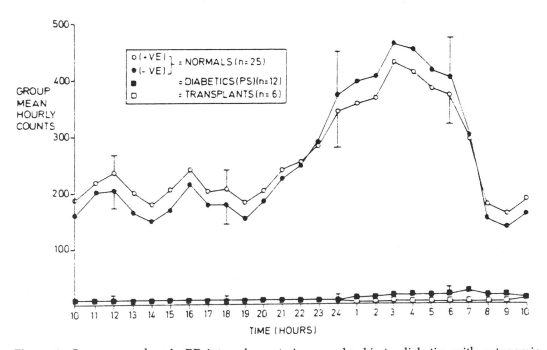

Figure 2. Group mean hourly RR interval counts in normal subjects, diabetics with autonomic damage and cardiac transplant patients (+VE: positive counts; -VE: negative counts). From Ewing et al.[32]

ment of brisk RR interval changes, such as MSSD, SDSD or the 'counts' method aim to evaluate parasympathetic activity which, of course, is directly responsible for rapid HR fluctuations, while SD covers all autonomic activity (including sympathetic) which the total variability of HR really expresses.

Heart Rate Variability Tests on the Frequency Domain

Frequency-domain analysis of HRV has been shown to offer a reliable quantification of several cyclic components of cardiac rhythmicity which are usually thought to depend on parasympathetic, sympathetic and other neuro-hormonal activity.[34] This chapter cannot take part in the active debate about what frequency-domain analysis of HRV really means, and which physiological activity can really be detected by the various cyclic components which can be obtained with it. The debate is amply dealt with in other chapters and elsewhere.[35-37] Here, we will limit ourselves to recalling some generally accepted concepts:

1. Power spectral analysis (PSA) of HRV is a sensitive method for detecting autonomic dysfunction, whether Fast Fourier Transform (FFT) or Autoregressive Mathematical Models are used.
2. It gives a reliable quantification of parasympathetic activity by calculating the square areas located at about 0.2 Hz of the spectra.
3. It gives some quantification of sympathetic activity by calculating the square areas located at about 0.1 Hz which are under both sympathetic and, to a lesser extent, parasympathetic control.
4. The ratio, or any other comparison between low-frequency (LF) (0.1 Hz) density components and high-frequency (HF) (0.2 Hz) density

components offer an acceptable indication of autonomic vagal-sympathetic balance in heart control.
5. Some very low-frequency (VLF) components (<0.03 Hz) are difficult to interpret and probably should be ignored for autonomic activity evaluation.

Some of the advantages HRV-PSA has over other time-domain methods are clear in the first four points listed above. Thus, apart from its debatably better sensitivity, HRV-PSA is of great interest to physicians studying autonomic diseases, because it can give a reliable quantification of sympathetic activity which other, more traditional approaches do not.[24] Moreover, among diabetologists there is great interest in investigating the vagal-sympathetic balance alterations which have recently been revealed to play an important role in the unexpected sudden deaths that are often observed in DAN patients.[38]

The above discussion serves to justify the recent introduction of frequency-domain HRV analysis into the study of diabetic neuropathy.[22-26]

In fact, HRV-PSA, as well as having shown that there is a reduction of both parasympathetic and sympathetic activity, has more importantly also shown an alteration in the vagal-sympathetic balance (Figures 3 and 4).[24] Moreover, in comparison with traditional cardiovascular reflex tests, HRV-PSA has been shown to be far more able to detect early sympathetic dysfunctions.[24] In a broader, critical study which compares HRV-PSA with time-domain autonomic tests, the conclusions drawn were slightly different from those described above, especially regarding which test correlates with which band of the spectra, or rather, exactly what time-domain and frequency-domain tests are exploring in terms of autonomic pathways.[25] Here, although the cited discrepancies could be explained by the fact that different mathematical models have been used (autoregressive and FFT, respectively) some important conclusions have been highlighted: a rearranged battery, including a reworked traditional HRV time-domain test and an HRV frequency-domain test should be used for an accurate diagnosis of autonomic dysfunction in diabetics.

HRV-PSA have also been used recently on the attempt to explain the high incidence of premature deaths in DAN.[39] In its wake has come an elegant study which shows how in DAN patients the well-known phenomenon of losing BP circadian rhythms is related to nocturnal cardiac sympathetic overactivity, detected by the LF/HF ratio as a measure of sympathovagal balance. In this same study the application of 24-hour HRV-PSA combined with 24-hour BP monitoring has led to the hypothesis of a major risk of cardiovascular accident in diabetics during the night-time, precisely when they show a reduction in BP fall and a contemporaneous sympathetic predominance in the heart (Figure 4).[40]

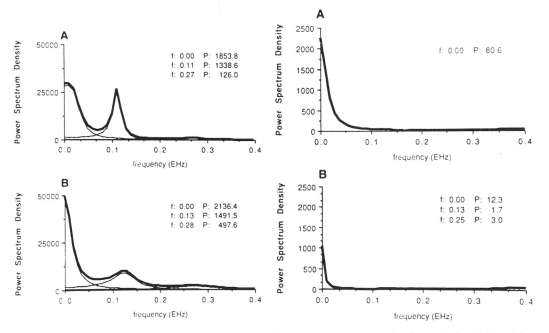

Figure 3. Power spectrum density of RR interval variation in a normal subject **(left side)** and in a diabetic patient with severe autonomic neuropathy **(right side)** standing **(A)** and lying **(B)**. Location of components' central frequencies, f, expressed in equivalent hertz (EHz) and their power, P, are also reported. From Bellavere et al.[24]

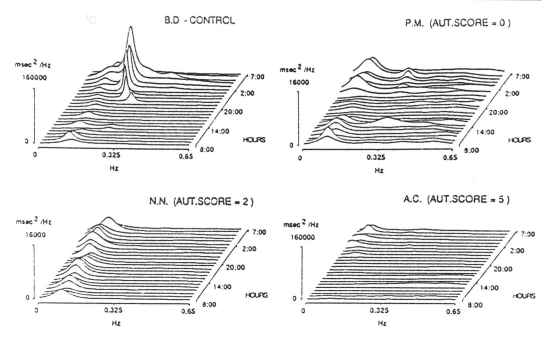

Figure 4. Examples of 24-hour pattern of LF and HF RR spectral components. B.D.: normal pattern in a normal subject, showing prevalence of the LF component during the day, whereas at night the HF component gradually increases reaching its highest level. A.C.: abnormal pattern of spectral components in a diabetic patient with definite cardiovascular test impairment (autonomic score = 5), showing, in addition to a lowering in total spectral power, persistence of the only sympathetic component during the night in the absence of detectable HF component. N.N.: blunted nocturnal increase in HF component and LF prevalence during the night in a diabetic patient with an early cardiovascular test impairment (autonomic score = 2). P.M.: presence of a normal trend in a diabetic petient with normal cardiovascular tests (autonomic score = 0), although an attenuation of HF nocturnal increase is already apparent. LF and HF are expressed in absolute units. From Spallone et al.[40]

Conclusions

In this chapter, the application of HRV tests to diabetes could seem to have been overemphasized. However, this reflects the real situation in clinical practice. In fact, DAN is so widely recognized and studied, that in almost all diabetic units there are physicians familiar with the various cardiovascular autonomic tests.

In reality, only a few of the papers on HRV tests in DAN have been mentioned here, just enough to support the line of argument and to show how these tests are used for diagnostic purposes.

Diabetologists need such tests in their daily attempts to create an objective 'picture' of each diabetic patient, with a reasoned prognosis and an outline of treatment.

There seems to be much less interest in the study of autonomic dysfunctions in noncardiological diseases, other than diabetes. It is well known that, as has already been discussed, various cardiovascular reflex tests have been applied to demonstrate autonomic involvement in a variety of disease, but, unlike in diabetology, they have not become a part of routine clinical practice. Furthermore, as far as I am aware, only a few papers outside the field of diabetology have applied the more advanced techniques such as HRV analysis on frequency domain.[14,41,42]

On the other hand, in recent years, anesthesiologists have become interested in HRV tests as a means of detecting patients at high risk for surgical intervention and there is an ongoing debate about the importance of such tests for patients undergoing general anesthesia.[43-45]

However, the seeming delay in applying HRV tests in a more generalized study of autonomic dysfunctions could be explained by the fact that they require a basic level of computer technology which is not yet available to all. But if we accept that HRV tests offer a reliable method for detecting autonomic dysfunctions, because these are present in many diseases, it is to be expected that some of the methodologies described above will be applied more and more often in the near future in all medical fields.

References

1. Weeler T, Watkins PJ. Cardiac denervation in diabetes. BMJ 1973; 4:584-586.
2. Ewing DJ, et al. Vascular reflexes in diabetic autonomic neuropathy. Lancet 1973; 7:1354-1356.
3. Ewing DJ, et al. The value of cardiovascular autonomic function tests: 10 years experience in diabetics. Diabetes Care 1985; 8:491-498.
4. Baldwa VS, Ewing DJ. Heart rate response to the valsalva manoeuvre. Reproducibility in normals and relation to variation in resting heart rate in diabetics. Br Heart J 1977; 39:641-644.
5. Bennett T, Hosking DJ, Hampton JR. Vasomotor responses to valsalva manoeuvre in normal subjects and in patients with diabetes mellitus. Br Heart J 1979; 42:422-435.
6. Sundkvist G, Almer LO, Lilja B. Respiratory influence on heart rate in diabetes mellitus. BMJ 1979; 1:924-925.
7. Ewing DJ, et al. Autonomic mechanisms in the initial response to standing. J Appl Physiol 1980; 49:809-814.
8. Bellavere F, et al. Standing to lying heart rate variation. A simple test in the diagnosis of the diabetic neuropathy. Diabet Med 1987; 4:41-43.
9. Duncan G, et al. Evidence of vagal neuropathy in chronic alcoholics. Lancet 1980; 2:1053-1057.
10. Johnson RH, Robinson BJ. Mortality in alcoholics with autonomic neuropathy. J Neurol Neurosurg Psychiatry 1988; 51:476-480.
11. Clark CV, Mapstone R. Autonomic neuropathy in ocular hypertension. Lancet 1985; 2:185-187.
12. Moore MV, Jeffcoate WJ, Haworth S. Autonomic neuropathy and the pathogenesis of glaucoma in diabetes mellitus. Diabet Med 1989; 6:717-719.
13. Vita G, et al. Uremic autonomic neuropathy. J Auton Nerv Syst 1990; 30:S179-S184.
14. Guzzetti S, et al. Effects of sympathetic activation on heart variability in chagas patients. J Auton Nerv Syst 1990; 30:S79-S82.
15. Iosa D, Massari DC, Dorsey FC. Chagas cardioneuromiopathy: effect of ganglioside treatment in chronic dysautonomic patients. A randomised, double blind, parallel placebo controlled study.Am Heart J 1991; 122:775-785.
16. Peterson HR, et al. Body fat and the activity of the autonomic nervous system. N Engl J Med 1988; 318:1077-1083.
17. Fedele D, et al. Impairment of cardiovascular autonomic reflexes in multiple symmetric lipomatosis. J Auton Nerv Syst 1984; 11:181-188.
18. Neubauer B, Gundersen JG. Analysis of heart rate variations in patients with multiple sclerosis. A simple measure of autonomic nervous disturbances using an ordinary ECG. J Neurol Neurosurg Psychiatry 1978; 41:417-419.
19. van Dijk JG, et al. Autonomic nervous system dysfunction in Parkinson's disease: relationships with age, medication, duration and severity. J Neurol Neurosurg Psychiatry 1993; 56:1090-1095.
20. Leden I, et al. Autonomic nerve function in rheumatoid arthritis of varying severity. Scand J Rheumatol 1983; 12:166-170.
21. Inukai T, et al. Parasympathetic nervous system activity in hypothyroidism determined by RR interval variations on electrocardiogram. J Intern Med 1990; 228:431-434.
22. Pagani M, et al. Spectral analysis of the heart rate variability in the assessment of autonomic diabetic neuropathy. J Auton Nerv Syst 1988; 23:143-153.
23. Freeman R, et al. Spectral analysis of heart rate in diabetic autonomic neuropathy. A comparison with standard tests of autonomic function. Arch Neurol 1991; 48:185-190.
24. Bellavere F, et al. Power spectral analysis of heart rate variations improves assessment of diabetic autonomic neuropathy. Diabetes 1992; 41:633-640.
25. Ziegler D, et al. Prevalence of cardiovascular autonomic dysfunction assessed by spectral analysis, vector analysis, and standard tests of heart rate variation and blood pressure response at various stages of diabetic neuropathy. Diabet Med 1992; 9:806-814.

26. Akinci A, et al. Heart rate in diabetic children: sensitivity of the time and frequency domain methods. Pediatr Cardiol 1993; 14:140-146.

27. Ewing DJ, et al. Abnormalities of ambulatory 24 hours heart rate in diabetes mellitus. Diabetes 1983; 32:101-105.

28. Murray A, et al. RR interval variations in young male diabetics. Br Heart J 1975; 37:882-885.

29. Gundersen HJC, Neubauer B. A long term diabetic autonomic nervous abnormality. Reduced variations in resting heart rate measured by a simple and sensitive method. Diabetologia 1977; 13:137-140.

30. Ewing DJ, et al. Cardiac autonomic neuropathy in diabetes: comparison of measures of R-R interval variation. Diabetologia 1981; 21:18-24.

31. Malpas SC, Maling TJB. Heart rate variability and cardiac autonomic function in diabetes. Diabetes 1990; 39:1177-1181.

32. Ewing DJ, Nielson JMM, Travis P. New method for assessing cardiac parasympathetic activity using 24 hour electrocardiograms. Br Heart J 1984; 50:396-402.

33. Bigger JT. Comparison of baroreflex sensitivity and heart period variability after miocardial infarction. Am J Cardiol 1989; 14:1511-1518.

34. Malliani A, et al. Cardiovascular neural regulation explored in the frequency domain. Circulation 1991; 84:482-492.

35. Malik M, Camm AJ. Heart rate variability: from facts to fancies. J Am Coll Cardiol 1993; 22:566-568.

36. Goldsmith RL, et al. Comparison of 24 hour parasympathetic activity in endurance trained and untrained young men. Am Coll Cardiol 1992; 20:552-558.

37. Pagani M, Lombardi F, Malliani A. Heart rate variability: disagreement on the markers of sympathetic and parasympathetic activity. J Am Coll Cardiol 1993; 22:951-953.

38. Bellavere F, et al. Prolonged QT period in diabetic autonomic neuropathy: a possible role in sudden cardiac death? Br Heart J 1988; 59:379-383.

39. Bernardi L, et al. Impaired circadian modulation of sympathovagal activity in diabetes. A possible explanation for altered temporal onset of cardiovascular disease. Circulation 1992; 86:1443-1445.

40. Spallone V, et al. Relationship between the circadian cardiac rhythms of blood pressure and sympathovagal balance in diabetic autonomic neuropathy. Diabetes 1993; 42:1745-1752.

41. Aharon Peretz J, et al. Increased sympathetic and decreased parasympathetic cardiac innervation in patients with Alzheimer disease. Arch Neurol 1992; 49:919-922.

42. Zahorska-Markiewicz B, et al. Heart rate variability in obesity. Int J Obesity 1993: 17:21-23.

43. Estefanous FG, et al. Analysis of heart rate variability to assess hemodynamic alterations following induction of anesthesia.J Cardiothorac Vasc Anesth 1992; 6:652-657.

44. Latson TW, O'Flaerthy D. Effects of surgical stimulation on autonomic reflex function: assessment by changes in heart rate variability. Br J Anesth 1993; 70:301-305.

45. O'Flaerthy D. Heart rate variability and anesthesia. Eur J Anesthesiol 1993; 10:419-432.

Chapter 39

Heart Rate Variability in the Fetus

Michael Hirsch, Jacob Karin, Solange Akselrod

Fetal heart rate (FHR), as well as adult heart rate (HR), basically originates from the inherent rhythmicity of the myocardial cells. The sinoatrial (SA) node takes the lead in eliciting the cardiac beat by depolarizing more frequently than any other element of the myocardium. Both sympathetic and parasympathetic components of the autonomic nervous system (ANS), act competitively on the SA node, accelerating or decelerating the rate, respectively. In the fetus, the resultant HR normally fluctuates around the mean by 5 to 15 bpm. These fluctuations have been described as beat-to-beat variation, short-term irregularity or heart rate variability (HRV).[1] Only the introduction of the electronic fetal monitoring in the 1960s enabled the tracing and appreciation of the subtle fluctuations existing in the basal HR. Clinically, a normal or average baseline variability is considered as a valid indicator of fetal well-being.

Clinical Characterization of Fetal Heart Rate Variability

Baseline FHR variability is generally assessed in stationary traces with steady baseline, which are encountered between periodic FHR changes (see Figures 1A-C). Periodic changes define gross temporal changes of FHR. These may appear as an increase in FHR associated mainly with fetal whole body movements—*accelerations*, or as a decrease in FHR either associated with uterine contractions (*type I and type II decelerations*), or as *variable decelerations* of an unsteady shape and relation to uterine contractions, which are usually linked with umbilical cord compression.[2]

The baseline variability includes (see examples in Figure 1): **short-term variability**—reflects the beat-to-beat changes due to the interval differences between successive R waves in the ECG signal; and **long-term variability**—defines the slow cycling effect

From: Malik M., Camm AJ (eds.): *Heart Rate Variability.* Armonk, NY. Futura Publishing Company, Inc., © 1995.

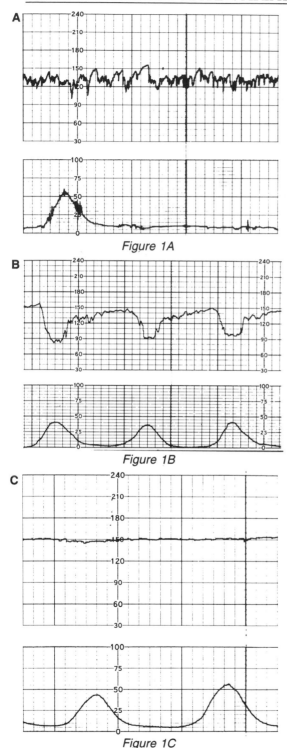

Figure 1A

Figure 1B

Figure 1C

Figures 1A-C. Examples of FHR variability (upper trace) and corresponding uterine contractions (lower trace). The time scale is 0.5 min/division. **A**: normal (to slightly increased) HRV, includes short- and long-term variability (also a few periodic changes in the middle of the trace). **B**: variable decelerations (periodic changes) whenever contractions occur. Short-term variability is reduced, long-term variability is still existing. **C**: absent HRV.

of RR over time. These changes are described in terms of frequency, and are normally in the range of 2 to 6 cycles per minute, with an amplitude of 6 to 10 bpm.

Visual assessment of variability involves both components and is usually expressed as *range* or *width* of variability band, oscillatory amplitude, etc. Clinically, the variability is defined as: absent 0 to 2 bpm, decreased 3 to 5 bpm, average 6 to 15 bpm, increased >15 bpm (see examples in Figure 1). An exaggeratedly increased variability-saltatory pattern >25 bpm, is usually pathological and generally indicates fetal hypoxia.

Long-term variability is less important in comparison to the short-term variability in determining the well-being of the fetus.[3] It may be preserved in a distressed fetus after the disappearance of the short-term variability and is usually expressed as an undulating baseline.

The Origin of Heart Rate Variability in the Fetus

Variability is the reflection of a healthy, well-developed ANS. As in the adult, it represents the interaction of the sympathetic and parasympathetic control systems. For an effective autonomic control of the fetal heart, there are several basic requirements: the growth of nerves into the heart and great vessels, the ability of the nerve terminals to produce active neurotransmitters, the development of an effector organ and the existence of functioning receptors in the effector organ. It seems that in the mammalian fetus, the ability of the effector organ to respond to a neurotransmitter precedes the release of neurotransmitters by the nerve terminals.[4]

Sympathetic innervation appears first in the SA region of the right atrium, next in the left atrium, then at the base of the ventricles, in the right ventricle, and finally in the apical region of the left ventricle.

Parasympathetic innervation of the mammalian fetus precedes the sympathetic system. In the human fetus, cholinesterase activity was detected as early as the 8th gestational week. The use of various vagal agonists and antagonists in diverse mammalian laboratory models have caused the expected pharmacological effects early during gestation.[4]

During pregnancy, a gradual decrease in the average FHR is a well-accepted observation.[5] Both short-term and long-term variability typically increase with the advance of gestation as the parasympathetic system matures.[6] This is further supported by showing that maternal injection of atropine has an increasing effect on the FHR as pregnancy advances.[7] The most consistent effect of atropine injection has been the loss of beat-to-beat variability.

This observation was traditionally attributed to the increase in parasympathetic control of the HR with the advance of gestation. However, in experiments performed on exteriorized, dennervated, 9 to 15 weeks of gestation fetal hearts, no difference in HR was found, when compared to hearts in-situ at the same gestational age.[8] Therefore, a presumption was made that the gradual reduction of the HR, at least at the beginning of pregnancy, is unrelated to the maturation of the parasympathetic innervation. It may rather be due to an intrinsic rhythmicity of the conductive system, principally the SA node, whereas the parasympathetic effect is of major significance only later during gestation.

The sympathetic component of the autonomic system most probably also contributes to increase HRV. This was shown by the appearance of increased variability in FHR traces obtained after maternal administration of ephedrine, a sympathetic stimulant.[9]

Nevertheless, the rapidity of HR response to transient vagal stimulation further emphasizes the major role of the para-

sympathetic autonomic control in affecting moment-to-moment short-term HRV.[10]

Various reflex mechanisms are thought to cause the parasympathetic system to produce HRV.[11-13] The baroreflex is functioning in term and preterm human newborns and probably also in the fetus,[14] and was shown to affect short-term HRV.[12] Chemoreceptors were found to react to acute hypoxemia by increasing HRV in the fetal monkey[15] or lamb.[11,16]

Other mechanisms, not essentially reflectory, were also reported to affect variability. In human fetuses, decreased HRV was shown to be associated with acidosis and low Apgar scores.[17] Barbiturates, narcotics and tranquilizers are known to reduce FHR variability.[18] Absence of fetal HRV may occur in situations complicated by fetal cardiac arrhythmias such as paroxysmal atrial tachycardia or complete heart block.[19]

Physiological Factors Modulating Fetal Heart Rate Variability

Several factors are known to modulate FHR variability throughout pregnancy. Short-term variability is governed mainly by the alternating stimulation and withdrawal of the parasympathetic nervous activity. This system matures with advancing gestational age.[20-22] A wandering baseline may reflect the early development of the long-term variability, which is also increasing with gestational age.[23,24]

However, there is no clear proof in the human fetus as to whether the short- or long-term fluctuations are directly related to one of the two basic control limbs, whether the short-term fluctuations are solely parasympathetic such as in the adult, or, whether sympathetic activity is reflected only in the long-term fluctuations. Even if an increase was observed in short-term fluctuations as a result of a sympathetic stimulus (ie, ephedrine), it is most probable that it caused, indirectly, an increase in parasympathetic activity, based on the observation in adults that sympathetic activation cannot cope with frequencies above 0.15 Hz.[25]

Enhanced variability is therefore considered to be produced by excessive vagal stimulation. This association is consistent with the frequent occurrence of bradycardia with increased variability. It is also more commonly found in the mature postdate fetus, who has a better developed parasympathetic system. Physiologically, enhanced variability has been noted during periods of increased fetal activity.[17] Increased uterine activity, mainly associated with head compression, will also show an increased variability due to the increase in parasympathetic tone.

Temporal correlation has been demonstrated between changes in HRV and the presence of fetal HR periodical changes. Beat-to-beat variations were reduced during accelerations and increased with decelerations. At any FHR level, episodes of fetal breathing were associated with a short-term variability relatively higher than during nonbreathing periods. This pattern is characterized by small, high-frequency (HF) fluctuations of the HR, which can be detected only in good quality FHR tracings obtained from fetal abdominal or scalp electrode electrocardiogram (ECG), but not by means of Doppler ultrasonography. The relatively smooth appearance of FHR acceleration could be, at least partly, attributed to the absence of breathing movements during this periodic change, in addition to being due to increased sympathetic tone associated with gross fetal movements. As already mentioned, short-term variability is inversely correlated with the baseline FHR.[26]

Clearly defined behavioral states, similar to those reported for the newborn,[27] were described in the fetus after the 36th gestational week.[28] During this period, the fetus spends approximately 90% of the time in active or quiet sleep. In active sleep, FHR is composed of numerous accelerations due to repeated gross fetal movements, and fetal HRV is relatively high. In addition, both irregular breathing and episodes of rapid eye movements are noted. During quiet sleep, breathing activity is regular, eye movements are absent and FHR presents a sporadic large acceleration and low oscillatory amplitude FHR variations. Consequently, the characteristic FHR pattern was suggested as a tool to differentiate fetal behavioral state using only HR recordings.[29,30] A similar concept was also advised for the neonate using visual inspection[31] or various mathematical formulations, to describe long- and short-term variability.[32]

Prior to 36 weeks of gestation (but after the 28th week) no definite behavioral state can be distinguished, since the various phenomena composing each state do not appear simultaneously. However, the particular FHR pattern of alternating high and low HRV, characterizing rest/activity cyclicity, can still be observed.[24,30,33]

The rest/activity cyclicity in HRV continues also during labor.[34] Close to term pregnancy, the FHR pattern of interchanging low and high HRV periods, resembles that of the newborn, with low HRV periods averaging an approximate duration of 20 minutes.[27,35,36]

Other fetal movements were also denoted to affect HRV. Fetal mouthing activity was clearly seen during rest periods as an episodic rhythmical movement of 1 to 3 Hz. The mouthing movements were responsible for the appearance of irregular baseline oscillations at a frequency of about 3 per minute. The rate of these oscillations corresponds to the burst rate of the mouthing movements. Around the 25th week, these mouthing bursts are of short duration, 1 to 2 seconds; later in pregnancy, they become longer, lasting from 2 to 20 seconds.[37,38] The mechanism by which the mouthing movements affect the HR is not yet resolved.[36]

Fetal HRV, as well as fetal breathing activity, and the incidence of HR accelerations, show a diurnal variation.[36,39] These diurnal changes are to a large extent considered to be of maternal origin. In fact, studies have shown that human newborns virtually miss all diurnal rhythmicity, probably due to immaturity of the responsible centers in the CNS.[27,35] Close to term pregnancy, there is a recognizable diurnal FHR rhythm, with a peak between 8 am and 9 am, and a nadir between 1 am and 4 am.[40] This rhythm seems to correlate with the simultaneous maternal HR. Furthermore, the diurnal variation in gross fetal movements and related FHR accelerations result in a doubling of the long-term variability around midnight relative to midday.[36]

Pathological Factors Affecting Fetal Heart Rate Variability

A decrease or absence of HRV may appear as a result of a variety of pathological states,[1,17,41] ie, fetal metabolic acidosis,[15,17,42] neurological abnormality,[43] or cardiac arrhythmia.[15] Diminished short-term variability was measured prior to intra-uterine fetal death.[44] A reduced HRV was found to be a better indicator of impending fetal death than late or variable decelerations.[45] A pattern of absent variability and elevated baseline rate has been associated with fetal brain death and inevitable neonatal death.[46] In an agonal-dying fetus, although baseline rate can remain in the normal range (120 to 160 bpm) until moments before death, variability will always be reduced in the acidotic/hypoxic fetus.[47,48] The FHR baseline is often, but not always, wandering in appearance. The majority of anencephalic fetuses demonstrate a diminution or absence in variability.[49,50] Hydrocephalous with absent variability usually indicates increased intracranial pressure.[51,52]

However other causes for absent or reduced variability may appear, such as marked prematurity,[53] drug effect,[54,55] fetal sleep,[36,56,57] fetal inactivity,[58,59] or even, a decrease in variability that accompanies a progressive increase in the baseline HR.[60] Thus, *a wide range of causes for reduced or absent variability is running from signaling a healthy fetus to warning for a dying fetus.* Therefore, it is no surprise that additional parameters are needed to assure the well-being status of the fetus. Furthermore, in tracings presenting absent variability, various characteristics, which are still in the normal range, cannot exclude a compromised fetal outcome. Normal baseline levels are not reassuring since normal baseline can be maintained in a terminally ill fetus just until moments before death. The fact that periodical changes do not appear, particularly those associated with hypoxia (ie, atypical variable or late decelerations), is not reassuring because in severe asphyxia, myocardial depression may be so marked that the fetal heart is unable to decelerate in response to further hypoxic changes.[51,61] However, the usual sequence of FHR manifestation during hypoxia is the following: late decelerations are the earliest sign, preceding changes in HRV or disappearance of accelerations.[62]

It was suggested that episodes characterized by low HRV may be further evaluated by fetal stimulation.[63-65] While shaking the fetus was found to be an unreliable means of external stimulation in periods of low HRV, a vibro-acoustic trigger or a high glucose content meal proved successful stimulants.[66] However, the ability to achieve such a diagnosis in utero, consistently enough to avoid a cesarean section for nonviable fetuses, awaits further studies and means.

Clinical Significance of Fetal Heart Rate Variability

Adequate beat-to-beat variability of the fetal heart is the most reliable fetal monitoring indicator of good fetal condition, especially when accompanied by periodic accelerations.[67-69] A good baseline variability even without HR accelerations, usually suggests a well-compensated state.[17,30] This has been demonstrated by the measurement of normal pH values under these circumstances.[70] During labor complicated by late decelerations,[17,71] better Apgar scores or fetal scalp pH were achieved in those fetuses preserving a good HRV. In another study,[72] the neonatal rate of respiratory distress syndrome and death, were found to occur nine-fold more frequently in those newborns who had a fetal HRV of less than 5 bpm prior to birth.

In growth-retarded fetuses,[72] the presence of FHR accelerations alone was of limited value for the anticipation of fetal deterioration. Alternatively, a measure of HRV was proposed as a tool to differentiate growth retarded fetuses at an increased risk.[58]

Standard Methods of Fetal Heart Rate Variability Estimation

Clinical evaluation of FHR variability is usually performed by visual assessment of the range of HR oscillations. A more precise way of estimating FHR variability can be achieved by applying a computerized quantification, based on mathematical expressions. Examples of such estimators are: the *short-term index* (the standard deviation of successive RR intervals) and the *interval difference index* (ID index) for short-term variations or the *long-term index* (the coefficient of variation of the RR intervals) and *long-term irregularity index* (LTI index), for long-term variations. These computations are performed usually for a predetermined period of time, generally 15 seconds. Evaluation and comparison of the different formulations have been widely reviewed.[74-77]

Standard Methods of Fetal Heart Rate Recording

Both phonocardiograms and Doppler ultrasound tachocardiometry were found less reliable for recording true beat-to-beat HR variability, when compared to direct (scalp electrode) or indirect (abdominal electrodes) fetal ECG. In phonocardiograms, an electronic demodulator has to eliminate one of the two consecutive heart sounds (normally the second), whereas the other heart sound is used for the computation of the FHR. However, depending on the relative strength of the heart sounds,

one is never sure which of the two sounds triggers the cardiotachometer, a fact that may artificially enhance the beat-to-beat variability.

Doppler-ultrasonography too, often results in an artificially increased beat-to-beat variability. Four separate waves are detected in association with opening or closure of the two semilunar and atrioventricular valves during each cardiac cycle. The tachometer circuitry is designed to trigger on only one of these waves during each cardiac cycle. Nevertheless, relative changes in the size of the reflected waves due to even minute changes in the fetal position, may result in triggering the cardiotachometer by any one of the four reflected waves, producing an exaggerated variability. Even the use of computerized methods of autocorrelation did not resolve this problem completely. Indeed, fetal breathing did not show any particular effect on the FHR baseline variability obtained by Doppler ultrasonography.[30] This is in opposition to findings obtained by using fetal electrocardiography for tracing the HRV, which usually reveals an increased short-term variability in association with fetal breathing movements during quiet sleep.[26,37,78] It hence seems likely that Doppler ultrasonography fails in detecting the HF fluctuations in FHR produced by respiration, even when the cardiotachometer is equipped with heavy micro-processor aid.[30]

There is thus a clear need for a highly accurate and reliable detector of instantaneous FHR, able to provide a beat-to-beat measure of FHR, not only at term but also during pregnancy and with an accuracy similar to that provided by the use of scalp ECG.

Abdominal Electrocardiogram Recordings and Algorithm for Fetal Heart Rate Detection

Phonocardiography and Doppler ultrasonography do not seem to provide an instantaneous HR accurate enough to enable a reliable spectral analysis of FHR fluctuations.[30] Such analysis could provide a quantitative insight into autonomic modulation of FHR, an estimate of autonomic balance during various fetal behavioral states, and, last but not least, a measure of the development of autonomic control as a function of gestational duration. In addition, if the breathing movements in the fetus do elicit HR modulation, similarly to the well-known respiratory sinus arrhythmia in the newborn, then, spectral analysis of FHR variability could possibly be used as an indicator of fetal breathing movements.

For this kind of application, a very precise FHR detection is required. Fetal ECG provided by a scalp electrode measurement allows fetal R-wave detection, at a level of accuracy similar to adult R-wave detection. Yet, the scalp electrode can only be connected during labor, after rupture of the membranes, and even then, it is evidently an invasive tool.

There is thus an obvious necessity for a method that would noninvasively provide a fetal ECG signal or at least, precisely detect fetal R-wave occurrence at prelabor stages of pregnancy. The ECG signal measured from the maternal abdomen is a good candidate, assuming that an efficient algorithm is available to separate the fetal from the maternal contribution.[79,80] Various research groups have invested their efforts in that direction.[81-83]

The maternal abdominal ECG signal (Figure 2) is a combination of the maternal and fetal cardiac contribution, with an amplitude ratio of at least an order of magnitude. In addition, it contains the contribution of a variety of noise sources, such as maternal muscle activity, contractions, electronic noise, etc. The extraction of the fetal complex is therefore an elaborate task, in particular when taking into consideration that very often the fetal heart beat coincides with some part of the maternal ECG complex (Figure 2).

Algorithm for the Detection of Fetal Complexes from Abdominal Electrocardiogram

We have developed and fine-tuned an algorithm for fetal ECG and FHR detection from the abdominal ECG.[79,80,84] This algorithm has been implemented in a dedicated, computer based system (Medco), which includes a very low noise amplifier and A/D converter. An example of the abdominal signal as monitored by this system is shown in Figure 2, following A/D conversion and without any signal processing. One can clearly observe the small fetal QRS complexes riding on top of the huge maternal contribution, while some of the fetal complexes may be completely buried behind the maternal QRS. Nonetheless, the algorithm succeeds in detecting all the fetal complexes (see Figure 2).

The core of our algorithm is based on a time-derivative approximation with variable parameter, which takes into account indirectly the difference in frequency content between maternal and fetal ECG.[79,80] A fast approximation of the second derivative of the sampled signal is computed, making use of an adjustable parameter to perform a combined filtration and derivation procedure. This filtration/derivation allows the creation of two sets of derivatives, the one excluding and the other including the fetal signal. Mathematical operations with these derivatives and a maternal template, allow the elimination of the maternal contribution and the subsequent detection of the fetal complexes.[79,80,84]

The abdominal ECG is digitized and the data of the first few seconds is processed to allow the on-line learning of the optimal parameters for further data analysis. During this learning period, automatic selection of the derivation parameters, of amplification factors and threshold values is performed, as well as the computation of a maternal template, followed by detection of fetal complexes (for verification purposes, the results of fetal R wave detection can be graphically displayed). Then, the algorithm is ap-

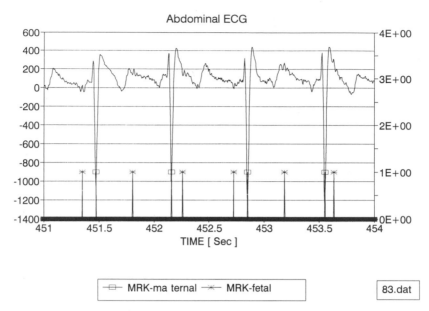

Figure 2. Example of abdominal ECG with indication of detection of fetal complexes by the FHR algorithm. Note that even when a fetal complex (F) is hidden by a maternal complex (M), it is accurately detected.

plied automatically and on-line, to the entire string of incoming abdominal ECG data. A series of instantaneous FHR values (as well as maternal HR) is created and displayed on-line, while at the end of the measurement an average fetal ECG complex is computed and displayed (Figures 3A-D and 4A and B).

Validation of Fetal Heart Rate Detection from Abdominal Electrocardiogram

In a consecutive series of 50 pregnant women (no incoming subject was skipped) monitored near term, the algorithm was successful in 42 women. In these 42 subjects, the average detection rate of the fetal complexes was 97%. Our experience seems to indicate that in about 20% of the near-term mothers, physiological factors (weight, fat layer, vernix, fetal size and position) are such, that abdominal ECG will not disclose the fetal ECG. In at least 80% of the mothers, the maternal abdominal signal will enable the successful detection of the fetal complex, even if the signal is noisy, even if the baseline is wandering, and even if the fetal com-

plex is superimposed on a maternal complex. A careful, beat-by-beat visual inspection of the detection, in all these recordings, indicates that in these mothers, almost not a single fetal beat was missed (95% accuracy regarding false negatives) or mislocated (97% accuracy regarding false positives).

The reliability of the fetal QRS detection is apparent when comparing the FHR obtained from the abdominal ECG (Medco) to FHR obtained from the scalp electrode (direct ECG-Corometrics), in a series of recordings performed in an additional group of women during labor. An excellent agreement between the two kinds of measurements of FHR is achieved in all cases.

Figure 3B shows the scalp ECG corresponding to the abdominal maternal signal in Figure 3A. Figure 3C displays the instantaneous FHR as extracted by the detection algorithm from the abdominal ECG, compared to the corresponding FHR as detected from the simultaneous scalp ECG trace. The correlation between the two curves is 0.94.

From these comparisons, one may thus conclude that the detection of the fetal com-

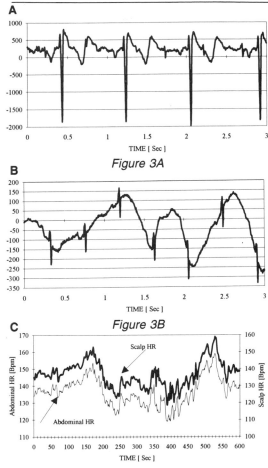

Figure 3A

Figure 3B

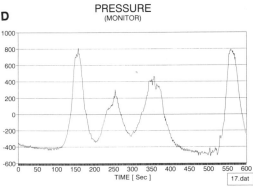

PRESSURE
(MONITOR)

17.dat

Figures 3A-D. A: 3 sec long example of abdominal ECGmeasured during labor (gestational age: 40 weeks). **B**: example of scalp ECG measured at an arbitrary time during the same recording session as displayed in Fig. 3A. **C**: FHR as detected from the noninvasive abdominal ECG(full scale left: 170) compared to invasive FHR from scalp ECG (full scale right: 160, so that the curves are slightly shifted), shown in Figs. 3A and B over 600 sec. Note the full agreement between the two FHR series. **D**: contractions simultaneous to data shown in Fig. 3C.

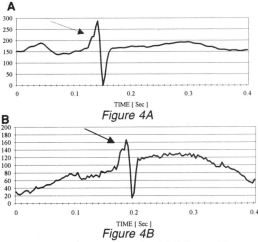

Figure 4A

Figure 4B

Figures 4A-B. A: average fetal ECG complex as created by a dedicated averaging algorithm, applied on the abdominal ECG signal shown in Fig. 3, following the detection of the fetal complexes. **B**: single fetal ECG complex as measured directly by scalp electrode (slightly noisier since not averaged), from the trace shown in Fig 3B. Note the close similarity in the features of the two fetal ECG complexes and the ability to display P, QRS and T-wave in the abdominal ECG.

plexes from the abdominal ECG is extremely accurate, and can provide a highly reliable FHR. The measurements shown in Figure 3 were made during the occurrence of contractions (Figure 3D), and nonetheless, the detection sensitivity was not impaired.

When computing an average ECG complex obtained from the abdominal signal with a single scalp fetal ECG complex, again a close agreement is observed (Figures 4A and B). The average complex displays all the intrabeat features (P, QRS and T waves) and allows the measurement of intracardiac conduction times, wave widths and wave shapes, well before birth. This might be of clinical value as an independent assessment of fetal congenital heart disease in addition to ultrasound imaging.

These examples demonstrate that at various stages of pregnancy (at least as early as the 24th week),[84] using the abdominal maternal ECG, both the fetal ECG complex and the fetal HR can be reliably obtained. The next step, spectral analysis of FHR variability is thus straightforward, applying the same variety of tools to FHR as presented in previous chapters of this book.

Spectral Analysis of Fetal Heart Rate Variability from Abdominal Electrocardiogram

Spectral analysis of FHR fluctuations can provide a more quantitative framework for the estimation of short- and long-term fluctuations, the specification of the dominant frequencies, as well as the typical power levels involved in fetal HRV. A wide range of criteria can be developed in order to assess in a more objective way, the various physiological and pathological fetal conditions described above.

A first step is to determine the normal pattern (or patterns) of FHR power spectra. From its dependence on gestational age, one can obtain insight into the development of the ANS.

Development of Fetal Autonomic Control from Fetal Heart Rate Spectral Analysis

A significant difference is observed between the young and the mature fetuses, indicating that fetal age (and thus development) may significantly affect the pattern of HRV power spectra.[84] Indeed, Figure 5

displays the results of spectral analysis of FHR, by showing the average spectral integrals (over 0.1 Hz bands) for a group of young fetuses (average gestational age: 23.5 weeks) and a group of mature fetuses (average age: 39.75 weeks). It is visible that young fetuses display more HRV power than older ones, most probably due to their less organized and more erratic neural activity.

The same study shows that both groups present significantly higher power during activity periods than during sleep states, and that in each state the younger fetuses display more HRV.[84] In addition, it seems that a respiratory peak can be observed mainly during sleep state of the fetuses (not during active state) and only using short-term traces of FHR (64 seconds). Spectral analysis of longer FHR traces (256 seconds), as typically used for adults, do not reveal a clear peak in the HF range. However, bearing in mind that the fetal breathing activity exists only for about 25% of the time,[85] and only for periods of 30 to 60 seconds, it is understandable why too long a trace might blur the respiratory peak if present. A peak in the HRV power spectrum at the frequency of respiration is observed in adults[86] around 0.3 Hz, while in newborns a relatively lower and often widespread peak is observed in the range of 0.4 to 0.8 Hz.[87] In the fetus the respiratory peak is even less

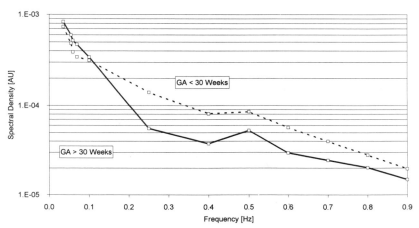

Figure 5. Average integrals (0.1 Hz wide) over HRV power spectra of 64 s subtraces from young pregnancies (gestational age: 24±0.8 weeks, n = 13) and mature pregnancies (gestational age: 39.75±1.5 weeks, n = 38). Note the higher power in the immature fetuses.

powerful and even more widely dispersed, around a 0.7 Hz center frequency.[88]

An 1/f relationship between spectral density and frequency is obtained for both gestational age groups. One may conclude that the general features of the power spectra of FHR traces are very similar to newborns, although in fetuses, the respiratory peak will often be very small, very smeared or absent. It seems that FHR power spectra can be used as a sensitive tool to estimate developmental or behavioral states.

Detection of Breathing Movements from Fetal Heart Rate Spectral Analysis

Though FHR, or more precisely, FHR variability is a very significant factor when testing fetal viability, more comprehensive information is required. The second, important indication of fetal stress is the existence or absence of breathing movements and their characteristics.[89-92] The reflection of fetal breathing movements was demonstrated in primate fetuses[93] invasively, and in human fetuses, when a direct measurement of fetal ECG was enabled during labor.[88]

Using a continuous way of analyzing FHR traces, by performing spectral analysis of short (64 seconds) partially overlapping traces, it is possible to display changes in autonomic activity as a function of time.[94,95] In particular, it is possible to investigate the changes as a function of time of some integral over the HF range. Such an integral (eg, over the 0.6 to 0.7 Hz range) could reflect the respiratory modulation of FHR, due to fetal breathing movements. In a study in which we measured abdominal maternal ECG (and subsequently detected FHR), simultaneously with the recording of breathing movements as observed by ultrasound imaging, we could investigate the possible correlation between the existence of fetal breathing movements and level of ANS activity in the HF range.[94,95] We found that in the 0.6 to 0.7 Hz range the ANS activity (most probably parasympathetic) is closely related with the initiation of breathing movements (Figure 6). Breathing movements appear to be initiated after an increase in the ANS activity in that frequency band. They continue for various amounts of time after the ANS has returned to baseline level. We also found some periodic elevations in ANS activity during nonbreathing periods. On the other hand, no fetal breathing was observed without some increase in HRV power in the HF range.

We therefore conclude that the fetal breathing movements are closely related to changes in fetal ANS activity which impinge on fetal HRV

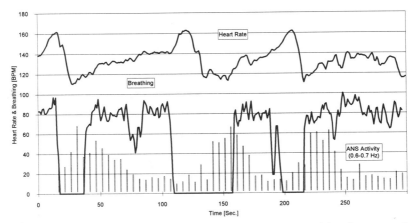

Figure 6. FHR, breathing movements and ANS activity (as expressed by the integral of the FHR power spectra, over the frequency band of 0.6 to 0.7 Hz). The data displays three clear episodes of breathing, which appear to be preceded by an enhancement of the autonomic activity in the frequency band of 0.6 to 0.7 Hz, located within the respiratory band (or HF range) of the FHR power spectrum.

and are reflected in the HF range of the FHR power spectrum. It even seems that the fetal breathing movements are a result of a surge in ANS activity and not the other way around.

The important conclusion of this study is that it seems possible to infer about breathing movements and to obtain an additional measure of fetal viability from the FHR power spectra, assuming that FHR is detected with high accuracy from abdominal or scalp ECG.

Summary

In general, a normal FHR baseline variability is the cardinal sign for the determination of the fetal status of well-being. Nevertheless, its appreciation in an objective way is extremely difficult when taking into account the variety of patterns obtained by FHR monitoring. The usual clinical approach today is the visual estimation of long- and short-term changes, as well as periodic changes. However, the clinical conclusions are far from being straightforward and unique, in particular in the suspicious cases.

On the other hand, the clinical importance of HRV is well accepted and beyond any doubt, for the estimation of fetal well-being, probably more than in any other medical field. Therefore, the use of spectral analysis of FHR, in conjunction with an accurate FHR detection, such as is made possible from a maternal abdominal ECG, may provide a new, quantitative insight in the various patterns of fetal HRV, related to fetal well-being, fetal behavioral states quiet or active sleep presence or absence of breathing movements) and fetal ANS development.

References

1. De Haan J, Van Bemmel JH, Versteeg B, et al. Quantitative evaluation of fetal heart rate patterns. Eur J Obstet Gynecol 1971; 1:95.

2. Cabaniss ML. Fetal Monitoring Interpretation. Philadelphia, Pa: JB Lippincott, 1993.

3. Boehm FH. FHR variability: key to fetal well-being. Contemp Obstet Gynecol 1977; 9:57.

4. Rudolph AM, Heymann MA. Control of the fetal circulation. In: Fetal and Neonatal Physiology; Proceeding of the Sir Joseph Barcroft Centenary Symposium. Cambridge, MA: Cambridge University Press, 1973; 89.

5. Ibarra-Polo AA, Guiloff E, Gomez-Rogers C. Fetal heart rate throughout pregnancy. Am J Obstet Gynecol 1972; 113:814-818.

6. Gagnon R, Campbell K, Hunse C, et al. Patterns of human fetal heart rate accelerations from 26 weeks to term. Am J Obstet Gynecol 1987; 157:743-748.

7. Schifferli PW, Caldyero-Barcia R. Effects of atropine and beta-adrenergic drugs on the heart rate of the human fetus. In: Boreus L (ed). Fetal Pharmacology. New York, NY: Raven Press, 1973.

8. Resch BA, Papp JG, Szontagh FE, et al. Comparison of spontaneous contraction rates of in situ and isolated fetal hearts in early pregnancy. Am J Obstet Gynecol 1974; 118:73-76.

9. Wright RG, Shnider SM, Levinson G, et al. The effect of maternal administration of ephedrine on fetal heart rate and variability. Obstet Gynecol 1981; 57:734-738.

10. de Haan J, Stolte LAM, Veth AFL, et al. Die bedeutung der schnellen oszillationen im kardiotachogramm des feten. In: Saling E, Dudenhausen JW (eds). Perinatale medizin, Bnd. III, Stuttgart, Thieme, 1972; 398-407.

11. Kardon MB, Peterson DF, Bishop VS. Beat-to-beat regulation of heart rate by afferent stimulation of the aortic nerve. Am J Physiol 1974; 227:598-600.

12. Fouron JC, Korcaz Y, Leduc B. Cardiovascular changes associated with fetal breathing. Am J Obstet Gynecol 1975; 123:868-876.

13. Dalton KJ, Dawes GS, Patrick JE. Diurnal, respiratory, and other rhythms of fetal heart rate in lambs. Am J Obstet Gynecol 1977; 127:414-424.

14. Moss AJ, Duffie ER, Emmanouilides G, et al. Blood pressure and vasomotor reflexes in the newborn infant. Pediatr 1963; 32:175-179.

15. Martin CB Jr. Regulation of the fetal heart rate and genesis of FHR patterns. Semin Perinatol 1978; 2:131-146.

16. Cohn HE, Sacks EJ, Heymann MA, et al. Cardiovascular responses to hypoxemia and acidemia in fetal lambs. Am J Obstet Gynecol 1974; 120:817-824.

17. Paul RH, Suidan AK, Yeh S, et al. Clinical fetal monitoring. VII. The evaluation and significance of intrapartum baseline FHR variability. Am J Obstet Gynecol 1975; 123:206-210.

18. Petrie RH. Effect of drugs and anesthetics on the fetal heart rate. Semin Perinatol 1978; 2:147-153.

19. Armstrong DH, Murata Y, Martin CB Jr, et al. Antepartum detection of congenital complete fetal heart block: a case report. Am J Obstet Gynecol 1976; 126:291-292.

20. Assali NS, Brinkman CR, Woods JR Jr, et al. Development of neurohumoral control of fetal, neonatal, and adult cardiovascular functions. Am J Obstet Gynecol 1977; 129:748-759.

21. Babaknia A, Niebyl JR. The effect of magnesium sulfate on fetal heart rate baseline variability. Obstet Gynecol 1978; 51(suppl):2s-4s.

22. Druzin ML, Fox A, Kogut E, et al. The relationship of the nonstress test to gestational age. Am J Obstet Gynecol 1985; 153:386-389.

23. Wheeler T, Cooke E, Murrills A. Computer analysis of fetal heart rate variation during normal pregnancy. Br J Obstet Gynaecol 1979; 86:186-197.

24. Visser GH, Dawes GS, Redman CW. Numerical analysis of the normal human antenatal fetal heart rate. Br J Obstet Gynaecol 1981; 88:792-802.

25. Rosenblueth A, Simeone FA. The interrelations of vagal and accelerator effects on the cardiac rate. Am J Physiol 1936; 110:42-55.

26. Dawes GS, Visser GH, Goodman JD, et al. Numerical analysis of the human fetal heart rate: modulation by breathing and movement. Am J Obstet Gynecol 1981; 140:535-544.

27. Prechtl HF. The behavioural states of the newborn infant (a review). Brain Res 1974; 76:185-212.

28. Nijhuis JG, Prechtl HF, Martin CB Jr, et al. Are there behavioural states in the human fetus? Early Hum Dev 1982; 6:177-195.

29. Timor-Tritsch IE, Dierker LJ, Hertz RH, et al. Studies of antepartum behavioral state in the human fetus at term. Am J Obstet Gynecol 1978; 132:524-528.

30. Pillai M, James D. The development of fetal heart rate patterns during normal pregnancy. Obstet Gynecol 1990; 76:812-816.

31. DeHaan R, Patrick J, Chess GF, et al. Definition of sleep state in the newborn infant by heart rate analysis. Am J Obstet Gynecol 1977; 127:753-758.

32. van Geijn HP, Jongsma HW, de Haan J, et al. Heart rate as an indicator of the behavioral state. Studies in the newborn infant and prospects for fetal heart rate monitoring. Am J Obstet Gynecol 1980; 136:1061-1066.

33. Dawes GS, Houghton CR, Redman CW, et al. Pattern of the normal human fetal heart rate. Br J Obstet Gynaecol 1982; 89:276-284.

34. Green KR, Natale R, Harrison CJ. Heart period variation and gross body and breathing movements after amniotomy in the human fetus. In: Rolfe P (ed). Fetal and Neonatal Physiological Measurements. Bath: Pitman Press, 1980; 250-256.

35. Junge HD. Behavioral states and state related heart rate and motor activity patterns in the newborn infant and the fetus antepartum—a comparative study. I. Technique, illustration of recordings, and general results. J Perinat Med 1979; 7:85-107.

36. Visser GH, Goodman JD, Levine DH, et al. Diurnal and other cyclic variations in human fetal heart rate near term. Am J Obstet Gynecol 1982; 142:535-544.

37. van Woerden EE, van Geijn HP, Swartjes JM, et al. Fetal heart rhythms during behavioural state 1F. Eur J Obstet Gynecol Reprod Biol 1988; 28:29-38.

38. van Woerden EE, van Geijn HP, Caron FJ, et al. Fetal mouth movements during behavioural states 1F and 2F. Eur J Obstet Gynecol Reprod Biol 1988; 29:97-105.

39. de Vries JI, Visser GH, Prechtl HF. The emergence of fetal behaviour. II. Quantitative aspects. Early Hum Dev 1985; 12:99-120.

40. Patrick J, Campbell K, Carmichael L, et al. Influence of maternal heart rate and gross fetal body movements on the daily pattern of fetal heart rate near term. Am J Obstet Gynecol 1982; 144:533-538.

41. Miller FC, Paul RH. Intrapartum fetal heart rate monitoring. Clin Obstet Gynecol 1978; 21:561-577.

42. De Haan J, Van Bemmel JH, Stolte LAM, et al. Quantitative evaluation of fetal heart rate patterns. II. The significance of fixed heart rate during pregnancy and labor. Eur J Obstet Gynecol 1971; 1:103.

43. van der Moer PE, Gerretsen G, Visser GH. Fixed fetal heart rate pattern after intrauterine accidental decerebration. Obstet Gynecol 1985; 65:125-127.

44. Street P, Dawes GS, Moulden M, et al. Short term variation in abnormal fetal heart rates records. Am J Obstet Gynecol 1991; 165:515-523.

45. Kubli F, Ruttgers H, Haller U, et al. Antepartum fetal heart rate. II. Baseline levels, baseline irregularity and decelerations with antepartum fetal death. Z Geburtshilfe Perinatol 1972; 76:309-323.

46. Nijhuis JG, Crevels AJ, van Dongen PW. Fetal brain death: the definition of a fetal heart rate pattern and its clinical consequences. Obstet Gynecol Surv 1990; 45:229-232.

47. Cetrulo CL, Schifrin BS. Fetal heart rate patterns preceding death in utero. Obstet Gynecol 1976; 48:521-527.

48. Parer JT. Fetal heart rate patterns preceding death in utero. In: Handbook of Fetal Heart Rate Monitoring. Philadelphia, Pa: WB Saunders, 1983; 147.

49. Peleg D, Goldman JA. Fetal heart patterns. A study of the anencephalic fetus. Obstet Gynecol 1979; 53:530-533.

50. Terao T, Kawashima Y, Noto H, et al. Neurological control of fetal heart rate in 20 cases of anencephalic fetuses. Am J Obstet Gynecol 1984; 149:201-208.

51. Dicker D, Gingold A, Peleg D, et al. Effect of intracranial pressure changes on the fetal heart rate. Study of a hydrocephalic fetus. Isr J Med Sci 1983; 19:364-367.

52. McCrann DJ Jr, Schifrin BS. Heart rate patterns of the hydrocephalic fetus. Am J Obstet Gynecol 1973;117:69-74.

53. Devoe LD. Antepartum fetal heart rate testing in preterm pregnancy. Obstet Gynecol 1982; 60:431-436.

54. Ayromlooi J, Tobias M, Berg P. The effects of scopolamine and ancillary analgesics upon the fetal heart rate recording. J Reprod Med 1980; 25:323-326.

55. Petrie RH, Yeh SY, Murata Y, et al. The effect of drugs on fetal heart rate variability. Am J Obstet Gynecol 1978; 130:294-299.

56. Hoppenbrouwers T, Combs D, Ugartechea JC, et al. Fetal heart rates during maternal wakefulness and sleep. Obstet Gynecol 1981; 57:301-309.

57. Sterman NB, Hoppenbrouwers T. The developement of sleep-waking and rest-activity patterns from fetus to adult in man. In: Sterman MB, McGinty DJ, Adinolfi AM (eds). Brain Development and Behaviour. New York, NY: Academic Press, 1971; 203-227.

58. Henson G, Dawes GS, Redman CW. Characterization of the reduced heart rate variation in growth-retarded fetuses. Br J Obstet Gynaecol 1984; 91:751-755.

59. Martin CB Jr. Behavioral states in the human fetus. J Reprod Med 1981; 26:425-432.

60. Roemer VM, Heinzl S, Peters FD, et al. Oscillation-frequency and baseline fetal heart rate in the last 30 minutes of labour. Br J Obstet Gynaecol 1979; 86:472-479.

61. Gaziano EP, Freeman DW. Analysis of heart rate patterns preceding fetal death. Obstet Gynecol 1977; 50:578-582.

62. Martin CB, de Haan J, Van der Wildt B, et al. Mechanism of late decelerations in the fetal heart rate. A study with autonomic blocking agents in fetal lambs. Eur J Obstet Gynecol Reprod Biol 1979; 9:361-373.

63. Divon MY, Braverman JJ, Guidetti DA, et al. Intrapartum vibratory acoustic stimulation of the human fetus during episodes of decreased heart rate variability. Am J Obstet Gynecol 1987; 57:1355-1358.

64. Ingemarsson I, Arulkumaran S, Paul RH, et al. Fetal acoustic stimulation in early labor in patients screened with the admission test. Am J Obstet Gynecol 1988; 158:70-74.

65. Zimmer EZ, Vadasz A, Reem Z. Intrapartum fetal vibratory acoustic stimulation during spontaneous and induced states of low activity and low heart rate variability. J Reprod Med 1990; 35:250-255.

66. Visser GH, Zeelenberg HJ, de Vries JI, et al. External physical stimulation of the human fetus during episodes of low heart rate variation. Am J Obstet Gynecol 1983; 145:579-584.

67. Earn AA. A proposed international scoring system for predicting fetal status derived from fetal heart rate patterns: compatible with current tests. (The fetal heart rate response as an aid in predicting perinatal status). Obstet Gynecol Surv 1980; 35:265-270.

68. Hon EH. Detection of asphyxia in utero-fetal heart rate. In: Gluck L (ed). Intra Uterine Asphyxia and the Developing Fetal Brain. Chicago, Ill: Yearbook Medical Publishers, 1977; 167.

69. Leveno KJ, Williams ML, DePalma RT, et al. Perinatal outcome in the absence of antepartum fetal heart rate acceleration. Obstet Gynecol 1983; 61:347-355.

70. Krebs HB, Petres RE, Dunn LJ, et al. II. Multifactorial analysis of intrapartum fetal heart rate tracings. Am J Obstet Gynecol 1979; 133:773-780.

71. Saling E. A new method for examination of the child during labor. Arch Gynaek 1962; 197:108-122.

72. Martin CB Jr, Siassi B, Hon EH. Fetal heart rate patterns and neonatal death in low birthweight infants. Obstet Gynecol 1974; 44:503-510.

73. Devoe LD, Castillo RA, Sherline DM. The nonstress test as a diagnostic test: a critical reappraisal. Am J Obstet Gynecol 1985; 152:1047-1053.

74. Yeh SY, Forsythe A, Hon EH. Quantification of fetal heart beat-to-beat interval differences. Obstet Gynecol 1973; 41:355-363.

75. Laros RK Jr, Wong WS, Heilbron DC, et al. A comparison of methods for quantitating fetal heart rate variability. Am J Obstet Gynecol 1977; 128:381-392.

76. Organ LW, Hawrylyshyn PA, Goodwin JW, et al. Quantitative indices of short- and long-term heart rate, variability. Am J Obstet Gynecol 1978; 130:20-27.

77. van Geijn HP, Jongsma HW, de Haan J, et al. Analysis of heart rate and beat-to-beat variability: interval difference index. Am J Obstet Gynecol 1980; 138:246-252.

78. Wheeler T, Gennser G, Lindvall R, et al. Changes in the fetal heart rate associated with fetal breathing and fetal movement. Br J Obstet Gynaecol 1980; 87:1068-1079.

79. Akselrod S, Karin J, Hirsh M. Computerized detection of fetal ECG from maternal abdominal signal. IEEE Comp Cardiol 1988; 88:261-264.

80. Karin J, Hirsh M, Akselrod S. Computerized Fetal Electrocardiography. VIII World Symposium on Cardiac Pacing and Electrophysiology; 1987; Israel; 553-560.

81. Nagel JH. Progresses in fetal monitoring by improved data acquisition. IEEE Eng in Med and Biol Mag 1984; 3:9.

82. Van Bemmel JH. Detection of fetal electrocardiogram by autocorrelation and crosscorrelations of envelopes. IEEE Trans Biomed Eng 1968; 15:17.

83. Longini RL, Reichert TA, Yu JMC, et al. Near-orthogonal basis functions: a real-time fetal ECG technique. IEEE Trans Biomed Eng 1977; 24:39.

84. Karin J, Hirsh M, Akselrod S. An estimate of fetal autonomic state by spectral analysis of fetal heart rate fluctuations. Pediatr Res 1993; 34(2):134-138.

85. Devoe LD, Ruedrich DA, Searle NS. Value of observation of fetal breathing activity in antenatal assessment of high risk pregnancy. Am J Obstet Gynecol 1989; 160:166-171.

86. Pomeranz B, MaCauley RJB, Caudill MA, et al. Assessment of autonomic function in humans by heart rate spectral analysis. Am J Physiol 1985; 248:H151-153.

87. Giddens DP, Kitney RI. Neonatal heart rate variability and its relation to respiration. J Theor Biol 1985; 113:759-780.

88. Divon MY, Sze-Ya Y, Zimmer EZ, et al. Respiratory sinus arrhythmia in the human fetus. Am J Obstet Gynecol 1985; 151:425-428.

89. Boddy K, Dawes GS. Fetal breathing. Br Med B 1975; 31:3-7.

90. Timor-Tritsch IE, Dieker LJ, Hertz RH, et al. Regular and irregular human fetal respiratory movement. Early Hum Dev 1980; 4:315-324.

91. Castle BM, Turnbull AC. The presence or absence of fetal breathing movements predicts the outcome of preterm labor. Lancet 1983; 2:471-473.

92. Devoe LD, Ruedrich DA, Searle NS. Value of observation of fetal breathing activity in antenatal assessment of high risk pregnancy. Am J Obstet Gynecol 1989; 160:166-171.

93. Myers MM, Fifer W, Haiken J, et al. Relationship between breathing activity and heart rate in fetal baboons. Am J Physiol 1990; 258:R1485-1497.

94. Karin J, Hirsh M, Sagiv C, et al. Fetal autonomic nervous system activity monitoring by spectral analysis of heart rate variations. IEEE Comp Cardiol 1992; 92:479-482.

95. Hirsh M, Karin J, Shechter B, et al. Detection of Fetal Breathing Activity in Real-time by Means of Spectral Analysis of Fetal Heart Rate Fluctuations. 2nd World Congress of Perinatal Medicine; 1993; 535-539.

Chapter 40

Ventricular Response in Patients with Sustained Atrial Fibrillation: Relation to the Underlying Cardiovascular Disease

Mark Walter Franz Schweizer, Kleber Gaspar Carvalho da Silva, Wolfgang Kübler, Johannes Brachmann

Introduction

Time- and frequency-domain measurements of heart period variability have been developed and used almost exclusively for the analysis of electrocardiograhic recordings during sinus rhythm.[1] However, the most frequent sustained cardiac rhythm beside sinus rhythm is atrial fibrillation.[2] Because atrial fibrillation is a common rhythm in patients suffering from a variety of cardiovascular diseases, the purpose of this study was to investigate, whether the underlying disease may exhibit an influence on the ventricular response during sustained atrial fibrillation. While undertaking this trial, some problems occurred. Frequency-domain analysis of heart period from minute segments during atrial fibrillation does not show distinct power in any frequency band, but it reveals widespread power spectra, which resemble to spectra from noise. There is no consistent interpretation of those widespread spectra as compared to spectra during sinus rhythm, where the low-frequency (LF) band may be associated to sympathetic and parasympathetic cardiac activity and the high-frequency (HF) band may be associated to parasympathetic cardiac activity.[3,4] Therefore, a meaningful physiological interpretation of heart period power spectra during atrial fibrillation is difficult to perform.

Time-domain measurements of heart period variability in the short and long time range are generally high, because beat-to-beat variabilty of heart period during atrial fibrillation is excessively high. What can easily be done instead also during atrial fi-

This study was supported by the Sonderforschungsbereich 320 "Herzfunktion und ihre Regulation" within the Deutsche Forschungsgemeinschaft. Dr. da Silva is a recipient of a grant from the National Bureau of Health of Brazil.
From: Malik M., Camm AJ (eds.): *Heart Rate Variability*. Armonk, NY. Futura Publishing Company, Inc., © 1995.

brillation, is the investigation of the frequency distribution of heart period. If there are major changes in ventricular response during atrial fibrillation in relation to an underlying disease or to different pharmacological treatment, one should expect that the frequency distributions should reveal different patterns. In addition, the average heart period and—as a measure of its variability—the standard deviation of heart period may give additional information about the time-dependent behavior of the atrioventricular node in atrial fibrillation.

This hypothesis was tested in patients with sustained atrial fibrillation under the condition of coronary artery disease, dilated cardiomyopathy, mitral valve insufficiency and systemic arterial hypertension.

Material and Methods

Patient Population

Patients with coronary artery disease build the main group. Sixty-four patients (52 men, 68±9 years and 12 females, 72±9 years) with coronary artery disease were enrolled in the study. All these patients were under pharmacological treatment, which consisted of beta-adrenergic blockers, digitalis, diuretics and nitrates. Coronary arteriograms had been performed in 31 patients and revealed one vessel coronary artery disease in 8 cases, two vessel coronary artery disease in 15 cases and three vessel disease in 8 cases. Four patients had suffered from a previous anterior and 12 patients from a previous posterior myocardial infarction (MI). One patient had previous anterior and posterior MI.

The second group encloses 34 patients (33 men, 58±9 years and 1 female, 71 years) with dilated cardiomyopathy. All patients were under common pharmacological treatment. The majority of the patients received angiotensin converting enzyme inhibitors and diuretics, as well as beta-blockers or calcium antagonists.

The third patient group is built of 27 individuals (19 men, 64±12 years and 8 females, 73±7 years) which suffer from systemic arterial hypertension. The last group with mitral valve insufficiency encloses 14 patients (9 men, 62±11 years and 5 females, 71±12 years).

All patients were on anticoagulation therapy and they were inpatients or outpatients of the Department of Cardiology at the Medical University Hospital of Heidelberg and they underwent long-term Holter electrocardiography from clinical indications.

Holter Analysis

The 24-hour Holter tapes were digitized using a GETEMED Cardioday 1000 Holter system (Kleinbeeren, Germany). The two channel electrocardiographic signals are digitized every 8 milliseconds and every QRS-complex is classified by means of a two channel Fast Fourier Transformation. In addition, every aberrant or premature QRS-complex is marked. By using this information, extra beats can be separated from normal beats during sinus rhythm. The accuracy of the measurement of the ventricular heart period (RR interval) is 8 milliseconds.

After digitization of the Holter tapes, the relative frequency distributions of heart period were calculated in 8-millisecond wide classes which ranged from 200 milliseconds to 1992 milliseconds. All heart periods were used for this calculation, irrespective whether the QRS-complexes were aberrant, normal or premature. Finally, the relative frequency distributions were averaged in every patient group and statistically compared with the nonparametric Wilcoxon, Mann and Whitney U-test for every distribution class.

In addition, the average heart period and its standard deviation were calculated for every hour of daytime and averaged for each patient group.

Assessment of Left Ventricular Pump Function

Left ventricular pump function was evaluated by echocardiography in all patients. A semiquantitative score, ranging from zero (normal) to four (seriously impaired) was used to measure left ventricular function.

Results

Relative Frequency Distributions of Heart Period

Figure 1 shows the relative frequency distributions from the patient groups with coronary artery disease and dilated cardiomyopathy. The abscissa was transformed from heart period to the corresponding heart rate (HR) for convenience. In the lower part of the figure, the significance level of the difference is shown for every distribution class. As one can easily see, the difference is only significant for ventricular rates greater than 115 per minute and for a small class which corresponds to a ventricular rate of 83 per minute. In other words, this means that ventricular rates greater than 115 per minute are significantly more frequent in patients with dilated cardiomyopathy as compared to patients with coronary artery disease.

Figure 2 shows the relative frequency distributions from the patient groups with coronary artery disease and mitral valve insufficiency. There were no significant differences.

Figure 3 shows the distributions for the patient groups with coronary artery disease and systemic arterial hypertension. Only between 132 per minute and 163 per minute ventricular rates were significantly more frequent in arterial hypertension as compared to coronary artery disease. However, the significance level is very tight to 5%.

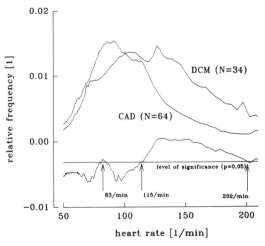

Figure 1. Mean relative frequency distributions of the beat-to-beat ventricular HR from 34 patients with dilated cardiomyopathy (DCM) and 64 patients with coronary artery disease (CAD) from 24-hour Holter recordings. All patients had sustained atrial fibrillation. The lower graph shows the significance level of the differences. If it is greater than the depicted 5% level of significance, the difference between the two distributions is statistically significant. Abscissa: HR; unit 1/min. Ordinate: Relative frequency; unit 1.

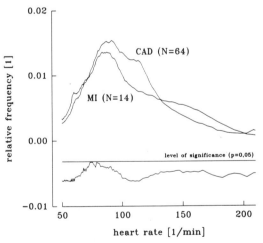

Figure 2. Mean relative frequency distributions of the beat-to-beat ventricular HR from 14 patients with mitral valve insufficiency (MI) and 64 patients with coronary artery disease (CAD) from 24-hour Holter recordings. All patients had sustained atrial fibrillation. The lower graph shows the significance level of the differences. If it is greater than the depicted 5% level of significance, the difference between the two distributions is statistically significant. Abscissa: HR; unit 1/min. Ordinate: Relative frequency; unit 1.

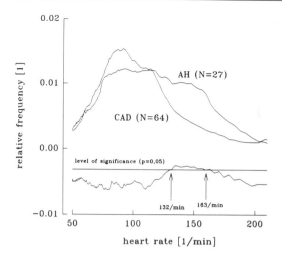

Figure 3. Mean relative frequency distributions of the beat-to-beat ventricular HR from 27 patients with systemic arterial hypertension (AH) and 64 patients with coronary artery disease (CAD) from 24-hour Holter recordings. All patients had sustained atrial fibrillation. The lower graph shows the significance level of the differences. If it is greater than the depicted 5% level of significance, the difference between the two distributions is statistically significant. Abscissa: HR; unit 1/min. Ordinate: Relative frequency; unit 1.

Mean Heart Period and its Standard Deviation

The hourly averaged heart period showed a circadian pattern in all patient groups. Mean heart period was lowest in the morning at approximately 10 o'clock and highest during nighttime at approximately 2 o'clock in the morning. The standard deviation of mean heart period was between 25% to 40% of mean heart period. However, there were no statistically significant differences between the patient groups.

Left Ventricular Pump Function

In coronary artery disease, the semiquantitative score of left ventricular pump function was on average 1.3, in dilated cardiomyopathy 2.5, in arterial hypertension 1.0 and in mitral valve insufficiency 0.6.

Discussion

In this study, differences in the ventricular response during atrial fibrillation were seen only in the relative frequency distributions between the patient groups with coronary artery disease, dilated cardiomyopathy and systemic arterial hypertension. However, from the hourly analysis of mean heart period and its standard deviation, there did not result significant differences. Despite the fact, that circadian patterns of mean heart period occurred, as has been previously reported,[5,6] we cannot conclude that the differences in frequency distribution of heart period occur at a certain hour of daytime, because in this case, one would expect some significant differences also in relation to time.

The frequency distribution of heart period contains no information about the time sequence of the heart periods and therefore, it is not a contradiction, that frequency distributions calculated from beat-to-beat heart periods may be statistically different in relation to the underlying cardiovascular disease, while the analysis in the time domain may not reveal differences, when the heart period is averaged every hour. However, the main finding, that the patient group with dilated cardiomyopathy showed significantly more frequent ventricular rates greater than 115 per minute, can be definitely interpreted in the sense, that ventricular cycle duration is more frequently shorter in dilated cardiomyopathy as compared to coronary artery disease. In addition, the patient group with dilated cardiomyopathy revealed impaired left ventricular function as compared to the patient group with coronary artery disease. This may be taken into consideration about the reasons for the more frequent fast ventricular rates in patients with dilated cardiomyopathy.

From the earliest reports about the investigation of ventricular response during atrial fibrillation,[7-11] there has been extensive discussion about the mechanisms that may be responsible for the behavior of ventricular cycle duration[12-15] during atrial fibrillation. Whether the 'pulse' in atrial fibrillation should be called irregular or not irregular at all times[16,17] appears—from a clinical point of view—less important than epidemiologic features of atrial fibrillation and prognosis.[18,19] The minimal value of heart period during atrial fibrillation is given by the functional refractory period of the atrioventricular node.[20] Concealed atrioventricular nodal conduction,[12,14] as well as postextrasystolic potentiation[13] or intermittent atrioventricular junctional rhythms,[15] or simple ventricular ectopy may all occur during atrial fibrillation and contribute to the ventricular cycle duration and its variability. In addition, different types of atrial fibrillation with different mean rates or intermittent atrial flutter may occur. This all may be present only during short periods.

In this study, we did not find significant differences in the variability of ventricular cycle duration between the investigated patient groups. However, we looked only at the hourly standard deviation of the ventricular cycle duration. A more detailed time related analysis perhaps would have been able to detect some intermittent characteristic patterns in ventricular response in relation to the underlying disease.

Conclusions

In atrial fibrillation, the ventricular rates in patients with dilated cardiomyopathy are more frequently faster as compared to patients with coronary artery disease. In mitral valve insufficiency and systemic arterial hypertension there were no significant major changes of ventricular rates as compared to coronary artery disease. The frequency distribution of heart period in 24 hours is a useful method to detect major differences in the ventricular response between patient groups with atrial fibrillation and different cardiovascular diseases. Time-related differences in ventricular response were not detectable on a hourly basis. However, more detailed analysis and the examination of intracardiac atrial and ventricular

electrocardiographic signals seems to be necessary in order to clarify the role of the atrioventricular node for the ventricular behavior during atrial fibrillation.

References

1. Kleiger RE, Bosner MS, Rottman JN, et al. Time-domain measurements of heart rate variability. J Amb Mon 1993; 6:1-18.10. Langendorf R, Pick A, Katz L. Ventricular response in atrial fibrillation: role of concealed conduction in the AV junction. Circulation 1965; 32:69-75.
2. The National Heart, Lung, and Blood Institute Working Group on Atrial Fibrillation. Atrial fibrillation: current understandings and research imperatives. J Am Coll Cardiol 1993; 22:1830-1834.
3. Lombardi F, Sandrone G, Pernpruner S, et al. Heart rate variability as an index of sympathovagal interaction after acute myocardial infarction. Am J Cardiol 1987; 60:1239-1245.
4. Malik M, Camm AJ. Heart rate variability: from facts to fancies. J Am Coll Cardiol 1993; 22:566-568.
5. Pitcher D, Papouchado M, James MA, et al. Twenty four hour ambulatory electrocardiography in patients with chronic atrial fibrillation. Br Med J 1986; 292:594.
6. Raeder EA. Circadian fluctuations in ventricular response to atrial fibrillation. Am J Cardiol 1990; 66:1013-1016.20. Rawles J. Atrial Fibrillation. London: Springer-Verlag, 1992.
7. Einthoven W, Korteweg AJ. On the variability of the size of the pulse in cases of auricular fibrillation. Heart 1915; 6:107-120.
8. Horbach L. Statistische Analyse der Reizüberleitung auf die Kammern bei Vorhofflimmern. Verh Deutsch Ges Kreislaufforsch 1965; 31:122-128.
9. Jordan H. Die zeitlichen Schwankungen der Herzschlagintervalle bei absoluter Arrhythmie. Archiv für Kreislaufforschung 1954; 21:40-49.
10. Langendorf R, Pick A, Katz L. Ventricular response in atrial fibrillation: role of concealed conduction in the AV junction. Circulation 1965; 32:69-75.
11. Söderström N. What is the reason for the ventricular arrhythmia in cases of auricular fibrillation? Am Heart J 1950; 40:212-223.
12. Fujiki A, Tani M, Mizumaki K, et al. Quantification of human concealed atrioventricular nodal conduction: relation to ventricular re-

sponse during atrial fibrillation. Am Heart J 1990; 120:598-603.

13. Hardmann SM, Noble MI, Seed WA. Postextrasystolic potentiation and its contribution to the beat-to-beat variation of the pulse during atrial fibrillation. Circulation 1992; 86:1223-1232.

14. Kirsh JA, Sahakian AV, Baerman JM, et al. Ventricular response to atrial fibrillation: role of atrioventricular conduction pathways. J Am Coll Cardiol 1988; 12:1265-1272.

15. Urbach JR, Grauman JJ, Straus SH. Quantitative methods for the recognition of atrioventricular junctional rhythms in atrial fibrillation. Circulation 1969; 39:803-817.

16. Meijler FL. The pulse in atrial fibrillation. Br Heart J 1986; 56:1-3.

17. Rawles JM, Rowland E. Is the pulse in atrial fibrillation irregularly irregular? Br Heart J 1986; 56:4-11.

18. Brand FN, Abbott RD, Kannel WB, et al. Characteristics and prognosis of lone atrial fibrillation. 30-year follow-up in the Framingham study. JAMA 1985; 254:3449-3453.

19. Kannel WB, Abbott RD, Savage DD, et al. Epidemiologic features of chronic atrial fibrillation. N Engl J Med 1982; 306:1018-1022.

Index